D1351519

owL

CRC Series in MODERN NUTRITION

Nutrient–Gene Interactions *in* Health *and* Disease

CRC SERIES IN MODERN NUTRITION
Edited by Ira Wolinsky and James F. Hickson, Jr.

Published Titles

Manganese in Health and Disease, Dorothy J. Klimis-Tavantzis

Nutrition and AIDS: Effects and Treatments, Ronald R. Watson

Nutrition Care for HIV-Positive Persons: A Manual for Individuals and Their Caregivers, Saroj M. Bahl and James F. Hickson, Jr.

Calcium and Phosphorus in Health and Disease, John J.B. Anderson and Sanford C. Garner

Edited by Ira Wolinsky

Published Titles

Practical Handbook of Nutrition in Clinical Practice, Donald F. Kirby and Stanley J. Dudrick

Handbook of Dairy Foods and Nutrition, Gregory D. Miller, Judith K. Jarvis, and Lois D. McBean

Advanced Nutrition: Macronutrients, Carolyn D. Berdanier

Childhood Nutrition, Fima Lifschitz

Nutrition and Health: Topics and Controversies, Felix Bronner

Nutrition and Cancer Prevention, Ronald R. Watson and Siraj I. Mufti

Nutritional Concerns of Women, Ira Wolinsky and Dorothy J. Klimis-Tavantzis

Nutrients and Gene Expression: Clinical Aspects, Carolyn D. Berdanier

Antioxidants and Disease Prevention, Harinda S. Garewal

Advanced Nutrition: Micronutrients, Carolyn D. Berdanier

Nutrition and Women's Cancers, Barbara Pence and Dale M. Dunn

Nutrients and Foods in AIDS, Ronald R. Watson

Nutrition: Chemistry and Biology, Second Edition, Julian E. Spallholz, L. Mallory Boylan, and Judy A. Driskell

Melatonin in the Promotion of Health, Ronald R. Watson

Nutritional and Environmental Influences on the Eye, Allen Taylor

Laboratory Tests for the Assessment of Nutritional Status, Second Edition, H.E. Sauberlich

Advanced Human Nutrition, Robert E.C. Wildman and Denis M. Medeiros

Handbook of Dairy Foods and Nutrition, Second Edition, Gregory D. Miller, Judith K. Jarvis, and Lois D. McBean

Nutrition in Space Flight and Weightlessness Models, Helen W. Lane and Dale A. Schoeller

Eating Disorders in Women and Children: Prevention, Stress Management, and Treatment, Jacalyn J. Robert-McComb

Childhood Obesity: Prevention and Treatment, Jana Pařízková and Andrew Hills

Alcohol and Coffee Use in the Aging, Ronald R. Watson

Handbook of Nutrition in the Aged, Third Edition, Ronald R. Watson

Vegetables, Fruits, and Herbs in Health Promotion, Ronald R. Watson

Nutrition and AIDS, Second Edition, Ronald R. Watson

Advances in Isotope Methods for the Analysis of Trace Elements in Man, Nicola Lowe and Malcolm Jackson

Nutritional Anemias, Usha Ramakrishnan

Handbook of Nutraceuticals and Functional Foods, Robert E. C. Wildman

The Mediterranean Diet: Constituents and Health Promotion, Antonia-Leda Matalas, Antonis Zampelas, Vassilis Stavrinos, and Ira Wolinsky

Vegetarian Nutrition, Joan Sabaté

Nutrient–Gene Interactions in Health and Disease, Naïma Moustaïd-Moussa and Carolyn D. Berdanier

Forthcoming Titles

Tryptophan: Biochemicals and Health Implications, Herschel Sidransky

Handbook of Nutraceuticals and Nutritional Supplements and Pharmaceuticals, Robert E. C. Wildman

Insulin and Oligofructose: Functional Food Ingredients, Marcel B. Roberfroid

Micronutrients and HIV Infection, Henrik Friis

Nutritional Aspects and Clinical Management of Chronic Diseases, Felix Bronner

CRC Series in MODERN NUTRITION

Nutrient–Gene Interactions *in* Health *and* Disease

Edited by Naïma Moustaïd-Moussa
Carolyn D. Berdanier

CRC Press
Boca Raton London New York Washington, D.C.

Library of Congress Cataloging-in-Publication Data

Nutrient-gene interactions in health and disease / edited by Naima Moustaïd-Moussa, Carolyn D. Berdanier.
      p. ; cm. -- (Modern nutrition)
  Includes bibliographical references and index.
  ISBN 0-8493-2216-2 (alk. paper)
     1. Nutrition. 2. Genetic regulation. 3. Gene expression. I. Moustaid-Moussa, Naima.
  II. Berdanier, Carolyn D. III. Modern nutrition (Boca Raton, Fla.)
  [DNLM: 1. Nutrition. 2. Adipose Tissue--metabolism. 3. Gene Expression Regulation.
 4. Vitamins--physiology. QU 145 N97017 2001]
  QP144.G45 N875 2001
  612.3'9--dc21

2001025109
CIP

Visit the CRC Press Web site at www.crcpress.com

© 2001 by CRC Press LLC

No claim to original U.S. Government works
International Standard Book Number 0-8493-2216-2
Library of Congress Card Number 2001025109
Printed in the United States of America   2 3 4 5 6 7 8 9 0
Printed on acid-free paper

Series Preface for Modern Nutrition

The CRC Series in Modern Nutrition is dedicated to providing the widest possible coverage of topics in nutrition. Nutrition is an interdisciplinary, interprofessional field par excellence. It is noted by its broad range and diversity. We trust the titles and authorship in this series will reflect that range and diversity.

Published for a scholarly audience, the volumes in the CRC Series in Modern Nutrition are designed to explain, review, and explore present knowledge and recent trends, developments, and advances in nutrition. As such, they will also appeal to the educated general reader. The format for the series will vary with the needs of the author and the topic, including, but not limited to, edited volumes, monographs, handbooks, and texts.

Contributors from any bona fide area of nutrition, including the controversial, are welcome.

We welcome the contribution of the volume Nutrient–Gene Interactions in Health and Disease edited by Naïma Moustaïd-Moussa and my long time, and much respected, colleague Carolyn D. Berdanier. This book is a worthy companion to two other CRC Press books on related subjects: *Nutrition and Gene Expression* edited by C.D. Berdanier and L.L. Hargrove and *Nutrients and Gene Expression, Clinical Aspects* edited by C.D. Berdanier. Taken together they make a splendid resource on the cutting edge topic of nutrient–gene interactions. This book will be useful to a broad spectrum of nutritionists and life scientists of all walks.

Ira Wolinsky, Ph.D.
University of Houston
Series Editor

Preface

A century ago biochemistry was in its infancy. Early biochemists were interested in the vital amines, later called vitamins, and how living cells work. In the 1930s biochemists and physiologists formed a scientific group devoted to identifying and understanding nutrient needs. Over the subsequent 60 years the essential nutrients were identified one by one and feeding studies were conducted to determine how much of each nutrient was required by a wide variety of species. Of interest was the fact that there was a high degree of inter-animal variability. In some instances the need for a given nutrient by one animal (including humans) could be twice that needed by another animal of the same age, sex, and breed. Researchers began to realize that this diversity in nutrient need was likely due to variations in the genetic backgrounds of the individual animals. Genetic diversity was utilized by animal and plant breeders to produce (through selective breeding) animals that efficiently use nutrients for specific purposes. Hence, rapidly growing, energy- and protein-efficient meat animals were produced that allowed farmers to bring their produce to market at a reduced feed cost. Chickens, for example, can be brought to market weight in half the time and feed expense by capitalizing on this selective breeding. These are but a few examples of nutrient–gene interactions using traditional methods of species improvement through selective breeding.

Today this method of species improvement has entered a new era. Techniques are now available to probe the genome to tease out those genetic messages that dictate nutrient need and tolerance. We have come to realize that optimal nutrient intake is determined by very specific genetic messages. This realization has meant that an entirely new approach to understanding nutrition is needed. With the completion of the whole genome sequence for several organisms including a draft of the human genome project, new genes with novel functions in nutritional diseases will be uncovered. With the advent of new technology, exploration of nutrient effects on gene expression will expand the identification of these new genes. The use of microarrays allows researchers to examine thousands of genetic messages simultaneously. Functional genomics and proteomics have given nutritionists a new way to examine nutrient response, especially with respect to nutrition-related diseases. Obesity, diabetes, heart disease, alcoholism, and anemia are but a few of the diseases that have both a nutrition component and a genetic one.

The present book and its two predecessors were compiled to update the reader on specific nutrient–gene interactions. The first book, edited by James Hargrove and Carolyn Berdanier, and entitled *Nutrition and Gene Expression*, was published in 1993. The second, *Nutrients and Gene Expression: Clinical Aspects*, edited by Berdanier, addressed some of the clinical conditions that arise as a result of nutrient–gene interactions. The present volume revisits the current basic science concerning nutrient-gene interactions. Reviews of examples of macronutrients and micronutrients as they affect gene expression are presented. The next volume will address nutrition from the functional genomics and proteomics point of view. We hope that you, the reader, enjoy reading about these important areas of research.

Naïma Moustaïd-Moussa
Carolyn D. Berdanier

Acknowledgments

We would like to dedicate this book to the American Society for Nutritional Sciences, especially to the Nutrient–Gene Interaction Research Interest Section and to our respective departments for promoting the field of molecular nutrition.

We would like to thank Dr. Ira Wolinsky, the series editor, who played a key role in getting the publisher's approval for this edition.

We express appreciation to our respective families, Hanna, Sami, and Zaina Moussa and Reese Berdanier for their love and patience during the preparation of this book, with special appreciation to Lynn Berdanier for her efforts in creating some of the figures.

Many thanks go to Marylenna Honeycutt and Margrethe Krogh for their secretarial help in preparing this book and to Kristin Morris for her editing assistance.

About the Authors

Naïma Moustaïd-Moussa, Ph.D. is associate professor of nutrition at the University of Tennessee in Knoxville, TN. She earned her B.S. in cell biology and physiology and her Ph.D. in endocrinology from the University of Paris in 1989. After a post-doctoral fellowship in molecular nutrition with emphasis on mechanisms of insulin regulation of lipogenic gene expression at Harvard School of Public Health, she joined the faculty at the Department of Nutrition at the University of Tennessee in Knoxville in 1993. She is a member of the North American Association for the Study of Obesity, the American Association for the Advancement of Sciences, and the American Association for Nutritional Sciences, where she serves on the program planning committee and as a current chair of the nutrient-gene interactions research interest section.

Her current research interests include the role of the endocrine function of adipocytes in obesity, nutritional and hormonal regulation of adipocyte gene transcription, and lipogenesis in humans. Her research has been funded by the American Diabetes Association, the American Heart Association, and the USDA.

Carolyn D. Berdanier, Ph.D. is professor emeritus at the University of Georgia in Athens, GA. She earned a B.S. from the Pennsylvania State University and M.S. and Ph.D. degrees from Rutgers University in 1966. After a post-doctoral fellowship with Dr. Paul Griminger at Rutgers, she served as a research nutritionist with the Nutrition Institute–Agricultural Research Service, U.S. Department of Agriculture. In 1975 she moved to the College of Medicine, University of Nebraska where she continued her research on nutrient–gene interactions. In 1977 she went to the University of Georgia where she served as head of the department of foods and nutrition. After 11 years she stepped down to pursue her interest in nutrient–gene interactions full time.

Her research has been supported by NIH, USDA, and various commodity groups. She is a member of the American Society for Nutritional Sciences, the Society for Experimental Biology and Medicine, the American Diabetes Association, and several honorary societies. She has served on the editorial bords of the *Journal of Nutrition*, *FASEB Journal*, *Nutrition Research*, and *Biochemical Archives*. Current research interests include studies on the role of nutrients in the control of mitochondrial gene expression.

Contributors

Gerard Ailhaud, Ph.D. Centre de Biochimie, Laboratoire Biologie du Dev. du tissue Adipeux, Faculte des Sciences, Parc Valrose, Nice, France

Fausto Andreola, Ph.D. Differentiation Control Section, LCCTP, NCI, NIH, Bethesda, Maryland

Carolyn Berdanier, Ph.D. Department of Family and Consumer Sciences, University of Georgia, Athens, Georgia

Kari J. Buck, Ph.D. Research Service, VA Medical Center, Portland, Oregon

Wenhong Cao, M.D. Division of Biological Psychiatry and Sarah W. Stedman Center for Nutritional Studies, Duke University Medical Center, Durham, North Carolina

Kate Claycombe, Ph.D. Nutritional Immunology Laboratory, Jean Mayer USDA Human Nutrition Research Center on Aging at Tufts University, Boston, Massachusetts

Elaine Collins, Ph.D. Department of Biochemistry, University of California, Riverside, California

Sheila Collins, Ph.D. Division of Biological Psychiatry and Sarah W. Stedman Center for Nutritional Studies, Duke University Medical Center, Durham, North Carolina

Kiefer W. Daniel, B.S. Division of Biological Psychiatry and Sarah W. Stedman Center for Nutritional Studies, Duke University Medical Center, Durham, North Carolina

Luigi M. De Luca, Ph.D. Differentiation Control Section, LCCTP, NCI, NIH, Bethesda, Maryland

Madhu Dhar, Ph.D. Oak Ridge National Laboratory and Graduate School of Genome Science and Technology, University of Tennessee, Oak Ridge, Tennessee

Tonya M. Dixon, B.S. Division of Biological Psychiatry and Sarah W. Stedman Center for Nutritional Studies, Duke University Medical Center, Durham, North Carolina

Helen B. Everts, Ph.D. Department of Family and Consumer Sciences, University of Georgia, Athens, Georgia

Daniel Fallon, B.S. Department of Biochemistry and Molecular Biology, University of Florida, Gainesville, Florida

Stephen Farmer, Ph.D. Department of Biochemistry, Boston University School of Medicine, Boston, Massachusetts

Christopher Fehr, M.D. Research Service, VA Medical Center, Portland, Oregon

Susan C. Frost, Ph.D. Department of Biochemistry and Molecular Biology, University of Florida, Gainesville, Florida

Valeria Giandomenico, Ph.D. Differentiation Control Section, LCCTP, NCI, NIH, Bethesda, Maryland

Fiona M. Herr, Ph.D. Department of Nutritional Sciences, Rutgers University, New Brunswick, New Jersey

Joseph B. Hwang, Ph.D. Department of Biochemistry and Molecular Biology, University of Florida, Gainesville, Florida

Jung Han Kim, Ph.D. The Jackson Laboratory, Bar Harbor, Maine

Suyeon Kim, M.S. Department of Nutrition, University of Tennessee, Knoxville, Tennessee

Young-Cheul Kim, Ph.D. Department of Biochemistry, University of Wisconsin, Madison, Wisconsin

Xingen Lei, Ph.D. Department of Animal Science, Cornell University, Ithaca, New York

Greg Marshall, B.S. Department of Biochemistry and Molecular Biology, University of Florida, Gainesville, Florida

Peter McCaffery, Ph.D. Differentiation Control Section, LCCTP, NCI, NIH, Bethesda, Maryland

Michael F. McEntee, D.V.M. Department of Pathology, University of Tennessee, College of Veterinary Medicine, Knoxville, Tennessee

Alexander Medvedev, Ph.D. Division of Biological Psychiatry and Sarah W. Stedman Center for Nutritional Studies, Duke University Medical Center, Durham, North Carolina

Simin Nikbin Meydani, D.V.M., Ph.D. Nutritional Immunology Laboratory, Jean Mayer USDA Human Nutrition Research Center on Aging at Tufts University, Boston, Massachusetts

Kristin Morris, M.S. Department of Nutrition, University of Tennessee, Knoxville, Tennessee

Ron F. Morrison, Ph.D. Boston University School of Medicine, Department of Biochemistry, Boston, Massachusetts

Naïma Moustaïd-Moussa, Ph.D. Department of Nutrition, University of Tennessee, Knoxville, Tennessee

Jürgen Naggert, Ph.D. The Jackson Laboratory, Bar Harbor, Maine

Anthony W. Norman, Ph.D. Department of Biochemistry, University of California, Riverside, California

James Ntambi, Ph.D. Department of Biochemistry, University of Wisconsin, Madison, Wisconsin

Hiroki Onuma, Ph.D. Division of Biological Psychiatry and Sarah W. Stedman Center for Nutritional Studies, Duke University Medical Center, Durham, North Carolina

Matthew T. Reilly, B.S. Research Service, VA Medical Center, Portland, Oregon

Catarina Sacristán, M.S. Nutritional Immunology Laboratory, Jean Mayer USDA Human Nutrition Research Center on Aging at Tufts University, Boston, Massachusetts

Hang Shi, B. Med. Department of Nutrition, University of Tennessee, Knoxville, Tennessee

Pamela J. Smith, M.D. Medical Nutrition R&D, Columbus, OH

Judith Storch, Ph.D. Nutritional Sciences, Rutgers University, New Brunswick, New Jersey

Yanxin Wang, Ph.D. Department of Nutrition, University of Tennessee, Knoxville, Tennessee

Jay Whelan, Ph.D. Department of Nutrition, University of Tennessee, Knoxville, Tennessee

Michael Zemel, Ph.D. Department of Nutrition, University of Tennessee, Knoxville, Tennessee

Bingzhong Xue, Ph.D. Department of Nutrition, University of Tennessee, Knoxville, Tennessee

Contents

1. **Dietary and Hormonal Regulation of the Mammalian Fatty Acid Synthase Gene** 1
   Kristin Morris, Yanxin Wang, Suyeon Kim and Naïma Moustaïd-Moussa

2. **Nutrition and Adipocyte Gene Expression** 25
   Ron F. Morrison and Stephen R. Farmer

3. **Regulation of the Stearoyl-CoA Desaturase Genes by Dietary Fat: Role of Polyunsaturated Fatty Acids** 49
   James M. Ntambi and Young-Cheul Kim

4. **Fatty Acids, White Adipose Tissue Development, and Adipocyte Differentiation** 63
   Gérard Ailhaud

5. **Acyl-CoA Synthetase 1 (ACS1): Regulation and Role in Metabolism** 77
   Pamela J. Smith

6. **Nutritional Regulation of Fatty Acid Transport Protein Expression** 101
   Judith Storch and Fiona M. Herr

7. **Alcohol and Gene Expression in the Central Nervous System** 131
   Matthew T. Reilly, Christoph Fehr, and Kari J. Buck

8. **Nutrient Control of Insulin-Stimulated Glucose Transport in 3T3-L1 Adipocytes** 163
   Joseph P. Hwang, Greg Marshall, Daniel Fallon, and Susan C. Frost

9. **Prohormone Processing and Disorders of Energy Homeostasis** 177
   Jung Han Kim and Jürgen K. Naggert

10. **The Agouti Gene in Obesity: Central and Peripheral Mechanisms, and Therapeutic Implications** 205
    Michael B. Zemel, Bingzhong Xue, and Hang Shi

11. Dietary Fats and APC-Driven Intestinal Tumorigenesis 231
    Jay Whelan and Michael F. McEntee

12. Body Weight Regulation, Uncoupling Proteins,
    and Energy Metabolism 261
    *Sheila Collins, Wenhong Cao, Tonya M. Dixon, Kiefer W. Daniel,
    Hiroki Onuma, and Alexander V. Medvedev*

13. Vitamin A and Gene Expression 283
    *Peter McCaffery, Fausto Andreola, Valeria Giandomenico,
    and Luigi M. De Luca*

14. Vitamin A and Mitochondrial Gene Expression 321
    Helen B. Everts and Carolyn D. Berdanier

15. Vitamin D and Gene Expression 349
    Anthony W. Norman and Elaine D. Collins

16. Vitamin E and Gene Expression 393
    Simin Nikbin Meydani, Kate J. Claycombe, and Catarina Sacristán

17. Differential Regulation and Function of Glutathione
    Peroxidases and Other Selenoproteins 425
    Xin Gen Lei

18. Ferritin: A Novel Human Ferritin Heavy-Chain MRNA
    is Predominantly Expressed in the Adult Brain 449
    Madhu S. Dhar

Index 459

1

Dietary and Hormonal Regulation of the Mammalian Fatty Acid Synthase Gene

Kristin Morris, Yanxin Wang, Suyeon Kim
and Naïma Moustaïd-Moussa

CONTENTS

1.1   Introduction 2
1.2   Organization and Function of the Multifunctional Fatty
      Acid Synthase 3
1.3   Structure of the Fatty Acid Synthase Gene 4
1.4   Fatty Acid Biosynthesis in Humans 5
1.5   Regulation of the Fatty-Acid Synthase Gene 5
1.6   *In Vivo* Effects of Fasting, Refeeding, and Aging 7
1.7   Effects of Insulin 8
        1.7.1   Insulin Responsive Sequences in the FAS Gene 8
        1.7.2   Transcription Factors 9
                1.7.2.1   Upstream Stimulatory Factors 9
                1.7.2.2   SREBP-1/ADD-1 9
1.8   Glucose Regulation of FAS Expression and Activity 11
1.9   Regulatory Effects of Polyunsaturated Fatty Acids 12
1.10 Effects of Glucagon and cAMP 13
1.11 Regulatory Effects of Thyroid Hormones 14
1.12 Insulin-Like Effects of Angiotensin II 15
1.13 Regulatory Effects of the Obesity Genes 15
        1.13.1 Leptin 15
        1.13.2 Agouti 16
1.14 Regulation of the FAS Gene by Other Factors 16
1.15 Conclusions and Implications 17
References 17

1.1 Introduction

Fatty acids in adipocytes can be derived from circulating lipoproteins via lipoprotein lipase, or they can be synthesized via *de novo* lipogenesis from carbohydrate precursors such as glucose. Excess glucose promotes lipogenesis by increasing the glycolytic flux and generating acetyl CoA. Acetyl CoA is the primary substrate for the synthesis of long-chain saturated fatty acids. These fatty acids are then used for esterification of α-glycerol phosphate-generating triacylglycerols, the major form of energy storage in adipose tissue.

Several enzymes contribute to lipogenesis. These enzymes include ATP-citrate lyase, which produces acetyl CoA from citrate; acetyl CoA carboxylase (ACC), which carboxylates acetyl CoA to generate malonyl CoA; fatty acid synthase (FAS), which catalyzes the synthesis of long-chain saturated fatty acids from acetyl CoA and malonyl CoA using NADPH generated by malic enzyme, glucose 6-phosphate dehydrogenase, 6-phosphogluconate, and citrate dehydrogenase (Fig. 1.1).

Fatty acid biosynthesis per se involves two of these enzymes, ACC and FAS. ACC catalyzes the first and rate-limiting step in *de novo* lipogenesis. The multifunctional FAS enzyme complex then catalyzes the following reaction:

$$\text{Acetyl CoA} + 7 \text{ Malonyl CoA} + 14 \text{ NADPH} + 14 \text{ H}^+$$
$$+ 7 \text{ ATP} + \text{H}_2\text{O} \longrightarrow \text{Palmitic Acid} + 8 \text{ CoA} + 14 \text{ NADP} + 7 \text{ ADP} + 7 \text{ P}_1$$

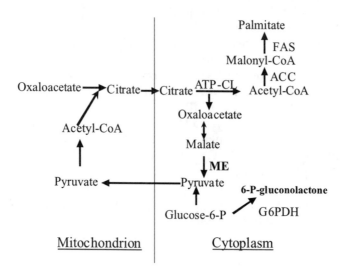

FIGURE 1.1
Key enzymes and intermediates of lipogenesis. ATP-CL, ATP-citrate lyase; FAS, fatty acid synthase; ACC, acetyl CoA carboxylase; ME, malic enzyme; G6PDH, glucose-6-phosphate dehydrogenase.

While ACC is subject to short-term regulation via allosteric modification of the enzyme, FAS is primarily regulated by the amount of mature protein.[1] FAS enzyme content generally correlates with the amount of FAS mRNA that is primarily controlled at the transcriptional level.[1,2] This review will focus on the mammalian FAS gene and its dietary and hormonal regulation.

1.2 Organization and Function of the Multifunctional Fatty Acid Synthase

The functional fatty acid synthase complex is a homodimer of two identical subunits with an apparent molecular mass of approximately 250 kD.[3] The multiple catalytic properties of FAS are responsible for the *de novo* synthesis of the long-chain fatty acid, palmitate. The structure of the rat and human FAS complexes is shown in Fig. 1.2. FAS involves seven different catalytic enzymes plus the acyl carrier protein, all of which are found in the FAS complex. These activities are arranged head-to-tail within discrete boundaries.[3] Such an arrangement facilitates the product of one reaction binding to the catalytic site and stimulating the activity of the subsequent enzyme activity. Free palmitate is the major fatty acid resulting from the catalytic activities of FAS *de novo*, accounting for 70% of all long-chain fatty acids synthesized by the fatty acid synthase complex.

Proceeding from the N-terminus of FAS, three domains containing the catalytic activities have been identified.[3] Domain I consists of the acetyl/malonyl transferase and β-ketoacyl synthase activities and is responsible for entry of the substrates, acetyl CoA and malonyl CoA, into the FAS enzyme complex by channeling them to the proper thiols. Domain II encodes the acyl carrier protein, which constitutes the eighth, albeit nonenzymatic, activity of the

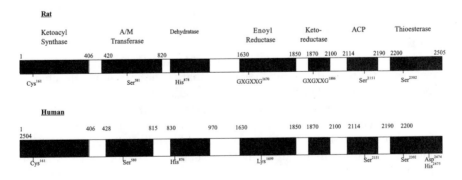

FIGURE 1.2
Structure of the rat and human fatty acid synthase multienzyme complex. Shown are the putative active sites of condensing enzyme (Cys[161]), acetyl/malonyl transacylases (Ser[580]), dehydratase (His[876]), and thioesterase (Ser[2302], Asp[2474], and His[2475]). Also shown: Point of attachment of 4'phosphopantetheine (Ser[2151]).

fatty acid synthase complex. β-ketoacyl reductase, enoyl reductase, and dehydratase activities are also found in the second domain. The third domain is situated at the carboxyl end of the protein and contains a single enzymatic activity, thioesterase. Dissociation of the native enzyme to individual monomers results in loss of palmitate synthesis even though six of the seven catalytic activities remain in the monomer.[3]

1.3   Structure of the Fatty Acid Synthase Gene

Fatty acid synthase is a multifunctional enzyme complex encoded by a single copy gene that produces a single mRNA species in mice, humans, and pigs and two mRNA species in rats, chickens, and geese.[4] This is consistent with the presence of two polyadenylation sites in the rat and avian sequences. The mammalian fatty acid synthase gene exhibits several characteristics consistent with mammalian genes: intron/exon junctions that follow GT/AG rules for splice sites, a 5′ flanking non-coding exon separated by a large intron from the second exon which contains the transcription initiation site.[4]

The murine fatty acid synthase was identified by differential screening of cDNA libraries derived from liver mRNA of rats that were fasted, or fasted rats then refed a high carbohydrate diet. Northern blot analysis identified a single 8.2-Kb mRNA species encoding the murine FAS.[5] This was consistent with the single mRNA species coding for FAS previously identified from the murine 3T3-L1 cell line.[5] One polyadenylation site was identified, in contrast to rat, goose, and duck sequences, which contains two polyadenylation signals, both of which are derived from a single gene.[6] Sequence comparison of the mouse cDNA found it to be 97% homologous to rat sequence.

FAS exhibits widespread tissue distribution in the mouse.[2, 3,5] The highest concentration of mRNA encoding for FAS is found in the liver, adipose tissue, and mammary glands.[5] However, FAS is also expressed at lower levels in other tissues.

Sequence analysis of goose FAS cDNA has found that it contains an additional 74 amino acids at its amino terminus that are not present in the chicken cDNA. This has been determined to be the result of a single nucleotide deletion in the 5′end of goose DNA that alters the reading frame without affecting the functional activity of the enzyme.[6]

The partial sequence of the human fatty acid synthase gene has also been reported,[7] and fundamental differences exist between the human and rodent or avian FAS gene. Three transcription initiation sites (Ti1, Ti2, and Ti3) were described in the human FAS gene, but only one of them (Ti1) was preceded by a classical TATA and CAAT boxes. Promoter II, situated upstream of Ti2, was shown to inhibit transcription from promoter I (upstream of Ti1).[7] Promoter 1 was shown to increase reporter gene activity in transfection assays, while promoter II represses this activity.[7]

1.4 Fatty Acid Biosynthesis in Humans

There are species differences in where lipogenesis occurs.[8] In rodents and humans, lipogenesis occurs in both adipose tissue and liver, while in birds, lipogenesis occurs primarily in the liver. In humans, the lipogenic capacity of the liver is significantly lower compared to other species. This is most likely attributable to the high fat content of the human diet. Rodents as well as other laboratory species are routinely fed low (~5 en %) fat diets. The major energy source in these diets is carbohydrate which, in turn, serves as the substrate for lipogenesis. Consistent with this, humans sustained parentally by high glucose solutions have much higher rates of lipogenesis than humans eating the typical Western diet.[9]

Despite its apparent low level, human lipogenesis has been shown to be regulated by several nutritional and hormonal factors including fasting, carbohydrates, and insulin.[10,11] Fasting inhibited the lipogenic effect of insulin by mechanisms involving both transport and metabolism of glucose.[10] In addition, when isolated human adipocytes were incubated with labeled glucose, 80% of intracellular radioactivity was incorporated into lipids.[11] *De novo* lipogenesis, measured by indirect calorimetry, was not detectable on low-carbohydrate diets but is increased on high-carbohydrate diets.[12] Results from these studies suggested that in depleted patients given hypercaloric high-carbohydrate diets, adipose tissue may account for up to 40% of whole body lipogenesis. In these subjects, total fat synthesis in adipose tissue was equal to or greater than in the liver on a per weight basis. Several studies have suggested that hepatic lipogenesis is a quantitatively minor pathway; however, these studies did not investigate adipose tissue lipogenesis.[13] A recent study confirmed that the liver plays a minor role in human lipogenesis and that adipose tissue is more likely the main site for *de novo* fatty acid synthesis in humans.[14] Using cultured human adipocytes, we demonstrated that insulin increases the expression of several lipogenic genes.[15] In addition, we found that human expression of FAS varies among adipose tissue depots, ranging from very low levels to very high levels that equal or surpass FAS expression in rodents (unpublished data) and that the combination of insulin and glucocorticoids leads to as much as 40% of glucose being converted to fatty acids (unpublished data).

1.5 Regulation of the Fatty Acid Synthase Gene

The rate of fatty acid biosynthesis is primarily determined by the availability of glucose.[16] Consuming a diet rich in carbohydrate elevates circulating glucose, which in turn signals the secretion of hormones which affect *de novo* synthesis of fatty acids.[16] Among these hormones, insulin and thyroid hormone (T3) are increased, and glucagon is decreased. Conversely, glucagon is decreased during feeding and elevated during starvation. Glucose, insulin, T3, agouti, and angiotensin II stimulate fatty acid synthesis and the expression of the fatty acid synthase gene while glucagon and polyunsaturated fatty acids (PUFA) downregulate FAS gene expression. We will review below the data available on the mechanisms of regulation of fatty acid synthase by these nutritional and hormonal factors.

The 5'-flanking region is critical for the regulation of FAS gene expression in cultured cells transfected with FAS-reporter fusion genes and in transgenic mice expressing this transgene. Several transcription factors, which bind specific cis-acting response elements in the FAS gene, mediate its dietary and hormonal regulation. Major regulatory sequences in the rat, human, and chicken genes are shown in Fig. 1.3 and are discussed in more detail in the following sections.

The cis-acting elements necessary for tissue-specific, nutritional, and hormonal regulation of FAS expression were identified using transgenic mice expressing FAS promoter linked to the chloramphenical acetyltransferase (CAT) reporter gene. The necessary sequences are contained mostly in the 2.1 kb of 5'-flanking DNA.[17] There is strong positive correlation between mRNA levels and the tissue-specific gene expression patterns of the reporter and the endogenous FAS in transgenic mice.[17] Fasting and refeeding, insulin, dibutyryl cAMP, and glucocorticoids regulated expression of the reporter gene and

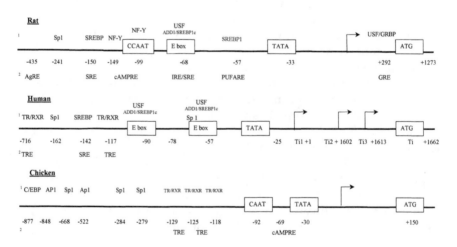

FIGURE 1.3

Major regulatory sequences in the rat, human, and chicken FAS gene. ADD1, adipocyte determination and differentiation factor; AgRE, agouti response element; cAMPRE, cAMP response element; CCAAT, inverted CCAAT box; C/EBP, CCAAT element binding protein; GRE, glucose response element; GRBP, glucose response element binding protein; NF, nuclear factor; PUFARE, polyunsaturated fatty acid response element; RXR, retinoid X receptor; SRE, sterol response element; SREBP, sterol response element-binding protein; TATA, TATA box, Ti: transcription initiation site; TRE: thyroid hormone response element, TR: thyroid hormone receptor; USF: upstream stimulatory factors.

[1] Transcription factors, [2] Response elements.

the endogenous FAS gene in a similar manner. In contrast, PUFAs such as menhaden oil, which is rich in long-chain n-3 fatty acids, dramatically suppressed endogenous FAS mRNA in both the liver and adipose tissue of transgenic mice compared to those fed oleic acid. However, CAT activities in the tissues of PUFA-treated mice were only 50% lower than in transgenic mice fed the oleic acid diet.[17] Thus, the stabilization of FAS mRNA that is observed during 3T3-L1 adipocyte differentiation and high-glucose or insulin treatment in HepG2 cells may also contribute to regulation of FAS mRNA levels by PUFA.[15,18,19] Alternatively, elements not contained in the first 2.1kb of the FAS 5′-flanking DNA may be necessary for full suppression of FAS transcription by PUFA. Identification of the cis-acting nucleotide sequences and trans-acting factors involved in the nutritional and hormonal regulation of the FAS gene will greatly facilitate the understanding of the underlying molecular mechanisms regulating expression of lipogenic genes.

1.6 *In Vivo* Effects of Fasting, Refeeding, and Aging

Fatty acid synthase is regulated in animals in response to nutrient and hormonal signals. Fasting in rodents results in decreased glucose conversion into fatty acids; when these animals are subsequently refed a low-fat, high-carbohydrate diet there is a rapid and efficient increase in production of fatty acids and triacylglycerols.[2] Such changes are mediated by hormonal changes in response to diet.[2] Changes in nutrient intake that increase circulating glucose levels elevate circulating insulin and thus promote lipogenesis. Conversely, dietary changes that lower circulating blood glucose levels invoke glucagon secretion and suppression of *de novo* lipogenesis. Suppression of FAS activity by glucagon is mediated by elevations in intracellular cAMP levels. The liver and adipose tissue undergo the most dramatic metabolic changes in response to fasting and refeeding.[2,5,17,20,21]

Activation of whole body lipogenesis and induction of the fatty acid synthase activity can be observed when animals are transitioned from a high-fat, low-carbohydrate diet to a low-fat, high-carbohydrate diet.[22] This can be mimicked by refeeding previously fasted animals.[22] Feeding a high-carbohydrate diet is accompanied by an increase in circulating insulin levels, both of which increase the transcriptional rate of fatty acid synthase, as well as other lipogenic genes.[22,23] Interestingly, this effect is attenuated by aging. While FAS mRNA was dramatically and rapidly induced by fat-free diets in young rats,[24] this response was much slower in aged rats, which did not exhibit significant elevations in FAS mRNA above fasting levels for 6 h. In addition to delaying transcriptional activation, maximum rates of gene transcription were not achieved until animals had been maintained on a fat-free diet for 24 h.[24] This implies that aging is a factor in the regulation of lipogenic gene transcription.[25]

1.7 Effects of Insulin

Feeding a low-fat, high-carbohydrate diet results in elevations in circulating insulin, which along with glucose, induce the enzymes of fatty acid synthesis including FAS, concomitant with suppression of the enzymes of fatty acid oxidation. FAS mRNA is low in animals made insulinopenic by administration of streptozotocin (STZ), a pancreatic β-cell toxin, compared to untreated animals. This effect is countered by insulin administration. Insulin treatment results in the rapid induction of FAS mRNA and gene transcription. Within 6 h of insulin administration to STZ-treated animals, FAS mRNA levels were induced to a level comparable to that observed when refeeding a low-fat, high-carbohydrate diet to previously fasted normal mice. Cyclohexamide, an inhibitor of protein synthesis, completely abolished the effect of insulin, demonstrating that transcriptional regulation of FAS by insulin requires ongoing protein synthesis.[26]

The murine 3T3-L1 adipocyte cell line is widely used to study regulation of lipogenic gene expression.[2] Insulin treatment of fully differentiated 3T3-L1 adipocytes upregulates FAS protein content and mRNA level. In contrast, treatment of 3T3-L1 adipocytes with dibutyryl cAMP dramatically reduced both FAS mRNA and the rate of enzyme synthesis.[20] Transcriptional regulation of FAS by insulin was observed in both rodent and human cultured adipocytes.[15,27] However, in human hepatoma HepG2 cells, glucose or insulin appear to increase FAS transcription by stabilizing FAS mRNA.[15,18]

Since FAS is not regulated allosterically but primarily at the transcriptional level, efforts have focused on identifying and characterizing regulatory sequences in the FAS gene, primarily in the 5′-flanking region, which may mediate hormonal and nutritional regulation of this gene. Insulin is the most extensively studied and best understood regulator of FAS gene expression.

1.7.1 Insulin Responsive Sequences in the FAS Gene

We generated constructs containing progressive deletions in the 5′-flanking region of the FAS gene linked to either the CAT or luciferase reporter genes. The constructs were then transfected into 3T3-L1 adipocytes.[28] In the presence of glucose and physiological concentrations of insulin, transfections of plasmids containing 5′deletions within –2100/–67 to +67, relative to the transcription start-site induced insulin responsiveness of the reporter gene.[28] However, deletions of the region between –67 and –25 abolished insulin responsiveness of the luciferase gene.[28] Additional observations led to the localization of the insulin responsive sequences (IRS) in the FAS gene in the –68/–52 region.[28] DNAse I footprinting analysis revealed a protected region from –68/–52. In addition, gel shift mobility assays demonstrate specific interactions between the protected region and nuclear factors isolated from mouse liver and 3T3-L1 nuclear extracts.[28] Finally, linking the heterologous

SV40 promoter to three tandem repeats corresponding to the −68/−52 region was sufficient to confer insulin responsiveness on the luciferase reporter gene (Fig. 1.3).[28] This mechanism may account for the stimulatory effects of carbohydrate feeding on the FAS gene. However, this does not preclude the existence of additional insulin responsive elements within the 5′-flanking region, which were indeed identified in upstream regions of the FAS promoter.[29]

1.7.2 Transcription Factors

1.7.2.1 Upstream Stimulatory Factors

An E-box DNA-binding motif (5′-CATGTG-3′) is located at −65/−60 bp within the IRS of the FAS gene.[29] This particular DNA sequence is recognized by upstream stimulatory factors 1 and 2 (USF1 and USF2), members of the basic helix-loop-helix family of transcription factors. This E-box sequence is important for basal- and insulin-stimulated activity of the FAS promoter. When deletions are introduced in the −73/−43 region in the first 150 bp of the 5′-flanking region, as much as 75% of basal promoter activity is lost. In addition to its role in basal transcription, interactions between USF transcription factors and the insulin responsive E-box of the FAS-IRS are functionally required for insulin regulation. Transfection assays demonstrated that mutations in the E-box sequence which abolish interactions with the USFs result in loss of insulin responsiveness. Furthermore, cotransfection of 3T3-L1 adipocytes with dominant negative USFs blunted the response of the FAS gene to insulin stimulation.[30]

Insulin regulates a wide variety of biological responses through a cascade of signaling events.[31] Insulin stimulation of the adipocyte FAS promoter is mediated by the phosphatidylinositol 3-kinase (PI3-K) pathway and protein kinase B (PKB)/Akt as the downstream effector in this cascade (Fig. 1.4).[32] In agreement with these studies, IRS-1/PI3-K/Akt activation has also been demonstrated to be essential for insulin stimulation of lipid synthesis in brown adipocytes.[33]

1.7.2.2 SREBP-1/ADD-1

Sterol regulatory element-binding proteins (SREBPs) are members of the basic-helix-loop-helix-leucine zipper (bHLH-Zip) family of transcription factors and regulate enzymes responsible for the synthesis of cholesterol, fatty acids, and triglycerides.[34] To date, three SREBP isoforms, SREBP-1a, -1c, and -2, have been identified and characterized. In addition to the USFs, SREBPs reportedly bind the FAS 5′-flanking DNA.[35] *In vitro*, SREBP binds to two regions of the FAS 5′-flanking DNA. The first region resides at −150/−140 bp and matches the SRE-1 sequence found in the LDL receptor 5′-flanking DNA. However, this region has proven dispensable for sterol regulation of FAS mRNA. The second SRE is within the FAS IRS and includes two tandem copies of SREBP binding sites that split the −65/−60 E-box.[35] Binding of a USF to

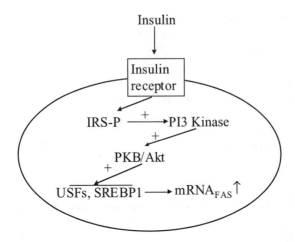

FIGURE 1.4

Proposed mechanism of insulin regulation of the fatty acid synthase gene. IRS-P: phosphory-lated insulin receptor substrate, PI3 Kinase: phosphatidylinositol 3 kinase, PKB: protein kinase B, USFs: upstream stimulatory factors, SREBP1: sterol response element binding protein 1, FAS: fatty acid synthase.

the –65/–60 E-box and SREBP to the flanking sites appears to be distinct pro-cesses.[30] Because the USF- and SREBP-binding sites overlap, distinct tran-scription factors may be utilized to regulate FAS gene transcription under different regulatory conditions. Overexpression of SREBP-1a in mice results in markedly elevated levels of FAS mRNA in hepatocytes and the concomitant accumulation of cholesterol and triglycerides in the liver.[36] However, feeding mice sterol-depleted or -enriched diets does not cause a consistent change in FAS mRNA level.[37] In HepG2 cells, FAS mRNA levels were decreased by ste-rols while overexpression of active SREBP stimulates FAS promoter activity.[38]

SREBP-2 is a relatively selective activator of cholesterol synthesis (as opposed to fatty acid synthesis) in liver and adipose tissue of mice and in cul-tured human cells, while SREBP-1c is a major mediator of insulin action on hepatic expression of glucokinase and lipogenic genes, including FAS.[38–40] Changes in the expression of lipogenic genes parallel changes in SREBP-1 expression.[36] The demonstration that hepatic expression of lipogenic genes is non-responsive to carbohydrate feeding in SREBP-1 knockout mice suggests a critical role for SREBP-1 in induction of hepatic lipogenesis.

SREBP-1c is also called adipocyte determination and differentiation factor (ADD1).[41] Insulin stimulates SREBP-1c expression at the level of transcrip-tion in cultured rat hepatocytes, while glucagon exerts an inhibitory effect on this gene.[42,43] The effect of insulin on stimulation of nuclear SREBP-1c has also been observed in adipocytes, both *in vivo* and *in vitro*.[42,43] Molecular dissec-tion of the FAS promoter has shown that ADD1/SREBP-1c acts through an E-box motif at nucleotides –64 to 59, which is identical to the region previously recognized as the major IRE.[28,42] In normal rats, the activation of this E-box is countered by the presence of a transcriptionally inactive sterol response element (SRE) binding site at 150, which limits the availability of nuclear ADD1/SREBPs. In obese Zucker *fa/fa* rats, overproduction of SREBP-1 can compensate for ADD1/SREBP-1 and bind to the inactive SRE, thus overcoming the negative effects of the inactive SRE.[44] Furthermore, ADD1/SREBP-1 regulation of FAS promoter activity in adipocytes was antagonized by dominant negative members of the HLH family in rat adipocytes and mature 3T3-L1 adipocytes.[45] In summary, SREBP-1c/ADD1 is a key transcription factor not only in fatty acid synthesis but in other aspects of lipid metabolism in both the liver and adipose tissue, acting in part via the insulin responsive E-box to regulate lipogenic gene transcription.

1.8 Glucose Regulation of FAS Expression and Activity

Since glucose increases circulating insulin levels, it is often difficult to differentiate between the effects of glucose metabolism and those of insulin in mediating the regulation of gene expression. Both glucose-dependent and glucose-independent effects of insulin have been reported.[16] A high level of glucose is not only required for insulin stimulation of FAS transcription but is also involved in stabilizing FAS mRNA as shown in studies using HepG2 cells and adipocyte differentiation studies.[18,19,46] In USF1 or USF2 knockout mice, induction of hepatic FAS gene expression by refeeding a carbohydrate-rich diet was severely delayed, whereas expression of SREBP-1 expression was almost normal. The insulin response was unchanged, suggesting USF transactivators, especially USF1/USF2 heterodimers, are essential to sustain dietary induction of the FAS gene in liver (Fig. 1.5).[47] ADD1/SREBP-1 has

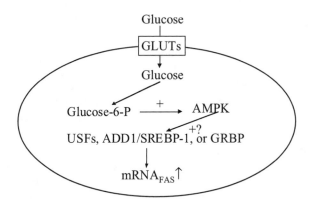

FIGURE 1.5
Proposed mechanism of glucose regulation of the fatty acid synthase gene. GLUTs: glucose transporter, AMPK: AMP-activated protein kinase, USFs: upstream stimulatory factors, ADD1/SREBP1: adipocyte determination and differentiation factor1/sterol response element binding protein 1, GRBP: glucose response binding protein, FAS: fatty acid synthase.

also been suggested to mediate glucose-induced expression of FAS as well as other hepatic genes (Fig. 1.5).[41,48] An upstream stimulatory factor (USF)-binding site at +292/+297 bp in the first intron was reported to be a positive regulatory element involved in glucose responsiveness of the FAS gene.[49]

Glucose-6-phosphate has been postulated to be the signaling molecule mediating glucose/insulin stimulation of several lipogenic genes including pyruvate kinase, spot 14, and FAS.[50,51] However, xyulose 5-phosphate, an intermediate in the pentose phosphate pathway, is also suggested to play this role.[50] Additionally, stimulation of FAS and S14 mRNA levels by glucose and xylitol in rat hepatocyte cultures is more closely correlated with changes in intracellular glucose 6-phosphate levels than xylulose 5-phosphate levels, supporting the hypothesis that glucose 6-phosphate is likely the critical metabolite for regulation of lipogenic gene expression by glucose.[51,52] However, the signaling pathway subsequent to glucose/glucose metabolites which mediate the transcriptional effects on gene expression, is still poorly understood. Glucose response-binding protein (GRBP) binds to the CACGTG motif of the glucose response element and has been identified as a transcription factor mediating the effects of glucose (Fig. 1.5). This protein is activated by high glucose concentrations *in vivo*.[50] Furthermore, the DNA-binding activity of GRBP was found to be inhibited by low glucose concentrations *in vivo* and by cAMP in cultured hepatocytes.[50]

1.9 Regulatory Effects of Polyunsaturated Fatty Acids

Polyunsaturated fatty acids of the n-3 and n-6 families are known to suppress hepatic mRNA levels of several lipogenic genes, including FAS.[53] With the exception of glucose-6-phosphate dehydrogenase, PUFAs exert their regulatory effects at the level of transcription.[53] PUFAs exert dominant negative effects on many of the genes of lipogenesis and are known to override the stimulatory effects of insulin, carbohydrates, and thyroid hormones. Furthermore, the direct effects of PUFAs on the liver do not require extrahepatic factors.

PUFAs are known to suppress hepatic gene expression through three distinct pathways: (1) a peroxisome proliferator activated receptor (PPAR)-dependent pathway, (2) a prostanoid pathway, and (3) a PPAR and prostanoid-independent pathway. Although fibrates and prostanoids have modest inhibitory effects on FAS gene expression, the PUFA-mediated suppression of this gene in the liver does not require either PPARα activation or cyclooxygenase conversion of PUFA to eicosanoids (Fig. 1.6).[54-56] However, the n-6 PUFA arachidonic acid inhibits several lipogenic genes, including FAS in 3T3-L1 adipocytes, through a prostanoid pathway.[57] Furthermore, cyclooxygenase products from non-parenchymal cells can act on parenchymal cells through a paracrine process and mimic the effect of n-6 PUFAs on lipogenic gene expression.[57]

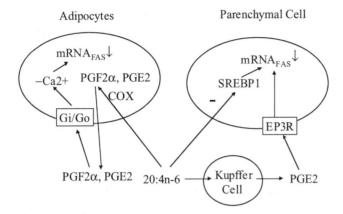

FIGURE 1.6
Proposed mechanism of polyunsaturated fatty acid regulation of the hepatic fatty acid synthase gene. FAS: fatty acid synthase, PGF2α: prostaglandin F2-α, PGE2: prostaglandin E2, COX: cyclooxygenase, 20:4n-6: arachidonic acid, SREBP1: sterol response element binding protein.

Several labs have investigated the mechanisms of PUFA regulation of FAS gene expression. Feeding PUFAs resulted in a decrease in the mature form of SREBP-1 in liver nuclei, which paralleled changes in FAS and ACC mRNA in wild-type mice. Studies using transgenic mice confirmed that the suppressive effect of PUFAs on hepatic FAS expression is due to a decrease in the mature form of SREBP-1 protein.[58] Other labs have also demonstrated the suppressive effects of dietary PUFAs on SREBP-1 expression mediate the subsequent regulation of FAS expression.[59,60] This has been confirmed by feeding fish oils, which downregulate the mature form of SREBP by decreasing SREBP-1c mRNA expression and leads to the concomitant decrease in hepatic FAS mRNA.[61,62] Studies using cultured hepatocytes linked fatty acid peroxidation to the effects of PUFAs on gene expression.[63] These findings suggest that the *in vivo* inhibitory effects of PUFAs on lipogenic genes could be mediated indirectly by a peroxidative mechanism. Further studies will be necessary to explore this signaling pathway in the liver.

1.10 Effects of Glucagon and cAMP

Fasting increases glucagon levels, which may contribute to downregulation of lipogenesis. Insulin presumably mediates the marked increase in the rate of FAS transcription that occurs subsequent to refeeding fasted animals. This elevation can be completely blocked by administration of glucagon or dibutyryl cAMP during the refeeding period. This implies that glucagon, via its second messenger cAMP, antagonizes the stimulatory effects of insulin on

FAS expression.[21] In support of this theory, *in vitro* studies using H4IIE hepatoma cells demonstrate that glucagon antagonizes the effect of insulin on FAS transcription by increasing intracellular levels of cAMP. Studies using the H4IIE hepatoma cell line with a CAT-linked FAS promoter, demonstrate that cAMP is an effective inhibitor of insulin-stimulated FAS transcription.[20] Progressive deletions of sequences from the FAS 5′-flanking region led to identification of a cAMP response element between −149 and +68. The FAS IRS was required for cAMP antagonism of insulin action.[16] An inverted CCAAT box was subsequently identified in the −99/−92 region of the FAS gene. Mutations in this region abolished cAMP responsiveness, suggesting this region is also responsible for mediating the effects of cAMP. Consistent with the localization of the FAS IRS to the −68/−52 bp region, insulin responsiveness was not affected by mutations in the −99/−92 region.[20] The identification of the cAMP response sequence of FAS as an inverted CCAAT box puts the FAS gene in a small group of cAMP-regulated genes that do not use the more common CREB- or ATF-1-binding sites for transcriptional regulation. In fact, the basal transcription factor NF-Y and related proteins bind to the inverted CCAAT box of the FAS promoter *in vitro*.[64]

1.11 Regulatory Effects of Thyroid Hormones

In addition to changes in the levels of circulating insulin and glucagon, thyroid hormone (T3) is also elevated during refeeding of fasted animals. Thyroid hormone stimulates FAS expression through a mechanism that is independent of insulin. Administration of thyroid hormone to rats for 7 days doubled FAS activity in liver.[65] Furthermore, hypothyroidism reduced hepatic FAS activity.[66] These effects can be demonstrated *in vitro* as well. FAS activity can be stimulated 2- to 3-fold in primary cultures of rat and chick embryo hepatocytes.[67–69] This is due to an increase in gene transcription and is accompanied by a 5-fold increase in FAS mRNA.

Adipocytes have also been demonstrated to be responsive to T3.[69] When mature 3T3-L1 adipocytes were treated with 10 nM T3, the relative rate of FAS synthesis, the steady-state mRNA level, and the transcriptional rate all increased within hours and could be sustained at this level for 24 h.[69] Thyroid hormone exerts its effects on FAS transcription by heterodimerization of ligand-bound thyroid hormone receptor (TR) with the retinoid receptor, RXR. The TR/RXR heterodimer binds to the consensus thyroid hormone response element (TRE) and promotes gene transcription.[70–72] Transfections of fusion constructs of the human FAS promoter linked to the luciferase reporter gene into cultured human cells have identified two TREs, TRE1 (GGGTTAcgtcCGGTCA at −716 to −731) and TRE2 (sequence GGGTCC, at −117 to −112).[73]

1.12 Insulin-Like Effects of Angiotensin II

In addition to its synthesis in the classical renin angiotensin system, the hypertensive hormone angiotensin II (AII) is secreted from adipose tissue.[74,75] In adipocytes, AII has an insulin-like effect and acts as a lipogenic hormone to increase fatty acid and triglyceride synthesis.[76] We have demonstrated that AII increases FAS enzyme activity and mRNA content by upregulating FAS gene transcription.[76] Recently, in an attempt to identify AII regulatory sequences in the FAS gene, we found that AII targets insulin regulatory sequences that were previously identified[28] as E-box motifs.[30] Furthermore, we found that ADD1 is a potential transcription factor mediating transcriptional regulation of the FAS gene by AII.[77]

1.13 Regulatory Effects of the Obesity Genes

1.13.1 Leptin

Leptin, the *ob* gene product, is a protein specifically secreted from adipose tissue, and is transported to the hypothalamus where it binds specific receptors resulting in a decrease in appetite.[78,79] Since its identification, leptin has been recognized as a hormone which induces satiety and increases basal energy expenditure. Food intake, specifically dietary carbohydrate, results in the rapid and specific induction of ob mRNA levels in rat adipose tissue.[80,81] The effects of leptin on FAS may be mediated by glucose, polyunsaturated fatty acids, or both. Administration of leptin to rats consuming a high-carbohydrate, fat-free diet suppressed the mRNA expression for several lipogenic enzymes compared to rats consuming a diet rich in corn oil. Corn oil, which is rich in polyunsaturated fatty acids, suppressed lipogenic enzyme expression while concomitantly increasing leptin expression.[79]

Using hepatocytes and adipocytes from Wistar fatty rats, Fukuda et al.[82] investigated the transcriptional regulation of the FAS gene by insulin/glucose, PUFAs, and leptin, and compared them to lean controls. The region of −57/−35 of the FAS gene, which has previously been identified as insulin responsive, was linked to the CAT-reporter gene containing a heterologous promoter and transfected into these cells.[28,82] In the presence of insulin, there was marked stimulation of reporter gene activity in hepatocytes from lean rats, but there was not a significant increase in hepatocytes from obese rats. Stimulation of the reporter gene by insulin was reduced in leptin-treated cells and in cells from lean rats containing an expression vector encoding leptin. However, leptin-treated cells from obese rats did not respond to insulin.

These effects were mediated by leptin-dependent reductions in the insulin-binding capacities of the hepatic and adipose tissue receptors.[82]

1.13.2   Agouti

Agouti is a paracrine factor normally secreted within hair follicles during the neonatal hair growth period. However, this hormone is also expressed in human adipose tissue,[83] suggesting its possible involvement in lipid and energy metabolism. The mechanism of the action of this hormone in both coat color and weight regulation is discussed in detail by Zemel et al. in Chapter 10 of this book. We will discuss only the transcriptional effects of agouti on the FAS gene.

We have demonstrated that agouti acts on adipocytes to increase lipogenesis via a calcium-dependent mechanism.[84] Obese viable yellow mice which over-express the agouti protein have significantly elevated levels of intracellular calcium and FAS gene expression compared to normal mice.[85] Furthermore, results from these studies determined that treatment of these animals with the calcium channel blocker, nifedipine, resulted in a dramatic increase in adipose FAS activity. This effect may be due, in part, to reduced plasma insulin levels in the nifedipine-treated viable yellow mice.[85] To test the possibility that increased FAS activity in adipose tissue of obese viable yellow mice was due to the direct effects of agouti, Jones et al. treated 3T3-L1 adipocytes *in vitro* with recombinant agouti protein.[86] Agouti treatment resulted in a 1.5-fold increase in FAS mRNA levels. In addition, FAS activity and triglyceride content were 3-fold higher in agouti-treated 3T3-L1 cells relative to controls. These effects were attenuated by simultaneous treatment with nifedipine. Together these data demonstrate that the agouti protein can directly increase lipogenesis in adipocytes via a calcium dependent mechanism.[86] Furthermore, we have identified an agouti-responsive region at the –435/–415 in the FAS promoter which is upstream of the previously identified insulin-responsive E-box.[87]

1.14   Regulation of the FAS Gene by Other Factors

Like glucagons and cAMP, growth hormone (GH) decreases FAS mRNA abundance by decreasing both gene transcription and mRNA stability.[88,89] GH-mediated inhibition of lipogenesis in adipocytes of growing pigs was due to decreased insulin sensitivity.[90] However, GH did not alter early events in the insulin signaling cascade, such as receptor binding and receptor kinase activation, suggesting that GH alters insulin signaling downstream of receptor activation.[90]

Other nutrients, including dietary protein and minerals, regulate FAS gene expression. Hepatic FAS mRNA abundance in Wistar fatty rats was significantly lower after feeding soybean protein compared to feeding casein.[91] The regulation of FAS by essential amino acids was also reported in HepG2 cells.[92] A deficiency of dietary copper is accompanied by a 2-fold increase in hepatic fatty-acid biosynthesis.[93] Dietary copper deficiency was demonstrated to increase hepatic FAS activity associated with a reduction in gene transcription. FAS gene transcription was suggested to be dependent on the hepatic thiol redox state.[93] This mechanism may mediate the effects of dietary copper on FAS activity and gene expression.

1.15 Conclusions and Implications

Despite the reduction in dietary fat consumption through massive promotion of low-fat foods, obesity has not ceased to increase.[94] This suggests that carbohydrates may be contributing to fat accumulation in humans. This is, in part, addressed by increased interest in the role of glycemic index in energy metabolism, obesity, and diabetes.

In a typical American diet (relatively high in fat), fatty acids would be derived primarily from lipoprotein triglycerides via the action of the lipoprotein lipase (LPL). As discussed in this chapter, although lipogenesis in humans has been considered as very limited for a long time, available studies clearly demonstrate that fatty acid biosynthesis is important enough in humans to be studied for its relevance to disorders of lipid metabolism. Limited data are available concerning regulation of genes of fatty acid biosynthesis in humans. Studies of the highly regulated fatty acid synthase gene as a marker in this pathway provide useful information on how lipogenesis may be regulated in humans. Inhibition of this enzyme has been shown to be beneficial for reductions of body weight[95] as well as tumorigenesis[96] (an aspect that we did not discuss in this chapter).

Thus, studies of this gene and other genes in fatty acid synthesis may bring additional insights into human diseases linked to abnormal fatty acid synthesis (such as cirrhosis, LPL deficiency).

References

1. Semenkovich, C. F., Regulation of fatty acid synthase., *Prog. Lipid Res.*, 36, 43, 1997.
2. Sul, H. S., Moustaïd, N., Sakamoto, K., Gekakis, N., Smas, C., and Jerkins, A., Nutritional and hormonal regulation of genes encoding enzymes involved in fat synthesis, In *Nutrition and Gene Expression*, Hargrove, J. L. and Berdanier, C., Eds., CRC Press, Boca Raton, 1993.

3. Smith, S., The animal fatty acid synthase: one gene, one polypeptide, seven enzymes, *FASEB J.*, 15, 1248, 1994.

4. Amy, C. M., Williams-Ahlf, B., Naggert, J., and Smith, S., Molecular cloning of the mammalian fatty acid synthase gene and identification of the promoter region, *Biochem. J.*, 27, 675, 1990.

5. Paulauskis, J. D. and Sul, H. S., Cloning and expression of mouse fatty acid synthase and other specific mRNA: developmental and hormonal regulation in 3T3-L1 cells, *J. Biol. Chem.*, 263, 7049, 1988.

6. Kameda, K. and Goodridge, A. G., Isolation and partial characterization of the gene for goose fatty acid synthase, *J. Biol. Chem.*, 266, 419, 1991.

7. Hsu, M.H., Chirala, S. S., and Wakil S. J., Human fatty acid synthase gene. Evidence for the presence of two promoters and their functional interaction, *J. Biol. Chem.*, 271, 13584, 1996.

8. Zelewski, M. and Swierczynski, J., Comparative studies on lipogenic enzyme activities in the liver of humans and some animal species, *Comp. Biochem. Physiol.*, 95, 469, 1990.

9. Tappy, L., Schwarz, J.M., Schneiter, P., Cayeux, C., Revelly, J. P., Fagerquist, C. K., Jequier, E., and Chiolero, R., Effects of isoenergetic glucose-based or lipid-based parenteral nutrition on glucose metabolism, *de novo* lipogenesis, and respiratory gas exchanges in critically ill patients, *Crit. Care Med.*, 26, 860, 1998.

10. Arner, P. and Engfeldt, P., Fasting-mediated alteration studies in insulin action on lipolysis and lipogenesis in obese women, *Am. J. Physiol.*, 253, E193, 1987.

11. Hjollund, E. and Pedersen, O., Transport and metabolism of D-glucose in human adipocytes. Studies of the dependence on medium glucose and insulin concentrations, *Biochem. Biophys. Acta.*, 937, 102, 1988.

12. Chascione, C., Elwyn, D. H., Davila, M., Gil, K. M., Askanazi, J., and Kinney, J. M., Effect of carbohydrate intake on *de novo* lipogenesis in human adipose tissue, *Am. J. Physiol.*, 253, E664,1987.

13. Hellerstein, M. K., Christiansen, M., Kaempfer, S., Kletke, C., Wu, K., Reid, J. S., Mulligan, K., Hellerstein, N. S., and Shackleton, C. H., Measurement of *de novo* hepatic lipogenesis in humans using stable isotopes, *J. Clin. Invest.*, 87, 1841, 1991.

14. Aarsland, A., Chinkes, D., and Wolfe, R. R., Hepatic and whole body fat synthesis in humans during carbohydrate overfeeding, *Am. J. Clin. Nutr.*, 65, 1774, 1997.

15. Claycombe, K. J., Jones, B. H., Standridge, M. K., Guo, Y., Chun, J. T., Taylor, J. W., and Moustaïd-Moussa, N., Insulin increases fatty acid synthase gene transcription in human adipocytes, *Am. J. Physiol.*, 274, R1253, 1998.

16. Ferre, P., Regulation of gene expression by glucose, *Proc. Nutr. Soc.*, 58, 621, 1999.

17. Soncini, M., Yet, S. F., Moon, Y., Chun, J. Y., and Sul, H. S., Hormonal and nutritional control of the fatty acid synthase promoter in transgenic mice, *J. Biol. Chem.*, 270, 30339, 1995.

18. Semenkovich, C. F., Coleman, T., and Goforth, R., Physiologic concentrations of glucose regulate fatty acid synthase activity in HepG2 cells by mediating fatty acid synthase mRNA stability, *J. Biol. Chem.*, 268, 6961, 1993.

19. Moustaïd, N. and Sul, H. S., Regulation of expression of the fatty acid synthase gene in 3T3-L1 cells by differentiation and triiodothyronine, *J. Biol. Chem.*, 266, 18550, 1991.

20. Rangan, V. S., Oskouian, B., and Smith, S., Identification of an inverted CCAAT box motif in the fatty acid synthase gene as an essential element for modification of transcriptional regulation by cAMP, *J. Biol. Chem.*, 271, 2307, 1996.
21. Lakshmanan, M. R., Nepokroeff, C. M., and Porter, J. W., Control of the synthesis of fatty acid synthetase in rat liver by insulin, glucagon, and adenosine 3′,5′cyclic monophosphate, *Proc. Natl. Acad. Sci. USA*, 69, 3516, 1972.
22. Towle, H. C. and Kaytor, E. N., Regulation of the expression of lipogenic genes by carbohydrate, *Ann. Rev. Nutr.*, 17, 405, 1997.
23. Girard, J., Ferre, P., and Foufelle, F., Mechanisms by which carbohydrates regulate expression of genes for glycolytic and lipogenic enzymes, *Ann. Rev. Nutr.*, 17, 325, 1997.
24. Jump, D. B. and Clarke, S. D., Regulation of gene expression by dietary fat, *Ann. Rev. Nutr.*, 19, 63, 1999.
25. Bois-Joyeux, B., Chanez, M., Aranda-Haro, F., and Peret, J., Age-dependent hepatic lipogenic enzyme activities in starved-refed rats, *Diabet Metab.*, 16, 290, 1990.
26. Oskouian, B., Rangan, V. S., and Smith, S., Transcriptional regulation of the rat fatty acid synthase gene: identification and functional analysis of positive and negative effectors of basal transcription, *Biochem. J.*, 317, 257, 1996.
27. Foufelle, F., Gouhot, B., Pegorier, J. P., Perdereau, D., Girard, J., and Ferre, P., Glucose stimulation of lipogenic enzyme gene expression in cultured white adipose tissue, *J. Biol. Chem.*, 267, 20543, 1992.
28. Moustaïd, N., Beyer, R. S., and Sul, H. S., Identification of an insulin response element in the fatty acid synthase promoter, *J. Biol. Chem.*, 269, 5629, 1994.
29. Wang, D. and Sul, H. S., Upstream stimulatory factors bind to insulin response sequence of the fatty acid synthase promoter, *J. Biol. Chem.*, 270, 28716, 1995.
30. Wang, D. and Sul, H. S., Upstream stimulatory factor binding to the E-box at -65 is required for insulin regulation of the fatty acid synthase promoter, *J. Biol. Chem.*, 272, 26367, 1997.
31. Hillgartner, F. B., Salati, L. M., and Goodridge, A. G., Physiological and molecular mechanisms involved in nutritional regulation of fatty acid synthesis, *Physiol. Rev.*, 75, 47, 1995.
32. Wang, D. and Sul, H. S., Insulin stimulation of the fatty acid synthase promoter is mediated by the phosphatidylinositol 3-kinase pathway: involvement of protein kinase B/Akt, *J. Biol. Chem.*, 273, 25420, 1998.
33. Valverde, A. M., Kahn, C. R., and Benito, M., Insulin signaling in insulin receptor substrate (IRS)-1-deficient brown adipocytes, *Diabetes*, 48, 2122, 1999.
34. Brown, M. S. and Goldstein, J. L., The SREBP pathway: regulation of cholesterol metabolism by proteolysis of a membrane-bound transcription factor, *Cell*, 89, 331, 1997.
35. Magana, M. M. and Osborne, T. F., Two tandem binding sites for sterol regulatory element binding proteins are required for sterol regulation of fatty acid synthase promoter, *J. Biol. Chem.*, 271, 32689, 1996.
36. Shimano, H., Horton, J. D., Hammer, R. E., Shimomura, I., and Brown, M. S., Overproduction of cholesterol and fatty acids causes massive liver enlargement in transgenic mice expressing truncated SREBP-1a, *J. Clin. Invest.*, 98, 1575, 1996.
37. Shimano, H., Yahagi, N., Amemiya-Kudo, A. H., Hasty, J.-I., Osuga, Y., Tamura, F., Shionoiri, Y., Iizuka, K., Ohashi, K., Harada, T., Gotoda, S., and Yamada, N., Sterol regulatory element-binding protein-1 as a key transcription factor for nutritional induction of lipogenic enzyme genes, *J. Biol. Chem.*, 274, 35832, 1999.

38. Bennett, M. K., Lopez, J. M., Sanchez, H. B., and Osborne, T. F., Sterol regulation of fatty acid synthase promoter. Coordinate feedback regulation of two major lipid pathways, *J. Biol. Chem.*, 270, 25578, 1995.

39. Kawabe, Y., Suzuki, T., Hayashi, M., Hamakubo, T., Sato, R., and Kodama, T., The physiological role of sterol regulatory element-binding protein-2 in cultured human cells, *Biochim. Biophys. Acta*, 1436, 307, 1999.

40. Foretz, M., Guichard, C., Ferre, P., and Foufelle, F., Sterol regulatory element binding protein-1c is a major mediator of insulin action on the hepatic expression of glucokinase and lipogenesis-related genes, *Proc. Natl. Acad. Sci. USA*, 96, 12737, 1999.

41. Foretz, M., Pacot, C., Dugail, I., Lemarchand, P., Guichard, C., Le Liepvre, X., Berthelier-Lubrano, C., Spiegelman, B., Kim, J. B., Ferre, P., and Foufelle, F., ADD1/SREBP-1c is required in the activation of hepatic lipogenic gene expression by glucose, *Mol. Cell. Biol.*, 19, 3760, 1999

42. Kim, J. B., Sarraf, P., Wright, M., Yao, K. M., Mueller, E., Solanes, G., Lowell, B. B., and Spiegelman, B. B., Nutritional and insulin regulation of fatty acid synthase and leptin gene expression through ADD1/SREBP1, *J. Clin. Invest.*, 101, 1, 1998.

43. Horton, J. D., Bashmakov, Y., Shimomura, I., and Shimano, H., Regulation of sterol regulatory element binding proteins in livers of fasted and refed mice, *Proc. Natl. Acad. Sci. USA*, 95, 5987, 1998.

44. Boizard, M., Le Liepvre, X., Lemarchand, P., Foufelle, F., Ferre, P., and Dugail, I., Obesity-related overexpression of fatty acid synthase gene in adipose tissue involves sterol regulatory element-binding protein transcription factors, *J. Biol. Chem.*, 273, 29164, 1998.

45. Moldes, M., Boizard, M., Liepvre, X. L., Feve, B., Dugail, I., and Pairault, J., Functional antagonism between inhibitor of DNA binding (Id) and adipocyte determination and differentiation factor 1/sterol regulatory element-binding protein-1c (ADD1/SREBP-1c) trans-factors for the regulation of fatty acid synthase promoter in adipocytes, *Biochem. J.*, 344, 873, 1999.

46. Hillgartner, F. B. and Charron, T., Glucose stimulates transcription of fatty acid synthase and malic enzyme in avian hepatocytes, *Am. J. Physiol.*, 274, E493, 1998.

47. Casado, M., Vallet, V. S., Kahn, V., and Vaulont, S., Essential *in vivo* role of upstream stimulatory factors for a normal dietary response of the fatty acid synthase gene in the liver, *J. Biol. Chem.*, 274, 20093, 1999.

48. Hasegawa, J.-I., Osatomi, K., Wu, R. F., and Uyeda, K., A novel factor binding to the glucose response elements of liver pyruvate kinase and fatty acid synthase genes, *J. Biol. Chem.*, 274, 1100, 1999.

49. Oskouian, B., Rangan, V. S., and Smith, S., Regulatory elements in the first intron of the rat fatty acid synthase gene. *Biochem. J.*, 324, 113, 1997.

50. Foufelle, F., Girard, J., and Ferre, P., Regulation of lipogenic enzyme expression by glucose in liver and adipose tissue: a review of the potential cellular and molecular mechanisms, *Adv. Enzyme Regul.*, 36, 199, 1996.

51. Morrieras, F., Foufelle, F., Foretz, M., Morin, J., Bouche, S., and Ferre, P., Induction of fatty acid synthase and S14 gene expression by glucose, xylitol and dihydroxyacetone in cultured rat hepatocytes is closely correlated with glucose 6-phosphate concentrations. *Biochem. J.*, 326, 345, 1997.

52. Doiron, B., Cuif, M.H., Chen, R., and Kahn, A., Transcriptional glucose signaling through the glucose response element is mediated by the pentose phosphate pathway, *J. Biol. Chem.,* 271, 5321, 1996.
53. Jump, D. B., Clarke, S. D., Thelen, A., Liimatta, M., and Ben, B., Dietary polyunsaturated fatty acid regulation of gene transcription, *Prog. Lipid Res.,* 35, 227, 1996.
54. Clarke, S. D., Turini, M., Jump, D. B., Abraham, S., and Reedy, M., Polyunsaturated fatty acid inhibition of fatty acid synthase transcription is independent of PPAR activation, *Z. Ernahrungswiss.,* 37,14, 1998.
55. Ren, B., Thelen, A. P., Peters, J. M., Gonzalez, F. J., and Jump, D. B., Polyunsaturated fatty acid suppression of hepatic fatty acid synthase and S14 gene expression does not require peroxisome proliferator-activated receptor α, *J. Biol. Chem.,* 272, 26827, 1997.
56. Mater, M. K., Thelen, A. P., and Jump, D. B., Arachidonic acid and PGE2 regulation of hepatic lipogenic gene expression, *J. Lipid Res.,* 40, 1045, 1999.
57. Mater, M. K., Pan. D., Bergen, W. G., and Jump, D.B., Arachidonic acid inhibits lipogenic gene expression in 3T3-L1 adipocytes through a prostanoid pathway, *J. Lipid Res.,* 39, 1327, 1998.
58. Jump, D. B., Thelen, A., and Mater, M., Dietary polyunsaturated fatty acids and hepatic gene expression, *Lipids,* 34, S209, 1999.
59. Yahagi, N., Shimano, H., Hasty, A.H., Amemiya-Kudo, M., Okazaki, H., Tamura, Y., Iizuka, Y., Shionoiri, F., Ohashi, K., Osuga, J.-I., Harada, K., Gotoda, T., Nagai, R., Ishibashi, S., and Yamada, N., A crucial role of sterol regulatory element-binding protein-1 in the regulation of lipogenic gene expression by polyunsaturated fatty acids, *J. Biol. Chem.,* 274, 35840, 1999.
60. Mater, M. K., Thelen, A. P., Pan, D.A., and Jump, D.B., Sterol response element-binding protein 1c (SREBP1c) is involved in the polyunsaturated fatty acid suppression of hepatic S14 gene transcription, *J. Biol. Chem.,* 274, 32725, 1999.
61. Xu, J., Nakamura, M. T., Cho, H. P., and Clarke, S. D., Sterol regulatory element binding protein-1 expression is suppressed by dietary polyunsaturated fatty acids, *J. Biol. Chem.,* 274, 23577, 1999.
62. Kim, H.-J., Takahashi, M., and Ezaki, O., Fish oil feeding decreases mature sterol regulatory element-binding protein 1 (SREBP-1) by down-regulation of SREBP-1c mRNA in mouse liver: a possible mechanism for down-regulation of lipogenic enzyme mRNAs, *J. Biol. Chem.,* 274, 25892, 1999.
63. Foretz, M., Foufelle, F., and Ferre, P., Polyunsaturated fatty acids inhibit fatty acid synthase and spot-14-protein gene expression in cultured rat hepatocytes by a peroxidative mechanism, *Biochem. J.,* 341, 371, 1999.
64. Roder, K., Wolf, S. S., Beck, K.-F., Sickinger, S., and Schweizer, M., NF-Y binds to the inverted CCAAT box, an essential element for cAMP-dependent regulation of the rat fatty acid synthase (FAS) gene, *Gene,* 184, 21, 1997.
65. Mariash, C. N., Kaiser, F. E., and Oppenheimer, J. H., Comparison of the response characteristics of four lipogenic enzymes to 3,5,3'-triiodothyronine administration: evidence for variable degrees of amplification of the nuclear 3,5,3'-triiodothyroine signal, *Endocrinology,* 106, 22, 1980
66. Diamant, S., Gorin, E., and Shafrir, E., Enzyme activities related to fatty acid synthesis in liver and adipose tissue of rats treated with triiodothyronine, *Eur. J. Biochem.,* 26, 553, 1972.

67. Swierczynski, J., Mitchell D. A., Reinhold, D. S., Salati, L. M., Stapleton, S. R., Klautky, S. A., Struve, A. E., and Goodridge, A. G., Triiodothyronine-induced accumulations of malic enzyme, fatty acid synthase, acetyl-coenzyme A carboxylase, and their mRNAs are blocked by protein kinase inhibitors. Transcription is the affected step, *J. Biol. Chem.,* 266, 17459, 1991.

68. Mariash, C. N., Kaiser, F. E., Schwartz, H. L., Towle, H. C., and Oppenheimer, J. H., Synergism of thyroid hormone and high carbohydrate diet in the induction of lipogenic enzymes in the rat. Mechanisms and implications, *J. Clin. Invest.,* 65, 1126, 1980.

69. Stapleton, S. R., Mitchell, D. A., Salati, L. M., and Goodridge, A. G., Triiodothyronine stimulates transcription of the fatty acid synthase gene in chick embryo hepatocytes in culture. Insulin and insulin-like growth factor amplify that effect, *J. Biol. Chem.,* 265, 18442, 1990.

70. Marks, M. S., Hallenbeck, P. L., Nagata, T., Segars, J. H., Appella, E., Nikodem, V. M., and Ozato, K., H-2RIIBP (RXR beta) heterodimerization provides a mechanism for combinatorial diversity in the regulation of retinoic acid and thyroid hormone responsive genes, *EMBO J.,* 11, 1419, 1992.

71. Umesono, K., Murakami, K. K., Thompson, C. C., and Evans, R. M., Direct repeats as selective response elements for the thyroid hormone, retinoic acid, and vitamin D3 receptors, *Cell,* 65, 1255, 1991.

72. Saatcioglu, F., Deng, T., and Karin, M., A novel cis element mediating ligand-independent activation by c-ErbA: implications for hormonal regulation, *Cell,* 75, 1095, 1993.

73. Xiong, S., Chirala, S. S., Hsu, M. H., and Wakil, S. J., Identification of thyroid hormone response elements in the human fatty acid synthase promoter, *Proc. Natl. Acad. Sci. USA,* 95, 12260, 1999.

74. Kim, S. K. and Moustaïd-Moussa, N., Secretory, endocrine and autocrine/paracrine function of the adipocyte, *J. Nutr.,* 130, 31105, 2000.

75. Jones, B. H., Standridge, M. K., Taylor, J. W., and Moustaïd, N., Angiotensinogen gene expression in adipose tissue: analysis of obese models and hormonal and nutritional control, *Am. J. Physiol.,* 273, R236, 1997.

76. Jones, B. H., Strandridge, M. K., and Moustaïd, N., Angiotensin II increases lipogenesis in 3T3-L1 and human adipose cells, *Endocrinology,* 138, 1512, 1997.

77. Kim, S., Dugail, I., Standridge, M., Claycombe, K., Chun, J., and N. Moustaïd-Moussa, The angiotensin II response element is the insulin response element in the adipocyte fatty acid synthase gene: the role of the ADDI/SREBP-1c, *Biochem. J.,* in press.

78. Rousseau, V., Becker, D. J., Ongemba, L. N., Rahier, J., Henquin, J. C., and Brichard, S. M., Developmental and nutritional changes of ob and PPAR gamma 2 gene expression in rat white adipose tissue, *Biochem. J.,* 321, 451, 1997.

79. Iritani, N., Sugimoto, T., and Fukuda, H., Gene expressions of leptin, insulin receptors and lipogenic enzymes are coordinately regulated by insulin and dietary fats, *J. Nutr.,* 130, 1183, 2000.

80. Thompson, M. P., Meal-feeding specifically induces obese mRNA expression, *Biochem. Biophys. Res. Commun.,* 224, 332, 1996.

81. Wang, J., Liu, R., Hawkins, M., Barzilai, N., and Rossetti, L., A nutrient-sensing pathway regulates leptin gene expression in muscle and fat, *Nature,* 93, 684, 1998.

82. Fukuda, H., Iritani, N., Sugimoto, T., and Ikeda, H., Transcriptional regulation of fatty acid synthase gene by insulin/glucose, polyunsaturated fatty acid and leptin in hepatocytes and adipocytes in normal and genetically obese rats, *Eur. J. Biochem.*, 260, 505, 1999.

83. Moussa, N. M. and Claycombe, K.J., The yellow mouse obesity syndrome and mechanisms of agouti-induced obesity, *Obes. Res.*, 7, 506, 1999.

84. Zemel, M. B., Nutritional and endocrine modulation of intracellular calcium: implications in obesity, insulin resistance and hypertension, *Mol. Cell Biochem.*, 188, 129, 1998.

85. Kim, J. H., Mynatt, R. L., Moore, J. W., Woychik, R. P., Moustaïd, N., and Zemel, M. B., The effects of calcium channel blockade on agouti-induced obesity, *FASEB J.*, 10, 1646, 1996.

86. Jones, B. H., Kim, J. H., Zemel, M. B., Woychik, R. P., Michaud, E. J., Wilkison, W. O., and Moustaïd, N., Upregulation of adipocyte metabolism by agouti protein: possible paracrine actions in yellow mouse obesity, *Am. J. Physiol.*, 270, E192, 1996.

87. Claycombe, K. J., Wang, Y., Jones, B. H., Kim, S., Zemel, M. B., Wilkinson, W. O., Chun, J., and Moustaïd-Moussa, N., Transcriptional regulation of the adipocyte fatty acid synthase gene by agouti: interaction with insulin, *Physiol. Genomics*, 3, 157, 2000.

88. Yin, D., Clarke, S. D., Peters, J. L., and Etherton, T. D., Somatotropin-dependent decrease in fatty acid synthase mRNA abundance in 3T3-F442A adipocytes is the result of a decrease in both gene transcription and mRNA stability, *Biochem. J.*, 331, 815, 1998.

89. Donkin, S. S., McNall, A. D., Swencki, B. S., Peters, J. L., and Etherton, T. D., The growth hormone-dependent decrease in hepatic fatty acid synthase mRNA is the result of a decrease in gene transcription, *J. Mol. Endocrinol.*, 16, 151, 1996.

90. Magri, K. A., Adamo, M., Leroith, D., and Etherton, T. D., The inhibition of insulin action and glucose metabolism by porcine growth hormone in porcine adipocytes is not the result of any decrease in insulin binding or insulin receptor kinase activity, *Biochem. J.*, 266, 107, 1990.

91. Iritani, N., Hosomi, H., Fukuda, H., Tada, K., and Ikeda, H., Soybean protein suppresses hepatic lipogenic enzyme gene expression in Wistar fatty rats, *J. Nutr.*, 126, 380, 1996.

92. Dudek, S. and Semenkovich, C. F., Essential amino acids regulate fatty acid synthase expression through an uncharged transfer RNA-dependent mechanism, *J. Biol. Chem.*, 270, 29323, 1995.

93. Wilson, J., Kim, S., Allen, K. G., Baillie, R., and Clarke, S. D., Hepatic fatty acid synthase gene transcription is induced by a dietary copper deficiency, *Am. J. Physiol.*, 272, E1124, 1997.

94. Popkin, B.M. and Doak, C.M., The obesity epidemic is a worldwide phenomenon, *Nutr. Rev.*, 56, 106,1998.

95. Loftus, T. M., Jaworsky, D. E., Frehwot, G. L., Townsend, C. A., Ronnett, G. V., Lane, M. D., and Kuhajda, F. P., Reduced food intake and body weight in mice treated with fatty acid synthase inhibitors, *Science*, 288, 2379, 2000.

96. Pizer, E. S., Jackisch, C., Wood, F. D., Pasternack, G. R., Davidson, N. E., and Kuhajda, F. P. Inhibition of fatty acid synthesis induces programmed cell death in human breast cancer cells, *Cancer Res.*, 56, 2745, 1996.

2

Nutrition and Adipocyte Gene Expression

Ron F. Morrison and Stephen R. Farmer

CONTENTS

2.1 Introduction 25
2.2 Pleiotropic Functions of the Adipocyte 26
2.3 Cascade of Transcriptional Events Mediating Adipogenesis 28
2.4 Nutritional Regulation of Adipocyte Gene Expression...........30
    2.4.1 Peroxisome Proliferator-Activated Receptors............31
        2.4.1.1 General Characteristics 31
        2.4.1.2 Natural and Synthetic Ligands 32
        2.4.1.3 Other Nutritional Considerations 34
    2.4.2 CCAAT/Enhancer-Binding Proteins 34
        2.4.2.1 General Characteristics 34
        2.4.2.2 Translational and Post-Translational Modifications 35
        2.4.2.3 Cooperative functions of C/EBPα...............................36
        2.4.2.4 Nutritional Considerations.................................36
    2.4.3 Adipocyte Determination and Differentiation
    Dependent Factor-1..37
        2.4.3.1 General Characteristics 37
        2.4.3.2 Nutritional Considerations.................................38
    2.4.4 Signal Transducers and Activators of Transcription...................39
        2.4.4.1 General Characteristics 39
        2.4.4.2 Nutritional Considerations.................................40
2.5 Perspectives and General Conclusions 40
References 41

2.1 Introduction

Excess adipose tissue, a condition commonly referred to as obesity, is associated with an increased risk of developing diabetes, hypertension, hyperinsulinemia, and cardiovascular disease.[1] Until recently, the adipocyte was viewed as a passive player in the development of obesity in much the way an oil can stores its contents. New discoveries implicating a more active role for the adipocyte in the regulation of energy homeostasis and body composition as well as other non-metabolic processes have given new incentives toward understanding the complexities of adipocyte differentiation. Current knowledge of this process includes a cascade of transcriptional events involving diverse families of transcription factors that cooperate to regulate, directly or indirectly, the gene expression necessary for the development and function of the mature adipocyte. Hormonal and nutritional signaling that impinges on these *trans*-acting factors provides a molecular link between extracellular mediators and adipocyte gene expression important for glucose and lipid homeostasis.

The contents of this chapter present three important aspects concerning nutrition and adipocyte gene expression. First, functions of the adipocyte are briefly discussed with the emphasis on defining this cell as a central mediator of lipid and glucose homeostasis as well as endocrine functions that are conveyed by its secretory products. Second, major transcription factor families considered to mediate adipocyte gene expression are presented in the context of a cascade of transcriptional events regulating the process of adipogenesis. Third, functional characteristics of these *trans*-acting factors are discussed in detail regarding mechanisms through which their transcriptional activities are modulated, as well as specific modes through which they function, singularly or cooperatively, to regulate adipocyte gene expression. Furthermore, current knowledge of the mechanisms through which dietary constituents and hormones mediate transcriptional activity and adipocyte gene expression will be discussed.

2.2   Pleiotropic Functions of the Adipocyte

As illustrated in Fig. 2.1, adipocyte functions can be generally grouped into three categories with potentially overlapping modalities. The classic role of this cell in lipid metabolism involves storage of energy in the form of triglycerides during times of plenty and its release as free fatty acids for vitally important processes such as myocardial contractions during times of need. The adipocyte is also central to glucose metabolism through the secretion of glycerol and fatty acids that play an important role in hepatic and peripheral glucose homeostasis. Furthermore, adipose tissue along with heart and skeletal muscle are the only tissues known to express and regulate the insulin-dependent glucose transporter, Glut4, that facilitates the entry of glucose into these cells and out of circulation postprandially. Emerging data suggest that the adipocyte also plays an important role in numerous processes through its secretory products and endocrine functions. In this regard, leptin has a wide

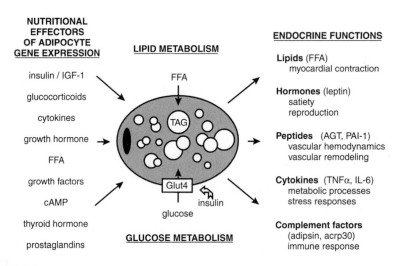

NUTRITIONAL EFFECTORS OF ADIPOCYTE GENE EXPRESSION

insulin / IGF-1

glucocorticoids

cytokines

growth hormone

FFA

growth factors

cAMP

thyroid hormone

prostaglandins

LIPID METABOLISM

FFA

TAG

Glut4

insulin

glucose

GLUCOSE METABOLISM

ENDOCRINE FUNCTIONS

Lipids (FFA)
myocardial contraction

Hormones (leptin)
satiety
reproduction

Peptides (AGT, PAI-1)
vascular hemodynamics
vascular remodeling

Cytokines (TNFα, IL-6)
metabolic processes
stress responses

Complement factors
(adipsin, acrp30)
immune response

FIGURE 2.1

Pleiotropic functions of the adipocyte. Adipocytes play major roles in lipid metabolism in the storage of free fatty acid (FFA) as triacylglycerol (TAG) and in glucose metabolism through expression of the insulin-dependent glucose transporter, Glut4. Endocrine functions include the secretion of angiotensinogen (AGT), plasminogen activator inhibitor type 1 (PAI-1), tumor necrosis factor α (TNFα), interleukin-6 (IL-6), adipsin and adipocyte complement related protein (acrp30). Various nutritional effectors of adipocyte gene expression and potential functions associated with secretory products from the adipocyte are illustrated.

spectrum of biological activities including a hormonal role in mediating satiety and possibly other effects on fertility, reproduction, and hematopoiesis. In addition to this hormone, adipose tissue secretes a variety of peptides, cytokines, and complement factors in which their various functions are linked inseparably to the adipocyte as a source for their production.[2]

While the adipocyte is vitally important to energy homeostasis, adipose tissue may also play a central role in many of the pathologies associated with obesity and its related disorders. Genetic mutations that alter the release of leptin from the adipocyte or suppress its interaction with receptors in the hypothalamus are well-known causes of obesity in mice. Cytokines and lipids released from adipose tissue may lead to a decrease in glucose utilization in skeletal muscle and enhance glucose production by the liver, both of which contribute to high levels of glucose in the peripheral circulation, a hallmark of non-insulin-dependent diabetes mellitus. Furthermore, cytokines from the adipocyte may play a role in activating various inflammatory responses that are considered important mediators of cardiovascular disease. In addition, the development of atherosclerotic lesions is likely to be compounded by hyperlipidemia contributed to by the release of fatty acids from fat-laden adipocytes.

Numerous hormones, cytokines, growth factors, and synthetic compounds have been investigated for their potential to modulate adipogenesis.[2] Regulation of adipocyte differentiation or adipocyte gene expression by any extracellular effector is likely to play a role in regulating any of the diverse adipocyte functions discussed above. A greater appreciation for the complexities of adipogenesis as well as newly ascribed adipocyte functions will lead to a greater understanding of the molecular mechanisms whereby nutrition may play an active role in lipid and glucose homeostasis through the regulation of adipocyte gene expression.

2.3 Cascade of Transcriptional Events Mediating Adipogenesis

Acquisition of function that develops during adipogenesis is estimated to involve both positive and negative changes in the expression of a great number of functional proteins.[3] While post-transcriptional regulation has been demonstrated, many of these changes occur at the gene expression level through a series of molecular events involving several transcription factor families that exhibit diverse modes of activation and function. The more prominent *trans*-acting factors currently considered to play a regulatory role in the process of adipogenesis[2-7] include peroxisome proliferator-activated receptor gamma (PPARγ) and members of the CCAAT/enhancer-binding proteins (C/EBPs), particularly, C/EBPα. Also included are members of the signal transducers and activators of transcription (STATs) and adipocyte determination and differentiation factor-1 (ADD-1), also known as sterol regulatory element binding protein-1c (SREBP-1c). Lesser understood roles for other transcription factors in mediating adipocyte gene expression have recently been reported[8] or reviewed elsewhere.[2]

Much of our knowledge concerning the sequence of transcriptional events mediating adipogenesis has evolved from cultured cell lines (e.g., 3T3-L1, 3T3-F442A) that differentiate from determined, fibroblastic-like cells into functionally mature adipocytes resembling those found in white adipose tissue, *in vivo*. A schematic of transcriptional events known to occur during differentiation of 3T3-L1 preadipocytes is illustrated in Fig. 2.2. Differentiation is initiated following exposure of post-confluent preadipocytes to a cocktail of mitogen and hormonal agents including fetal bovine serum, insulin (at concentrations known to activate the IGF-1 receptor), dexamethasone (a synthetic glucocorticoid), and methylisobutylxanthine (an agent that increases cAMP levels). Among the earliest transcriptional events following exposure to these inducers is the dramatic, but transient elevation in C/EBPβ and C/EBPδ gene expression.[9] While ectopic expression of these C/EBPs in non-progenitor fibroblasts results in significant adipocyte conversion,[10-12] their early and transient expression in lieu of the delayed and sustained expression of most adipocyte genes led to the hypothesis that these C/EBPs play a role in regulating the expression of other transcription factors that initiate and/or maintain the gene expression constituting the adipocyte phenotype. Considerable evidence now

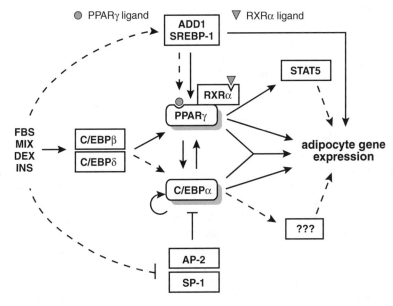

FIGURE 2.2
Cascade of transcriptional events mediating adipocyte differentiation. Activation of adipocyte differentiation culminates in the expression of PPARγ and C/EBPα that regulate, directly or indirectly, much of the gene expression necessary for the functionally mature adipocyte. Broken lines represent transcription factor interactions or pathways that are poorly understood.

suggests that these trans-acting factors contribute to the process of adipogenesis, at least in part, by transactivating the expression of PPARγ[10,13] and possibly C/EBPα.[14] The kinetics of expression, gain- and loss-of-function studies, and identification of functional consensus sequences in the promoters of many adipocyte genes position PPARγ and C/EBPα as central regulators of adipogenesis (discussed below). Evidence suggests that the expression of PPARγ and C/EBPα is continuously maintained despite the ensuing decay of C/EBPβ and C/EBPδ, primarily through cross-regulation.[15] While data suggest that C/EBPα has the capacity to autoregulate its own expression,[14,16,17] a recent study indicates that this is probably not the case for PPARγ, as ectopic PPARγ expression was not capable of activating endogenous gene expression in C/EBPα deficient fibroblasts.[18] Once expressed, PPARγ and C/EBPα transactivate much of the adipocyte gene program as a function of either *trans*-acting factor alone or through the cooperative efforts of both (discussed below).

Additional early events are known to be important for the activation of PPARγ and C/EBPα gene expression. For example, exposure of preadipocytes to mitogens and hormonal agents that induce differentiation also leads to an early upregulation of ADD-1/SREBP-1c gene expression.[19] It has been postulated that this SREBP family member plays a role in upregulating PPARγ gene expression.[20] Moreover, evidence suggests that

ADD-1/SREBP-1c may be involved in gene expression that leads to the production of endogenous PPARγ ligands needed for transcriptional activity.[21] Other studies have demonstrated that undifferentiated preadipocytes express a number of inhibitory proteins that must be repressed or functionally inactivated for the process of differentiation to proceed. For example, exposure of preadipocytes to the differentiation agents leads to repression of AP-2α and Sp1 transcriptional activity, events that are necessary for C/EBPα gene expression.[22–24] Inhibitory molecules may function to maintain the preadipocyte phenotype until hormonal and nutritional conditions are supportive for adipocyte differentiation. Similar paradigms are now considered dogma in cell proliferation pathways where numerous proteins serve checkpoint functions regulating commitment to cell cycle progression.

Although PPARγ and C/EBPα play a regulatory role in the development of the mature adipocyte, only a limited number of the exhaustive list of genes encoding for proteins mediating adipocyte function are known to contain active consensus sequences for either PPARγ or C/EBPα. It is conceivable that these potent adipogenic transcription factors modulate the expression of other genes, indirectly, through the activation of intermediary *trans*-acting factors. In this regard, recent evidence indicates that the differentiation-dependent induction of STAT1, STAT5A, and STAT5B, are regulated downstream of PPARγ in the differentiation paradigm.[25] Although upregulated in a differentiation-dependent fashion, the precise function of STATs in modulating adipogenesis has yet to be determined. While future studies will undoubtedly identify other unknown transcription factors downstream of PPARγ and C/EBPα, activation of STAT expression represents the only known regulation of *trans*-acting factors by either of these adipogenic mediators.

2.4   Nutritional Regulation of Adipocyte Gene Expression

Nutrition has long been considered to play an active role in signaling metabolic tissues about the need for energy storage vs. energy expenditure. Until recently, the molecular mechanisms whereby these signals may regulate adipocyte gene expression to ensure energy homeostasis have been poorly understood. Even less has been known concerning the role of nutrition in regulating gene expression which leads to alterations in energy balance that culminate in pathological states such as diabetes, hyperlipidemia, and obesity. The following discussion will address specific characteristics regarding transcription factor families considered important mediators of adipocyte gene expression. Our understanding of the mechanisms whereby lipid-related compounds along with the hormone insulin may mediate the activity of these trans-acting factors *in vitro* and *in vivo* will be included.

2.4.1 Peroxisome Proliferator-Activated Receptors

2.4.1.1 General Characteristics

The peroxisome proliferator-activated receptors (PPARs) belong to the super-family of nuclear hormone receptors whose transcriptional activities depend on binding of specific ligands to the receptors and heterodimerization with other members of this superfamily prior to DNA binding and transactivation. The three known PPAR family members, PPARα, PPARγ, and PPARδ, bind similar peroxisome proliferator response elements (PPREs), but exhibit different transactivating functions that are mediated, in part, by tissue distribution, ligand specificity, and coactivator recruitment.[7] PPARγ presents a more restricted pattern of expression than PPARα and PPARδ.[26] This receptor has two isoforms, γ1 and γ2,[27,28] which are derived from the same gene by alternative promoter usage and splicing.[29,30] Both isoforms are expressed predominantly in adipocytes of brown and white adipose tissue. In mice and humans, PPARγ1 and PPARγ2 are also expressed at lower levels in skeletal muscle to an extent that is not likely due to adipose contamination.[31,32] The PPARγ1 isoform is also expressed in a variety of other cell types including macrophages[33] and epithelial cells of the breast, bladder, and colon.[34,35] Binding of either PPARγ isoform to the promoter of a target gene is dependent upon association with its obligate heterodimeric partner, retinoic X receptor alpha (RXRα).[36]

Numerous studies have demonstrated an upstream, regulatory role for PPARγ in mediating the process of adipogenesis. The expression of PPARγ kinetically precedes the onset of most adipocyte gene expression and characteristic lipid accumulation.[12] Functional PPREs have been identified in the promoters of several adipocyte genes including the fatty acid binding protein, aP2, lipoprotein lipase (LPL), and phosphoenolpyruvate carboxykinase (PEPCK).[7] Ectopic expression of PPARγ in non-progenitor fibroblasts[29] and myoblasts[37] in combination with adipogenic inducers and synthetic ligands or activators for PPARγ has been shown to result in nearly complete morphological and biochemical adipocyte differentiation. Synthetic ligands specific for PPARγ also have been shown to enhance the hormonally induced differentiation of 3T3-L1[38] and 3T3-F442A[39] preadipocytes.

Several loss-of-function studies also support a regulatory role for PPARγ during adipogenesis. For example, expression of a dominant negative mutant of PPARγ in primary human preadipocytes has been shown to block differentiation mediated by a standard induction cocktail that included a synthetic ligand for PPARγ.[40] Synthetic compounds that bind to the receptor and exhibit little[41] or no[42] PPARγ agonist activity *in vitro* are known to block the ability of adipogenic cell lines to undergo hormone-mediated cell differentiation in the absence of exogenous ligands. Gene ablation studies have been complicated by early embryonic lethality due to placental defects. Supplementing PPARγ null embryos with wild-type placentas via aggregation with tetraploid embryos produced one mouse that survived to term before dying of other complications. This study reported that brown adipose tissue was absent in the neonate, but the contribution of PPARγ to white adipose tissue could not be determined because death occurred before the normal development of this tissue.[43] Heterozygous PPARγ-deficient mice, generated by the same technique, survived birth and were described as having smaller adipocytes and a decreased fat mass.[44] Another means of circumventing the placental defect was approached by generating chimeric mice from wild-type and PPARγ null cells. In this study, little or no contribution of null cells to adipose tissue was observed.[45] The requirement of PPARγ for adipose tissue development is further supported by the reduced capacity of embryonic stem cells[45] or mouse embryo fibroblasts[44] to differentiate *in vitro* under strong adipogenic conditions. Collectively, the results from gain- and loss-of-function studies provided strong evidence supporting an obligatory role for PPARγ in adipocyte differentiation, *in vitro* and *in vivo*.

2.4.1.2 Natural and Synthetic Ligands

PPARs, originally classified as orphan receptors without identified ligands, are now considered to be receptors activated and bound by a broad range of both natural and synthetic molecules (Fig. 2.3). Compounds that are able to

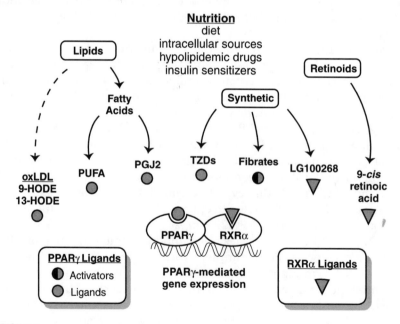

FIGURE 2.3
Natural and synthetic ligands modulating PPARγ-RXRα transcriptional activity. Lipid-related molecules, such as metabolites of oxidized low-density lipoproteins (oxLDL), polyunsaturated fatty acids (PUFA), and prostaglandin J2 (PGJ2) are natural ligands for PPARγ. Synthetic ligands or activators of PPARγ include various insulin-sensitizing and hypolipidemic drugs such as thiazolidinediones (TZDs) and fibrates. The natural ligand for RXRα, 9-*cis*-retinoic acid, is derived from retinoids and vitamin A. Unknown involvement of specific ligands in adipocyte gene expression are represented by broken lines.

induce PPAR-mediated transactivation, but not yet proven to directly bind to the receptor are called activators. Ligands, on the other hand, are molecules that interact with the ligand-binding domain of the receptor and modulate transcriptional activity. Prior to the discovery of these receptors, a variety of diverse agents such as fibrate hypolipidemic drugs, phthalate ester plasticizers, and herbicides were observed to cause a massive proliferation in peroxisomes in rodent hepatocytes.[46] The observation that nutrients, such as high-fat diets, could also induce perixosome proliferation, coupled with the knowledge that most of the major pathways of lipid metabolism are mediated by PPAR-regulated genes led to the discovery that various fatty acids and their metabolites function as natural ligands for PPARs. Several long-chain, polyunsaturated fatty acids (PUFA) bind to PPARγ *in vitro* and can stimulate lipid lowering and enhanced insulin sensitivity effects similar to those reported for synthetic PPAR ligands.[47] Fibrates,[48,49] fatty acids,[29,49,50] and eicosanoids (i.e., arachidonic acid metabolites)[51,52] can induce differentiation of cultured preadipocytes presumably through enhancing PPARγ activity, suggesting that PUFAs and various prostaglandins, especially 15-deoxy prostaglandin J2 (PGJ2),[53-55] function as natural PPARγ ligands in the adipocyte. The uptake of oxidized low-density lipoproteins (oxLDL) through scavenger receptors has been shown to enhance the expression of PPARγ in macrophages known as foam cells residing within atherosclerotic lesions of the arterial wall. In these cells, lipid components of oxLDL, 9-hydroxyoctadecadienoic acid (9-HODE), and 13-HODE also function as endogenous ligands of PPARγ.[56,57] While it is unknown if these molecules serve any role in the adipocyte, these data support the notion that lipid-related compounds are most likely the natural ligands for PPARγ. The fatty acids and lipid metabolites that have thus far been characterized as natural ligands have weaker binding kinetics than ligands for other nuclear hormone receptors with Kd values in the micromolar vs. nanomolar range. While these kinetics have generated some concern as to the physiological role of these ligands, it should be noted that the level of plasma fatty acids is sufficiently high for PPARγ activation. With this notion in mind, it has been postulated that it may not be a requirement for lipids, whose concentrations are naturally high and higher still in lipid overload, to bind PPARγ with high affinity.[58]

A synthetic class of compounds known as thiazolidinediones (TZDs) selectively bind PPARγ with high affinity (nanomolar range) and potently enhance transcriptional activity.[59] Interestingly, these compounds were developed and used as lipid-lowering and insulin-sensitizing agents before the discovery that they are also potent ligands for PPARγ. As antidiabetic agents, TZDs appear to work by either mimicking or enhancing insulin action without stimulating β-cell insulin secretion[60] and have been demonstrated as very effective in improving insulin sensitivity and glucose tolerance in diabetic patients.[61-63] Studies using various animal models of obesity and diabetes have also reported that these synthetic compounds are effective in lowering hyperglycemia and hyperinsulinemia and improving insulin sensitivity.[64-66] The notion that TZDs produce these effects through

modulating PPARγ activity is strongly supported by the observed close correlation between the relative binding kinetics of TZDs to PPARγ and their
antidiabetic action *in vivo*.[54,59] It is interesting to note that synthetic ligands
(e.g., LG100268) for RXR-α, obligatory heterodimeric partner PPARγ,
enhance the insulin-sensitizing effects of TZDs when administered to
obese, insulin-resistant mice.[67,68] In fact, the combination of PPARγ and
RXRα ligands appears to induce a greater transcriptional activation than
either ligand alone,[69] suggesting that a combination of synthetic ligands
may be more efficacious in the treatment of hyperlipidemia and insulin
resistance. The physiological role of the natural ligand for RXRα, 9-*cis*-ret-
inoic acid, derived from retinoids and vitamin A, in mediating adipocyte
gene expression has not been investigated extensively.

2.4.1.3 *Other Nutritional Considerations*

It is not surprising that PPARγ, which plays a significant role in mediating
adipogenesis, is regulated during altered states of nutrition and obesity. Elevated levels of PPARγ2 mRNA in adipose tissue of human obese patients
have been reported where there was a strong positive correlation between the
ratio of PPARγ2/γ1 and body mass index.[32] Restricting caloric intake for 10%
weight loss in these patients resulted in a 25% decrease in PPARγ2 mRNA
that reverted to pretreatment levels after 4 weeks of weight maintenance.[32]
Similar nutritional effects were observed in mice where high-fat diets or fasting were shown to produce a 50% increase or 80% decrease in adipose
PPARγ2 mRNA levels, respectively.[31] These nutritionally linked changes in
mRNA levels suggest the possibility that PPARγ gene expression may be regulated, directly or indirectly, by hormones such as insulin. This notion is supported by the observation that PPARγ mRNA levels are suppressed in
insulin-dependent diabetic mice and can be partially restored with insulin
treatment.[31] While cause and effect have not been established, it could be
hypothesized that hormonally-mediated changes in gene expression in conjunction with nutrient-mediated changes in transcriptional activity position
PPARγ as an important molecular link between changes in diet and the effect
on gene expression modulating energy homeostasis.

2.4.2 CCAAT/Enhancer-Binding Proteins

2.4.2.1 *General Characteristics*

The CCAAT/enhancer-binding proteins (C/EBPs) belong to a large family
of transcription factors containing a leucine zipper motif that functions in
forming homo- or hetero-dimeric complexes with other C/EBP family
members. Three of these family members, C/EBPα, C/EBPβ, and C/EBPδ,
are expressed in both brown and white adipocytes as well as a variety of
other cell types and have been implicated as major role players in regulating the gene expression necessary for adipocyte differentiation.[4,70–72]

C/EBPα is expressed immediately prior to the transcription of a number of adipocyte-specific genes. Analyses of the upstream regulatory regions of aP2, stearoyl CoA desaturase 1 (SCD1), Glut4, PEPCK, leptin, and the insulin receptor have revealed functional C/EBP consensus sequences in the proximal promoters.[2] Ectopic expression of C/EBPα in 3T3-L1 preadipocytes has been shown to be sufficient for inducing adipogenesis without the use of external hormonal inducers.[73] Furthermore, ectopic expression of C/EBPα or C/EBPβ has resulted in potent induction of adipogenesis in non-progenitor fibroblasts under adipogenic conditions.[10,11,74] The observation that antisense expression of C/EBPα inhibits differentiation of cultured preadipocytes provides further evidence supporting a regulatory role for C/EBPs during adipogenesis.[16] Mice targeted for C/EBPα gene ablation die within 8 h postpartum due, in part, to hypoglycemia since administration of glucose can rescue these animals for up to 40 h.[75] Within this time frame, lipid droplets appeared in white and brown adipose tissue of control animals. In contrast, C/EBPα deficient mice are suppressed in their ability to develop brown adipocytes and completely devoid of characteristic white adipose tissue. Gene ablation studies that target both C/EBPβ and C/EBPδ also demonstrate a reduced propensity for adipogenesis, with deficient animals developing markedly less adipose tissue compared to wild-type littermates.[76] Collectively, these data demonstrate a prominent role for C/EBP family members during the development of adipocyte differentiation, *in vitro* and *in vivo*.

2.4.2.2 Translational and Post-Translational Modifications

Translational and post-translational modifications are thought to play a regulatory role in C/EBP transcriptional activity. Both C/EBPα and C/EBPβ genes give rise to multiple protein isoforms through the regulated use of alternate translational start sites.[17] The first and third in-frame AUG of C/EBPα yields two proteins of 42 kDa and 30 kDa, where the former is more efficient at inducing adipogenesis and the post-mitotic growth arrest associated with terminal differentiation.[17,77] Changes in the ratio of C/EBPα isoforms during the course of differentiation has led to the notion that regulated alternate translational products may have a role in regulating C/EBP function.[17] Similar changes have been observed for alternate translational products of C/EBPβ proteins, 32 kDa and 20 kDa, referred to as liver activator protein (LAP) and liver inhibitor protein (LIP), respectively. In this case, the truncated 20-kDa isoform lacks a transactivation domain and functions as a dominant negative when heterodimerized with other C/EBPs.[78] Post-translational modification may also be an important mode of regulating C/EBP functional activity where C/EBPα protein is phosphorylated on as many as six amino acid residues in fully differentiated adipocytes.[79] Signaling pathways that lead to selective dephosphorylation of specific sites may serve an important function in regulating adipocyte gene expression (discussed below).

2.4.2.3   Cooperative functions of C/EBPα

Although PPARγ and C/EBPα are considered the most prominent adipogenic transcription factors, much evidence now suggests that complete adipocyte differentiation requires cooperation of their transcriptional activities.
While many adipocyte genes may be regulated by one or the other of these
transcription factors, the promoters of aP2 and PEPCK contain functional
binding sites for both PPARγ and C/EBPα. One approach to understanding
the unique contribution between these *trans*-acting factors is to ectopically
express one under conditions not permissive for the other and examine the
effect on adipogenesis or adipocyte function. For example, differentiation of
3T3-L1 preadipocytes by the standard induction cocktail does not require
supplement of exogenous PPARγ ligands for complete differentiation. In contrast, differentiation of C/EBPα-defective NIH-3T3 fibroblasts ectopically
expressing PPARγ is dependent upon exogenous ligands unless C/EBPα and
PPARγ are co-expressed.[80] These data indicate that the state of PPARγ ligand
independence is mediated, directly or indirectly, by C/EBPα. Cooperation is
also noted in studies where PPARγ was ectopically expressed in C/EBPα
knockout mouse embryo fibroblasts[18] or in NIH-3T3 fibroblasts that are
defective for C/EBPα expression.[81] Under potent adipogenic conditions
including PPARγ ligand supplement, fibroblasts in either case formed characteristic lipid droplets and expressed many genes associated with adipocyte
differentiation. However, these fibroblasts were insulin resistant regarding
glucose uptake. Rescue of this defect with co-expression of C/EBPα clearly
demonstrates synergy among these adipogenic transcription factors within a
program of events involving many proteins necessary for the complex process of insulin sensitivity. Similar studies in PPARγ-deficient fibroblasts
ectopically expressing C/EBPα will provide additional information regarding the cooperation and unique functions of these adipogenic transcription
factors once cells become available.

2.4.2.4   Nutritional Considerations

Numerous studies have demonstrated a positive correlation between Glut4
and C/EBPα gene expression, suggesting that acquisition of insulin sensitivity in the adipocyte is tightly coupled to the function of this transcription factor. Adipose tissue Glut4 gene expression increases and decreases during
states of high-fat feeding and fasting, respectively,[82] suggesting that both
gene expression and transporter localization to the membrane may be under
hormonal control. While the effects of fasting and refeeding on C/EBPα gene
expression *in vivo* have not been reported, it could be hypothesized that a
coordinate change in C/EBPα would occur under similar nutritional conditions. It has been shown that C/EBPα mRNA is overexpressed in adipose tissue of obese Zucker rats, suggesting a possible role for this *trans*-acting factor
in regulating lipid-related gene expression associated with obesity.[83] Para-
doxically, insulin has been shown to cause a coordinate decrease in both
Glut4 gene expression and C/EBPα activity when exposed to fully differen-

tiated 3T3-L1 adipocytes in culture. The kinetics of repression and the functional C/EBP-binding site in the Glut4 promoter lead to the possibility that the effects of insulin on Glut4 gene expression in culture are mediated by coordinate changes in C/EBPα activity. It has been reported that the mechanism by which insulin induces this repression on C/EBPα transcriptional activity may involve at least three mechanisms: suppression of C/EBPα gene expression, rapid dephosphorylation of C/EBPα protein, and inactivation of C/EBPα through induction of the dominant negative form of C/EBPβ (i.e., LIP).[79,84,85] Additional evidence suggests that insulin stimulates the dephosphorylation of C/EBPα through inactivation of glycogen synthase kinase 3.[86] While these results are unlikely to account for the positive effects of insulin on transporting glucose into the adipocyte postprandially, they may provide a transcriptional mechanism coupling the disease states of hyperinsulinemia and insulin resistance. Further studies *in vitro* and *in vivo* are required to ascertain the physiological effects of nutrition on C/EBPα-mediated gene expression.

2.4.3 Adipocyte Determination and Differentiation Dependent Factor-1

2.4.3.1 *General Characteristics*

Sterol regulatory element binding proteins (SREBPs) are known to modulate transcription of numerous genes encoding proteins that function in both cholesterol and fatty acid metabolism.[87] The SREBP family consists of three proteins, designated SREBP-1a, -1c, and -2, that are encoded by two independent genes. In humans and mice, SREBP-1a and SREBP-1c are produced from a single gene using alternate transcription start sites. Adipocyte determination and differentiation dependent factor-1 (ADD-1), cloned independently from a rat adipocyte cDNA library,[88] is homologous to human SREBP-1c. SREBPs contain two transmembrane domains that anchor the protein to the endoplasmic reticulum in an inactive state (Fig. 2.4). When sterol levels are low, two proteolytic events result in the cleavage and release of the cytoplasmic N-terminal fragment that translocates to the nucleus, binds to the promoters of target genes, and regulates transcription.[89,90] The functional fragment of SREBPs (i.e., amino terminus) contains a basic-helix-loop-helix leucine zipper domain that exhibits dual specificity for classic E-box motifs as well as non-E-box sterol regulatory elements (SREs). While all three SREBPs are capable of activating similar gene expression, evidence suggests that regulation of gene expression important in fat metabolism is primarily mediated by SREBP-1a and ADD-1/SREBP-1c. SREBP-2 is more associated with cholesterol metabolism.[91] Adipose tissue, *in vivo*, predominantly expresses ADD-1/SREBP-1c over other forms of SREBPs.

A role for ADD-1 in adipogenesis was indicated when ectopic expression of a constitutively active form was shown to enhance adipocyte gene expression in non-progenitor NIH-3T3 fibroblasts under differentiation conditions. In addition, expression of a dominant negative form of this *trans*-acting factor

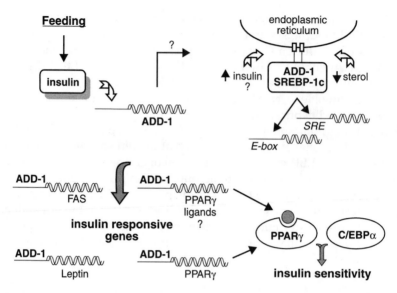

FIGURE 2.4
Potential role of ADD-1 in mediating insulin action in the adipocyte. Insulin activation of cell surface receptors leads to an increase in ADD-1 gene expression through an unidentified mechanism. This protein is initially processed as an inactive molecule that is tethered to the endoplasmic reticulum. Following proteolytic cleavage, the amino terminus of ADD-1 translocates to the nucleus and activates insulin-responsive gene expression. Gene targets for ADD-1 also include PPARγ and potentially genes mediating the production of endogenous PPARγ ligand. Gene programs leading to insulin sensitivity with regard to glucose uptake are mediated by the cooperative efforts of both PPARγ and C/EBPα.

suppressed 3T3-L1 preadipocyte differentiation.[92] As discussed above, it appears that ADD-1 functions, in part, through cooperation with PPARγ by increasing its expression[20] and by regulating the production of a lipid ligand[21] that modulates its transcriptional activity (Fig. 2.4). In a parallel fashion to PPARγ, ADD-1/SREBP-1c also functions directly in the transcription of several genes important for lipid homeostasis, such as fatty acid synthase (FAS) and leptin.[93] While ablation of the SREBP-1 gene (mice lacking both SREBP-1a and SREBP-1c) has been reported to have little effect on white adipose tissue mass, redundancy of function (i.e., SREBP-2 expression) has not been ruled out.[94]

2.4.3.2 *Nutritional Considerations*

New insights into the role of ADD-1 in mediating the hormonal effects of insulin in both adipocytes and hepatocytes have recently been reported.[95] This anabolic hormone is generally considered the major regulator of energy homeostasis during the feed state. Insulin action at the level of the adipocyte includes regulation of insulin-sensitive processes such as uptake of glucose from the circulation as well as activation of numerous lipogenic genes important for energy storage. Although insulin-responsive elements have been identified in the promoters of many anabolic genes, the identification of adipogenic transcription factors through which insulin may mediate gene expression has been elusive. Recent reports indicate that the mRNA levels of ADD-1 and two of its transcriptional target genes, FAS and leptin, decrease in adipose tissue when animals are fasted and increase upon refeeding (Fig. 2.4). These nutritional effects can be duplicated in culture through exposure to insulin.[93] Interestingly, the insulin-responsive element in the FAS promoter contains an E-box motif that binds ADD-1.[93,96]

Analogous studies have been reported for cultured hepatocytes where insulin directly stimulates ADD-1 mRNA accumulation.[97] Furthermore, the expression of a dominant negative form of ADD-1 in hepatocytes blocks the ability of insulin to induce the expression of insulin-responsive genes. In addition, the expression of a dominant positive mutant of ADD-1 stimulates the expression of these insulin-responsive genes in hepatocytes even in the absence of insulin.[98] As discussed above, hepatic ADD-1 is initially tethered to the endoplasmic reticulium in an inactive form until proteolytic cleavage is induced by a decrease in cellular sterol levels. If ADD-1 is initially synthesized in an inactive form in adipocytes as well as hepatocytes, it will be interesting to determine if elevated insulin levels also mediate the release of ADD-1 in a fashion similar to that induced by low sterol levels (Fig. 2.4). It appears that ADD-1/SREBP-1c is positioned to mediate insulin action in the mature adipocyte directly through regulating insulin-responsive gene expression important for carbohydrate and lipid homeostasis as well as indirectly through the transcriptional activities of PPARγ and C/EBPα that are essential for the establishment of insulin sensitivity during adipogenesis (Fig. 2.4).

2.4.4 Signal Transducers and Activators of Transcription

2.4.4.1 *General Characteristics*

Signal transducers and activators of transcription (STATs) comprise a family of cytoplasmic proteins that are activated and mediate gene expression in response to extracellular effectors that target receptors with intrinsic kinase activity or receptors to which Janus kinases (JAKs) are bound.[99] Ligand-mediated dimerization of the receptor results in phosphorylation of the associated kinase, which subsequently phosphorylates the cytoplasmic tail of the receptor, which then serves as a docking site for STAT recruitment. The receptor-bound STAT is phosphorylated, then dimerizes with other STAT proteins and translocates to the nucleus to mediate specific gene expression. The seven known STAT family members are constitutively expressed in a variety of tissues in an inactive form until receptor-mediated phosphorylation events occur. The expression of three members of this family, STAT1, STAT5A, and STAT5B, is upregulated during differentiation of cultured preadipocytes in a coordinate fashion with the expression of PPARγ and C/EBPα.[100,101] While the function of STATs during adipocyte differentiation is still unclear, gene ablation of STAT5A and STAT5B produces animals with markedly less white adipose tissue compared to wild-type littermates, demonstrating a significant role for these proteins during adipogenesis.[102]

2.4.4.2 Nutritional Considerations

Differentiation-dependent expression and loss-of-function studies suggest that the upregulation of specific STAT proteins is likely to be an important regulated process during adipogenesis. It should be emphasized that activation of these inducible STATs (discussed above) and the constitutively expressed STATs (i.e., STAT3 and STAT6) in the adipocyte may also function as a regulatory mechanism in mediating adipocyte gene expression before, during, and after the process of differentiation. The notion that numerous cytokines, growth factors, and hormones are known to regulate STAT activity in other cell types[99] and that these extracellular effectors have pronounced effects on gene expression in the mature adipocyte[2,103] suggests that some of these effects may be mediated by one or more STAT proteins. For example, interferon-γ, leukemia inhibitory factor, and oncostatin-M induce significant tyrosine phosphorylation and prominent translocation of STAT3 into the nucleus following acute treatment in mature 3T3-L1 adipocytes.[104,105] Furthermore, growth hormone stimulates a dramatic activation of STAT5A and STAT5B in fully differentiated 3T3-L1[104,105] and 3T3-F442A[106] adipocytes. In contrast, interleukin-4 induces STAT6 tyrosine phosphorylation and DNA binding, but only in undifferentiated preadipocytes.[107]

A recent study also reports that STAT3 is phosphorylated in subconfluent preadipocytes and during postconfluent mitotic clonal expansion that follows induction of differentiation, suggesting a possible role for STAT3 during proliferative phases of adipogenesis.[108] The *in vivo* effects of fasting and refeeding or obesity on STAT expression or activation in adipose tissue are not currently available. It would not be unexpected, however, to find that various dietary aspects of nutrition also regulate STATs. In differentiated 3T3-L1 adipocytes, acute insulin treatment results in serine phosphorylation of STAT3.[105,109] The relevance of this post-translational event are yet to be determined since insulin does not appear to affect the expression, activation, and translocation of any STAT protein in cultured adipocytes, including STAT3.[104,105] The function of highly regulated STAT expression and activation during physiological and pathological states of lipid and glucose homeostasis will become clearer following the completion of studies addressing the effects of nutrition and the identification of gene targets of STATs in the adipocyte.

2.5 Perspectives and General Conclusions

Over the last decade, there has been tremendous development in our understanding of the mechanisms by which nutrients direct changes in gene expression. In addition to the well-characterized hormonal signaling of the fed state imparted by insulin, it now appears that the diet contains biological molecules (fatty acids, eicosanoids, vitamins) that can activate intracellular receptors in much the same way as steroid hormones. These nuclear hormone receptors provide a direct link between the availability of nutrients and the gene expression mediating fuel storage and utilization. The discovery that nuclear receptors can modulate adipogenesis through a transcriptional mechanism has opened a new field of research in adipocyte biology and is consistent with dietary factors being important modulators of gene expression, *in vivo*. Lipid-related molecules that bind to these receptors can no longer be regarded simply as biological substrates for energy metabolism, but rather as mediators that signal for changes in gene expression important for energy homeostasis. As the link between nutrients and the regulation of gene expression has been poorly understood, these findings represent a breakthrough in the molecular understanding of the relationship between dietary intake and energy homeostasis.

Although our knowledge concerning the transcriptional control of adipocyte gene expression has advanced significantly over the last few years, there are many questions still unanswered. Currently, we position PPARγ and C/EBPα as the most prominent transcription factors mediating adipogenesis. The direct mechanism whereby these *trans*-acting factors, independently and/or cooperatively, activate gene expression important for adipocyte function and their roles in regulating the expression of intermediary transcription factors will undoubtedly represent a focus of future investigations. The increasing list of adipocyte functions beyond the storage of triglycerides will require an evolving definition of adipocyte differentiation and, consequently, the cascade of transcriptional events mediating adipogenesis. Analysis of the mechanisms whereby hormonal and nutritional signaling impinges on the adipogenic transcription factors will provide an important link between the cellular environment and regulation of gene expression important for glucose and lipid homeostasis.

References

1. Spiegelman, B. M. and Flier, J. S., Adipogenesis and obesity: rounding out the big picture, *Cell*, 87, 377, 1996.
2. Gregoire, F. M., Smas, C. M., and Sul, H. S., Understanding adipocyte differentiation, *Physiol. Rev.*, 78, 783, 1998.
3. Cornelius, P., MacDougald, O. A., and Lane, M. D., Regulation of adipocyte development, *Annu. Rev. Nutr.*, 14, 99, 1994.
4. MacDougald, O. A. and Lane, M. D., Transcriptional regulation of gene expression during adipocyte differentiation, *Annu. Rev. Biochem.*, 64, 345, 1995.
5. Brun, R. P., Kim, J. B., Hu, E., Altiok, S., and Spiegelman, B. M., Adipocyte differentiation: a transcriptional regulatory cascade, *Curr. Opin. Cell Biol.*, 8, 826, 1996.

6. Morrison, R. F. and Farmer, S. R., Insights into the transcriptional control of adipocyte differentiation, *J. Cell. Biochem.*, 32/33, 59, 1999.

7. Rosen, E. D., Walkey, C. J., Puigserver, P., and Spiegelman, B. M., Transcriptional regulation of adipogenesis, *Genes Dev.*, 14, 1293, 2000.

8. Reusch, J. E., Colton, L. A., and Klemm, D. J., CREB activation induces adipogenesis in 3T3-L1 cells, *Mol. Cell. Biol.*, 20, 1008, 2000.

9. Cao, Z., Umek, R. M., and McKnight, S. L., Regulated expression of three C/EBP isoforms during adipose conversion of 3T3-L1 cells, *Genes Dev.*, 5, 1538, 1991.

10. Wu, Z., Xie, Y., Bucher, N. L. R., and Farmer, S. R., Conditional ectopic expression of C/EBPβ in NIH3T3 cells induces PPARγ and stimulates adipogenesis, *Genes Dev.*, 9, 2350, 1995.

11. Yeh, W.-C., Cao, Z., Classon, M., and McKnight, S. L., Cascade regulation of terminal adipocyte differentiation by three members of the C/EBP family of leucine zipper proteins, *Genes Dev.*, 9, 168, 1995.

12. Wu, Z., Xie, Y., Morrison, R. F., Bucher, N. L. R., and Farmer, S. R., PPARγ induces the insulin-dependent glucose transporter GLUT4 in the absence of C/EBPα during the conversion of 3T3 fibroblasts into adipocytes, *J. Clin. Invest.*, 101, 22, 1998.

13. Clarke, S. L., Robinson, C. E., and Gimble, J. M., CAAT/enhancer binding proteins directly modulate transcription from the peroxisome proliferator-activated receptor gamma 2 promoter, *Biochem. Biophys. Res. Comm.*, 240, 99, 1997.

14. Christy, R. J., Kaestner, K. H., Geiman, D. E., and Lane, M. D., CCAAT/enhancer binding protein gene promoter: binding of nuclear factors during differentiation of 3T3-L1 preadipocytes, *Proc. Natl. Acad. Sci. USA*, 88, 2593, 1991.

15. Shao, D. and Lazar, M. A., Peroxisome proliferator activated receptor gamma, CCAAT/enhancer-binding protein alpha, and cell cycle status regulate the commitment to adipocyte differentiation, *J. Biol. Chem.*, 272, 21473, 1997.

16. Lin, F. T. and Lane, M. D., Antisense CCAAT/enhancer-binding protein RNA suppresses coordinate gene expression and triglyceride accumulation during differentiation of 3T3-L1 preadipocytes, *Genes Dev.*, 6, 533, 1992.

17. Lin, F. T., MacDougald, O. A., Diehl, A. M., and Lane, M. D., A 30-kDa alternative translation product of the CCAAT/enhancer binding protein alpha message: transcriptional activator lacking antimitotic activity, *Proc. Natl. Acad. Sci. USA*, 90, 9606, 1993.

18. Wu, Z., Rosen, E. D., Brun, R., Hauser, S., Adelmant, G., Troy, A. E., McKeon, C., Darlington, G. J., and Spiegelman, B. M., Cross-regulation of C/EBP alpha and PPAR gamma controls the transcriptional pathway of adipogenesis and insulin sensitivity, *Mol. Cell*, 3, 151, 1999.

19. Ericsson, J., Jackson, S. M., Kim, J. B., Spiegelman, B. M., and Edwards, P. A., Identification of glycerol-3-phosphate acyltransferase as an adipocyte determination and differentiation factor 1- and sterol regulatory element-binding protein-responsive gene, *J. Biol. Chem.*, 272, 7298, 1997.

20. Fajas, L., Schoonjans, K., Gelman, L., Kim, J. B., Najib, J., Martin, G., Fruchart, J. C., Briggs, M., Spiegelman, B. M., and Auwerx, J., Regulation of peroxisome proliferator-activated receptor gamma expression by adipocyte differentiation and determination factor 1/Sterol regulatory element binding protein 1: implications for adipocyte differentiation and metabolism, *Mol. Biol. Cell*, 19, 5495, 1999.

21. Kim, J. B., Wright, H. M., Wright, M., and Spiegelman, B. M., ADD1/SREBP1 activates PPARγ through the production of endogenous ligand, *Proc. Natl. Acad. Sci. USA*, 95, 4333, 1999.

22. Tang, Q. Q., Jiang, M. S., and Lane, M. D., Repression of transcription mediated by dual elements in the CCAAT/enhancer binding protein alpha gene, *Proc. Natl. Acad. Sci. USA*, 94, 13571, 1997.

23. Jiang, M. S., Tang, Q. Q., McLenithan, J., Geiman, D., Shillinglaw, W., Henzel, W. J., and Lane, M. D., Derepression of the C/EBPalpha gene during adipogenesis: identification of AP-2 alpha as a repressor, *Proc. Natl. Acad. Sci. USA*, 95, 3467, 1998.

24. Tang, Q. Q., Jiang, M. S., and Lane, M. D., Repressive effect of Sp1 on the C/EBPα gene promoter: role in adipocyte differentiation, *Mol. Cell. Biol.*, 19, 4855, 1999.

25. Stephens, J. M., Morrison, R. F., Wu, Z., and Farmer, S. R., PPARγ ligand-dependent induction of STAT1, STAT5A, and STAT5B during adipogenesis, *Biochem. Biophys. Res. Commun.*, 262, 216, 1999.

26. Braissant, O., Foufelle, F., Scotto, C., Dauca, M., and Wahli, W. Differential expression of peroxisome proliferator-activated receptors (PPARs): tissue distribution of PPAR-alpha, -beta, and -gamma in the adult rat, *Endocrinology*, 137, 354, 1996.

27. Tontonoz, P., Hu, E., Graves, R. A., Budavari, A. I., and Spiegelman, B. M., mPPAR gamma 2: tissue-specific regulator of an adipocyte enhancer, *Genes Dev.*, 8, 1224, 1994.

28. Zhu, Y., Alvares, K., Huang, Q., Rao, M. S., and Reddy, J. K., Cloning of a new member of the peroxisome proliferator-activated receptor gene family from mouse liver, *J. Biol. Chem.*, 268, 26817, 1993.

29. Tontonoz, P., Hu, E., Devine, J., Beale, E. G., and Spiegelman, B. M., Stimulation of adipogenesis in fibroblasts by PPARγ2, a lipid-activated transcription factor, *Cell*, 79, 1147, 1994.

30. Zhu, Y., Qi, C., Korenberg, J. R., Chen, X. N., Noya, D., Rao, M. S., and Reddy, J. K., Structural organization of mouse peroxisome proliferator-activated receptor gamma (mPPAR gamma) gene: alternative promoter use and different splicing yield two mPPAR gamma isoforms, *Proc. Natl. Acad. Sci. USA*, 92, 7921, 1995.

31. Vidal-Puig, A., Jimenez-Linan, M., Lowell, B. B., Hamann, A., Hu, E., Spiegelman, B., Flier, J. S., and Moller, D. E., Regulation of PPAR gamma gene expression by nutrition and obesity in rodents, *J. Clin. Invest.*, 97, 2553, 1996.

32. Vidal-Puig, A. J., Considine, R. V., Jimenez-Linan, M., Werman, A., Pories, W. J., Caro, J. F., and Flier, J. S., Peroxisome proliferator-activated receptor gene expression in human tissues. Effects of obesity, weight loss, and regulation by insulin and glucocorticoids, *J. Clin. Invest.*, 99, 2416, 1997.

33. Ricote, M., Li, A., Willson, T., Kelly, C., and Glass, C., The peroxisome proliferator-activated receptor-gamma is a negative regulator of macrophage activation, *Nature*, 391, 79, 1998.

34. Mueller, E., Sarraf, P., Tontonoz, P., Evans, R. M., Martin, K. J., Zhang, M., Fletcher, C., Singer, S., and Spiegelman, B. M., Terminal differentiation of human breast cancer through PPARγ, *Mol. Cell*, 1, 465, 1998.

35. Lefebvre, A. M., Paulweber, B., Fajas, L., Woods, J., McCary, C., Colombel, J. F., Najib, J., Fruchart, J. C., Datz, C., Vidal, H., Desreumaux, P., and Auwerx, J., Peroxisome proliferator-activated receptor gamma is induced during differentiation of colon epithelium cells, *J. Endocrinol.*, 162, 331, 1999.

36. Mangelsdorf, D. J. and Evans, R. M., The RXR heterodimers and orphan receptors, *Cell*, 83, 841, 1995.

37. Hu, E., Tontonoz, P., and Spiegelman, B. M., Transdifferentiation of myoblasts by the adipogenic transcription factors PPARγ and C/EBPα, *Proc. Natl. Acad. Sci. USA*, 92, 9856, 2000.

38. Kletzien, R. F., Clarke, S. D., and Ulrich, R. G., Enhancement of adipocyte differentiation by an insulin-sensitizing agent, *Mol. Pharmacol.*, 41, 393, 2000.

39. Sandouk, T., Reda, D., and Hofmann, C., Antidiabetic agent pioglitazone enhances adipocyte differentiation of 3T3-F442A cells, *Am. J. Physiol.*, 264, C1600-C16082000.

40. Gurnell, M., Wentworth, J. M., Agostini, M., Adams, M., Collingwood, T. N., Provenzano, C., Browne, P. O., Rajanayagam, O., Burris, T. P., Schwabe, J. W., Lazar, M. A., and Chatterjee, V. K., A dominant-negative peroxisome proliferator-activated receptor gamma (PPARgamma) mutant is a constitutive repressor and inhibits PPARgamma-mediated adipogenesis, *J. Biol. Chem.*, 275, 5754, 2000.

41. Oberfield, J. L., Collins, J. L., Holmes, C. P., Goreham, D. M., Cooper, J. P., Cobb, J. E., Lenhard, J. M., Hull-Ryde, E. A., Mohr, C. P., Blanchard, S. G., Parks, D. J., Moore, L. B., Lehmann, J. M., Plunket, K., Miller, A. B., Milburn, M. V., Kliewer, S. A., and Willson, T. M., A peroxisome proliferator-activated receptor gamma ligand inhibits adipocyte differentiation, *Proc. Natl. Acad. Sci. USA*, 96, 6102, 1999.

42. Wright, H. M., Clish, C. B., Mikami, T., Hauser, S., Yanagi, K., Hiramatsu, R., Serhan, C. N., and Spiegelman, B. M., A synthetic antagonist for the peroxisome proliferator-activated receptor gamma inhibits adipocyte differentiation, *J. Biol. Chem.*, 275, 1873, 2000.

43. Barak, Y., Nelson, M. C., Ong, E. S., Jones, Y. Z., Ruiz-Lozano, P., Chien, K. R., Koder, A., and Evans, R. M., PPAR gamma is required for placental, cardiac, and adipose tissue development, *Mol. Cell*, 4, 585, 1999.

44. Kubota, N., Terauchi, Y., Miki, H., Tamemoto, H., Yamauchi, T., Komeda, K., Satoh, S., Nakano, R., Ishii, C., Sugiyama, T., Eto, K., Tsubamoto, Y., Okuno, A., Murakami, K., Sekihara, H., Hasegawa, G., Naito, M., Toyoshima, Y., Tanaka, S., Shiota, K., Kitamura, T., Fujita, T., Ezaki, O., Aizawa, S., and Kadowaki, T., PPAR gamma mediates high-fat diet-induced adipocyte hypertrophy and insulin resistance, *Mol. Cell*, 4, 597, 1999.

45. Rosen, E. D., Sarraf, P., Troy, A. E., Bradwin, G., Moore, K., Milstone, D. S., Spiegelman, B. M., and Mortensen, R. M., PPAR gamma is required for the differentiation of adipose tissue *in vivo* and *in vitro*, *Mol. Cell*, 4, 611, 1999.

46. Schoonjans, K., Staels, B., and Auwerx, J., Role of the peroxisome proliferator-activated receptor (PPAR) in mediating the effects of fibrates and fatty acids on gene expression, *J. Lipid Res.*, 37, 907, 1996.

47. Xu, H. E., Lambert, M. H., Montana, V. G., Parks, D. J., Blanchard, S. G., Brown, P. J., Sternbach, D. D., Lehmann, J. M., Wisely, G. B., Willson, T. M., Kliewer, S. A., and Millburn, M. V., Molecular recognition of fatty acids by peroxisome proliferator-activated receptors, *Mol. Cell*, 3, 397, 1999.

48. Gharbi-Chihi, J., Teboul, M., Bismuth, J., Bonne, J., and Torresani, J., Increase of adipose differentiation by hypolipidemic fibrate drugs in Ob 17 preadipocytes: requirement for thyroid hormones, *Biochim. Biophys. Acta,* 1177, 8, 1993.
49. Amri, E. Z., Bertrand, B., Ailhaud, G., and Grimaldi, P., Regulation of adipose cell differentiation. I. Fatty acids are inducers of the aP2 gene expression, *J. Lipid Res.,* 32, 1449, 1991.
50. Chawla, A. and Lazar, M. A., Peroxisome proliferator and retinoid signaling pathways co-regulate preadipocyte phenotype and survival, *Proc. Natl. Acad. Sci. USA,* 91, 1786, 1994.
51. Negrel, R., Gaillard, D., and Ailhaud, G., Prostacyclin as a potent effector of adipose-cell differentiation, *Biochem. J.,* 257, 399, 1989.
52. Gaillard, D., Negrel, R., Lagarde, M., and Ailhaud, G., Requirement and role of arachidonic acid in the differentiation of pre-adipose cells, *Biochem. J.,* 257, 389, 1989.
53. Yu, K., Bayona, W., Kallen, C. B., Harding, H. P., Ravera, C. P., McMahon, G., Brown, M., and Lazar, M. A., Differential activation of peroxisome proliferator-activated receptors by eicosanoids, *J. Biol. Chem.,* 270, 23975, 1995.
54. Forman, B. M., Tontonoz, P., Chen, J., Brun, R. P., Spiegelman, B. M., and Evans, R. M., 15-Deoxy-delta 12, 14-prostaglandin J2 is a ligand for the adipocyte determination factor PPAR gamma, *Cell,* 83, 803, 1995.
55. Kliewer, S. A., Lenhard, J. M., Willson, T. M., Patel, I., Morris, D. C., and Lehmann, J. M., A prostaglandin J2 metabolite binds peroxisome proliferator-activated receptor gamma and promotes adipocyte differentiation, *Cell,* 83, 813, 1995.
56. Tontonoz, P., Nagy, L., Alvarez, J. G. A., Thomazy, V. A., and Evans, R. M., PPARγ promotes monocyte/macrophage differentiation and uptake of oxidized LDL, *Cell,* 93, 241, 1998.
57. Nagy, L., Tontonoz, P., Alvarez, J. G. A., Chen, H., and Evans, R. M., Oxidized LDL regulates macrophage gene expression through ligand activation of PPARγ, *Cell,* 93, 229, 1998.
58. Krey, G., Braissant, O., L'Horset, F., Kalkhoven, E., Perroud, M., Parker, M. G., and Wahli, W., Fatty acids, eicosanoids, and hypolipidemic agents identified as ligands of peroxisome proliferator-activated receptors by coactivator-dependent receptor ligand assay, *Mol. Endocrinol.,* 11, 779, 1997.
59. Lehmann, J. M., Moore, L. B., Smith-Oliver, T. A., Wilkison, W. O., Wilson, T. M., and Kliewer, S. A., An antidiabetic thiazolidinedione is a high affinity ligand for peroxisome proliferator-activated receptor γ (PPARγ), *J. Biol. Chem.,* 270, 12953, 1995.
60. Saltiel, A. R. and Olefsky, J. M., Thiazolidinediones in the treatment of insulin resistance and type II diabetes, *Diabetes,* 45, 1661, 1996.
61. Iwamoto, Y., Kuzuya, T., Matsuda, A., Awata, T., Kumakura, S., Inooka, G., and Shiraishi, I., Effect of new oral antidiabetic agent CS-045 on glucose tolerance and insulin secretion in patients with NIDDM, *Diabetes Care,* 14, 1083, 1991.
62. Suter, S. L., Nolan, J. J., Wallace, P., Gumbiner, B., and Olefsky, J. M., Metabolic effects of new oral hypoglycemic agent CS-045 in NIDDM subjects, *Diabetes Care,* 15, 193, 1992.
63. Nolan, J. J., Ludvik, B., Beerdsen, P., Joyce, M., and Olefsky, J., Improvement in glucose tolerance and insulin resistance in obese subjects treated with troglitazone, *N. Engl. J. Med.,* 331, 1188, 1994.

64. Fujiwara, T., Yoshioka, S., Yoshioka, T., Ushiyama, I., and Horikoshi, H., Characterization of new oral antidiabetic agent CS-045. Studies in KK and ob/ob mice and Zucker fatty rats, *Diabetes,* 37, 1549, 1988.
65. Fujiwara, T., Wada, M., Fukuda, K., Fukami, M., Yoshioka, S., Yoshioka, T., and Horikoshi, H., Characterization of CS-045, a new oral antidiabetic agent, II. Effects on glycemic control and pancreatic islet structure at a late stage of the diabetic syndrome in C57BL/KsJ-db/db mice, *Metab. Clin. Exp.,* 40, 1213, 1991.
66. Lee, M. K., Miles, P. D., Khoursheed, M., Gao, K. M., Moossa, A. R., and Olefsky, J. M., Metabolic effects of troglitazone on fructose-induced insulin resistance in the rat, *Diabetes,* 43, 1435, 1994.
67. Mukherjee, R., Davies, P. J., Crombie, D. L., Bischoff, E. D., Cesario, R. M., Jow, L., Hamann, L. G., Boehm, M. F., Mondon, C. E., Nadzan, A. M., Paterniti, Jr., J. R., and Heyman, R. A., Sensitization of diabetic and obese mice to insulin by retinoid X receptor agonists, *Nature,* 386, 407, 1997.
68. Mukherjee, R., Jow, L., Croston, G. E., and Paterniti, Jr. J. R., Identification, characterization, and tissue distribution of human peroxisome proliferator-activated receptor (PPAR) isoforms PPARgamma2 versus PPARgamma1 and activation with retinoid X receptor agonists and antagonists, *J. Biol. Chem.,* 272, 8071, 1997.
69. Barroso, I., Gurnell, M., Crowley, V. E., Agostini, M., Schwabe, J. W., Soos, M. A., Maslen, G. L., Williams, T. D., Lewis, H., Schafer, A. J., Chatterjee, V. K., and O'Rahilly, S., Dominant negative mutations in human PPARgamma associated with severe insulin resistance, diabetes mellitus and hypertension, *Nature,* 402, 880, 1999.
70. Lane, M. D., Lin, F. T., MacDougald, O. A., and Vasseur-Cognet, M., Control of adipocyte differentiation by CCAAT/enhancer binding protein alpha (C/EBP alpha), *Int. J. Obes. Relat. Metab. Disord.,* 20 (3) S91, 1996.
71. Mandrup, S. and Lane, M. D., Regulating adipogenesis, *J. Biol. Chem.,* 272, 5367, 1997.
72. Darlington, G. J., Ross, S. E., and MacDougald, O. A., The role of C/EBP genes in adipocyte differentiation, *J. Biol. Chem.,* 273, 30057, 1998.
73. Lin, F. T. and Lane, M. D., CCAAT/enhancer binding protein alpha is sufficient to initiate the 3T3-L1 adipocyte differentiation program, *Proc. Natl. Acad. Sci. USA,* 91, 8757, 1994.
74. Freytag, S. O., Paielli, D. L., and Gilbert, J. D., Ectopic expression of the CCAAT/enhancer-binding protein alpha promotes the adipogenic program in a variety of mouse fibroblastic cells, *Genes Dev.,* 8, 1654, 1994.
75. Wang, N. D., Finegold, M. J., Bradley, A., Ou, C. N., Abdelsayed, S. V., Wilde, M. D., Taylor, L. R., Wilson, D. R., and Darlington, G. J., Impaired energy homeostasis in C/EBP alpha knockout mice, *Science,* 269, 1108, 1995.
76. Tanaka, T., Yoshida, N., Kishimoto, T., and Akira, S., Defective adipocyte differentiation in mice lacking the C/EBPβ and/or C/EBPδ gene, *EMBO J.,* 16, 7432, 1997.
77. Hendricks-Taylor, L. R. and Darlington, G. J., Inhibition of cell proliferation by C/EBP alpha occurs in many cell types, does not require the presence of p53 or Rb, and is not affected by large T-antigen, *Nucleic Acids Res.,* 23, 4726, 1995.
78. Descombes, P. and Schibler, U., A liver-enriched transcriptional activator protein, LAP, and a transcriptional inhibitory protein, LIP, are translated from the same mRNA, *Cell,* 67, 569, 1991.

79. Hemati, N., Ross, S. E., Erickson, R. L., Groblewski, G. E., and MacDougald, O. A., Signaling pathways through which insulin regulates CCAAT/enhancer binding protein alpha (C/EBPalpha) phosphorylation and gene expression in 3T3-L1 adipocytes. Correlation with GLUT4 gene expression, *J. Biol. Chem.*, 272, 25913, 1997.

80. Brun, R. P., Tontonoz, P., Forman, B. M., Ellis, R., Chen, J., Evans, R. M., and Spiegelman, B. M., Differential activation of adipogenesis by multiple PPAR isoforms, *Genes Dev.*, 10, 974, 1996.

81. El-Jack, A. K., Hamm, J. K., Pilch, P. F., and Farmer, S. R., Reconstitution of insulin-sensitive glucose transport in fibroblasts requires expression of both PPARgamma and C/EBPalpha, *J. Biol. Chem.*, 274, 7946, 1999.

82. Kahn, B. B., Dietary regulation of glucose transporter gene expression: tissue specific effects in adipose cells and muscle, *J. Nutr.*, 124, 1289S, 1994.

83. Rolland, V., LeLiepure, X., Houbiguian, M. L., Lavau, M., and Dugail, I., C/EBP alpha expression in adipose tissue of genetically obese Zucker rats, *Biochem. Biophys. Res. Commun.*, 207, 761, 1995.

84. MacDougald, O. A., Cornelius, P., Liu, R., and Lane, M. D., Insulin regulates transcription of the CCAAT/enhancer binding protein (C/EBP) alpha, beta, and delta genes in fully-differentiated 3T3-L1 adipocytes, *J. Biol. Chem.*, 270, 647, 1995.

85. Hemati, N., Erickson, R. L., Ross, S. E., Liu, R., and MacDougald, O. A., Regulation of CCAAT/enhancer binding protein alpha (C/EBP alpha) gene expression by thiazolidinediones in 3T3-L1 adipocytes, *Biochem. Biophys. Res. Comm.*, 244, 20, 1998.

86. Ross, S. E., Erickson, R. L., Hemati, N., and MacDougald, O. A., Glycogen synthase kinase 3 is an insulin-regulated C/EBPalpha kinase, *Mol. Cell. Biol.*, 19, 8433, 1999.

87. Brown, M. S. and Goldstein, J. L., The SREBP pathway: regulation of cholesterol metabolism by proteolysis of a membrane-bound transcription factor, *Cell*, 89, 331, 1997.

88. Tontonoz, P., Kim, J. B., Graves, R. A., and Spiegelman, B. M., ADD1: a novel helix-loop-helix transcription factor associated with adipocyte determination and differentiation, *Mol. Cell. Biol.*, 13, 4753, 1993.

89. Wang, X., Sato, R., Brown, M. S., Hua, X., and Goldstein, J. L., SREBP-1, a membrane-bound transcription factor released by sterol-regulated proteolysis, *Cell*, 77, 53, 1994.

90. Brown, M. S. and Goldstein, J. L., Sterol regulatory element binding proteins (SREBPs): controllers of lipid synthesis and cellular uptake, *Nutr. Rev.*, 56, S1, 1998.

91. Yokoyama, C., Wang, X., Briggs, M. R., Admon, A., Wu, J., Hua, X., Goldstein, J. L., and Brown, M. S., SREBP-1, a basic-helix-loop-helix-leucine zipper protein that controls transcription of the low density lipoprotein receptor gene, *Cell*, 75, 187, 1993.

92. Kim, J. B. and Spiegelman, B. M., ADD1/SREBP1 promotes adipocyte differentiation and gene expression linked to fatty acid metabolism, *Genes Dev.*, 10, 1096, 1996.

93. Kim, J. B., Sarraf, P., Wright, M., Yao, K. M., Mueller, E., Solanes, G., Lowell, B. B., and Spiegelman, B. M., Nutritional and insulin regulation of fatty acid synthetase and leptin gene expression through ADD1/SREBP1, *J. Clin. Invest.*, 101, 1, 1998.

 94. Shimano, H., Shimomura, I., Hammer, R. E., Herz, J., Goldstein, J. L., Brown, M. S., and Horton, J. D., Elevated levels of SREBP-2 and cholesterol synthesis in livers of mice homozygous for a targeted disruption of the SREBP-1 gene, *J. Clin. Invest.*, 100, 2115, 1997.
 95. Flier, J. S. and Hollenberg, A. N., ADD-1 provides major new insights into the mechanisms of insulin action, *Proc. Natl. Acad. Sci. USA*, 96, 14191, 2000.
 96. Sul, H. S., Latasa, M. J., Moon, Y., and Kim, K. H., Regulation of the fatty acid synthase promoter by insulin, *J. Nutr.*, 130, 315S, 2000.
 97. Foretz, M., Pacot, C., Dugail, I., Lemarchand, P., Guichard, C., LeLiepure, X., Berthelier-Lubrano, C., Spiegelman, B., Kim, J. B., Ferre, P., and Foufelle, F., ADD1/SREBP-1c is required in the activation of hepatic lipogenic gene expression by glucose, *Mol. Cell. Biol.*, 19, 3760, 1999.
 98. Foretz, M., Guichard, C., Ferre, P., and Foufelle, F., Sterol regulatory element binding protein-1c is a major mediator of insulin action on the hepatic expression of glucokinase and lipogenesis-related genes, *Proc. Natl. Acad. Sci. USA*, 96, 12737, 1999.
 99. Darnell, Jr. J. E., STATs and gene regulation, *Science*, 277, 1630, 1997.
100. Stephens, J. M., Morrison, R. F., and Pilch, P. F., The expression and regulation of STATs during 3T3-L1 adipocyte differentiation, *J. Biol. Chem.*, 271, 10441, 1996.
101. Stewart, W. C., Morrison, R. F., Young, S. L., and Stephens, J. M., Regulation of signal transducers and activators of transcription (STATs) by effectors of adipogenesis: coordinate regulation of STATs 1, 5A, and 5B with peroxisome proliferator-activated receptor-gamma and C/AAAT enhancer binding protein-alpha, *Biochim. Biophys. Acta*, 1452, 188, 1999.
102. Teglund, S., McKay, C., Schuetz, E., van Deursen, J. M., Stravopodis, D., Wang, D., Brown, M., Bodner, S., Grosveld, G., and Ihle, J. N., Stat5a and Stat5b proteins have essential and nonessential, or redundant, roles in cytokine responses, *Cell*, 93, 841, 1998.
103. Hwang, C. S., Loftus, T. M., Mandrup, S., and Lane, M. D., Adipocyte differentiation and leptin expression, *Annu. Rev. Cell Dev. Biol.*, 13, 231, 1997.
104. Balhoff, J. P. and Stephens, J. M., Highly specific and quantitative activation of STATs in 3T3-L1 adipocytes, *Biochem. Biophys. Res. Commun.*, 247, 894, 1998.
105. Stephens, J. M., Lumpkin, S. J., and Fishman, J. B., Activation of signal transducers and activators of transcription 1 and 3 by leukemia inhibitory factor, oncostatin-M, and interferon-gamma in adipocytes, *J. Biol. Chem.*, 273, 31408, 1998.
106. Smit, L. S., Vanderkuur, J. A., Stimage, A., Han, Y., Luo, G., Yu-Lee, L.Y., Schwartz, J., and Carter-Su, C., Growth hormone-induced tyrosyl phosphorylation and deoxyribonucleic acid binding activity of Stat5A and Stat5B, *Endocrinology*, 138, 3426, 1997.
107. Deng, J., Hua, K., Lesser, S. S., Greiner, A. H., Walter, A. W., Marrero, M. B., and Harp, J. B., Interleukin-4 mediates STAT6 activation in 3T3-L1 preadipocytes but not adipocytes, *Biochem. Biophys. Res. Commun.*, 267, 516, 2000.
108. Deng, J., Hua, K., Lesser, S. S., and Harp, J. B., Activation of signal transducer and activator of transcription-3 during proliferative phases of 3T3-L1 adipogenesis, *Endocrinology*, 141, 2370, 2000.
109. Ceresa, B. P. and Pessin, J. E., Insulin stimulates the serine phosphorylation of the signal transducer and activator of transcription (STAT3) isoform, *J. Biol. Chem.*, 271, 12121, 1996.

3

Regulation of the Stearoyl-CoA Desaturase Genes by Dietary Fat: Role of Polyunsaturated Fatty Acids

James M. Ntambi and Young-Cheul Kim

CONTENTS

3.1 Introduction 49
3.2 Regulation of SCD Expression by Polyunsaturated Fatty Acids 51
3.3 Mechanisms of Polyunsaturated Fatty Acid Control of SCD
      Gene Expression..53
      3.3.1 Transcriptional Control 53
      3.3.2 Post-Transcriptional Control 56
3.4 Conclusions and Future Direction..57
References 58

3.1 Introduction

When dietary intake of fat is insufficient for daily requirements, animals derive fatty acids mainly from *de novo* synthesis by the fatty acid synthase complex (FAS) which catalyzes the condensation of acetyl-CoA, and malonyl-CoA producing palmitate (C16:0) as the major end product.[1] Palmitate then serves as a substrate for the microsomal malonyl-CoA dependent elongase to produce stearate (C18:0). Because stearate and, to a lesser extent, palmitate are to be stored,[2] the end product of this pathway is usually oleate (C18:1Δ9) and palmitoleate (C16:1Δ9) which are synthesized by the stearoyl-CoA desaturase (SCD) (Fig. 3.1). This enzyme is the terminal component of a multicomponent complex which includes cytochrome b_5 and an NAD(P)H-dependent cytochrome b_5 reductase. In the presence of molecular oxygen this complex catalyzes the desaturation of methylene-interrupted fatty acyl-CoA substrates by the insertion of a double bond between carbons 9 and 10.[3]

0-8493-2216-2/01/$0.00+$1.50
© 2001 by CRC Press LLC

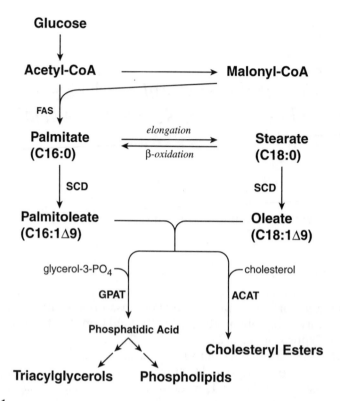

FIGURE 3.1

Pathway for synthesis of palmitioleic and oleic acids from palmitate and stearate and their incorporation into triacylglycerols, phospholipids, and cholesterol esters. The sites for the action of SCD are depicted. SCD: stearoyl-CoA desaturase; FAS: fatty acid synthase; GPAT: glycerol-3-phosphate acyltransferase; ACAT: acyl-CoA:cholesterol acyl transferase; G-3-PO$_4$: glycerol-3-phosphate

Although several substrates including vaccenic acid[4] are used by the SCD, the main substrates are palmitoyl- and stearoyl-CoA which are converted to palmitoleoyl- and oleoyl-CoA, respectively.[3] The overall rate of the desaturation reaction is limited by the terminal component, the SCD, and it is the SCD that shows changes in expression in response to dietary changes, hormonal imbalance, developmental processes, temperature changes, metals, alcohol, peroxisomal proliferators, and phenolic compounds.[5–6] Changes in SCD activity in tissues are reflected in the composition of cell membrane phospholipids, cholesterol esters, and triglycerides, and therefore, regulation of SCD is of considerable physiological importance and has the potential to affect a variety of key physiological variables including insulin sensitivity, metabolic rate, adiposity, atherosclerosis, cancer, and obesity.

The mouse and rat genome contain two well-characterized structural genes (SCD1 and SCD2) that are highly homologous at the nucleotide and amino acid level and encode the same functional protein.[7–9] Both genes are structurally similar with 5 exons and 6 introns with translated region present in every exon. Recently, a single human SCD gene that is highly homologous to the mouse SCD1 and SCD2 genes was cloned and characterized.[10] Other SCD cDNAs and genes have been isolated from different species including yeast,[11] ovine,[12] and hamster,[13] and their regulation is currently being studied. Despite the fact that both mouse SCD genes are structurally similar, sharing ~87 % nucleotide sequence identity in the coding regions, their 5' flanking regions differ resulting in divergent tissue-specific gene expression. The physiological significance of having two or more mouse or rat SCD isoforms and their tissue distribution is not currently known but could be related to the substrate specificity of each SCD isoform or the means by which cells compartmentalize lipid biosynthesis for specific functions.[14] Many mechanisms may exist for regulating the expression of the SCD genes by nutritional, hormonal, developmental, and environmental factors in normal and disease states. It is the goal of this chapter to discuss the recent advances of the regulation of the mouse SCD genes by dietary fat, emphasizing the role of polyunsaturated fatty acids. Several reviews provide excellent coverage of the role of polyunsaturated fatty acids in the regulation of other genes involved in lipid and carbohydrate metabolism.[15-17]

3.2 Regulation of SCD Expression by Polyunsaturated Fatty Acids

The ω-3 and ω-6 polyunsaturated fatty acids (PUFAs) are essential fatty acids that cannot be synthesized by mammals and therefore can be obtained from plant sources. These fatty acids have been shown to reduce the expression of SCD[18] and many enzymes involved in lipid and carbohydrate metabolism.[17] By reducing the expression of these enzymes, it is believed that PUFAs control the *de novo* synthesis of saturated, monounsaturated, and polyunsaturated fatty acids. It would, therefore, appear that in a normal healthy animal receiving adequate amounts of the essential fatty acids, *de novo* fatty acid synthesis would be suppressed. Only when the animal ingests carbohydrate over and above its energy requirements is the repressive effect of PUFAs overcome and the lipogenic enzymes induced. The inhibitory effects of PUFAs on lipogenesis may explain the results of stable isotope experiments which show that *de novo* fatty acid synthesis in humans who consume recommended American diets that are relatively rich in polyunsaturated fatty acids is minor.[19] In support of this observation, when humans are fed diets that are fat free and rich in fructose there is indeed induction of lipogenesis. [20]

The specific regulation of SCD activity by PUFAs may be central to the overall repression of lipogenesis. The SCD catalyzes the first regulatory step in the formation of long-chain unsaturated fatty acids such as (n-9)-eicosatrienoic acid (20:3 n-9).[21] Accumulation of 20:3 n-9 is associated with reduction of ω-3 and ω-6 PUFAs of membrane phospholipids[21] and is the hallmark of essential fatty acid deficiency in humans.[21] Therefore, an attractive explanation for the unique suppression of lipogenesis by ω-3 and ω-6 PUFAs is their ability to suppress the formation and accumulation of ω-9 fatty acids by inhibiting SCD gene expression in order to maintain the proper phospholipid membrane composition. If not suppressed, enrichment of membrane phospholipids with ω-9 fatty acids would occur at the expense of the essential fatty acids and would compromise several cellular functions including hormone binding, signal transduction, accelerated heat loss, increased transdermal water loss, and impaired fetal and neonatal growth.[15] In the shorter term, PUFAs would inhibit the expression of the SCD first, thus limiting the net synthesis of palmitoleoyl- and oleoyl-CoA resulting in an accumulation of palmitoyl-CoA and stearoyl-CoA. These saturated fatty acyl-CoAs would then feedback inhibit acetyl-CoA carboxylase and fatty acid synthase thereby inhibiting general fatty acid biosynthesis.

The regulation of SCD by PUFAs may occur at several levels. Some evidence has been provided that some PUFAs, such as sterculic acid and thia fatty acids, directly inhibit the SCD activity.[22,23] However, studies of liver, lymphocyte, brain, and adipocytes indicate that the effects of PUFAs on SCD activity are mainly at the level of SCD gene expression.[24-36] Under normal dietary conditions, mouse and rat SCD2 mRNA is expressed constitutively at high levels in the brain, is not expressed in liver, and its expression in kidney, adipose, and lung tissue is slightly increased by shifting mice from a diet containing unsaturated fatty acids to a fat-free diet.[8] The tissue distribution and expression of the mouse and rat SCD1 mRNA differ markedly from that of SCD2, being constitutive in adipose tissue, and are markedly induced in liver in response to feeding of a high-carbohydrate fat-free diet.[7-8,24,36] The increase in SCD1 mRNA in response to feeding of a high-carbohydrate fat-free diet was due to both insulin and carbohydrate.[36] Studies conducted in mice showed that when the fat-free high-carbohydrate diet was supplemented with various triglycerides containing linoleic (18:2n-6), arachidonic (20:4n-6), and linolenic (18:3n-3) acids, the hepatic SCD1 mRNA expression was repressed whereas triglycerides containing saturated (i.e., 18:0 and 16:0) and monounsaturated fatty acids (16:1n-9 and 18:1n-9) had very little effect.[24] Similar results have been obtained with primary hepatocytes and mouse cell lines.[27,33] Using a diabetic mouse model it was shown that induction of SCD mRNA expression by insulin could be repressed by PUFAs, showing that the mechanism of PUFA repression of the SCD gene is insulin independent.[26]

The repression of SCD gene expression by PUFAs is not liver specific. PUFAs repress the expression of SCD mRNA in adipose tissue of both lean and obese Zucker rats.[30] Interestingly, the SCD mRNA content was much higher in obese rats compared to normal rats both with and without PUFA supplementation.[30] In the 3T3-L1 adipocyte cell line, arachidonic acid, linoleic, linolenic, and eicosapentaenoic acid (EPA) decreased SCD1 mRNA in a dose-dependent manner.[25] The regulation of SCD gene expression by PUFAs has also been observed in the brain, and cells of the immune system,[31–32,37] indicating that PUFA regulation of SCD gene expression is far more widespread than originally thought.

It is not known whether the PUFAs have to be metabolized first in order to repress SCD gene expression. Inhibiting eicosonoid synthesis did not prevent the PUFA suppression of SCD1 gene expression in adipocytes and lymphocytes, suggesting that the oxidative metabolism of arachidonic acid to eicosonoids is not involved in the arachidonic acid-mediated decrease of SCD1 mRNA expression[28,31] Furthermore, as indicated above, the desaturase gene expression is repressed by a range of PUFAs, some of which do not give rise to eicosonoids, suggesting that repression of SCD mRNA expression is PUFA specific. The basic requirement for a dietary fatty acid to inhibit expression of lipogenic genes had been proposed to contain 18 carbons and possess at least 2 double bonds, one between position 9 and 10 and the other between 12 and 13.[15–16] However, recently it has been demonstrated that the *trans*-10, *cis*-12 isomer of conjugated linoleic acid (CLA) also represses SCD mRNA expression in liver,[35] although this fatty acid does not contain a double bond at position 9. It contains instead double-bonds at positions 6 and 8 from the ω-carbon. The only double bond position that CLA and other PUFAs share is at position 6. The inhibitory effects PUFAs have on the expression of the SCD1 mRNA levels may, therefore, be related to the position and orientation of just one of the double bonds present in these fatty acids. This information could become important in determining the PUFA structure that is required to inhibit gene expression. Many mechanisms may exist for regulating the tissue-specific expression of the SCD genes by PUFAs but recent investigations show that PUFAs repress the SCD gene expression mainly at the level of gene transcription and mRNA stability.[5,24–25,27–28,32–34,38]

3.3 Mechanisms of Polyunsaturated Fatty Acid Control of SCD Gene Expression

3.3.1 Transcriptional Control

PUFA-mediated suppression of SCD1 expression in liver and primary hepatocytes and of SCD2 expression in lymphocytes was shown to be largely due to a decrease in their rates of gene transcription.[5,24,27–28,32–34,38] Therefore, many recent studies have focused on the hypothesis that a *cis*-acting PUFA responsive element (PUFA-RE) exists in the promoters of SCD genes to which a transcription factor binds blocking transcription. Using deletion analysis, the SCD1 and SCD2 PUFA-REs were localized to a 60-bp region in each of their promoters.[38] This is the only region of high sequence homology within the promoters of the two SCD genes.[8] The PUFA-REs of the rat S14 and pyruvate kinase genes have also been mapped[39,40] and were found to share homologous sequences.

```
                                                    SRE              NF-Y
                                                 ‾‾‾‾‾‾‾‾‾‾      ‾‾‾‾‾‾‾‾‾‾
SCD2 -188  GGGAGGAGGGGGGGCGGAGCTGGAGGCAGAGGGAACAGCAGATTGTGCAGAGCCAATGA
           :::::::: :  :: : :::: :::::::::::::::::::::::::  :: :::::::::
SCD1 -459  GGGAGGAGAGACGGAGAAGCTAGAGGCAGAGGGAACAGCAGATTGCGCCTAGCCAATGG
                              ‾‾‾‾‾‾‾‾‾‾‾‾‾‾‾‾‾‾‾‾‾‾‾‾‾‾‾‾‾‾‾‾‾‾
                              PUFA-RE


                                             NF-Y
                                        ‾‾‾‾‾‾‾‾‾‾
           GAGCAGCAGGACGAGGTGGTACCAAATTCCCATCGGCCAATGACTAGCCAG -77
           : :::::::: ::::::: ::::::::: : : :::::::::: :: : :
           AAAAGGCAGGACAAGGTGGCACCCAAATTCTCTTTGGCCAATGACAAGACGG -349
           ‾‾‾‾‾‾‾‾‾‾‾‾‾‾‾‾‾‾‾‾
           PUFA-RE
```

FIGURE 3.2

The nucleotide sequence similarity of the 110-bp segment in the 5′-flanking region of the mouse SCD2 and SCD1 genes showing the binding sites for the sterol regulatory element-binding protein (SRE) and the CCAAT box-binding factor or nuclear factor Y (NF-Y). The polyunsaturated fatty acid response element is underlined (PUFA-RE).

However, these PUFA-REs are not homologous to those of SCD1 or SCD2. A novel *cis* element in the PUFA-RE of the SCD1 and SCD2 genes (Fig. 3.2) that functions as a sterol regulatory element (SRE) has been identified.[41] This sequence (5′AGCAGATTGTG3′), shown to bind purified sterol regulatory element-binding protein (SREBP), is distinct from previously described SREs. It does not contain the direct repeat nor does it contain a functional E-box,[41] but 5 and 48 base pairs 3′ of the SRE are two conserved 5′-CCAAT-3′ boxes for the binding of NF-Y (Fig. 3.2). Mutation of either the SRE or the NF-Y binding site attenuates the transriptional regulation of the SCD genes in response to PUFAs. Based on these observations it has been hypothesized that PUFAs repress SCD genes by inhibiting the formation of an SREBP-NF-Y complex on the DNA.[42] However, the involvement of these two transcription factors in maximum PUFA repression of the SCD gene has been difficult to assess since mutations in the CCAAT and SRE motifs reduce dramatically the basal promoter activities of the two genes.[42]

　　SREBPs are transcription factors first isolated as a result of their properties for binding to the SRE and conferring sterol regulation to genes involved in cholesterol synthesis.[43] SREBPs are inserted into the membrane of the endoplasmic reticulum envelope in a wide variety of tissues. In sterol-deficient cells, proteolytic cleavage of SREBPs releases their N-terminal mature forms from the membrane, enabling them to enter the nucleus where they bind to SREs and activate the transcription of genes involved in cholesterol, triglyceride, and fatty acid biosynthesis.[44-47] The promoters of a number of the lipogenic genes known to be inhibited by PUFAs contain elements to which SREBP and either NF-Y or Sp1 bind.[48-49] It has been demonstrated that the mRNAs of all of these genes, including SCD, are increased in the livers of transgenic mice that overexpress mature SREBPs.[45–47] Thus, the SREBPs appear to play a pivotal role in the expression of lipogenic genes. The nuclear abundance of SREBP-1 and mRNA has been found to be reduced by fasting and greatly increased by refeeding a high-carbohydrate diet.[50] In addition, changes in the nuclear content of SREBP-1 resulting from starving–refeeding displayed a temporal pattern that is similar to the pattern observed for several lipogenic genes.[50] In light of these observations it was postulated that PUFAs coordinately suppress the transcription of hepatic genes by suppressing the expression of SREBP-1.[51]

PUFAs are potent ligand activators of a family of nuclear transcription factors termed peroxisome proliferator-activated receptors (PPARs) and have, therefore, been hypothesized to be the endogenous activators of this receptor.[16] The dominant PPAR in liver is PPARα, and fatty acid activation appears to coordinately induce genes encoding enzymes involved in fatty acid oxidation and ketogenesis.[52,53] Both peroxisome proliferators and PUFAs[16,54] repress lipogenic genes, such as S14 and FAS, but the direct involvement of PPARs in the PUFA suppression of these genes has not been demonstrated.[55,56] However, one possibility is that PUFA activation of PPARα could lead to the suppression of SREBP that is common to several lipogenic genes and in this way indirectly lead to the inhibition of lipogenic gene expression. Such a mechanism would provide a unifying explanation for how PUFAs induce genes of hepatic lipid oxidation and concomitantly suppress genes of lipogenesis. When rats were fed the fat-free diets supplemented with n-6 and n-3 PUFAs, the hepatic level of SREBP as well as FAS and SCD were dramatically reduced while as expected the expression of the acyl-CoA oxidase was increased.[51,57] It has, therefore, been speculated that PUFAs repress SREBP-1 by a PPARα-dependent mechanism. Consistent with this hypothesis, Xu et al.[51] found that feeding rats the potent PPARα-specific activator WY-14,643 reduced the abundance of hepatic SREBP-1 mRNA to the level comparable with that found in rats fed diets containing PUFA. Taken together, one would speculate that the PUFA-activated PPARα might repress SCD1 gene transcription as well. Unexpectedly, studies on the effects of peroxisome proliferators on SCD1 gene expression have shown that PUFA and peroxisome proliferators had opposing effects on the SCD1 mRNA levels in mouse liver.[58] Therefore, unlike the S14, FAS and SREBP-1 genes, peroxisome proliferators induced the expression of the SCD1 gene. In addition, transient transfection experiments localized the SCD1 peroxisome proliferator response element (PPRE) to an area of the SCD1 promoter that is distinct from the PUFA-RE.[58] This indicates that different mechanisms account for the transcriptional regulation of the SCD1 gene by peroxisome proliferators and PUFAs and suggests that PUFA-repression of the SCD genes may proceed through an SREBP-independent mechanism.

PUFAs and oleic acid have been shown *in vitro* to reduce the activity of promoters with SREs by inhibiting the proteolytic maturation of SREBP.[59] These studies suggest that the mature form of SREBP participates in the repression of the SCD gene transcription by PUFA. However, oleic acid could not reduce the transcription of the SCD genes both *in vivo* and *in vitro*.[24,27] Cotransfection of the

SCD1 promoter with expression vectors of the mature form of SREBP leads to activation of the SCD1 and SCD2 promoter activity and no repression is observed in the presence of cholesterol, consistent with the role of cholesterol in inhibiting the maturation of SREBP. However, unlike the case of cholesterol, activation of the SCD promoter by mature form of SREBP remains sensitive to PUFA repression (T. Drews and J. M. Ntambi, unpublished). Thus, SREBP maturation does not seem to exhibit the selectivity required to explain PUFA control of SCD gene transcription, suggesting that PUFA may utilize a different protein to repress SCD1 and SCD2 transcription. This protein is probably not NF-Y because cotransfection of a dominant negative form of NF-Y reduces the basal activity of the SCD promoter but the residual activity remains sensitive to PUFA repression.[42] In addition, the SREBP or the NF-Y elements on their own do not mediate PUFA repression in a heterologous promoter context,[58] but PUFA repression is observed only when the entire 60 bp PUFA-RE is used in a heterologous promoter context.[58] Therefore, although there are indications that SREBP maturation and binding of the SREBP and NF-Y to the PUFA-RE are involved in PUFA repression, there is strong evidence for the existence of an SREBP-independent mechanism involving a putative PUFA-binding protein through which PUFA repress SCD gene expression.

3.3.2 Post-Transcriptional Control

Studies on the SCD genes in mature adipocytes and in yeast have shown that the effect of PUFA on these genes could be at the level of mRNA stability.[28,60] When added to cultures of fully differentiated 3T3-L1 adipocytes, arachidonic acid decreased the SCD1 mRNA half-life from 8 to 4 h.[28] By contrast, oleic acid and stearic acid did not affect SCD1 mRNA stability. Therefore, this response is unique to PUFAs. Arachidonic acid also decreased the stability of the SCD2 mRNA transcript in adipocytes (A. Sessler and J. M. Ntambi, unpublished). Although transcriptional regulation could not be ruled out completely, changes in transcriptional rates were not detected, suggesting that transcriptional regulation does not play a significant role in PUFA suppression of SCD gene expression in mature adipocytes.[28] The observed reduction in enzyme activity (60%) could be completely accounted for by decreases in SCD1 mRNA levels (80%). Thus, there appears to be no additional downregulation occurring post-translationally. Therefore, in contrast to what occurs in hepatocytes, changes in mRNA stability are the major determinant of SCD1 mRNA abundance in adipocytes in response to PUFA. Interestingly, it has been recently found that changes in SREBP mRNA abundance in liver of rats fed PUFAs and the specific PPARα activator WY-14,643 were not accompanied by changes in SREBP gene transcription, suggesting that PUFA and WY-14,643 reduced the hepatic content of SREBP-1 mRNA possibly by accelerating the rate of SREBP mRNA degradation. In this respect the regulation of SREBP mRNA expression in liver would be similar to that of SCD in adipocytes.

Destabilization of SCD mRNA in adipocytes may be regulated through mRNA sequences in the 3′-untranslated region (UTR). The mouse, rat, and human SCD cDNAs contain an unusually long 3′-UTR.[7–9,10] The role of such a long 3′-noncoding stretch is currently unknown, though it contains several structural motifs (e.g., AUUUA) characteristic of mRNA destabilization sequences.[61] Four of these sequences are clustered close to the 3′-end of the coding region. Because these AU-rich elements (ARE) play active roles in the selective degradation of several mRNAs in response to various factors, these sequences could be possible targets of PUFA effects on SCD1 and SCD2 mRNA in adipocytes. In yeast, PUFAs act through sequences in the 5′-UTRs to decrease the Δ9-desaturase gene 1 (OLE1) mRNA stability.[60] Northern blot analysis shows that the single human SCD gene gives rise to two mRNA transcripts of 3.9 and 5.2 kb which arise as a consequence of the two polyadenlyation signals indicating that the two differently expressed transcripts encode the same SCD polypeptide.[10] The function of the polyadenylation is not known but could be in addition to the transcriptional control, a means by which the two transcripts differ in stability or translatability thus allowing for rapid and efficient changes in cellular environment.[10]

The work on SCD gene regulation by PUFA in adipocytes and SREBP in liver suggests that PUFAs regulate gene expression through different mechanisms in different tissue types, the reasons for which are not yet understood. How PUFAs may alter the stability of SREBP and SCD transcripts remains to be determined. However, it is interesting to note that significant quantities of PPARα are located in the cytosol of some cells, suggesting that PPARα could regulate gene expression by influencing both transcriptional and post-transcriptional events.[51] The ongoing search for the possible protein mediators that destabilize SCD1 and SREBP mRNA should provide further definition to the molecular basis of PUFA regulation of lipogenic gene expression.

3.4   Conclusions and Future Direction

PUFAs can control the synthesis of monounsaturated fatty acids in liver and other tissues by regulating the expression of the SCD genes. In this way PUFAs can affect the membrane fluidity and the metabolic state of cells. The role of SREBP in mediating the transcriptional regulation of SCD gene expression by PUFA needs more study as does the possible role of PPARα in mediating SCD and SREBP mRNA stability. Several lipogenic genes such as FAS and S14 are expressed at very low levels in humans but the SCD mRNA expression is high in several human tissues. This makes sense because some of the saturated fatty acids ingested in the diet have to be desaturated to maintain the correct saturated to monounsaturated fatty acid ratio required to preserve membrane fluidity of the cells. The regulation of the SCD gene may, therefore, be more important than that of other

58 — Nutrient–Gene Interactions in Health and Disease

lipogenic genes considering the multitude of human diseases linked to abnormal synthesis of monounsaturated fatty acids. Further studies will be required to elucidate the mechanisms by which PUFAs alter cellular monounsaturated fatty acids to determine the impact of SCD gene regulation in various human disease states.

Acknowledgments: The authors wish to to thank Dr. Steven Clarke and Donald Jump for useful discussions. The research on which this chapter is based was supported by USDA Hatch grant #3784 and support from the Graduate School of the College of Agriculture and Life Sciences of the University of Wisconsin-Madison and department of biochemistry of the University of Wisconsin-Madison.

References

1. Bloch, K. and Vance, D., Control mechanisms in the synthesis of saturated fatty acids, *Annu. Rev. Biochem.*, 46, 263, 1977.
2. McGilvery, R. W., *A Functional Approach*, 2nd ed. Saunders, Philadelphia, 1979.
3. Enoch, H. G., Catala, A., and Strittmatter, P., Mechanism of rat liver microsomal stearyl-CoA desaturase: studies of the substrate specificity, enzyme-substrate interactions, and the function of lipid, *J. Biol. Chem.*, 251, 5095, 1976.
4. Griinari, J. M. and Bauman, D. E., *Advances in Conjugated Linoleic Acid Research*, Vol. 1, AOCS Press, Champaign, IL, 1999, 180.
5. Ntambi, J. M., Regulation of stearoyl-CoA desaturase, *Prog. Lipid. Res.*, 34, 139, 1995.
6. Tocher, D. R., Leaver, M. J., and Hodgson, P. A., Recent developments in the molecular biology and biochemistry of fatty acyl desaturases, *Prog. Lipid Res.*, 37, 73, 1998.
7. Ntambi, J. M., Buhrow, S. A., Kaestner, K. H., Christy, R. J., Sibley, E., Kelly, Jr. T. J., and Lane, M. D., Differentiation-induced gene expression in 3T3-L1 preadipocytes: Characterization of a differentially expressed gene encoding stearoyl-CoA desaturase, *J. Biol. Chem.*, 263, 17291, 1988.
8. Kaestner, K. H., Ntambi, J. M., Kelly, Jr. T. J., and Lane, M. D., Differentiation-induced gene expression: A second differentially expressed gene encoding stearoyl-CoA desaturase, *J. Biol. Chem.*, 264, 14755, 1989.
9. Mihara, K., Structure and regulation of rat liver microsomal stearoyl-CoA desaturase gene, *J. Biochem.*, 108, 1022, 1990.
10. Zhang, L., Ge, L., Parimoo, S., Stenn, K., and Prouty, S. M., 1999 Human stearoyl-CoA desaturase: alternative transcripts generated from a single gene by usage of tandem polyadenylation sites, *Biochem. J.*, 340, 255, 1999.
11. Stukey, J. E., McDonough, V. M., and Martin, C. E., The OLE1 gene of *saccharomyces cervisiae* encodes the delta 9 fatty acid desaturase and can be functionally replaced by the rat stearoyl-CoA desaturase gene, *J. Biol. Chem.*, 265, 20144, 1990.
12. Ward, R. J., Travers, M. T., Richards, S. E., Vernon, R. G., Salter, A M., Buttery, P. J., and Barber, M. C., Stearoyl-CoA desaturase mRNA is transcribed from a single gene in the ovine genome, *Biochim. Biophys. Acta*, 1391, 145, 1998.

13. Ideta, R. Seki, T., and Adachi, K., Sequence analysis and characterization of FAR-17c, an androgen-dependent gene in the flank organs of hamsters, *J. Dermatol. Sci.*, 9, 94, 1995.

14. Vance, J. E., Eukaryotic lipid-biosynthetic enzymes: the same but not the same, *TIBS*, 23, 423, 1998.

15. Clarke, S. D. and Jump, D. B., Regulation of gene transcription by polyunsaturated fatty acids, *Prog. Lipid Res.*, 32, 139, 1993.

16. Clarke, S. D. and Jump, D. B., Polyunsaturated fatty acid regulation of hepatic gene transcription, *Lipids*, 31, S-7, 1996.

17. Sul, H. S. and Wang, D., Nutritional and hormonal regulation of enzymes in fat synthesis: Studies of fatty acid synthase and mitochondrial glycerol-3-phosphate acyltransferase gene transcription, *Annu. Rev. Nutr.*, 18, 331, 1998.

18. Jeffcoat, R. and James, A. T., The control of stearoyl-CoA desaturase by dietary linoleic acid, *FEBS Letters*, 85, 114, 1978.

19. Hellerstein, M. K., De novo lipogenesis in humans: metabolic and regulatory aspects, *Eur. J. Clin. Nutr.*, 53, S53, 1999.

20. Hirsch, J., Hudgins, C., Leibel, R. L., and Rosenbaum, M., Diet composition and energy balance in humans, *Am. J. Clin. Nutr.*, 67, 551S, 1998.

21. Hyman, B.T., Stoll, L.L., and Spector, A. A., Accumulation of (n-9)-eicosatrienoic acid in confluent 3T3-L1 and 3T3 cells, *J. Biol. Chem.*, 256, 8863, 1981.

22. Khoo, D. E. Fermor, B., Miller, J., Wood, C. B., Apostolov, K., Barker, W., Williamson, R. C. N., and Habib, N. A., Manipulation of body fat composition with sterculic acid can inhibit mammary carcinomas *in vivo*, *Brit. J. Cancer*, 63, 97, 1991.

23. Hovik, K. E., Spydevold, O. S., and Bremer, J., Thia fatty acids as inhibitors and substrates of stearoyl-CoA desaturase, *Biochem. Biophys. Acta*, 1349, 251, 1997.

24. Ntambi J. M., Dietary regulation of stearoyl-CoA desaturase 1 gene expression in mouse liver, *J. Biol. Chem.*, 267, 10925, 1992.

25. Sessler A. M. and Ntambi, J. M., Polyunsaturated fatty acid regulation of gene expression, *J. Nutr.*, 128, 923, 1998.

26. Waters, K. M., James M., and Ntambi, J. M., Polyunsaturated fatty acids inhibit hepatic stearoyl-CoA desaturase 1 gene in diabetic mice, *J. Lipids*, 31, S-33, 1996.

27. Ntambi, J. M., Sessler, A. M., and Takova, T., A model cell line for studying stearoyl-CoA desaturase gene regulation by insulin and polyunsaturated fatty acids, *Biochem. Biophys. Res. Commun.*, 220, 990, 1996.

28. Sessler, A. M., Kaur, N., Paulta, J. P., and Ntambi, J. M., Regulation of stearoyl-CoA desaturase 1 mRNA stability by polyunsaturated fatty acids in 3T3-L1 adipocytes, *J. Biol. Chem.*, 271, 29854, 1996.

29. Ntambi, J. M., Regulation of stearoyl-CoA desaturase by polyunsaturated fatty acids and cholesterol, *J. Lipid Res.*, 40, 1549, 1999.

30. Jones, B., Maher, M. A., Banz, W. J., Zemel, M. B., Whelan, J., Smith, P., and Moustaïd, N., Adipose tissue stearoyl-CoA desaturase mRNA is increased by obesity and decreased by polyunsaturated fatty acids, *Am. J. Physiol.*, 34, E44, 1996.

31. Tebbey, P. W. and Buttke, T. M., Stearoyl-CoA desaturase gene expression in lymphocytes, *Biochem. Biophys. Res. Commun.*, 186, 531, 1992.

32. Tebbey, P. W. and Buttke, T. M., Arachidonic Acid regulates unsaturated fatty acid synthesis in lymphocytes by inhibiting stearoyl-CoA desaturase gene expression, *Biochem. Biophys. Acta*, 1171, 27, 1992.

33. Landschulz, K. T., Jump, D. B., MacDougald, O. A., and Lane, M. D., Transcriptional control of the stearoyl-CoA desaturase-1 gene by polyunsaturated fatty acids, *Biochem. Biophys. Res. Commun.*, 200, 763, 1994.

34. Ntambi, J. M., Cellular differentiation and dietary regulation of gene expression, *Prostaglandins, Leukotrienes Essen. Fatty Acids*, 52, 117, 1995.

35. Lee, K. N., Pariza M. W., and Ntambi, J. M., Conjugated linoleic acid decreases hepatic stearoyl-CoA desaturase mRNA, *Biochem. Biophys. Res. Commun.*, 248, 817, 1998.

36. Waters, K. M. and Ntambi, J. M., Insulin and dietary fructose induce stearoyl-CoA desaturase 1 gene expression in liver of diabetic mice, *J. Biol. Chem.*, 269, 27773, 1994.

37. DeWillie, J.W. and Farmer, S. J., Postnatal dietary fat influences mRNAs involved in mylenatin, *Develop. Neurosci.*, 14, 61, 1992.

38. Waters, K. M., Miller, C. W., and Ntambi, J. M., Localization of a polyunsaturated fatty acid response region in stearoyl-C-A desaturase gene. 1, Biophys. Biochem. Acta, 1349, 33, 1997.

39. Jump, D. B., Clarke, S. D., MacDougald, O. A., and Thelen, A., Polyunsaturated fatty acids inhibit S14 gene transcription in rat liver and cultured hepatocytes, *Proc. Natl. Acad. Sci. USA*, 90, 8454, 1993.

40. Liimatta, M., Towle, H. C., Clarke, S., and Jump, D. B., Dietary polyunsaturated fatty acids interfere with the insulin/glucose activation of L-type pyruvate kinase gene transcription, *Mol. Endo.*, 8, 1147, 1994.

41. Tabor, D. E., Kim, J. B., Spiegelman, B. M., and Edwards, P. A., Transcriptional activation of the stearoyl-CoA desaturase 2 gene by sterol regulatory element-binding protein/adipocyte determination and differentiation factor 1, *J. Biol. Chem.*, 273, 22052, 1998.

42. Tabor, D. E., Kim, J. B., Spiegelman, B. M., and Edwards, P. A., Identification of conserved cis-elements and transcription factors required for sterol-regulated transcription of stearoyl-CoA desaturase 1 and 2, *J. Biol. Chem.*, 274, 20603, 1999.

43. Brown, M. S. and Goldstein, J. L., The SREBP pathway: Regulation of cholesterol metabolism by proteolysis of a membrane-bound transcription factor, *Cell*, 89, 331, 1977.

44. Korn, B. S., Shimomura, I., Bashmakov, Y., Hammer R. E., Horton, J. D., Goldstein, J. L., and Brown, M. S., Blunted feed back suppression of SREBP processing by dietary cholesterol in transgenic mice expressing sterol-resistant SCAP (D443N), *J. Clin. Invest.*, 102, 2050, 1998.

45. Shimomura, I., Shimano, H., Korn, B. S., Bashmakov, Y., and Horton, J. D., Nuclear sterol regulatory element-binding proteins activate genes responsible for the entire program of unsaturated fatty acid biosynthesis in transgenic mouse liver, *J. Biol. Chem.*, 273, 35299, 1998.

46. Horton, J. D., Shimomura, L., Brown, M. S., Hammer, R. E., Goldstein, J. L., and Shimano, H., Activation of cholesterol synthesis in preference to fatty acid synthesis in liver and adipose tissue of transgenic mice overexpressing sterol regulatory element binding protein, *J. Clin. Invest.*, 101, 2331, 1998.

47. Pai, J., Guryev, O., Brown M. S., and Goldstein, J. L., Differential stimulation of cholesterol and unsaturated fatty acids in cells expressing individual nuclear sterol regulatory element-binding proteins, *J. Biol. Chem.*, 273, 26138, 1998.

48. Mantovani, R. and Edwards, P. A., Synergistic activation of transcription by nuclear factor Y and sterol regulatory element binding protein, *J. Lipid Res.*, 39, 767, 1998.

49. Dooley, K. M., Millinder, S., and Osborne, T. F., Sterol regulation of 3-hydroxy-3-methylglutaryl-coenzyme A synthase gene through a direct interaction between sterol regulatory element binding protein and the trimeric CCAAT-binding factor/nuclear factor Y, *J. Biol. Chem.*, 273, 1349, 1998.

50. Horton, J. D., Bashmakov, Y., Shimomura, I., and Shimano, H., Regulation of sterol regulatory element binding proteins in livers of fasted and refed mice, *Proc. Natl. Acad. Sci. USA.* 95, 5987, 1998.

51. Xu, J., Nakamura, M. N., Cho, H. P., and Clarke, S. D., Sterol regulatory element binding protein-1 expression is suppressed by dietary polyunsaturated fatty acids, *J. Biol. Chem.*, 274, 23577, 1999.

52. Power, G. W. and Newsholme, E. A., Dietary fatty acids influence the activity and metabolic control of mitochondrial carnitine palmitoyltransferase 1 in rat heart and skeletal muscle, *J. Nutr.*, 127, 2142, 1997.

53. Brandt, J. M., Djouadi, F., and Kelly, D. P., Fatty acids activate transcription of the muscle carnitine palmitoyltransferase I gene in cardiac myocytes via the peroxisome proliferator-activated receptor α, *J. Biol. Chem.*, 273, 23786, 1998.

54. Bing, R., Thelen, A., and Jump, D. B., Peroxisome proliferator-activated receptor a inhibits hepatic S14 gene transcription, *J. Biol. Chem.*, 271, 17167, 1996.

55. Bing, R., Thelen, A. P., Peters, J. M., Gonzalez, F. J., and Jump, D. B., Polyunsaturated fatty acid suppression of hepatic fatty acid synthase and S14 gene expression does not require peroxisome proliferator-activated receptor a, *J. Biol. Chem.*, 272, 26827, 1997.

56. Clarke, S. D., Turini, M., and Jump, D. B., Polyunsaturated fatty acids regulate lipogenic and peroxisomal gene expression by independent mechanisms, *Prostaglandins, Leukotrienes, Essen. Fatty Acids*, 57, 65, 1997.

57. Kim, J. H., Takahashi, M., and Ezaki, O., Fish oil feeding decreases mature sterol regulatory element-binding protein 1 (SREBP-1) by down-regulation of SREBP-1c mRNA in mouse liver, *J. Biol. Chem.*, 274, 25892, 1999.

58. Miller, C. W. and Ntambi, J. M., Peroxisome proliferators induce mouse liver stearoyl-CoA desaturase 1 gene expression, *Proc. Natl. Acad. Sci. USA*, 93, 9443, 1996.

59. Worgall, T. S., Sturley, S. L., Soe, T., Osborne, T. F., and Deckelbaum, R. J., Polyunsaturated fatty acids decrease expression of promoters with sterol regulatory elements by decreasing levels of sterol regulatory element-binding protein, *J. Biol. Chem.*, 273, 25537, 1998.

60. Gonzalez C. I. and Martin, C. E., Fatty acid responsive control of mRNA stability: unsaturated fatty acid-induced degradation of the saccharomyces OLE1 transcript, *J. Biol. Chem.*, 271, 25801, 1996.

4

Fatty Acids, White Adipose Tissue Development, and Adipocyte Differentiation

Gérard Ailhaud

CONTENTS

4.1 Introduction 63
4.2 WAT Development: Relationships with Amount and Type
of Dietary Fats 64
4.3 Fatty Acids and Regulation of Gene Expression in Preadipose
and Adipose Cells 65
4.4 Fatty Acids and Adipocyte Differentiation 67
4.5 Molecular Sensors of Fatty Acids and Fatty Acid Metabolites
in Preadipose and Adipose Cells 68
4.6 Conclusions..70
References 72

4.1 Introduction

In adult animals and humans dietary fat intake is now widely recognized to be associated with gain of fat body mass.[1,2] During development, evidence also exists that a fatty diet is associated with fat body mass and obesity.[3,4] It has been proposed that the large percentage of lipids in many foods overwhelm fat-induced satiety signals.[5] Since changes in dietary fat fail to promote acutely fat oxidation, increase in fat stores follows.[6] In humans under normal dietary conditions and in contrast to rodents, adipose tissue relies on the exogenous supply of fatty acids (FA) from chylomicrons for triglyceride synthesis,[7] although *de novo* fatty acid synthesis is likely taking place in white adipose tissue (WAT) in lipoprotein lipase (LPL)-deficient patients,[8] as has been reported in LPL-knockout mice.[9] The available evidence indicates that WAT is the primary target of FA originating from triglyceride-rich lipoprotein particles.

0-8493-2216-2/01/$0.00+$1.50

Until the late 1980s, it was thought that FA were only playing the role of substrates for complex and neutral lipid synthesis. In the last 10 years, however, it has become clear that both amount and type of dietary fat were important in regulating fat pad weight through hyperplasia and/or hypertrophy. It has also become clear that FA and some of their metabolites are active as signal transducing molecules[10] and are implicated in the differentiation of precursor cells into adipocytes.[11,12] Important molecular sensors of FA have been characterized in the recent years as nuclear *trans*-acting factors of the steroid hormone super-family, termed peroxisome proliferator-activated receptors (PPARs).[13] The properties and mechanisms of PPAR action have provided an important link not only between FA and adipocyte differentiation *in vitro* but also between high-fat intake and augmented development of adipose tissue *in vivo*. This review intends to present these various points and to discuss some nutritional issues.

4.2 WAT Development: Relationships with Amount and Type of Dietary Fats

High-fat diets were shown to induce in adult mice and rats an increase in the cellularity of various adipose depots which takes place by hypertrophy often accompanied by hyperplasia.[14,15] Dietary fats induce adipose tissue growth independent of caloric intake.[16] However, intake of diets enriched in saturated fats as compared to diets enriched in unsaturated fats has led to conflicting results. With similar caloric intake, hypertrophy of perirenal and epididymal adipose tissues was lower with high-fat diets enriched in mono- and polyunsaturated FA than with high-fat diets enriched with saturated FA.[17–20] In another study, hyperplasia appeared to be involved: The role of dietary fats (45% calories as fat) was analyzed in 1-month-old male Sprague-Dawley rats fed for 5 to 7 weeks with either beef tallow (high saturated fat), safflower oil (high polyunsaturated fat), or corn starch. When fed *ad libitum* and compared to corn starch fed rats, dietary saturated fats induced expansion of inguinal retroperirenal fat pads through increased adipocyte number.[18] Similarly, in 1-month-old male Sprague-Dawley rats fed for 12 weeks (26% calories as fat) with perilla oil (high in α-linolenic acid), beef tallow, olive oil, or safflower oil, perilla oil was shown to lower the growth of epididymal and perirenal fat pads that was associated with hypoplasia and mainly hypotrophy as compared to the other dietary fats.[21]

It has been reported recently that 5-week-old fa/fa rats but not Fa/? rats exhibit a greater reduction in body weight gain and a larger increase in heat production when the animals were fed (65% calories as fat) for 8 weeks with soybean oil (high in linoleic acid) than when they were fed with palm oil (high in palmitic acid).[19] More recently,[20] mother rats were fed diets (45% calories as fat) containing either coconut oil resembling milk fat (high in lauric, myristic, and palmitic acids) and termed COD or safflower oil (high in oleic and linoleic acids) and termed SOD and mated to provide Fa/Fa and Fa/fa lean offsprings as well as fa/fa obese offsprings. Suckling rats were analyzed at 17 days of age, whereas additional 28-day-old male rats were maintained after weaning on the same diet as their mothers until 12 weeks of age. Interestingly, although inguinal fat pad weight were similar in the 17-day-old pups, fat cell number was higher in the inguinal fat pad of the three genotypes in SOD pups, whereas fat cell size was higher in COD pups. The enhanced neutral lipid accumulation is consistent with the increased activities of lipoprotein lipase (LPL), fatty acid synthase (FAS), and malic enzyme (ME) in COD pups as compared to SOD pups. In the 12-week-old rats, when analyzing inguinal, retroperitoneal, and epididymal fat pads, fat cell number was nearly 2-fold higher in SOD rats than in COD rats of the three genotypes, whereas fat cell size was significantly higher in COD rats in fa/fa rats only, again consistent with increased LPL, FAS, and ME activities observed in COD rats.

Thus, despite a similar quantitative fat intake, these data indicate qualitative differences with respect to dietary fatty acid composition regardless of the genotype, where long-chain polyunsaturated FA (18:1ω9, C18:2ω6, and C18:3ω3) appear to favor hyperplasia through enhanced adipose cell differentiation, whereas long-chain saturated FA (C12:0, C14:0 and C16:0) appear to favor hypertrophy through enhanced triglyceride accumulation. In other words, the development of adipose tissue soon after birth and in the few weeks after birth is sensitive to fatty acid composition and amount of ingested fats. Nevertheless, even at later ages, fat depots remain able to respond to dietary fats in a site-specific manner. When 50-day old Wistar rats are fed for 4 weeks with high-fat diets (40% calories as fat) enriched with ω3 polyunsaturated FA, i.e., eicosapentaenoic acid or docosahexaenoic acid, a lower weight gain of the internal retroperitoneal depot was observed as compared to the subcutaneous depot, consistent with a lower expression of lipid-related genes in the internal depot.[22] The mechanisms for such differences remain unclear but should implicate metabolic differences among FA (oxidation for energy requirements, esterification processes for complex and neutral lipid biosynthesis, desaturation and elongation, eicosanoid and leukotriene formation). The mechanisms should also implicate differences *in vivo* between FA and FA metabolites as signal transducing molecules reported to trigger *in vitro* adipogenesis, i.e., the differentiation of precursor cells into adipocytes (*vide infra*).

4.3 Fatty Acids and Regulation of Gene Expression in Preadipose and Adipose Cells

The first line of evidence that FA were involved in the process of adipose cell differentiation was obtained after purification and characterization of the main adipogenic component of fetal bovine serum because the latter was originally used extensively to grow and differentiate preadipose into adipose cells. This main component of serum was characterized as being arachidonic acid (AA).[23] Both the long-term adipogenic effect as assayed by glycerol-3-phosphate dehydrogenase (GPDH) activity and the short-term intracellular production of cAMP induced by AA were blocked by cyclooxygenase inhibitors such as aspirin or indomethacin, suggesting strongly that some prostanoid(s) was involved in these responses. Prostacyclin (PGI_2), under the form of its stable analogue (carba)prostacyclin ($cPGI_2$), was then found to induce short- and long-term effects of AA.[24] The adipogenic effect of carbacyclin could be extended to the differentiation of rat and human adipose precursor cells in primary culture.[25] Other analogues of PGI_2, such as 6β-PGI_1 and iloprost, although less potent than $cPGI_2$, were also active.[26] It is interesting to note that glucocorticoids which were able to increase AA mobilization and its metabolism to PGI_2 in Ob1171 preadipose cells also behaved as strong adipogenic hormones.[27]

Antibodies directed against PGI_2 were shown to strongly diminish the adipogenic effect induced by AA in 5F medium. Thus, PGI_2 secreted into the culture medium of Ob1771 preadipocytes upon exposure to AA behaved as an autocrine/paracrine effector of adipose cell differentiation.[26]

The second line of evidence in preadipose and adipose cells that FA were important regulators of the process of adipose cell differentiation was obtained when it was shown that long-chain FA could act as transcriptional regulators of lipid-related genes, as first reported for the gene encoding the adipocyte lipid-binding protein (ALBP), also termed adipocyte fatty acid-binding protein (a-FABP) or aP2 protein.[10] The accumulation of aP2 protein was parallel to that of aP2 mRNA. The transcriptional effect of exogenous FA was observed in culture in glucose-supplemented preadipose cells as well as in glucose-free adipose cells, that is under conditions where endogenous fatty acid synthesis remained low. Long-chain FA (LCFA) (saturated, mono- and polyunsaturated) were able to activate within a few hours the aP2 gene but also the gene encoding for the acyl-CoA synthase-1 (ACS1).[11,28] Thus the expression of two key proteins involved, respectively, in FA transport and activation was regulated at the gene level by FA. Metabolism of FA was not required as α-bromopalmitate, a non-metabolized LCFA in preadipose cells, was more potent than natural LCFA in activating the aP2 gene at a transcriptional level.[29] This effect of α-bromopalmitate could be extended to cultured adipose precursor cells from rat adipose tissue in a serum-free, chemically defined medium, thus excluding any specific effect of FA in cells from preadipocyte clonal lines and any synergy of FA with serum components.[11] The transcriptional effect of FA occurred early in preadipose cells and was confined to some but not to all lipid-related genes, i.e., to the fatty acid translocase (FAT) gene as an early marker of differentiation[30] and also the ACS1 and aP2 genes among intermediate markers, but the genes encoding for late markers such as GPDH and adipsin were not affected.[10,11] In addition to transcriptional effects of

FA, a stabilizing effect of FA was also assumed in adipose cells because aP2 mRNA accumulation appeared accompanied only by a weak increase in the transcription of the aP2 gene.[31]

At odds with this observation, a destabilization effect of FA in adipose cells appears to take place. When exposed to AA, the half-life of SCD1 mRNA[32] and that of GLUT4 mRNA[33] were decreased in 3T3-L1 cells by 67 and 43%, respectively. Both ω3 (AA, linolenic acid, and eicosapentaenoic acid) and ω6 polyunsaturated FA (linoleic acid) led to a decrease in SCD1 mRNA stability.[32] The transcriptional effects of FA in adipose cells are well described for the PEPCK gene[34] but, in some instances, the mechanisms by which FA regulate the expression of the products of lipid-related genes in preadipose and adipose cells appear more complex than anticipated. Preadipose cells are known to express LPL constitutively. However, when preadipose and adipose cells were exposed to LCFA or α-bromopalmitate, a rapid (2 to 8 h) and dose-dependent increase (up to 6-fold) in LPL mRNA occurred, primarily due to increased transcription which is accompanied by a decrease in LPL cellular activity. Under these conditions, secretion of active LPL was nearly abolished. Removal of LCFA led to full recovery of LPL activity and secretion. Thus, FA appeared to exert their main biological effects at translational and post-translational levels to regulate secreted active LPL.[35] This suggests that the regulation of LPL by LCFA may be important *in vivo* with regard to the fine tuning of FA entry into preadipocytes during adipocyte formation and in adipocytes during fasting/feeding periods.

4.4 Fatty Acids and Adipocyte Differentiation

The involvement of FA as inducers of the differentiation of preadipose to adipose cells was first reported in cultured cells of Ob1771 and 3T3-F442A clonal lines.[11,12] The triggering effect of FA took place in preadipose cells, and the adipogenic action of FA did not require their metabolism as the non-metabolized α-bromopalmitate was more effective than metabolized natural LCFA. Of note is the fact that the synthetic ω3 AA was less efficient than the natural ω6 AA in promoting terminal differentiation (R. Négrel, personal communication). When compared to control adipogenic conditions, a brief exposure of preadipose cells (1 to 3 days) to LCFA was sufficient to bring a maximal effect and led within 1 to 2 weeks to hyperplasia, an increase in the number of differentiated cells and to hypertrophy, an increase in triglyceride accumulation accompanied by enhanced overexpression of terminal differentiation-related genes.[11,12]

In other words, in the appropriate hormonal milieu, a hyperplastic phenomenon could be observed *in vitro* upon short exposure of precursor cells to exogenous, unprocessed LCFA. For instance, under these conditions, the concentration of unbound α-bromopalmitate in the external milieu should be very low.[36] After its uptake and intracellular traffic, it is likely that its transient increased concentration within the nucleus should remain very low as part may remain bound within the cytosol of preadipose cells by the epidermal fatty acid-binding protein (eFABP).[37] If this were so, this low rise in FA concentration would remain sufficient to activate directly or indirectly the expression of lipid-related genes (*vide infra*).

4.5 Molecular Sensors of Fatty Acids and Fatty Acid Metabolites in Preadipose and Adipose Cells

Like retinoic acid and fibrates, FA are amphipatic carboxylates. As retinoic acid binds specifically and activates specific nuclear receptors, it was hypothesized that fibrates and FA could act in a similar way via new members of the nuclear receptor families. PPARα, a member of the nuclear steroid hormone receptor superfamily activated by fibrates was first cloned from mouse liver.[38] PPARα as well as other PPAR isoforms were thereafter identified from cDNA libraries obtained from various organs of different species.[30,39–47] Evidence was obtained that peroxisome proliferators and FA can activate PPARα in transactivation assays.[40] With one exception,[48] PPARα could not be detected in preadipose cells, in contrast to PPARδ and trace levels of PPARγ. Once differentiated, PPARδ remained present in adipose cells, whereas PPARγ was then expressed at high levels.[30] PPARγ was shown to be predominantly, but not exclusively, expressed in adipose tissue; PPARδ and PPARα showed a more widespread tissue distribution although a higher expression was observed in lipid-synthesizing tissues (adipose tissue, liver, intestine).[30,44]

All the PPAR isoforms are active as heterodimers with retinoic X receptor α (RXRα) by recognizing *cis*-acting sequences (DR-1, direct repeat, 1 base spacer).[13] By direct comparison of the various PPARs expressed at low levels in transfected NIH-3T3 fibroblasts, the adipogenic potential of PPARγ and to a lesser degreee that of PPARα was shown, whereas that of PPARδ was not observed.[49] However, using a direct approach with 3T3-C2 fibroblasts, the critical role of this nuclear receptor in adipogenesis has been recently shown: no PPARγ expression, and no subsequent adipocyte formation, can take place unless prior activation of PPARδ by natural LCFA or α-bromopalmitate in the presence of a specific agonist of PPARγ, i.e., the thiazolidinedione BRL49653. Treatment of PPARδ-expressing fibroblasts with FA stimulated the expression of the early FAT gene. Of note is the fact that the most potent effector was (carba)prostacyclin (EC_{50} ~ 20 nM) whereas the most specific agonist ligands of PPARγ, i.e., BRL49653 and 15d-PGJ$_2$,[50,51] were inactive.[52] The data strongly suggest that active PPARδ led to PPARγ expression which, upon activation, promoted the formation of adipose cells. The key initial role in adipose cell differentiation of PPARδ as primary target appears consistent with recent experiments showing that a dominant-negative form of PPARδ impairs the expression of PPARγ and the differentiation of Ob1771 and 3T3-F442A pread-ipose cells (P. Grimaldi, personal communication).

The sequential promotion of adipose cell differentiation by PPARδ and PPARγ emphasizes their role as nuclear sensors of FA and FA metabolites. Until recently it was uncertain whether FA, fatty acid metabolites, and several exogenous substances such as fibrates were mere activators of PPARs by displacing intracellularily the natural ligands of PPARs or whether these effectors could indeed bind to the nuclear receptors. Binding of FA and FA metabolites as well as that of fibrates and other amphipatic carboxylates to PPARα, PPARδ and PPARγ has been shown using various indirect approaches.[53-55] Very recently the direct proof of FA binding to PPARs has been elegantly brought by direct binding assays and X-ray cristallography.[56,57] PPARα and PPARδ bind saturated and unsaturated long-chain FA whereas PPARγ bind most efficiently polyunsaturated FA and only weakly monounsaturated FA. The crystal structure of PPARγ[58] and that of PPARδ[57] provide amazing insight into the ability of PPARs to interact with a variety of synthetic compounds (fibrates, thiazolidinediones) and natural compounds, including $FA_3 \geq C14$ of varying degrees of unsaturation. However, it should be pointed out that despite these remarkable observations, the nature of the FA and/or that of the FA metabolites, which are the actual ligands of PPARδ and PPARγ within the nucleus of preadipose and adipose cells, remains to be shown.

Among FA metabolites, circumstantial evidence favors prostacyclin as a putative ligand involved in the activation of PPARδ in preadipose cells as

1. Prostacyclin (PGI_2) is produced by preadipose cells in which PPARδ is expressed simultaneously as does the cell surface IP receptor which binds prostacyclin specifically.[58]

2. Using authentic target cells, i.e., preadipose cells, PGI_2 and its stable analogue $cPGI_2$ behave as adipogenic hormones whereas other prostaglandins such as PGD_2, PGJ_2, Δ^{12}-PGJ_2 and 15d-Δ^{12-14}-PGJ_2 are inactive.[59]

3. In preadipose cells (carba)prostacyclin regulates the expression of several genes including a-FABP, angiotensinogen, and the uncoupling protein UCP-2. This effect of $cPGI_2$ could *not* be mimicked by PGE_1, 6-keto-PGE_1, or BMY45778 despite the fact that they are all ligands of the cell surface IP receptor, altering cAMP and calcium levels. Once the cells are differentiated, the cell surface responses induced by PGI_2 or $cPGI_2$ disappear, but $cPGI_2$ remains able to regulate the expression of these genes in adipose cells.[60]

4. Prostacyclin analogues, especially (carba)prostacyclin, transactivate all PPAR isoforms in the expected range of concentrations (0.025 to 10 μM).[48]

5. (Carba)prostacyclin induces adipogenesis in transfected fibroblasts expressing PPARα or PPARγ within the same range of concentrations as in transactivation assays.[49]

6. In PPARδ-expressing fibroblasts, (carba)prostacyclin shows the unique ability to substitute for a combination of a PPARδ activator (α-bromopalmitate) and a PPARγ ligand (BRL49653) for the promotion of adipose differentiation ($EC_{50} \sim 20$ nM).[52]

7. (Carba)prostacyclin is indeed a ligand of PPARδ.[53]

Although of interest, these data cannot rule out that the natural ligand(s) of PPARδ differ from prostacyclin, but it should be stressed that this prostaglandin is the only metabolite of arachidonic acid currently characterized in preadipose cells with PGE_2 and trace levels of $PGE_{2\alpha}$.[61] Moreover, PGI_2 has been shown recently to upregulate via the IP receptor in preadipose cells the expression of C/EBPβ and δ, which plays a key role in adipose tissue development by regulating, in turn, like PPARδ (see above), the expression of PPARγ.[62-65] The above observations emphasize a role of prostacyclin via PPARδ in the early events of adipose cell differentiation and underline that the role played by PPARs can hardly be envisioned *independently* from the site of synthesis and/or the availability of their natural ligands.

4.6   Conclusions

Taken together, current *in vitro* data suggest two complementary roles of LCFA in the development of adipose tissue (Fig. 4.1). The intensity and duration of the flux of dietary LCFA entering adipose tissue, proportionate to the amount of ingested fat, is assumed to alter transiently the intracellular concentrations of LCFA and/or their metabolites within the nucleus. In preadipose cells PPARδ, which binds both saturated and unsaturated FA and appears as their primary target, leads to the rapid expression of PPARγ. In adition, AA arising from both the diet and the elongation/desaturation processes of the essential linoleic acid, is the substrate entering the lipoxygenase and cyclooxygenase pathways. Among AA metabolites, prostacyclin appears unique in its ability to promote terminal differentiation of preadipose to adipose cells.[52,59] Prostacyclin via the cell surface receptor IP triggers the expression of C/EBPβ and δ critical for PPARγ and C/EBPα expression and adipose tissue formation,[62-65] but it could also bind directly to PPARδ.[53] If that were so, among unsaturated FA, AA would specifically

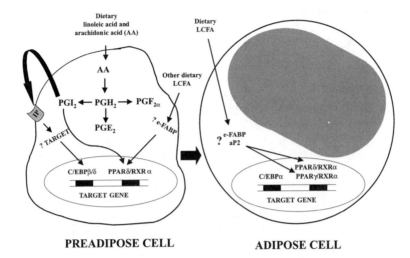

PREADIPOSE CELL   **ADIPOSE CELL**

FIGURE 4.1

Putative role of fatty acids (FA) and arachidonic acid (AA) metabolites in preadipose and adipose cells. This scheme assumes that LCFA from exogenous origin trigger terminal differentiation as no significant FA synthesis takes place in preadipose cells.[10] Once differentiated, LCFA from endogenous origin (not shown) and exogenous origin should be implicated in adipocyte hypertrophy. Prostacyclin (AA metabolite) interacts with the IP receptor present in preadipose cells only and regulates C/EBP§ and CEBPδ gene expression. As prostacyclin production and IP receptor expression cease in adipose cells, only PPARδ and PPARγ would then act as molecular sensors of FA.

and indirectly favor differentiation via prostacyclin, consistent with data showing that a high-fat diet enriched in linoleic acid favors adipose tissue hyperplasia in pups and young rats.[20]

Once differentiated adipose cells cease the production of prostacyclin (unless stimulated by angiotensin II)[66] and cease to express the IP receptor.[67] The differentiated cells still express PPARδ but now express PPARγ in addition to C/EBPα. At that stage, the nature of the ligands of PPARδ and PPARγ in adipose cells remains unknown. According to their binding properties, it is assumed that PPARγ would then be preferentially activated by mono- and polyunsaturated FA, whereas PPARδ would be activated by saturated, mono- and polyunsaturated FA. Although both PPARs act as nuclear sensors of FA and could potentially regulate adipocyte hypertrophy, PPARγ should play a key role in maintaining the adipose state through the regulation of its expression by adipocyte differentiation and determination of factor-1 (ADD-1)/sterol regulating binding protein-1 (SREBP-1),[68] and its cross-regulation with C/EBPα.[69]

Acknowledgments: The contribution of Prof. R. Négrel over the years and that of all the members of the laboratory are gratefully acknowledged. Thanks are due to Dr. P. Grimaldi for careful reading of the manuscript and for helpful discussion.

References

1. Romieu, I., Willett W. C., Stampfer, M. J., Colditz, G. A., Sampson, L., Rosner, B., Henneckens, C. H., and Speizer, F. E., Energy intake and other determinants of relative weight, *Am. J. Clin. Nutr.*, 47, 406, 1988.
2. Tucker, L. A. and Kano, M. J., Dietary fat and body fat: a multivariate study of 205 adult females, *Am. J. Clin. Nutr.*, 56, 616, 1992.
3. Nguyen, V. T., Larson, D. E., Johnson, R. K., and Goran, M. J., Fat intake and adiposity in children of lean and obese parents, *Am. J. Clin. Nutr.*, 63, 507, 1996.
4. Klesges, R. C., Klesges, L. M., Eck, L. H., and Shelton, M. L., A longitudinal analysis of accelerated weight gain in preschool children, *Pediatrics*, 95, 126, 1995.
5. Blundell, J. E., Cotton, J. R., Delargy, H., Green, S., Greenough, A., King, N. A., and Lawton, C. L., The fat paradox: fat-induced satiety signals versus high fat overconsumption, *Int. J. Obes.*, 19, 832, 1995.
6. Schutz, Y., Flatt, J. P., and Jequier, E., Failure of dietary fat intake to promote fat oxidation: a factor favoring the development of obesity, *Am. J. Clin. Nutr.*, 5, 307, 1989.
7. Goldberg, J. J., Lipoprotein lipase and lipolysis: central roles in lipoprotein metabolism and atherogenesis, *J. Lipid Res.*, 37, 693, 1996.
8. Brun, L. D., Gagne, C., Julien P., Tremblay, A., Moorjani, S., Bouchard, C., and Lupien, P. J., Familial lipoprotein lipase-activity deficiency: study of total body fatness and subcutaneous fat tissue distribution, *Metabolism*, 38, 1005, 1989.
9. Weinstock, P. H., Levak-Frank, S., Hudgins, L. C., Radner, H., Friedman, J. M., Zechner, R., and Breslow, J. L., Lipoprotein lipase controls fatty acid entry into adipose tissue, but fat mass is preserved by endogenous synthesis in mice deficient in adipose tissue lipoprotein lipase, *Proc. Natl. Acad. Sci. USA*, 94, 10261, 1997.
10. Amri, E. Z., Bertrand, B., Ailhaud, G., and Grimaldi, P., Regulation of adipose cell differentiation. I. Fatty acids are inducers of the aP2 gene expression, *J. Lipid Res.*, 32, 1449, 1991.
11. Ailhaud, G., Abumrad, N., Amri, E. Z., and Grimaldi, P. A., New insights in the process of differentiation of pre-adipose cells: the role of fatty acids as signal transducing molecules, in *Obesity in Europe 1993*, Ditschuneit, H., Gries, F. A., Hauner, H., Schusdziarra, V., and Wechsler, J. G., Eds., Libbey, London, 1994, 51.
12. Amri, E. Z., Ailhaud, G., and Grimaldi, P. A., Fatty acids as signal transducing molecules: involvement in the differentiation of preadipose to adipose cells, *J. Lipid Res.*, 35, 930, 1994.
13. Schoonjans, K., Staels, B., and Auwerx, J., Role of the peroxisome proliferator-activated receptor (PPAR) in mediating the effects of fibrates and fatty acids on gene expression, *J. Lipid Res.*, 37, 907, 1996.
14. Faust, I. M., Johnson, P. R., Stern, J. S., and Hirsch, J., Diet-induced adipocyte number increase in adult rats: a new model of obesity, *Am. J. Physiol.*, 235, E279, 1978.
15. Klyde, B. J. and Hirsch, J., Increased cellular proliferation in adipose tissue of adult rats fed a high-fat diet, *J. Lipid Res.*, 20, 705, 1979.
16. Oscai, L. B., Brown, M. M., and Miller, W. C., Effect of dietary fat on food intake, growth and body composition in rats, *Growth*, 48, 415, 1984.

17. Parrish, C. C., Pathy, D. A., and Angel, A., Dietary fish oils limit adipose tissue hypertrophy in rats, *Metabolism*, 39, 217, 1990.
18. Shillabeer, G. and Lau, D. C. W., Regulation of new fat cell formation in rats: the role of dietary fats, *J. Lipid Res.*, 35, 592, 1994.
19. Loh, M. Y., Flatt, W. P., Martin, R. J., and Hausman, D. B., Dietary fat type and level influence adiposity development in obese but not lean Zucker rats, *Proc. Soc. Exp. Biol. Med.*, 218, 38, 1998.
20. Cleary, M. P., Phillips, F. C., and Morton, A. A., Gentoype and diet effects in lean and obese Zucker rats fed either safflower or coconut oil diets, *Proc. Soc. Exp. Biol. Med.*, 220, 153, 1999.
21. Okuno, M., Kajiwara, K., Imai, S., Kobayashi, T., Honna, N., Maki, T., Suruga, K., Goda, T., Takase, S., Muto, Y., and Moriwaki, H., Perilla oil prevents the excessive growth of visceral adipose tissue in rats by downregulating adipocyte differentiation, *J. Nutr.*, 127, 1752, 1997.
22. Raclot, T., Groscolas, R., Langin, D., and Ferre, P., Site-specific regulation of gene expression by n-3 polyunsaturated fatty acids in rat white adipose tissues, *J. Lipid Res.*, 38, 1963, 1997.
23. Gaillard, D., Négrel, R., Lagarde, M., and Ailhaud, G., Requirement and role of arachidonic acid in the differentiation of preadipose cells, *Biochem. J.*, 257, 389, 1989.
24. Négrel, R., Gaillard, D., and Ailhaud, G., Prostacyclin as a potent effector of adipose differentiation, *Biochem. J.*, 257, 399, 1989.
25. Vassaux, G., Gaillard, D., Ailhaud, G., and Négrel, R., Prostacyclin is a specific effector of adipose cell differentiation: its dual role as a cAMP- and Ca2+-elevating agent, *J. Biol. Chem.*, 267, 11092, 1992.
26. Catalioto, R. M., Gaillard, D., Maclouf, J., Ailhaud, G., and Négrel, R., Autocrine control of adipose cell differentiation by prostacyclin and $PGF_{2\alpha}$, *Biochim. Biophys. Acta*, 1091, 364, 1991.
27. Gaillard, D., Wabitsch, M., Pipy, B., and Négrel, R., Control of terminal differentiation of adipose precursor cells by glucocorticoids, *J. Lipid Res.*, 32, 569, 1991.
28. Suzuki, H., Kawarabayasi, Y., Kondo, J., Abe, T., Nishikawa, K., Kimura, S., Hashimoto, T., and Yamamoto, T., Structure and regulation of rat long-chain acyl-CoA synthetase, *J. Biol. Chem.*, 265, 8681, 1990.
29. Grimaldi, P., Knobel, S. M., Whitesell, R. R., and Abumrad, N. A., Induction of aP2 gene by nonmetabolized long chain fatty acids, *Proc. Natl. Acad. Sci. USA*, 89, 10930, 1992.
30. Amri, E. Z., Bonino, F., Ailhaud, G., Abumrad, N. A., and Grimaldi, P. A., Cloning of a protein that mediates transcriptional effects of fatty acids in preadipocytes. Homology to peroxisome proliferator-activated receptors, *J. Biol. Chem.*, 270, 2367, 1995.
31. Distel, R. J., Robinson, G. S., and Spiegelman, B. M., Fatty acid regulation of gene expession: transcriptional and post-transcriptional mechanisms, *J. Biol. Chem.*, 267, 5937, 1992.
32. Sessier, A. M., Karur, N., Palta, J. P., and Ntambi, J. M., Regulation of stearoyl-CoA desaturase 1 mRNA stability by polyunsaturated fatty acids in 3T3-L1 adipocytes, *J. Biol. Chem.*, 271, 29854, 1996.
33. Long, S. D. and Pekala, P. H., Regulation of GLUT4 gene expression by arachidonic acid, *J. Biol. Chem.*, 271, 1138, 1996.

34. Antras-Ferry, J., Le Bigot, G., Robin, P., and Forest, C., Stimulation of phospho-enolpyruvate carboxykinase gene expression by fatty acids, *Biochem. Biophys. Res. Commun.,* 203, 385, 1994.
35. Amri, E. Z., Teboul, L., Vannier, C., Grimaldi, P. A., and Ailhaud, G., Fatty acids regulate the expression of lipoprotein lipase gene and activity in preadipose and adipose cells, *Biochem. J.,* 314, 541, 1996.
36. Abumrad, N., Harmon, C., and Ibrahimi, A., Membrane transport of long-chain fatty acids: evidence for a facilitated process, *J. Lipid Res.,* 39, 2309, 1998.
37. Ibrahimi, A., Teboul, L., Gaillard, D., Amri, E., Ailhaud, G., Young, P., Cawthorne, M. A., and Grimaldi, P., Evidence for a common mechanism of action for fatty acids and thiazolidinedione antidiabetic agents on gene expression in preadipose cells, *Mol. Pharmacol.,* 46, 1070, 1994.
38. Isseman, I. and Green, S., Activation of a member of the steroid hormone receptor superfamily by peroxisome proliferators, *Nature,* 347, 645, 1990.
39. Dreyer, C., Krey, G., Keller, H., Givel, F., Helftenbein, G., and Wahli, W., Control of peroxisomal β-oxidation pathway by a novel family of nuclear hormone receptors, *Cell,* 68, 879, 1992.
40. Gottlicher, M., Widmark, E., Li, Q., and Gustafsson, J. A., Fatty acids activate chimera of the clofibric acid-activated receptor and the glucocorticoid receptor, *Proc. Natl. Acad. Sci. USA,* 89, 4653, 1992.
41. Schmidt, A., Endo, N., Rutledge, S. J., Vogel, R., Shinar, D., and Rodan, G. A., Identification of a new member of the steroid hormone receptor superfamily that is activated by a peroxisome proliferator and fatty acids, *Mol. Endocrinol.,* 6, 1634, 1992.
42. Zhu, Y., Alvares, K., Huang, Q., Rao, M. S., and Reddy, J. K., Cloning of a new member of the peroxisome proliferator activated receptor gene family from mouse liver, *J. Biol. Chem.,* 268, 26817, 1993.
43. Chen, F., Law, S. N., and O'Malley, B. W., Identification of two mPPAR related receptors and evidence for the existence of the five subfamily members, *Biochem. Biophys. Res. Commun.,* 196, 671, 1993.
44. Tontonoz, P., Hu, E., Graves, R. A., Budavari, A. I., and Spiegelman, B. M., mPPARγ2: tissue-specific regulator of an adipocyte enhancer, *Genes Dev.,* 8, 1224, 1994.
45. Kliewer, S. A., Forman, B. M., Blumberg, B., Ong, E. S., Borgmeyer, U., Mangelsdorf, D. J., Umesono, K., and Evans, R. M., Differential expression and activation of a family of murine peroxisome proliferator-activated receptors, *Proc. Natl. Acad. Sci. USA,* 91, 7355, 1994.
46. Greene, M. E., Blumberg, B., McBride, O. W., Yi, H. F., Kronquist, K., Kwan, K., Hsieh, L., Greene, G., and Nimer, S. D., Isolation of the human peroxisome proliferator activated receptor gamme cDNA: expression in hematopoietic cells and chromosomal mapping, *Gene Expr.,* 4, 281, 1995.
47. Aperlo, C., Pognonec, P., Saladin, R., Auwerx, J., and Boulukos, K., Isolation and characterization of the hamster peroxisomal proliferator activated receptor hPPARγ, a member of the nuclear hormone receptor superfamily, *Gene,* 162, 297, 1995.
48. Yu, K., Bayona, W., Kallen, C. B., Harding, H. P., Ravera, C. P., McMahon, G., Brown, M., and Lazar, M. A., Differential activation of peroxisome proliferator-activated receptors by eicosanoids, *J. Biol. Chem.,* 270, 23975, 1995.

49. Brun, R. P., Tontonoz, P., Forman, B. M., Ellis, R., Chen, J., Evans, R. M., and Spiegelman, B. M., Differential activation of adipogenesis by multiple PPAR isoforms, *Genes Dev.*, 10, 974, 1996.

50. Forman, B. M., Tontonoz, P., Chen, J., Brun, R. P., Spiegelman, B. M., and Evans, R. M., 15-deoxy-$\Delta^{12,14}$ prostaglandin J2 is a ligand for the adipocyte determination factor PPARγ, *Cell*, 83, 803, 1995.

51. Kliewer, S. A., Lenhard, J. M., Willson, T. M., Patel, I., Morris, D. C., and Lehman, J. M., A prostaglandin J2 metabolite binds peroxisome proliferator-activated receptor γ and promotes adipocyte differentiation, *Cell*, 83, 813, 1995.

52. Bastié, C., Holst, D., Gaillard, D., Jehl-Pietri, C., and Grimaldi, P. A., Expression of peroxisome proliferator-activated receptor PPARδ promotes induction of PPARγ and adipocyte differentiation in 3T3C2 fibroblasts, *J. Biol. Chem.*, 274, 21920, 1999.

53. Forman, B. M., Chen, J., and Evans, R. M., Hypolipidemic drugs, polyunsaturated fatty acids, and eicosanoids are ligands for peroxisome proliferator-activated receptors, *Proc. Natl. Acad. Sci. USA*, 94, 4312, 1997.

54. Kliewer, S. A., Sundseth, S. S., Jones, S. A., Brown, P. J., Wisely, G. B., Koble, C. S., Devchand, P., Wahli, W., Willson, T. M., Lenhard, J. M., and Lehmann, J. M., Fatty acids and eicosanoids regulate gene expession through direct interactions with peroxisome proliferator-activated receptors α and γ, *Proc. Natl. Acad. Sci. USA*, 94, 4318, 1997.

55. Krey, G., Braissant, O., L'Horset, F., Kalkhoven, E., Perroud, M., Parker, G. M., and Wahli, W., Fatty acids, eicosanoids, and hypolipidemic agents identified as ligands of peroxisome proliferator-activated receptors by coactivator-dependent receptor ligand assay, *Mol. Endo.*, 11, 779, 1997.

56. Nolte, R. T., Wisely, G. B., Westin, S., Cobb, J. E., Lambert, M. H., Kurokawa, R., Rosenfeld, M. G., Willson, T. M., Glass, C. K., and Milburn, M. V., Ligand binding and co-activator assemby of the peroxisome proliferator-activated receptor γ, *Nature*, 395, 137, 1998.

57. Xu, H. E., Lambert, M. H., Montana, V. G., Parks, D. J., Blanchard, S. G., Brown, P. J., Sternbach, D. D., Lehmann, J. M., Wisely, G. B., Willson, T. M., Kliewer, S. A., and Milburn, M. V., Molecular recognition of fatty acids by peroxisome proliferator-activated receptors, *Mol. Cell*, 3, 397, 1999.

58. Wise, H. and Jones, R. L., Focus on prostacyclin and its novel mimetics, *TIPS*, 17, 17, 1996.

59. Ailhaud, G., Cell surface receptors, nuclear receptors and ligands that regulate adipose tissue development, *Clin. Chim. Acta*, 286, 181, 1999.

60. Aubert, J., Ailhaud, G., and Négrel, R., Evidence for a novel regulatory pathway activated by (carba)prostacyclin in preadipose and adipose cells, *FEBS Lett.*, 397, 117, 1996.

61. Négrel, R. and Ailhaud, G., Metabolism of arachidonic acid and prostaglandin synthesis in Ob17 preadipocyte cell line, *Biochem. Biophys. Res. Commun.*, 98, 768, 1981.

62. Wu, Z., Xie, Y., Bucher, N. L. R., and Farmer, S. R., Conditional ectopic expression of C/EBPβ in NIH-3T3 cells induces PPARγ and stimulates adipogenesis, *Genes Dev.*, 9, 2350, 1995.

63. Wu, Z., Bucher, N. L. R., and Farmer, S. R., Induction of peroxisome proliferator-activated receptor γ during the conversion of 3T3 fibroblasts into adipocytes is mediated by C/EBPβ, C/EBPδ, and glucocorticoids, *Mol. Cell. Biol.*, 16, 4128, 1996.

64. Tanaka, T., Yoshida, N., Kishimoto, T., and Akira, S., Defective adipocyte differentiation in mice lacking the C/EBPβ and/or C/EBPδ gene, *EMBO J.,* 16, 7432, 1997.

65. Moitra, J., Mason, M. M., Olive, M., Krylov, D., and Gavrilova, O., Marcus-Samuels, B., Feigenbaum, L., Lee, E., Aoyama, T., Eckhaus, M., Reitman, M. L., Vinson, C., Life without white fat: a transgenic mouse, *Gene Dev.,* 12, 3168, 1998.

66. Darimont, C., Vassaux, G., Ailhaud, G., and Negrel, R., Differentiation of preadipose cells: paracrine role of prostacyclin upon stimulation of adipose cells by angiotensin II, *Endocrinology,* 135, 2030, 1994.

67. Bšrglum, J. D., Pedersen, S. B., Ailhaud, G., Négrel, R., and Richelsen, B., Differential expression of prostaglandin receptors during adipose cell differentiation, *Prostaglandins Other Lipid Mediat.,* 57, 305, 1999.

68. Fajas, L., Schoonjans, K., Gelman, L., Kim, J. B., Najib, J., Martin, G., Fruchart, J. C., Briggs, M., Spiegelman, B. M., and Auwerx, J., Regulation of peroxisome proliferator-activated receptor γ expression by adipocyte differentiation and determination factor 1/sterol regulatory element binding protein 1: implications for adipocyte differentiation and metabolism, *Mol. Cell. Biol.,* 19, 5495, 1999

69. Wu, Z., Rosen, E. D., Brun, R., Hauser, S., Adelmant, G., Troy, A. E., McKeon, C., Darlington, G. J., and Spiegelman, B. M., Cross-regulation of C/EBPα and PPARγ controls the transcriptional pathway of adipogenesis and insulin sensitivity, *Mol. Cell,* 3, 151, 1999.

5

Acyl-CoA Synthetase 1 (ACS1): Regulation and Role in Metabolism

Pamela J. Smith

CONTENTS

5.1   ACS1: Structure and Function...77
5.2   ACS1 Gene Expression: Tissue Distribution
      and Developmental Regulation 79
5.3   The ACS Gene Family 81
5.4   Nutritional and Hormonal Regulation of ACS1 Gene Expression.......82
5.5   Disease State-Specific Regulation of ACS1 Gene Expression...............87
References 94

5.1   ACS1: Structure and Function

The Acyl-CoA synthetase 1 (ACS1) (EC6.2.1.3)[1] gene encodes a key gate-keeper enzyme in long-chain fatty acid metabolism. ACS1 catalyzes the activation of free long-chain (C12–18) fatty acids to long-chain acyl-CoA esters, the requisite initial step in the cellular utilization of long-chain fatty acids. Both endogenous and exogenous long-chain fatty acids must be activated by ACS1 to their CoA esters before they can be utilized for triacylglycerol synthesis or for fatty acid oxidation.

ACS1 is a member of a growing family of acyl-CoA synthetases which displays a range of substrate specificities. ACS1 was the first mammalian acyl-CoA synthetase to be purified and to be cloned. ACS1 was originally purified to homogeneity from rat liver by Tanaka et al.[2] in 1979 from both the microsomal and mitochondrial fractions. All properties of the enzymes isolated from the mitochondrial and microsomal fractions were identical and they have, therefore, been regarded as the same enzyme. The purified rat liver ACS1 enzyme was determined to have a specific activity of 26 to 29 units/mg protein at 35°C and most efficiently catalyzes the activation of saturated fatty acids with 10 to 18 carbon atoms and unsaturated fatty acids with 16 to 20 carbon atoms. The purified enzyme absolutely requires adenosine tri-phosphate (ATP), Mg^{2+}, fatty acid, and CoA for activity; *in vitro* analysis confirmed that the enzyme catalyzes the stoichiometric conversion of ATP, fatty acid, and CoA to adenosine monophosphate (AMP), inorganic phosphate (PPi), and acyl-CoA. The reaction proceeds in two steps: first, ACS reacts with the carboxyl group of the fatty acid and with ATP to form an acyl-AMP and free PPi in the presence of Mg^{2+}; then the ACS enzyme catalyzes the formation of acyl-CoA and free AMP from acyl-AMP and CoA.[3]

ACS1 has also been demonstrated to have important pharmacologic substrates. The profen (2-arylproprionate) class of non-steroidal anti-inflammatory drugs, which includes the widely used compounds ibuprofen and naproxen, are administered as racemic mixtures. The unidirectional chiral inversion from the inactive (R) to the active (S) enantiomer occurs by activation of the 2-arylpropionic acid by forming an acyl-CoA thioester intermediate, which is catalyzed by ACS1.[4,5] The subsequent epimerization and hydrolysis steps in the activation process are not enantioselective. It has been suggested that profens might alter lipid biochemistry, e.g., as a substrate which competes with long-chain fatty acids for ACS1, thereby inhibiting β-oxidation and/or lipogenesis.[6] The hypolipidemic xenobiotic carboxylic acid agents of the fibrate class of peroxisome proliferators (e.g., clofibrate, gemfibrozil, ciprofibrate, bezafibrate) are also substrates for ACS1 and are competitive as substrates with natural long-chain fatty acids.[7] It is thought that the induction of peroxisome proliferation in rodent livers by these compounds requires their activation to the acyl-CoA thioester.[7,8] Although there is some evidence for the existence of other ACS isoenzymes as activators of the profens and xenobiotic carboxylic acids,[9,10] most laboratories have found that ACS1 accounts for all activity toward these substrates.

Further progress in characterizing the structure of ACS1 was achieved by Suzuki et al.,[3] who reported the sequence of the rat ACS1 messenger RNA (mRNA), which they identified by using a polyclonal antibody raised against the purified enzyme to screen an expression recombined DNA (cDNA) library prepared from rat liver. The rat liver ACS1 mRNA encodes a polypeptide of 699 amino acids, 78 kDa in length. The protein is organized into five regions: an NH2 terminus, two luciferase-like regions, a linker connecting the luciferase regions, and a COOH terminus. Further studies in which ACS1 was overproduced in *E. coli* and purified to homogeneity have permitted rigorous characterization of the specific activity and substrate specificities of ACS1 *in vitro*: ACS1 has a specific activity of 26.2 µmol.min-1.mg-1; results confirmed that among saturated fatty acids the most preferred substrates were palmitic, myristic, pentadecanoic, and stearic acids, and the most preferred unsaturated fatty acids were palmitoleate, oleate, and linoleate.[11] Increasing concentrations of Mg^{2+} will increase the relative substrate preference of ACS1 for both oleic acid and arachidonic acid as well increasing the overall Vmax of the enzyme.[12] More recently, evidence has emerged indicating that ACS1 is the enzyme that activates the branched-chain fatty acid phytanic acid in peroxisomes where it undergoes α-oxidation to pristanic acid.[13]

Mutational analysis revealed that all five regions of ACS1 were required for functional activity; deletion of any region abolished enzyme activity.[11] The similarities among both prokaryotic and eukaryotic acyl-CoA synthetases indicate a common ancestry; and there is a common 25-amino acid consensus sequence near the COOH terminus (DGWLHTGDIGXWXPXGXLKIIDRKK) that is common to all ACS genes.[14] Site-directed mutational analysis has demonstrated that this ACS signature motif is essential for catalytic activity and appears to compose part of the fatty acid binding site since several site-specific mutations within the sequence affected substrate specificity with respect to chain length.[14] This region is thought to project into the cytoplasm, at least when ACS is associated with microsomal, peroxisomal, and outer mitochondrial membranes.[2]

Studies of the subcellular localization of ACS1 have demonstrated that it is abundant in mitochondria and microsomes and is also found in peroxisomes.[2,15,16] In heart, ACS activity is more than 80% associated with the mitochondrial fraction, wherease in adipose tissue ACS is predominantly associated with the microsomal fraction.[1] These tissue-specific differences in subcellular compartmental distribution undoubtedly reflect primary organ functions; e.g., the heart prefers fatty acid for fuel substrate, which it metabolizes by mitochondrial β-oxidation, whereas a major adipose tissue function is lipid synthesis and storage, with adipocyte lipogenic enzymes coordinately regulated and associated with microsomal membranes.

Another recent study has provided evidence for the association of ACS1 with adipocyte plasma membranes, where it has been proposed to play a role in facilitating fatty acid uptake.[17] Several studies have given evidence that ACS1 is an integral membrane protein.[15-17] The amino acid sequence predicted by the rat liver ACS1 cDNA contains a potential membrane spanning region.[3] Biochemical studies using proteases as probes for exposed domains performed by Hesler et al. delineated the transverse plane topography of ACS1 in the mitochondrial outer membrane.[16] These studies determined that ACS is a transmembrane enzyme with crucial domains on both sides of the outer membrane, and that one protease-sensitive essential domain which is involved in CoA binding is localized to the cytosolic surface of the membrane. Other studies of the peroxisomal localization of ACS1 using proteolytic enzymes also demonstrated that the enzymatic site of ACS1 is on the cytoplasmic surface in peroxisomal membranes as well.[15]

5.2   ACS1 Gene Expression: Tissue Distribution and Developmental Regulation

Tissue distribution of ACS1 has been studied by several groups. ACS1 is expressed most abundantly in tissues that are specialized to utilize long-chain fatty acids to synthesize triacylglycerol or for β-oxidization of long-chain fatty acids. The enzyme is most abundant in liver, adipose tissue, heart, and muscle,[18] but it is expressed in a wide range of tissues including lung, brain, intestine, kidney, adrenal, testis, pancreatic β-cells,[19] and probably is responsible for the ACS activity in certain blood leukocytes, e.g., neutrophils.[20] ACS1 expression in lung and small intestine is only about 10% of that in liver, heart, and epididymal adipose tissue.[3]

Developmental expression patterns have not been well characterized, but ACS1 is not expressed in proliferating or confluent 3T3-L1 preadipocytes cultured in standard medium supplemented with fetal bovine serum.[21,22] However, when adipocyte differentiation is induced by the standard differentiation treatment with dexamethasone and 1-methyl-3-isobutyl-xanthine (MIX), ACS mRNA is strongly induced by day 3 and reaches maximal abundance by day 5.[21,22] Insulin-like growth factor I (IGF-I) is essential for activation of the ACS1 gene during adipose differentiation; in fact, cDNA sequences for ACS1 were first cloned by differential screening of cDNA libraries constructed from 3T3-L1 preadipocytes and from adipocytes differentiated by treatment with IGF-I in medium containing serum which had been depleted of insulin, corticosteroids, and growth factors.[21,22]

Although preadipocytes do not synthesize large amounts of lipids as adipocytes do, the ability to activate long-chain fatty acids is still essential for other cellular functions such as membrane synthesis or protein acylation. Another enzyme that is 60% homologous to ACS1 has recently been identified in proliferating adipocytes and in intestinal epithelial cells: ACS5 consists of 683 amino acids, and it differs from ACS1 in that its substrate preference is for C16–C18 unsaturated fatty acids, although it utilizes a wide range of fatty acids similar to those that are substrates for ACS1.[23] Unlike ACS1, ACS5 mRNA expression levels do not change during adipose differentiation.[23] However, in the Caco-2 human intestinal cell line, acyl-CoA synthetase activity increased approximately 40% during the differentiation of Caco-2 cells *in vitro*, and the incorporation of palmitic acid into triacylglycerol increased nearly 2-fold.[24] It is not known which ACS isozyme is induced during Caco-2 cellular differentiation. Thus, cellular requirements for activated long-chain fatty acids apparently can be handled by one or more isoforms of acyl-CoA synthetase with overlapping ranges of substrate specificity, or one ACS may compensate for the absence of another under certain metabolic circumstances, e.g., during preadipocyte proliferation. However, in some circumstances a given cell type may contain only one form of ACS or may require a specific form for viability. Triacsin C, a compound produced by some bacteria, is an 11-carbon alkenyl chain with a terminal N-hydroxytriazene moiety and is a potent and specific inhibitor of ACS1 enzyme activity.[20] Triacsin C has been shown to inhibit the proliferation of several cultured mammalian cell lines including Vero, HeLa, and Raji (Burkitt lymphoma) cells.[25] Inhibition of ACS activity in blood neutrophils by triacsin C *in vitro* also prevented the induction of peroxide generation and degranulation.[20]

5.3   The ACS Gene Family

The family of known mammalian acyl-CoA synthetases has grown rapidly. ACS2 is expressed in different tissues than ACS1; ACS2 mRNA is most abundantly expressed in brain.[11] Its specific activity is 7.4 μmol.min-1.mg-1 (compared to 26.2 μmol.min-1.mg-1 for ACS1), but its substrate preferences are the same as ACS1.[11] ACS3 is a recently identified isozyme that preferentially utilizes laurate, myristate, arachidonate, and eicosapentaenoate.[26] ACS3 is most abundant in brain, but it is also detectable in lung, adrenal gland, kidney, and small intestine.[27] It consists of 720 amino acids and has two major forms of 79 and 80 kDA which arise from alternative translation initiation sites, i.e., the first and second in-frame AUG sites. Both have the same activities toward palmitate and myristate. The 80-kDA ACS3 isoform was found to be abundant in rat cerebrum, primarily compartmentalized to microsomes; only trace amounts of the 79-kDA polypeptide were detected.[17] ACS4 has been identified as an acyl-CoA synthetase that preferentially utilizes arachidonate and eicosapentaenoate and has a low affinity for palmitate.[28] It is 68% homologous to ACS3 and contains 670 amino acids. Although it is detectable in a wide range of tissues, it is most abundantly expressed in steroidogenic cells of the adrenal gland, corpus luteum and stromal luteinized cells of ovary, and Leydig cells of testis in the rat. The human homologs of ACS1,[28a] ACS2,[29] and ACS4[30] have been identified.

The multiplicity of mammalian long-chain acyl-CoA synthetases is mirrored by the system in the yeast *Saccharomyces cerevisiae*, which may be even more complex, or may predict additional isoforms for which mammalian homologs may eventually be characterized. Like mammalian ACS isozymes, these yeast ACS enzymes display a variable range of specificities: Faa1p prefers C12:0-C16:0; Faa2p is active toward a wider range of substrates and prefers C9:0-C13:0; Faa3p prefers C16 and C18 fatty acids with a cis-double bond at C-9-C-10.[31] A unique feature of *S. cerevisiae* long-chain acyl-CoA synthetases is that only Faa1 and Faa4 have the ability to activate imported exogenous long-chain saturated and unsaturated fatty acids.[32,33] Although functional separation of these fatty acid pools by specific mammalian ACS isozymes has been suggested, their existence has not yet been definitively demonstrated.

Genomic sequences for rat ACS1 have been partially characterized, and results revealed multiple promoters that generate several mRNA transcripts which display 5′-end heterogeneity and which are expressed in a tissue specific manner.[34] Three promoters (A, B, and C) span 20 kb of 5′-genomic sequence and each generates a unique exon 1 which is spliced to exon 2; exon 1 is 5′-UTR and the protein coding region begins and is completely contained within exon 2. Exon 1A is the major species of ACS1 exon 1 usage in rat liver. It is abundant in adipose tissue and is also found in heart. Exon 1B is detectable at low levels in liver isolated from animals treated with an agent that induces liver peroxisome proliferation, but it is not found in normal liver. Form 1C ACS mRNA is the major transcript in heart. It is expressed in low levels in normal liver but is strongly induced in liver by a peroxisome proliferating agent. The C promoter contains E1 and E3 sequences that are commonly found in the 5′-flanking regions of inducible peroxisomal β-oxidation genes.[34]

5.4   Nutritional and Hormonal Regulation of ACS1 Gene Expression

Acyl-CoA synthetase 1 was originally considered to be a constitutive enzyme because early studies found little or no change in enzyme activity measured under various nutritional conditions. Studies with pharmacologic agents sometimes produced conflicting results. The lack of conclusive evidence for physiologic regulation of ACS1 may have been due to the instability of the enzyme in membrane preparations. The isolation and characterization of ACS1 cDNA sequences have made it possible to obtain much more extensive and definitive information about the regulation of ACS1 gene expression.

Nutritional regulation of ACS1 gene expression in rat liver was demonstrated by Suzuki et al. by refeeding animals fasted for 48 h with either a high-carbohydrate or high-fat diet.[3] The fasting/carbohydrate refeeding protocol has been widely used to identify and characterize genes regulated by insulin, e.g., lipogenic genes such as fatty acid synthase.[35] Refeeding with either high carbohydrate or high fat diets produced a 7- to 8-fold increase in ACS1 mRNA levels in liver, in contrast to unchanged levels of expression in rats refed standard chow diet, which indicates that both increased exogenous fatty acid delivery and *de novo* lipogenesis induces ACS1 gene expression.[3] These results also suggested that ACS would be positively regulated by insulin. The fasting–carbohydrate refeeding protocol is widely regarded as a nutritional method for decreasing circulating insulin levels during fasting and then stimulating maximal insulin release during high carbohydrate refeeding.[35,36] Schoonjians et al. observed that fasted neonatal rats had 37-fold lower levels of liver ACS1 mRNA compared to fed rats.[36] In contrast, both groups found minimal decrease in liver ACS1 mRNA levels in fasted adult rats previously fed on standard chow. They also found that the during weaning there was a transient decrease in liver ACS1 mRNA expression, which they proposed might be due to either or both decreased caloric and decreased lipid intake. Lee et al. found modestly decreased ACS1 mRNA only in adipose tissue of starved adult rats,[37] whereas Memon et al. found dramatically decreased ACS1 mRNA expression in adipose tissue only in Syrian hamsters fasted for 24 h.[38] Furthermore, rats fasted for 24 h have been observed to have 18% decreased adipocyte mitochondrial ACS1 enzyme activity[39] and 25% decreased activity in adipocyte homogenates.[40]

The first evidence for hormonal regulation of ACS1 was developed by R. M. Bell and coworkers:[41] They incubated isolated rat fat cells with 400 µU/ml of insulin for 60 min. and measured the specific activity of ACS and found an approximately 2-fold increase in ACS1 activity, which was maximal at 2 min. and stable during the 60 min. of incubation.[41] The mechanism for this effect of insulin on ACS1 enzyme activity is still not known, but it is possible that regulation is mediated by phosphorylation/dephosphorylation since the ACS1 amino acid sequence contains several potential serine phosphorylation sites.

More recently, we have demonstrated that physiologically relevant subnanomolar concentrations of insulin rapidly and maximally induced a 2.4-fold increase in ACS1 gene transcription *in vitro* in cultured 3T3-L1 adipocytes, which does not require protein synthesis[42] (Fig. 5.1). Moreover, ACS1 was more sensitive to the stimulatory action of insulin than two other lipogenic enzyme genes, lipoprotein lipase, and stearoyl-CoA desaturase (Fig. 5.2). ACS1 mRNA expression in adipocytes is dependent on one or more hormones and/or growth factors found in serum; when adipocyte cultures are incubated in serum-free medium, ACS1 mRNA levels decrease significantly within 24 h.[42] Addition of 0.5 nM insulin for 24 h resulted in at least a 2.3-fold increase in ACS1 mRNA levels. We have also demonstrated induction of ACS1 expression by insulin *in vivo* in mesenteric adipose tissue of streptozocin-diabetic mice.[43] Previously, Saggerson and Carpenter observed that streptozocin-diabetes caused a decline in epididymal adipose ACS1 enzyme activity that was significantly restored 2 h after administration of insulin.[44]

Genes whose expression is positively regulated by insulin are very often negatively regulated by counterregulatory hormones such as corticosteroids. Fasting, the nutrient-deprived state, is associated with increased circulating levels of corticosteroids and elevated intracellular concentrations of 3',5'-cyclic monophosphate (cAMP). Therefore, we also characterized the responses of ACS1 to these agents in cultured 3T3-L1 adipocytes. The 3T3-L1 adipocyte system is widely used as an *in vitro* model of insulin action in the control of cellular processes such as lipid and carbohydrate synthesis and metabolism. Terminally differentiated 3T3-L1 adipocytes were pre-incubated in serum-free medium for 24 h followed by treatment with 7 nM dexamethasone for 24 h. Dexamethasone treatment downregulated ACS1 mRNA expression and gene transcription significantly below basal levels.[42] The effect on ACS1 gene expression of 1-methyl-3-isobutylxanthine (MIX), which raises intracellular cAMP, was also evaluated in 3T3-L1 adipocytes. Adipocyte cultures maintained in Dulbeco's Modified Eagles (DME) media supplemented with 10% fetal bovine serum display maximal levels of ACS1 gene transcription and mRNA expression. Addition of MIX ranging in concentration from 0.05 mM to 0.5 mM for 24 h inhibited both ACS1 gene transcription and mRNA expression in a dose-dependent manner; at 0.5 mM MIX the expression of ACS1 mRNA and gene transcription were almost abolished.[42]

Nutritionally replete states, e.g., carbohydrate feeding, are associated with increased circulating levels of triiodothyronine (T3).[45] We also characterized the effect of T3 on ACS1 gene expression in 3T3-L1 adipocytes. Adipocytes

(A)

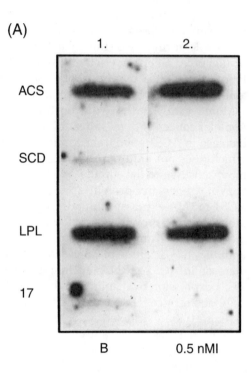

B   0.5 nMI

FIGURE 5.1

(A) Effect of physiological concentration of insulin (0.5 nM) on transcription rate of the native ACS gene in 3T3-L1 adipocytes, and comparison with LPL and SCD-1. Nuclei were isolated from fully differentiated 3T3-L1 adipocytes preincubated for 24 h in serum-free medium + 0.1% BSA (slot blot 1) followed by treatment with 0.5 nM insulin for 24 h (slot blot 2), and nuclear transcription run-assays were performed. Equal aliquots of ^{32}P-labeled transcripts (5×10^6 counts/min) were hybridized with excess denatured pBluescript, pACS, pSCD-1, pLPL, and pC.17 plasmid DNA fixed to each nitrocellulose slot blot. Vector sequences (negative control) were not detectable on the autoradiographs and thus are not shown. Autoradiographs are representative of 3 separate experiments. (B) Effect of inhibition of protein synthese on stimulation of ACS gene transcription wihout hormones. Adipocyte cultures were preincubated for 24 h without hormones. Cultures were then treated with 0.1 nmM cycloheximide (cyc) for 1 h (slot blot 1) before μM insulin was added for 45 min (slot blot 2). Vector sequences (negative control) were not detectable. Autoradiographs are representative of 4 separate experiments. (From Kansara et al., *Am. J. Physiol.*, 270, E875, 1996. With permission.)

(B)

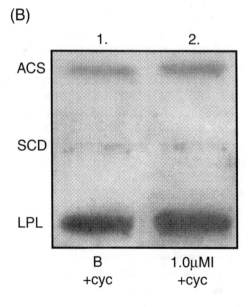

B   1.0μMI
+cyc   +cyc

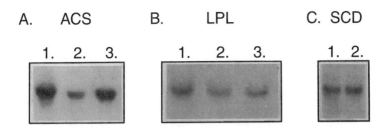

FIGURE 5.2
Effect of insulin on acyl-CoA synthetase (ACS) mRNA expression in 3T3-L1 adipocytes and comparison with lipoprotein lipase (LPL) and stearoyl-CoA desaturase (SCD-1) mRNA levels; Northern analysis. Total cellular RNA was prepared from fully differentiated 3T3-L1 adipocytes treated for 24 h with 0.5 nM insulin after 24 h of preincubation in Dulbecco's modified Eagle's medium (DMEM) supplemented with 0.1% bovine serum albunin (BSA) from control cultures maintained in standard medium, DMEM + 10% fetal bovine serum (FBS). The RNA, 10 μg per lane, was subjected to denaturing agarose gel electrophoresis. Blots were probed with ^{32}P-labeled randomly primed ACS, LPL, and SCD-1 cDNA inserts excised from recombinant pBluescript plasmids. The autoradiograph in (A) is representative of 6 independent experiments, and those in (B) and (C) of 3 independent experiments. (A) Effect of 0.5 nM insulin on ACS mRNA levels. Lane 1, DMEM + 10 FBS (F); lane 2, DMEM + 0.1% BSA (B); lane 3, DMEM + 0.1% BSA + 0.5 nM insulin (I). (B) Effect of 0.5 nM insulin on LPL mRNA abundance. Lane 1, DMEM + 10 FBS; lane 2, DMEM + 0.1% BSA; lane 3, DMEM + 0.1% BSA + 0.5 nM insulin. (C) Effect of 0.5 nM insulin on SCD-1 mRNA abundance. Lane 1, DMEM + 0.1% BSA; lane 2, DMEM + 0.1% BSA + 0.5 nM insulin. (From Kansara et al., *Am. J. Physiol.*, 270, E875, 1996. With permission.)

were pre-incubated in serum-free medium to reduce ACS1 gene expression to basal unstimulated levels. Cultures were then incubated with 10 nM T3 for 24 h. Both ACS1 gene transcription and mRNA levels were strongly induced, 2.8-fold and 2.4-fold, respectively[42] (Fig. 5.3). We have also confirmed induction of ACS1 mRNA *in vivo* in mice 24 h after injection with T3.[46]

Long-chain fatty acids are major regulators of ACS1 gene expression. Schoonjans et al. have conducted elegant studies characterizing the ACS1 gene promoter and the molecular signal transduction pathways by which ACS1 gene expression is activated by fatty acids and the related xenobiotic carboxylic acid compounds known as peroxisome proliferators and used as lipid lowering agents.[47] Treatment of cultured Fa-32 rat hepatoma cells and primary hepatocyte cultures for 48 h with 100 uM α-linolenic acid resulted in a 9-fold induction of the C isoform of ACS1 mRNA. Fatty acids are metabolized so rapidly that the maximum possible activating effects of fatty acids on ACS1 gene expression are most accurately measured by using nonmetabolized fatty acids such as α-bromopalmitate, which at 100 μM induced a 21-fold increase in ACS1 mRNA in cultured hepatocytes.[47] The peroxisome proliferator fenofibrate (500 μM) induced the C isoform of ACS1 mRNA 29-fold in cultured hepatocytes, and the A-isoform also increased.[47] Regulation of ACS1 gene expression by fibrates has also been demonstrated to occur in a tissue-specific manner. Fenofibrate induced a rapid transient approximately 7-fold increase in adipose ACS1 mRNA expression that peaked at 24 h in rats fed fenofibrate (0.5% w/w, approximately 0.5 g/kg/day) for 14 days,[48] while ACS1 expression in kidney

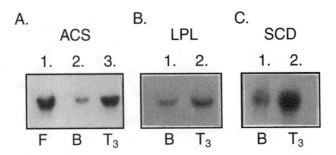

FIGURE 5.3
Effect of triiodothyronine (T_3) on ACS mRNA levels and gene transcription; comparison with LPL and SCD-1. (A) Effects of T_3 on ACS, LPL, and SCD-1 mRNA abundance. Total cellular RNA was isolated from 3T3-L1 adipocytes, treated with 10 nM T_3 for 24 h, and subjected to Northern analysis. Representative autogradiographs for ACS are the result of 3 independent experiments, for LPL, of 5 independent experiments and for SCD-1, duplicate experiments. For ACS, lane 1, DMEM + 10% FBS; lane 2, DMEM + 0.1% BSA; lane 3, DMEM 0.1% BSA + 10 nM T_3; for LPL, lane 1, DMEM +0.1% BSA; lane 2, DMEM + 0.1% BSA + nM T_3; for SCD-1, lane 1, DMEM +0.1 % BSA; lane 2, DMEM +0.1% BSA + 10 nM T_3. (B) Effects of T_3 on ACS, LPL, and SCD-1 gene transcription. Nuclei were isolated from adipocytes preincubated for 24 h in hormone-free medium (DMEM +0.1% BSA; slot blot 1) followed by addition of 10 nM T_3 for 24 h (slot blot 2). Run-on transcription assays were performed. Vector sequences (negative control) were not detectible and hence not shown. Autoradiographs are representative of 4 independent assays of ACS and LPL gene transcription and 2 assays of SCD-1 gene transcription. (From Kansara et al., *Am. J. Physiol.*, 270, E877, 1996. With permission.)

was induced less strongly (maximum 3-fold)[49] and in heart, skeletal muscle, and intestine ACS1 gene expression was relatively insensitive to fenofibrate.[48] ACS1 enzyme activity in liver and adipose tissue also increased in a dose-dependent manner that correlated with the increase in mRNA levels.[48]

After demonstrating that the induction of ACS1 gene expression by fenofibrate and fatty acids (10- and 3.5-fold, respectively) was mediated at the transcriptional level in a manner that was independent of protein synthesis, Schoonjans et al. characterized the ACS1 promoter region to identify the sequences in the ACS1 gene that mediate responsiveness of the ACS1 gene to fatty acids and fibrates.[47] Compounds that function as peroxisome proliferators in rodents are well-known to induce multiple genes involved in fatty acid metabolism, especially genes encoding enzymes for fatty acid oxidation, e.g., acyl-CoA oxidase. The basal expression of several of these enzymes is lower in mutant peroxisome proliferator-activated receptor (PPARα)-null mice.[50] The signal transduction pathway mediating the effects of peroxisome proliferators has also been well characterized. Nuclear receptor proteins of the PPARα class have been found to activate these fatty-acid oxidation genes by binding to a consensus sequence, the PPRE (peroxisome proliferator response element) that was initially identified in the acyl-CoA oxidase gene.[51] Since long-chain fatty acids must be activated by the ACS1 enzyme before they can undergo oxidation, and since ACS gene expression is stimulated by peroxisome proliferator compounds, PPARα would likely be involved in mediating ACS1 induction by fibrates and fatty acids. Schoonjans et al. prepared plasmids containing sequences corresponding to the A, B, and C promoter regions placed upstream of the CAT (chloramphenicol acyl-transferase) reporter gene and transiently co-transfected the ACS1 reporter plasmids into Fa-32 hepatocytes with a PPARα expression plasmid in the presence of 500 uM fenofibric acid.[47] Only the C promoter CAT construct was induced by the fibrate, and was therefore further characterized by progressive 5′ deletion mutagenesis to position 282 upstream of the translation initiation site. All constructs were inducible by fenofibric acid and PPARα, indicating that the PPAR response element resided within the 282 nucleotides immediately 5′ to the translation start site. Computer homology search identified a potential PPRE localized around positions −175 and −154. This sequence (<u>TGACTGATGCCCTGAAAGACCT</u>) contained 3 copies of a motif similar to the consensus steroid hormone receptor binding half-site TGACCT arranged in direct repeats. When this sequence was site-specifically mutated in reporter constructs, responsiveness to fenofibric acid was lost. This sequence was also demonstrated to be specifically bound by complexes of PPARα and its obligate heterodimeric partner, the RXR (rexinoid) orphan nuclear hormone receptor.[47] Additional experiments demonstrated that the ACS1-C promoter PPRE is a lower affinity PPRE than the acyl-CoA oxidase PPRE.

It is of significant interest that co-transfection of another PPAR isoform, PPARγ, with the ACS1 reporter plasmid in the presence of fenofibric acid yields a similar level of induction of the reporter gene. In fact, the ACS1 gene PPRE oligonucleotide bound PPARγ-RXR heterodimers as well as it bound PPARα-RXR heterodimers.[47] Many fatty acids have been shown to bind both the PPARα and PPARγ receptor isoforms, often with differences in affinity for one over the other.[52] Generally they have higher affinity for PPARα, but several have nearly as high affinity for PPARγ as for PPARα, (i.e., IC50 values of 2.2 μM or lower for PPARγ and 1.2 μM or lower for PPARα); these include dihomo-γ-linolenic, arachidonic, and eicosapentanoic acid.[52] Other fatty acids that have significantly high affinity for PPARγ (e.g., < 6.5 μM IC50) include palmitioleic, oleic, linoleic, and α-linolenic acids; all display high affinity for PPARα (IC50 < 2.0 μM). All of these fatty acids, with the possible exception of arachidonic acid, which has its own isoform (ACS4), are good substrates for ACS1, which prefers C10–16 saturated fatty acids and C16–20 unsaturated fatty acids. These fatty acids would also be likely to regulate ACS1 gene expression through either or both PPARα and PPARγ isoforms, depending on the concentration of these PPARs and their co-activators in specific tissues.

5.5 Disease State-Specific Regulation of ACS1 Gene Expression

The cytokine tumor necrosis factor-alpha (TNFα) is an important physiological mediator of feeding behavior and lipid metabolism as well as functioning as a key pro-inflammatory signaling molecule released from macrophages in response to endotoxin (lipopolysaccharide [LPS]).[53] TNFα is also produced by adipocytes and has been implicated as a mediator of insulin resistance by inhibiting insulin signaling and by acting as a lipolytic and anti-lipogenic cytokine to oppose insulin action.[54] TNFα has also been observed to de-differentiate adipocytes *in vitro*.[53,55] Studies in 3T3-L1 adipocytes demonstrated that incubation with 5 nM TNFα for 24 h resulted in 75 to 90% downregulation of ACS1 mRNA, with a similar decline in the rate of ACS1 gene transcription[22] (Fig. 5.4). Several other lipogenic enzymes are similarly regulated by TNFα, e.g., lipoprotein lipase[56] and stearoyl-CoA desaturase.[22]

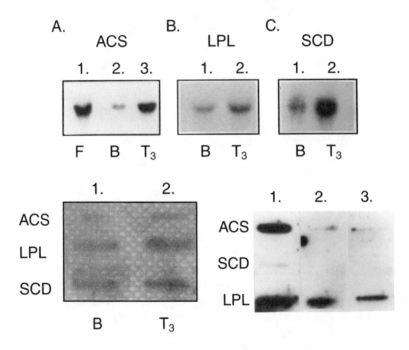

FIGURE 5.4
Effect of TNFα on the transcription rates of the ACS, SCD-1, and LPL genes. (From Weiner et al., *J. Biol. Chem.*, 266, 23527, 1991. With permission.)

The endotoxin (LPS)-stimulated release of the cytokines TNFα and interleukin-1 (IL-1) into the circulation results in increased hepatic lipid synthesis and inhibition of hepatic fatty acid oxidation.[38] Adipose triglyceride storage decreases and heart and muscle uptake of fatty acids decreases as well.[38] Studies by Memon et al. of the effects of *in vivo* administration of LPS, TNFα, and IL-1 on ACS1 mRNA expression and enzyme activity demonstrated that very low concentrations of LPS (1 to 100 µg/100 g body weight) potently inhibited ACS1 mRNA expression in liver, adipose tissue, heart, and muscle[38] (Fig. 5.5). Hepatic ACS1 mRNA was decreased by 90% 4 h after LPS administration (100 µg/100 g body weight) and was decreased in adipose tissue by

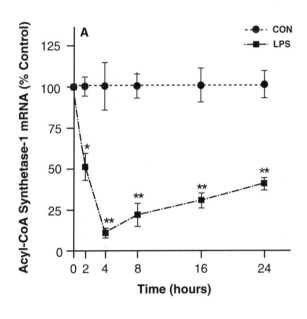

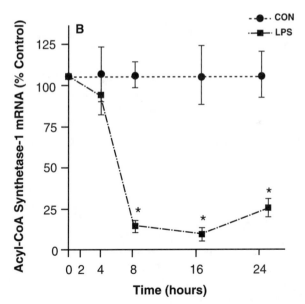

FIGURE 5.5

Time course of endotoxin (lipopolysaccharid (LPS)) effect on mRNA levels of ACS 1 in liver (A) and adipose tissue (B). Syrian hamsters were injected i.p. either with saline (controls) or LPS (100 μg/100 g body wt.), and food was removed from both groups. At the indicated times, animals were euthanized and tissues were harvest for RNA isolation. ACS 1 mRNA levels were determined by Northern blotting. Values are means SE; *n* = 5 for each time point. (A) *P < 0.002; **P < 0.001; (B) *P < 0.001. (From Memon et al., *Am. J. Physiol.*, 275, E66, 1998. With permission.)

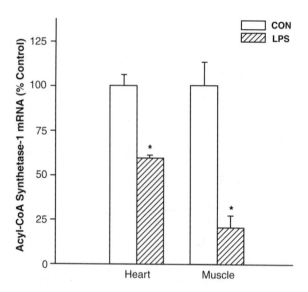

FIGURE 5.5 (CONTINUED)
(C) Effect of TNFα on the transcription rates of the ACS, SCD-1, and lipoprotein lipase genes. on ACS1 mRNA levels in heart and muscle. Syrian hamsters were injected i.p, either with saline (controls) or LPS (100 μg/100 g body wt.), and food was removed from both groups. Sixteen hours later animals were euthanized and tissues were harvested for RNA isolation. ACS1 mRNA levels were determined by Northern blotting. Values are means SE; $n = 4$ for each group. *$P < 0.001$. (From Memon et al., *Am. J. Physiol.*, 275, E68, 1998. With permission.)

the same amount after 8 h, despite little change at 4 h; 16 h after LPS treatment ACS1 mRNA was 40% decreased in heart and 80% in muscle.[38] Similar results were obtained with administration of TNFα or IL-1 alone or in combination at concentrations that have previously been shown to mimic the metabolic effects of LPS. Administration of LPS also resulted in significant decreases in ACS1 activity in heart (38%), muscle (51%), and adipose tissue (54%) (Fig. 5.5). ACS1 activity was only 20% decreased in liver homogenates despite the very large mRNA decrease; however, LPS produced a 61% decrease in mitochondrial ACS1 activity and a 55% increase in microsomal activity. This compartmental shift or differential activation of the ACS1 enzyme is consistent with the lipogenic hepatic metabolic response to LPS because triacylglycerol synthesis is predominantly localized to microsomes and fatty acid oxidation to mitochondria. These effects appeared to be mediated primarily by interleukins-1 (IL-1).

A similar differential localization of ACS1 activity has been observed in livers of *ob/ob* mice, which are a null mutant for leptin production and are widely studied as an animal model of obesity, insulin resistance, and Type II diabetes.[57] In *ob/ob* mice 34% of hepatic ACS1 enzyme activity was associated with mitochondria and 66% with microsomes, in contrast to 61% mitochondrial association and 39% with microsomes in lean control animals[55] (Fig. 5.6). Adipose ACS1 mRNA expression was also higher in *ob/ob* animals.[57] These data are consistent with the increased hepatic production of the

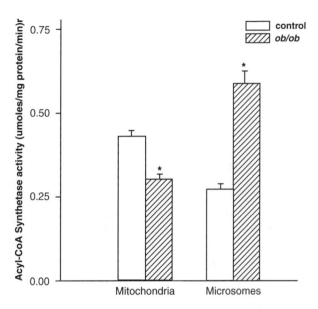

FIGURE 5.6
Mitochondrial and microsomal ACS activity in liver of *ob/ob* mice and their control litter-mates. Mice were killed and livers were obtained. Mitochondrial and microsomal fractions were isolated by differential centrifugation, and ACS activity was measured. Data are means SE, *n* = 5 for each group. *P < 0.001. (From Memon et al., *Diabetes*, 48, 126, 1999. With permission.)

triglyceride-rich lipoproteins and increased adipose lipid stores that are characteristic of the *ob/ob* phenotype.

In another leptin mutant, the hyperphagic Zucker (*fa/fa*) rat, ACS1 activity and mRNA have been shown to be 3.3- and 3.9-fold higher, respectively, in abdominal subcutaneous adipose tissue than in lean controls, and mesenteric ACS1 activity and mRNA concentrations were elevated 2.0- and 2.2-fold, respectively.[58] These data are consistent with the greatly increased adipose lipid synthesis and storage characteristic of the Zucker (*fa/fa*) rat. Liver ACS1 activity and mRNA levels were only modestly increased, but another previous study reported that in Zucker (*fa/fa*) liver acyl-CoA is much more utilized for esterification to triacylglycerol than for β-oxidation (80 vs. 20%, respectively), compared with lean control rats (40 vs. 60%).[59] These observations are also consistent with a subcompartmental shift of ACS1 enzyme activity from mitochondria to microsomes.[59] The mechanisms for the increased expression of the ACS1 gene in these animal models is unknown. Potential regulatory signals could include hyperinsulinemia, elevated free fatty-acid levels, and/or the lack of suppression by the defective leptin pathway. The Otsuka Long-Evans Tokushima Fatty (OLETF) rat is another model of obesity and insulin resistance that is characterized by visceral fat accumulation and hyperlipidemia prior to the onset of insulin resistance; at this stage, hepatic ACS activity and mRNA expression are also elevated.[60] In another hyperphagic animal model of obesity, the VMH (ventromedial hypthalamus)-lesioned rat, ACS mRNA concentrations and enzyme activity are significantly elevated in both subcutaneous and mesenteric adipose tissue, which is consistent with any or all of these pathways as well.[61]

Excessive levels of free fatty acids and/or long-chain acyl-CoAs have been suggested as a major mechanism for several abnormalities that are characteristic of Type II diabetes, e.g., impaired glucose-stimulated insulin secretion, elevated basal levels of insulin, and impaired suppression of hepatic gluconeogenesis. We tested the effect of inhibiting ACS1 enzyme activity on basal and glucose-stimulated insulin secretion in the cultured βTC3 pancreatic β-cell line in the presence or absence of elevated levels of long-chain fatty acid. Treatment with 2 mM palmitic acid for 4 days induced ACS1 mRNA expression 2.4-fold and produced a 3.5-fold increase in basal insulin secretion. Treatment with the ACS1 inhibitor Triacsin C (50 μM) for the last 24 h completely abolished the increase in insulin secretion.[62] Treatment of the cultured βTC3 cells with Triacsin C (50 μM) resulted in a 75 to 85% inhibition of glucose stimulated insulin secretion.[62] In contrast, Newgard and co-workers found no effect of a lower concentration of Triacsin C (10 μM) on glucose-stimulated insulin secretion in the INS-1 insulinoma line despite a 47% decrease in long-chain acyl-CoA and a potent inhibition of fatty acid oxidation.[19]

Inhibition of insulin secretion by long-chain acyl-CoA has been proposed to be mediated by effects on malonyl-CoA levels[63] or on intracellular Ca++ flux that triggers insulin release.[64] However, long-chain acyl-CoA levels must also be at a level permissive for budding and eventual exocytosis of insulin secretory vesicles.[65] It is possible that intracellular concentrations of long-chain acyl-CoA required to affect insulin secretion may vary among these regulatory mechanisms. The potential role and mechanisms of action of ACS1 in mediating metabolic defects in Type II diabetes that are associated with abnormal lipid metabolism clearly require more study.

The thiazolidenedione class of ligands that specifically activates PPARγ has been demonstrated to induce the expression of the ACS1 gene and several other genes involved in fatty acid uptake in adipose tissue.[49] The compound BRL49653, which is a high-affinity thiazolidinedione ligand for PPARγ, induced ACS1 mRNA 9-fold by 4 days of treatment. This coordinate induction has been proposed to lead to increased adipose fatty acid uptake, resulting in a free fatty acid "steal" from muscle that may improve insulin sensitivity and glucose metabolism.[66] However, ACS1 enzyme activity was not measured in these studies, and therefore, the ultimate effect of thiazolidinediones on ACS1 enzyme function has not been definitively characterized.

A recent study reports that the major metabolite of troglitazone, its sulfoconjugate derivative (M1) noncompetitively inhibits ACS1 enzyme in both mitochondria and microsomes, and thereby inhibits hepatic long-chain fatty acid oxidation and triglyceride synthesis.[67] Presumably the same effect would occur in adipose tissue, and if that were the case, an increase in ACS1 mRNA would be a compensatory feedback response to increased substrate accumulation due to insufficient available active enzyme. Another recent study reports that troglitazone treatment of cultured pancreatic islets from Zucker diabetic fatty rats (ZDF) resulted in decreased fatty acid esterification and increased oxidation with a 38% decrease in ACS1 mRNA.[68] The inconsistencies among these studies are puzzling and serve to emphasize the need for further study of the regulation of tissue-specific expression of the ACS1 gene and gene product, especially in metabolic disease states, in order to understand its role in the pathophysiology of diseases that are major causes of morbidity and mortality, such as Type II diabetes, obesity, and dyslipidemias.

Last, the endproducts of the reaction catalyzed by ACS1, long-chain acyl-CoA esters, have been proposed to regulate multiple cellular processes in addition to insulin secretion, as discussed by Faergeman and Knudsen in their recent review.[69] Acyl-CoA esters have been observed *in vitro* to regulate many enzymes involved in lipid and energy metabolism. However, only acetyl-CoA carboxylase is inhibited and AMP-activated kinase is stimulated by nanomolar concentrations of long-chain acyl-CoA esters. A number of important metabolic enzymes are inhibited *in vitro* by micromolar concentrations of acyl-CoA esters, e.g., HMG CoA reductase, carnitine palmitoyltransferase I, (CPT I), long chain acyl-CoA dehydrogenase, hormone-sensitive lipase, adenine nucleotide translocase (ANT), glucokinase, glucose-6-phosphatase, and pyruvate dehydrogenase. However, it is not yet known whether these effects are physiologically relevant because intracellular concentrations of long-chain acyl-CoA under normal conditions are likely to be well under 200 nM, and probably below 10 nM. It has been proposed, however, that long-chain acyl-CoAs can be donated directly from a binding protein, e.g., acyl-CoA binding protein (ACBP) and fatty acid binding protein (FABP), since it has been observed that the acyl-CoA–ACBP complex can donate acyl-CoA to the acyl-CoA:lysophopholipid acyl transferase for β-oxidation in red blood cells.

In *E. coli*, long-chain acyl-CoA esters regulate gene transcription by preventing the binding of the fadR gene product to the fadB gene promoter, a regulon by which fatty acid biosynthesis and degradation are coordinately regulated. It is not known whether long-chain acyl-CoAs regulate transcription in a similar manner in mammals, but there is evidence that long-chain acyl-CoA esters may also be involved in regulating transcription of genes for lipid biosynthesis and metabolism in yeast. Both saturated and unsaturated long-chain acyl-CoA esters have been demonstrated to inhibit the binding of T3 to its nuclear receptor in rat liver (K_i approximately 0.45 μM) more efficiently than the corresponding nonesterified fatty acids. Since T3 induces lipogenic enzymes, this action of long-chain acyl-CoA esters would provide negative feedback regulation when lipid synthesis and stores are sufficient.

Long-chain acyl-CoA esters have also been linked to the etiology of the insulin resistance that is a key feature of Type II diabetes and is also characteristic of obesity. For instance, high-fat feeding has been shown to induce insulin resistance in muscle, and there was a strong inverse correlation between glucose uptake and long-chain acyl-CoA concentrations in rat quadriceps muscle during a hyperinsulinemic glucose clamp study.[70] Furthermore, although hyperinsulinemia significantly suppressed circulating free fatty acid in these high fat-fed rats, skeletal muscle intracellular fatty acid availability was not reduced, with long-chain fatty acyl-CoA esters remaining 2.3-fold above control levels.[71] Further research is urgently needed to delineate the role of ACS1 and its acyl-CoA ester endproducts in the pathophysiology of insulin resistance. It has also been suggested that disregulated ACS1 activity may be involved in triggering some of the pro-inflammatory[20,72] and pro-oxidant[73] pathways that have been etiologically linked to the premature development of atherosclerosis in people with Type II diabetes.

In summary, we have described the structure of ACS1 as a member of an extensive gene family of long-chain acyl-CoA synthetases that are specialized by substrate specificity ranges and tissue and species distribution. The long-chain acyl-CoA synthetase 1 enzyme catalyzes an essential step in the activation of long-chain fatty acids for incorporation into lipid or for their metabolism. The expression of the ACS1 gene and its activity are tightly regulated by nutrients such as saturated and unsaturated long-chain fatty acids; by hormones such as insulin, T3, and corticosteroids; by cytokines such as TNFα; and by ligands for the peroxisome proliferator-activated receptor (PPAR) family of nuclear steroid hormone receptors.

ACS1 has been demonstrated to act not only on naturally occurring long-chain fatty acids but also on pharmacologic substrates such as xenobiotic carboxylic acids, which include the peroxisome proliferator class of fibrate lipid-lowering compounds, and the profen (2-arylproprionate) class of nonsteroidal anti-inflammatory drugs such as naproxen. The ACS1 enzyme, which is membrane bound and requires ATP, CoA, and Mg^{2+}, catalyzes a reaction that results in an endproduct, long-chain acyl-CoA, which itself is considered to have an important role in the regulation of multiple diverse cellular processes. These functions include coordinate feedback regulation of lipid, carbohydrate, and energy biosynthesis and metabolism; modulation of pancreatic insulin secretion and skeletal muscle sensitivity to insulin; and effects on atherogenic pro-inflammatory and pro-oxidant pathways.

Contrary to initial biochemical characterization of ACS1 as serving a constitutive cellular function, much evidence has emerged in recent years from studies utilizing recombinant technology that reveals an important and complex multifactorial regulatory role for acyl-CoA synthetase 1 and its long-chain acyl-CoA endproducts in health and disease.

References

1. Kornberg, A. and Pricer, Jr., W. E., Enzymatic synthesis of the coenzyme A derivatives of long chain fatty acids, *J. Biol. Chem.*, 204, 329, 1953.
2. Tanaka, T., Hosaka, K., Hoshimaru, M., and Numa, S., Purification and properties of long-chain acyl-Coenzyme A synthetase from rat liver, *Eur. J. Biochem.*, 98, 165, 1979.

3. Suzuki, H., Kawarabayasi, Y., Kondo, J., Abe, T., Nishikawa, K., Kimura, S., Hashimoto, T., and Yamamoto, T., Structure and regulation of rat long-chain acyl-CoA synthetase, *J. Biol. Chem.*, 265, 8681, 1990.
4. Knights, K. M., Drew, R., and Meffin, P. J., Enantiospecific formation of fenoprofen coenzyme A thioester *in vitro*, *Biochem. Pharmacol.*, 37, 3539, 1988.
5. Brugger, R., Garcia, A. B., Reichel, C., Waibel, R., Menzel, S., Brune, K., and Geisslinger, G., Isolation and characterization of rat liver microsomal R-ibuprofenoyl-CoA synthetase, *Biochem. Pharmacol.*, 52, 1007, 1996.
6. Mayer, J. M., Roy-De Vos, M., Audergon, C., Testa, B., and Etter, J. C., Interactions of anti-inflammatory 2-arylpropionates (profens) with the metabolism of fatty acids: *in vitro* studies, *Int. J. Tiss. Reac.*, 16, 59, 1994.
7. Amigo, L., McElroy, M. C., Morales, M. N., and Bronfman, M., Subcellular distribution and characteristics of ciprofibroyl-CoA synthetase in rat liver, *Biochem. J.*, 284, 283, 1992.
8. Tomaszewski, K. E., and Melnick, R.L., *In vitro* evidence for involvement of Co-A thioesters in peroxisome proliferation and hypolipidaemia, *Biochim. Biophys. Acta*, 1120, 118, 1994.
9. Roberts, B. J., MacLeod, J. K., Singh, I., and Knights, K. M., Kinetic characteristics of rat liver peroxisomal nafenopin-CoA ligase, *Biochem. Pharmacol.*, 49, 1335, 1995.
10. Knights, K. M. and Roberts, B. J., Xenobiotic acyl-CoA formation: evidence of kinetically distinct hepatic microsomal long-chain fatty acid and nafenopin-CoA ligases, *Chem. Biol. Interact.*, 90, 215, 1994.
11. Iijima, H., Fujino, T., Minekura, H., Suzuki, H., Kang, M. J., and Yamamoto, T., Biochemical studies of two rat acyl-CoA synthetases, ACS1 and ACS2, *Eur. J. Biochem.*, 242, 186, 1996.
12. Saunders, C., Voigt, J. M., and Weis, M. T., Evidence for a single non-arachidonic acid-specific fatty acyl-CoA synthetase in heart which is regulated by Mg^{2+}, *Biochem. J.*, 313, 849, 1996.
13. Watkins, P. A., Howard, A. E., Gould, S. J., Avigan, J., and Mihalik, S. J., Phytanic acid activation in rat liver peroxisomes is catalyzed by long-chain acyl-CoA synthetase, *J. Lipid Res.*, 37, 2288, 1996.
14. Black, P. N., Zhang, Q., Weimar, J. D., and DiRusso, C. C., Mutational analysis of a fatty acyl-coenzyme A synthetase signature motif identifies seven amino acid residues that modulate fatty acid substrate specificity, *J. Biol. Chem.*, 272, 4896, 1997.
15. Lazo, O., Contreras, M., and Singh, I., Topographical localization of peroxisomal acyl CoA ligases: differential localization of palmitoyl-CoA and lignoceroyl-CoA ligases, *Biochemistry*, 29, 3981, 1990.
16. Hesler, C. B., Olymbios, C., and Haldar, D., Transverse-plane topography of long-chainacyl-CoA synthetase in the mitochondrial outer membrane, *J. Biol. Chem.*, 265, 6600, 1990.
17. Gargiulo, C. E., Stuhlsatz-Krouper, S. M., and Schaffer, J. E., Localization of adipocyte long-chain fatty acyl-CoA synthetase at the plasma membrane, *J. Lipid Res.*, 40, 881, 1999.
18. Brindley, D. N., Metabolism of triacylglycerols, in *Biochemistry of Lipids and Membranes*, Vance, D. E. and Vance, J. E., Eds., Menlo Park, California, 1985, chap. 7.
19. Antinozzi, P.A., Segall, L., Prentki, M., McGarry, J. D., and Newgard, C. B., Molecular or pharmacologic perturbation of the link between glucose and lipid metabolism is without effect on glucose-stimulated insulin secretion, *J. Biol. Chem.*, 273, 16146, 1998.

20. Korchak, H. M., Kane, L. H., Rossi, M. W., and Corkey, B. E., Long chain acyl coenzyme A and signaling in neutrophils; an inhibitor of acyl coenzyme A synthetase, triacsin C, inhibits superoxide anion generation and degranulation by human neutrophils, *J. Biol. Chem.,* 269, 30281, 1994.

21. Smith, P. J., Wise, L. S., Berkowitz, R., Wan, C., and Rubin, C. S., Insulin-like growth factor-I is an essential regulator of the differentiation of 3T3-L1 adipocytes, *J. Biol. Chem.,* 263, 9402, 1988.

22. Weiner, F. R., Smith, P. J., Wertheimer, S., and Rubin, C. S., Regulation of gene expression by insulin and tumor necrosis factor-α in 3T3-L1 cells; modulation of the transcription of genes encoding acyl-CoA synthetase and stearoyl-CoA desaturase-1, *J. Biol. Chem.,* 266, 23525, 1991.

23. Oikawa, E., Iijama H., Suzuki, T., Sasano, H., Kamatake, A., Nagura, H., Kang, M. J., Fujino, T., Suzuki, H., and Yamamoto, T. T., A novel acyl-CoA synthetase, ACS5, is expressed in intestinal epithelial cells and proliferating preadipocytes, *J. Biochem.,* 124, 679, 1998.

24. Trotter, P. J. and Storch, J., Fatty acid esterification during differentiation of the human intestinal cell line Caco-2, *J. Biol. Chem.,* 268, 10017, 1993.

25. Tomoda, H., Igarashi, K., Cyong, J.-C., and Omura, S., Evidence for an essential role of long chain acyl-CoA synthetase in animal cell proliferation, *J. Biol. Chem.,* 266, 4214, 1991.

26. Fujino, T., Man-Jong, K., Minekura, H., Suzuki, H., and Yamamoto, T. T., Alternative translation initiation generates acyl-CoA synthetase 3 isoforms with heterogeneous amino termini, *J. Biochem.,* 122, 212, 1997.

27. Fujino, T., Kang, M. J., Suzuki, H., Iijima, H., and Yamamoto, T., Molecular characterization and expression of rat acyl-CoA synthetase 3, *J. Biol. Chem.,* 271, 16748, 1996.

28. Kang, M. J., Fujino, T., Sasano, H., Minekura, H., Yabuki, N., Nagura, H., Iijima, H., and Yamamoto, T. T., A novel arachidonate-preferring acyl-CoA synthetase is present in steroidogenic cells of the rat adrenal, ovary, and testis, *Proc. Natl. Acad. Sci. USA,* 94, 2880, 1997.

28a. Ghosh, B., Barbosa, E., and Singh, I., Molecular cloning and sequencing of human palmitoyl-CoA ligase and its tissue specific expression, *Mol. Cell. Biochem.,* 151, 77, 1995.

29. Cantu, E. S., Sprinkle, T. J., Ghosh, B., and Singh, I., The human palmitoyl-CoA ligase (FACL2) gene maps to the chromosome 4q34-q35 region by fluorescence in situ hybridization (FISH) and somatic cell hybrid panels, *Genomics,* 28, 600, 1995.

30. Piccini, M., Vitelli, F., Bruttini, M., Pober, B. R., Jonsson, J. J., Villanova, M., Zollo, M., Borsani, G., Ballabio, A., and Renieri, A., FACL4, a new gene encoding long-chain acyl-CoAsynthetase 4, is deleted in a family with Alport syndrome, elliptocytosis, and mental retardation, *Genomics,* 47, 350, 1998.

31. Knoll, L. J., Johnson, D. R., and Gordon, J. I., Biochemical studies of three Saccharomyces cerevisiae acyl-CoA synthetases, Faa1p, Faa2p, and Faa3p, *J. Biol. Chem.,* 269, 16348, 1994.

32. DiRusso, C. C. and Black, P. N., Long-chain fatty acid transport in bacteria and yeast. Paradigms for defining the mechanism underlying this protein-mediated process, *Mol. Cell. Biochem.,* 192, 41, 1999.

33. Choi, J. Y. and Martin, C. E., The Saccharomyces cerevisiae FAT1 gene encodes an acyl-CoA synthetase that is required for maintenance of very long chain fatty acid levels, *J. Biol. Chem.,* 274, 4671, 1999.

34. Suzuki, H., Watanabe, M., Fujino, T., and Yamamoto, T., Multiple promoters in rat acyl-CoA synthetase gene mediate differential expression of multiple transcripts with 5'-end heterogeneity, *J. Biol. Chem.*, 270, 9676, 1995.

35. Paulauskis, J. D. and Sul, H. S., Cloning and expression of mouse fatty acid synthase and other specific mRNAs; developmental and hormonal regulation in 3T3-l1 cells, *J. Biol. Chem.*, 263, 7049, 1988.

36. Schoonjans, K., Staels, B., Grimaldi, P., and Auwerx, J., Acyl-CoA synthetase mRNA expression is controlled by fibric-acid derivatives, feeding and liver proliferation, *Eur. J. Biochem.*, 216, 615, 1993.

37. Lee, J.-J., Smith, P. J., and Fried, S .K., Mechanisms of decreased lipoprotein lipase activity in adipocytes of starved rats depend on duration of starvation, *J. Nutr.*, 128, 940, 1998.

38. Memon, R. A., Fuller, J., Moser, A. H., Smith, P. J., Feingold, K. R., and Grunfeld, C., *In vivo* regulation of acyl-CoA synthetase mRNA and activity by endotoxin and cytokines, *Am. J. Physiol.*, 275 (Endocrinol. Metab. 38), E64, 1998.

39. Moore, K. H., Dandurand, D. M., and Kiechle, F. L., Fasting induced alterations in mitochondrial palmitoyl-CoA metabolism may inhibit adipocyte pyruvate dehydrogenase activity, Int. *J. Biochem.*, 24, 809, 1992.

40. Lawson, N., Pollard, A. D., Jennings, R. J., Gurr, M. I., and Brindley, D. N., The activities of lipoprotein lipase and of enzymes involved in triacylglycerol synthesis in rat adipose tissue, *Biochem. J.*, 200, 285, 1981.

41. Jason, C. J., Polokoff, M. A., and Bell, R. M., Triacylglycerol synthesis in isolated fat cells; an effect of insulin on microsomal fatty acid coenzyme A ligase activity, *J. Biol. Chem.*, 251, 1488, 1976.

42. Kansara, M. S., Mehra, A. K., Von Hagen, J., Kabotyansky, E., and Smith, P. J., Physiological concentrations of insulin and T3 stimulate 3T3-L1 adipocyte acyl-CoA synthetase gene transcription, *Am. J. Physiol.*, 270 (Endocrinol. Metab. 33), E873, 1996.

43. Kansara, M., Von Hagen, J., and Smith, P. J., Tissue specific regulation of acyl-CoA synthetase gene expression by insulin *in vivo, Diabetes*, 45, (Suppl. 2), 226A, 1996.

44. Saggerson, E.D. and Carpenter, C.A., Effects of streptozotocin-diabetes and insulin administration *in vivo* or *in vitro* on the activities of five enzymes in the adipose-tissue triacylglycerol-synthesis pathway, *Biochem. J.*, 243, 289, 1987.

45. Moustaïd, N. and Sul, H. S., Regulation of expression of the fatty acid synthase gene in 3T3-L1 cells by differentiation and triiodothyronine, *J. Biol. Chem.*, 266, 18550, 1991.

46. Kansara, M., Von Hagen, J., and Smith, P. J., Tissue specific regulation of acyl-CoA synthetase gene expression by triiodothyronine *in vivo, Tenth Int. Congr. Endocrinol.*, Vol. 1, 426, 1996.

47. Schoonjans, K., Watanabe, M., Suzuki, H., Mahfoudi, A., Krey, G., Wahli, W., Grimaldi, P., Staels, B., Yamamoto, T., and Auwerx, J., Induction of the acyl-Coenzyme A synthetase gene by fibrates and fatty acids is mediated by a peroxisome proliferator response element in the C promoter, *J. Biol. Chem.*, 270, 19269, 1995.

48. Schoonjians, K., Staels, B., Grimaldi, P., and Auwerx, J., Acyl-CoA synthetase mRNA is controlled by fibric-acid derivatives, feeding and liver proliferation, *Eur. J. Biochem.*, 216, 615, 1993.

49. Martin, G., Schoonjans, K., Lefebvre, A.-M., Staels, B., and Auwerx, J., Coordinate regulation of the expression of the fatty acid transport protein and acyl-CoA synthetase genes by PPARα and PPARγ activators, *J. Biol. Chem.,* 272, 28210, 1997.

50. Aoyama, T., Peters, J. M., Iritani, N., Nakajima, T., Furihata, K., Hashimoto, T., and Gonzalez, F. J., Altered constitutive expression of fatty acid-metabolizing enzymes in mice lacking the peroxisome proliferator-activated receptor alpha (PPARalpha), *J. Biol. Chem.,* 273, 5678, 1998.

51. Krey, G., Braissant, O., L'Horset, F., Kalkhoven, E., Perroud, M., Parker, M. G., and Wahli, W., Fatty acids, eicosonoids, and hypolipidemic agents identified as ligands of peroxisome proliferator-activated receptors by coactivator-dependent receptor ligand assay, *Mol. Endocrinol.,* 11, 779, 1997.

52. Xu, E. E., Lambert, M. H., Montana, V. G., Parks, D. J., Blanchard S. G., Brown, P. J., Sternback, D. D., Lehmann, J. M., Wisely, G. B., Willson, T. M., Kliewer, S. A., and Miburn, M. V., Molecular recognition of fatty acids by peroxisome proliferator-activated receptors, *Mol. Cell,* 3, 397, 1999.

53. Torti, F. M., Dieckmann, B., Cerami, A., and Ringold, G., A macrophage factor inhibits adipocyte gene expression: an *in vitro* model of cachexia, *Science,* 229, 867, 1985.

54. Hotamisligil, G. S. and Spiegelman, B. M., Tumor necrosis factor α: a key component of the obesity-diabetes link, *Diabetes,* 43, 1271, 1994.

55. Beutler, B. and Cerami, A., Cachectin and tumor necrosis factor as two sides of the same biological coin, *Nature,* 320, 584, 1986.

56. Zechner, R., Newman, T. C., Sherry, B., Cerami, A., and Breslow, I. L., Recombinant human cachectin/tumor necrosis factor but not interleuken-1 alpha downregulates lipoprotein lipase gene expression at the transcriptional level in mouse 3T3-L1 adipocytes, *Mol. Cell. Biol.,* 8, 2394, 1988.

57. Memon, R. A., Fuller, J., Moser, A. H., Smith, P. J., Grunfeld, C., and Feingold, K. R., Regulation of putative fatty acid transporters and acyl-CoA synthetase in liver and adipose tissue in ob/ob mice, *Diabetes,* 48, 121, 1999.

58. Shimomura, I., Tokunaga, K., Jiao, S., Funahashi, T., Keno, Y., Kobatake, T., Kotani, K., Suzuki, H., Yamamoto, T., Tarui, S., and Matsuzawa, Y., Marked enhancement of acyl-CoA synthetase activity and mRNA, paralleled to lipoprotein lipase mRNA, in adipose tissues of Zucker obese rats (fa/fa), *Biochim. Biophys. Acta.,* 1124, 112, 1992.

59. Azain, M. J., Fukuda, N., Chao, F. F., Yamamota, M., and Ontko, J., A., Contribution of fatty acid and sterol synthesis to triglyceride and cholesterol secretion by the perfused rat liver in genetic hyperlipemia and obesity, *J. Biol. Chem.,* 260, 174, 1985.

60. Kuriyama, H., Yamashita, S., Shimomura, I., Funahashi, T., Ishigami, M., Aragane, K., Miyaoka, K., Nakamura, T., Takemura, K., Man, Z., Toide, K., Nakayama, N., Fukuda, Y., Lin, M. C., Wetterau, J. R., and Matsuzawa, Y., Enhanced expression of hepatic acyl-coenzyme A synthetase and microsomal triglyceride transfer protein messenger RNAs in the obese and hypertriglycer-idemic rat with visceral fat accumulation, *Hepatology,* 27, 557, 1998.

61. Shimomura, I., Takahashi, M., Tokunaga, K., Keno, Y., Nakamura, T., Yamashita, S., Takemura, K., Yamamoto, T., Funahashi, T., and Matsuzawa, J., Rapid enhancement of acyl-CoA synthetase, LPL, and GLUT-4 mRNAs in adipose tissue of VMH rats, *Am. J. Physiol.,* 270 (*Endocrinol. Metab. 33*), E995, 1996.

62. Von Hagen, J., Kansara, M., and Smith, P.J., The role of acyl-CoA synthetase and fatty acids in the regulation of insulin secretion, *Diabetes*, 46, (Suppl. 1), Abstr. 0315, 80A, 1997.

63. Prentki, M., Vischer, S., Glennon, M. C., Regazzi, R.l., Deeney, J. T., and Corkey, B. E., Malonyl-CoA and long chain acyl-CoA esters as metabolic coupling factors in nutrient-induced insulin secretion, *J. Biol. Chem.*, 267, 5802, 1992.

64. Deeney, J. T., Tornheim, K., Korchak, H. M., Prentki, M., and Corkey, B. E., Acyl-CoA esters modulate intracellular Ca⁺⁺ handling by permeabilized clonal pancreatic β-cells, *J. Biol. Chem.*, 267, 19840, 1992.

65. Glick, B. S. and Rothman, J. E., Possible role for fatty acyl-Coenzyme A in intracellular transport, *Nature*, 326, 309, 1987.

66. Martin, G., Schoonjans, K., Staels, B., and Auwerx, J., PPARγ activators improve glucose homeostasis by stimulating fatty acid uptake in the adipocytes, *Atherosclerosis*, 137, Suppl. S75, 1998.

67. Fulgencio, J.-P., Kohl, C., Girard, J., and Pegorier, J.-P., Troglitazone inhibits fatty acid oxidation and esterification, and gluconeogenesis in isolated hepatocytes from starved rats, *Diabetes*, 45, 1556, 1996.

68. Shimabukuro, M., Zhou, Y.T., Lee, Y., and Unger, R.H., Troglitazone lowers islet fat and restores beta cell function of Zucker diabetic fatty rats, *J. Biol. Chem.*, 273, 3547, 1998.

69. Faergeman, N.J. and Knudsen, J., Role of long-chain acyl-CoA esters in the regulation of metabolism and in cell signalling, *Biochem. J.*, 323, 1, 1997.

70. Oakes, N. D., Bell., K. S., Furler, S. M., Camilleri, S., Saha, A. K., Ruderman, N. B., Chisholm, D. J., and Kraegen, E. W., Diet-induced muscle insulin resistance in rats is ameliorated by acute dietary lipid withdrawal or a single bout of exercise: parallel relationship between insulin stimulation of glucose uptake and suppression of long-chain fatty acyl-CoA, *Diabetes*, 46, 2022, 1997.

71. Oakes, N. D., Cooney, G. J., Camilleri, S., Chisholm, D. J., and Kraegen, E. W., Mechanisms of liver and muscle insulin resistance induced by chronic high-fat feeding, *Diabetes*, 46, 1768, 1997.

72. Namatame, I., Tomoda, H., Arai, H., Inoue, K., and Omura, S., Complete inhibition of mouse macrophage-derived foam cell formation by triacsin C, *J. Biochem. Tokyo*, 125, 319, 1999.

73. Bakker, S. J., Ijzerman, R. G., Teerlink, T., Westerhoff, H. V., Gans, R. O., and Heine, R. J., Cytosolic triglycerides and oxidative stress in central obesity: the missing link between excessive atherosclerosis, endothelial dysfunction, and failure? *Atherosclerosis*, 148, 17, 2000.

6

Nutritional Regulation of Fatty Acid Transport Protein Expression

Judith Storch and Fiona M. Herr

CONTENTS

6.1 Introduction 102
6.2 Mechanism of Fatty Acid Flux across the Plasma Membrane 102
    6.2.1 FABPpm 103
    6.2.2 Fatty Acid Translocase (FAT/CD36) 104
    6.2.3 Fatty Acid Transport Protein (FATP) 105
    6.2.4 Other Putative Transporters: Caveolin-1 and FA
            Receptor (FAR) 105
6.3 Intracellular Fatty Acid-Binding Proteins 106
6.4 Nutritional Regulation of Fatty Acid Transport Proteins 107
    6.4.1 Regulation of Membrane-Associated Fatty Acid
            Transporter Expression 107
    6.4.2 Regulation of Intracellular FABP Expression 108
            6.4.2.1 LFABP 109
            6.4.2.2 IFABP 110
            6.4.2.3 AFABP 111
            6.4.2.4 HFABP 111
            6.4.2.5 Other FABPs 112
6.5 Molecular Mechanism of Fatty Acid Regulation
     of Transport Proteins 113
    6.5.1 Peroxisome Proliferator-Activated Receptors 113
    6.5.2 Mode of Action — Ligand Binding and Cofactor Proteins 115
    6.5.3 The Effect of PPARs on Fatty Acid Transport Proteins 116
            6.5.3.1 Membrane Fatty Acid Transport Proteins 116
            6.5.3.2 Intracellular FABPs 117
6.6 Concluding remarks 118
References 120

0-8493-2216-2/01/$0.00+$1.50

6.1 Introduction

The typical Western diet contains abundant triacylglycerol (TG), with average daily intakes of 90 to 100 gm.[1] The gastrointestinal tract efficiently digests the TG and absorbs the high levels of fatty acids produced, making fatty acid flux of great importance in the absorptive enterocyte. Several other cell types are also notable for high levels of fatty acid metabolism and transport, including the hepatocyte, muscle cell, and adipocyte. Virtually all other cell types, though not necessarily considered to be particularly active in lipid metabolism, must also process fatty acids for energy production, membrane phospholipid synthesis, and intracellular signal transduction. Thus, fatty acid transport into cells and within cells is a critical process that contributes to the utilization and function of this important nutrient. Perhaps not surprisingly, the intake of dietary lipid has been shown, in turn, to influence the expression of proteins involved in fatty acid transport.

Cellular proteins that are designated as fatty acid transport proteins consist of two types: transmembrane proteins and intracellular cytoplasmic proteins. It is generally thought that the former are involved in uptake and efflux of fatty acids across the plasma membrane (and, perhaps, organellar membranes, although little information in this regard is available), while the latter are involved in intracellular fatty acid transport and targeting. In this chapter, an overview of the basic biochemical and functional properties of the fatty acid transport proteins will be presented, followed by discussion of the nutritional regulation of expression of these two classes of proteins.

6.2 Mechanism of Fatty Acid Flux across the Plasma Membrane

The diverse metabolic roles of long-chain fatty acids in the maintenance of intracellular energy stores, post-translational modification of proteins, and the synthesis of membrane lipids have led to careful examination of how these lipophilic compounds traverse the plasma membrane of cells. Historically, two distinct mechanisms have been proposed: a diffusion-driven flux across the membrane and protein-mediated transport mechanisms. The diffusion mechanism holds that unbound unesterified fatty acids bind to the outer leaflet of the membrane bilayer, become protonated, and then flip to the inner leaflet.[2,3] However, kinetic evidence has suggested that a diffusional mechanism may be too slow to accommodate the high cellular requirements for FA,[4] and numerous other studies support a protein-mediated uptake process. For example, fatty acid uptake to cells has been shown to be rapid, temperature sensitive, and saturable, and can be inhibited by FA analogs,

TABLE 6.1

Fatty Acid Transport Proteins

	Tissue Distribution	**Size**	**Ref.**
Membrane Associated			
FABPpm	Liver, heart, adipose, intestine	40 kDa	10
FAT/CD36	Heart, skeletal muscle, adipose, intestine	88 kDa	15
FATP	Adipose, brain, skeletal muscle, heart	63 kDa	9
Caveolin-1	3T3-LI adipocytes, fibroblasts, endothelial, etc.	22 kDa	30
FAR	Heart	56 kDa	32
Intracellular			
LFABP	Liver, small intestine	14 kDa	150, 151
IFABP	Small intestine	15 kDa	152
HFABP	Muscle, brain, mammary gland, kidney, adrenals, ovaries, testis	15 kDa	153
AFABP	Adipose, monocytes	15 kDa	154, 155
BFABP	Central nervous system	15 kDa	40, 156
KFABP	Epidermis, adipose, mammary, testis	15 kDa	41, 157
MFABP (myelin P2)	Central and peripheral nerve myelin	15 kDa	158

blocked by specific antibodies, and inhibited by proteases.[5–9] These investigations have led to the identification of a series of membrane-associated proteins thought to be involved in FA transport across the plasma membrane (Table 6.1). It is currently thought that these high-affinity protein-mediated transport systems work in conjunction with a low-affinity diffusional process to affect fatty acid influx and/or efflux across the plasma membrane of cells. The following discussions will focus on FA transporters identified in mammalian systems.

6.2.1 FABPpm

Stremmel and Berk identified the first membrane-associated fatty acid carrier protein from a solubilized rat hepatocyte plasma membrane preparation using substrate affinity chromatography.[6] A 40-kDa protein was purified based on its specific binding to an oleate-agarose column and was named FABPpm. This protein was also shown to reversibly bind a variety of unesterified long-chain FA. Interestingly, FABPpm was determined to be a membrane-bound form of the mitochondrial enzyme, aspartate aminotransferase (mAspAT).[10] FABPpm is expressed on the plasma membrane of a variety of tissues, predominantly the liver, heart, adipose, and intestine.[10,11]

Other than ligand-binding properties, direct evidence for the involvement of FABPpm in cellular fatty acid transport has been obtained via a series of antibody studies. Incubation of hepatocytes, myocytes, or adipocytes with anti-FABPpm (or anti-mAspAT) led to approximately 50% reductions in [^{3}H]-FA uptake into these cells.[10–12] In addition, expression of FABPpm in both *Xenopus laevis* oocytes and 3T3 fibroblast cells corresponded with a marked increase in FA uptake rates for these cell systems.[11,13] Transfection of the fibroblasts resulted in a saturable, high-affinity uptake process which was inhibited by anti-FABPpm antibodies, thus demonstrating that FABPpm plays some direct role in modulating FA flux across the plasma membrane of 3T3 fibroblasts.[11,14]

6.2.2 Fatty Acid Translocase (FAT/CD36)

Abumrad and colleagues employed a series of reactive sulfo-*N*-succinimidyl fatty acid derivatives in identifying an 88-kDa protein involved in FA uptake in rat adipocytes, designated as fatty acid translocase (FAT).[8] The radiolabeled protein was purified and its cDNA isolated from a rat adipocyte library, and was found to be the rat homolog of human CD36, a thrombospondin-binding protein first isolated in 1989.[15] FAT/CD36 is a large glycoprotein with two putative transmembrane domains. It can bind native long-chain FA with high affinity but does not bind medium-chain FA, in accordance with the specificity of FA transport in adipocytes.[16,17] Inspection of the amino acid sequence has highlighted a region of similarity between a 150 residue extracellular domain of FAT/CD36 and the fatty acid-binding domain of the intracellular heart fatty acid-binding protein (HFABP, see below), suggesting a potential region for FA binding to FAT.[16,18] FAT mRNA expression is associated with cells that have a high metabolic capacity for long-chain FA utilization, with levels highest in adipose, cardiac muscle, skeletal muscle, intestine, and spleen.[15] In adipocytes, FAT/CD36 expression is induced during adipocyte differentiation.[19]

A direct role for FAT/CD36 in FA transport across the membrane has been supported by several different experimental approaches. For example, anti-CD36 antibodies inhibit the uptake of arachidonic acid into platelets.[20] In addition, transfection of Ob17PY fibroblasts, which lack CD36, with the gene for CD36 results in an increased rate of long-chain FA uptake and subsequent metabolism of the FA. The magnitude of the increased uptake correlates with levels of expressed CD36 and the uptake is a saturable, high-affinity process.[21] Diminished levels of CD36, secondary to antisense expression, resulted in diminished FA uptake rates,[22] and patients with a congenital absence of CD36 displayed defective FA uptake into the heart.[23] Recently, mice lacking expression of CD36 were shown to have decreased fatty acid uptake into adipocytes, and myocytes isolated from the knockouts were found to have decreased oleate transport rates at low FA:albumin ratios.[24] These studies provide the most direct evidence thus far that FAT/CD36 plays an integral role in cellular fatty acid flux and metabolism.

6.2.3   Fatty Acid Transport Protein (FATP)

A third putative FA transport protein was identified from adipocytes by Schaffer and Lodish using expression cloning.[9] A cDNA library constructed from 3T3-L1 adipocytes was transfected into COS7 fibroblast cells, which were then screened for their ability to incorporate a fluorescently labeled fatty acid analog by fluorescence-activated sorting. This approach led to the identification of a cDNA that encodes a 63-kDa protein that was named fatty acid transport protein (FATP).[9] Hydropathy modeling of the predicted amino acid sequence of FATP identified 4 to 6 potential transmembrane regions [9] and immunohistochemistry has demonstrated that the protein is localized to the cell surface.[9,25] Recent evidence suggests that FATP represents a large evolutionarily conserved gene family found to be functional long-chain fatty acid transporters in such diverse organisms such as *Fugu rubripes*, *Drosophila melanogster*, and *Caenorhabditis elegans*.[26] In humans there are at least six FATP homologue genes that demonstrate tissue specific expression.[26] FATP contains a highly conserved ATP-binding and hydrolysis domain that is essential for its FA transport activity,[27] and displays 40% identity with very-long chain acyl-CoA synthetase.[19,27] Studies wherein its yeast homolog, FAT1, was disrupted, demonstrated that FAT1 has cellular acyl-CoA synthetase activity against very-long and long-chain fatty acids and its disruption results in the accumulation of very-long chain fatty acids.[28] Still, the role of coenzyme activation in FATP-mediated fatty acid transport across the membrane is not fully understood. FATP mRNA levels are highest in tissues with high FA requirements: brain, adipose tissue, skeletal and heart muscle.[9] Specific involvement of FATP in FA transport has been supported by studies on stably transfected fibroblast cell lines, in which a marked increase in the specific and saturable uptake of fluorescently labeled long-chain FA[9] was observed, indicating a role for FATP in FA flux.

6.2.4   Other Putative Transporters: Caveolin-1 and FA Receptor (FAR)

Two additional putative transporters have been identified but not well characterized. First, in studies of 3T3-L1 preadipocyte differentiation, Trigatti et al.[7] and Gerber et al.[29] used a photoreactive fatty acid analog to identify proteins with high affinities for lipids. A 22-kDa plasma membrane protein was labeled by 11-m-diazirinophenoxy[11-^{3}H]undecanoate in a specific and saturable manner. Subsequent immunohistochemical studies demonstrated that this protein was caveolin-1,[30] a structural component of membrane caveolae, involved in receptor-mediated transport.[31] Second, a 56-kDa protein which exhibits high affinity for binding to fatty acids has been purified from rat cardiac sarcolemmal membranes and has been named fatty acid receptor (FAR). Initial biochemical characterization of FAR revealed it to be a single, amphiphilic polypeptide with high-affinity binding for long-chain FA.[32,33] Additional information on this protein is not available but there is some speculation in the literature that it may, in fact, be FATP.[19] Functional involvement of caveolin-1 and FAR in cellular fatty acid flux is currently uncertain.

6.3   Intracellular Fatty Acid-Binding Proteins

The intracellular fatty acid-binding proteins (FABPs) are 14 to 15-kDa proteins that were discovered in the early 1970s as abundant cytoplasmic proteins that bind long-chain fatty acids *in vitro*.[34,35] (See Table 6.1.) FABPs from intestine (IFABP),[34,36] liver (LFABP),[34,35] and heart (HFABP)[37] were the first of the family to be well characterized. A specific FABP has also been purified from another lipid-active tissue, adipose tissue (AFABP),[38] as well as from several other tissues such as nervous system and skin (BFABP, KFABP).[39–41] It is now known that the FABPs encompass a growing list of related proteins, some of which bind small hydrophobic ligands other than, or in addition to, fatty acids.[42–44] Information on their tissue distribution, ligand-binding affinities and specificities, and developmental regulation[18,42,45,46] has led to the rather broad hypothesis that the FABPs are important in intracellular lipid metabolism and transport. The function of the FABPs in intracellular transport and targeting has recently been reviewed.[47]

Equilibrium binding analyses and structural studies clearly demonstrate that most FABPs bind long-chain fatty acids (C_{16}–C_{20}) with high affinity and a molar stoichiometry of 1:1.[48–51] The most prominent exception is LFABP, which binds other acyl ligands as well as long-chain fatty acids, and binds fatty acids at a molar ratio of 2:1.[52–57] Sensitive fluorimetric assays have demonstrated previously unrecognized differences in equilibrium binding affinities of various FABPs for different fatty acids. For example, lower ligand binding affinities for the adipocyte FABP relative to other FABPs have been reported.[58] Affinities of most of the FABPs are generally highest for palmitate, oleate, and stearate, and increased water solubility of polyunsaturated long-chain fatty acids is reflected by higher K_d values.[58,59]

X-ray crystallography and nuclear magnetic resonance (NMR) spectroscopy have been used to obtain high-resolution structures for several of the FABPs. All of the proteins appear to have the same basic tertiary structure, being composed of 10 antiparallel β-strands which form a barrel-like configuration containing the ligand-binding cavity, with the barrel capped by two short α-helical segments.[18] The helices and the closely appositioned β-turns are often referred to as the portal region of the FABP, where it is hypothesized that ligands enter and exit the binding cavity. Despite their similar tertiary structures and their interactions with long-chain fatty acids, abundant circumstantial evidence suggests that different FABPs may have different intracellular functions. Unlike other intracellular lipid-binding proteins such as the acyl CoenzymeA-binding protein (ACBP) and several phospholipid transport proteins, which do not exhibit singular tissue-specific forms, the FABP family has diverged to express a large number of tissue-specific homologues. Indeed, in the intestinal absorptive cell high and approximately equivalent levels of two separate FABPs are expressed,[60] further suggesting a functional specificity for different family members. Differences in ligand-binding properties, fatty acid transfer mechanisms, and different patterns of tissue specificity and developmental expression provide further indication of functional diversity.[47,58,61]

6.4 Nutritional Regulation of Fatty Acid Transport Proteins

As might be anticipated from their roles in nutrient metabolism, it is likely that both the plasma membrane and intracellular classes of fatty acid transport proteins are modulated by nutritional factors. In the case of the transmembrane transporters, that link is only beginning to be explored. More information is available for the intracellular FABPs. With the likelihood very high for functional diversity among the various intracellular FABPs, it is perhaps not surprising that they are not coordinately regulated by nutritional factors, as will be shown below.

6.4.1 Regulation of Membrane-Associated Fatty Acid Transporter Expression

Extensive studies examining the effect of diet on the levels of putative membrane transporters have not yet been published. Studies employing whole animal models, however, have provided some information regarding overall regulation of these proteins. For example, FABPpm expression is markedly elevated in the white adipose tissue of Zucker diabetic and obese (*fa/fa*) rats.[62] These rats have lost insulin sensitivity and therefore an increased level of FABPpm mRNA in these animals indicates insulin is a negative regulator of FABPpm expression. The insulin effect in these animals appears to be tissue sensitive, as there was no difference in FABPpm levels in the liver of these rats.[62] No information regarding the presence or absence of an insulin-responsive element (IRE) upstream of the FABPpm coding region is available to date. FABPpm levels are also affected by the FA utilization requirements of the tissue. FABPpm levels have been shown to increase in oxidative skeletal muscle during fasting, a metabolic state that necessitates high FA utilization.[63] In addition, studies in humans have demonstrated that the protein is induced in skeletal muscle with prolonged endurance training, again concomitant with an increased need for FA utilization.[64-66]

Similar to FABPpm, FATP mRNA levels can also be increased markedly by nutrient depletion. This marked increase was observed in murine adipose tissue and has been attributed to an insulin effect at the level of transcription, with insulin downregulating FATP mRNA.[67] An insulin-responsive element (IRE) for FATP has been identified, and is similar to other known insulin-responsive regulatory sequences.[67,68] In accordance with the presence of an insulin-control element, FATP expression is elevated in the adipose tissue of the insulin-resistant Zucker diabetic and obese *fa/fa* rats.[62] FATP expression is also under the control of peroxisome proliferating agents, which include fatty acids, and will be discussed below.

FAT/CD36 expression is also altered in a diabetic state. For example, CD36 protein levels are increased several-fold in NOD diabetic mice[69] and CD36 mRNA levels are slightly elevated in the Zucker diabetic and obese rats, although not to the extent that the FABPpm and FATP mRNA levels are increased.[62] Further clarification of the regulatory relationship between FAT/CD36 expression and insulin is required.[19] The distribution of FAT mRNA along the gastro-colic axis is greatest in the jejunum, the main site of fatty acid absorption, and its mRNA levels are regulated by the intake of dietary fat. Specifically, high fat diets administered to rats increase FAT mRNA levels, with a diet rich in long-chain fatty acids increasing levels most dramatically.[70] The effect of dietary fats may be due directly to the action of a series of fatty acid-responsive nuclear receptors. Indeed, both fatty acids and other lipophilic compounds such as peroxisome proliferators induce FAT mRNA expression,[71,72] and the gene appears to be regulated directly by these ligands, as will be discussed below.

6.4.2 Regulation of Intracellular FABP (IFABP) Expression

From their earliest identification approximately 30 years ago, the FABPs have been proposed as central to the cellular disposition of dietary lipid, in that tissues with high rates of fatty acid uptake, metabolism, and storage have high FABP levels.[46,73] Particularly supportive of the relationship between diet and FABP expression is the intestinal distribution of LFABP and IFABP, from duodenum-to-colon and crypt-to-villus tip, which correlates well with the distribution of dietary lipid absorption and intracellular processing.[74-76] It would, therefore, seem logical to examine the influence of diet, particularly the amount and type of dietary fat, on the abundance of FABP protein in various lipid-active tissues. Although a limited number of studies in rodents have examined effects of dietary fat and carbohydrate on FABP levels, primarily on the two major gastrointestinal FABPs, liver FABP and intestinal FABP, surprisingly little information which directly addresses the nutritional regulation of the FABPs is available. This could be due to the relatively modest effects of diets that have been reported, which may have dampened enthusiasm for further investigation. The abundance of the FABP protein itself in various cell types is likely to contribute to the modest scale of nutritional regulation. Several of the FABPs have been estimated to comprise as much as 6% of soluble protein.[77-80] It would seem, therefore, that increases of manyfold would not be expected. Further, the turnover rate for the LFABP was found to be relatively slow, with a half-life of 3.1 days, thus making acute regulation by dietary influence less likely.[81] It should be kept in mind, nevertheless, that owing to their great abundance even modest changes, as expressed on a percentage or "fold" basis, represent quite large changes in absolute amounts of FABP.

6.4.2.1   Liver FABP

Of all the FABPs, the nutritional regulation of LFABP levels has been the most extensively investigated. Studies for the most part have examined dietary fat level rather than fat type, and have demonstrated a positive correlation between lipid intake and liver and intestinal LFABP levels. In comparison to a chow-based 5% fat diet, high fat diets consisting of 20 to 38% vegetable oil consumed for 3 to 4 weeks increased the level of liver FABP by 40% in liver, 30% in jejunum, and 50% in the ileum.[73] Since the ileal abundance of LFABP in control animals is approximately one third that of jejunal LFABP, it was reasoned that the larger relative change in the distal small intestine represents an adaptive response so as to increase the ability of the intestine to absorb and process the additional lipid, whereas the already high levels of LFABP expression in proximal intestine are only modestly increased by additional dietary fat.[73] Studies in Zucker rats[82] and pigs[83] have also found that high fat diets increase hepatic LFABP levels. Recently, Veerkamp and van Moerkerk examined the effects of diets containing 5 to 40% of energy as fat, and the results suggested a dose-dependent increase in LFABP content, with approximately 25% greater liver levels on the highest fat intake. A comparison of diets containing 10% of calories as corn oil (high n-6 PUFA), menhaden oil (high n-3 PUFA), or lard (high SFA) showed no differences in liver LFABP level.[84]

Few studies have reported the regulation of LFABP mRNA levels by diet. In the adult hamster, Lin and colleagues found that a high fat diet resulted in approximately 80% and 40% increases in LFABP mRNA in liver and intestine, respectively.[85] Poirier et al.[86] also found that proximal small intestinal LFABP mRNA and protein levels were elevated following sunflower oil feeding. Interestingly, they found similar effects after infusing very small quantities of linoleic acid, the primary fatty acid found in sunflower oil. Changes in LFABP expression as a function of development indirectly suggest that the LFABP gene is induced by dietary fat content. The mRNA for LFABP in the liver and intestine increases markedly at birth, concomitant with the onset of suckling and a high-fat maternal diet.[87] A 20-fold increase in LFABP protein level between fetal and adult liver has also been shown; however, an abrupt increase in mRNA at birth was not observed.[88]

In contrast to the effects of a high fat diet, fasting decreases LFABP expression. A 48-hour fast resulted in a marked decrease in liver content of LFABP, in parallel with total protein, such that the relative abundance of LFABP remained unchanged.[81,89] A decline in hepatic LFABP and its mRNA following a 3-day fast has also been shown using immunocytochemistry and *in situ* hybridization, respectively.[90] Interestingly, fasting did not cause a relative decrease in LFABP levels in the intestine. Furthermore, it resulted in the appearance of LFABP in villus crypt cells, from which it is typically absent.[76,91] It has been suggested that the increased expression in crypt cells could be secondary to the increased plasma concentrations of fatty acid that accompany the starved state.[91,92]

A protocol of fasting followed by high carbohydrate refeeding, well known to cause the rapid induction of many lipogenic enzymes, resulted in little change in the cytosolic concentration of LFABP,[81] in accord with its relatively long half-life. Consistent with these results, a 60% sucrose diet fed for several weeks did not alter liver LFABP levels.[73] The fact that LFABP levels increase secondary to a high fat diet, and do not respond to a lipogenic diet, implies that LFABP expression may be regulated by exogenous fatty acid but not endogenous fatty acid.[73] Nevertheless, insulin, which is lipogenic, appears to be involved in the expression of LFABP, as streptozotocin-diabetic rats were found to have decreased LFABP expression.[93,94] Effects of insulin may be indirect, given that an insulin-responsive promoter element has not been identified in the LFABP gene.

As will be shown below, the regulation of LFABP expression by lipid is likely mediated via peroxisomal proliferator activated receptor (PPAR) transcription factors. Among the ligands that are now known to bind to these nuclear hormone receptors are long-chain fatty acids, thereby providing a mechanism by which the ligand modulates expression of its binding protein. Nevertheless, intestinal isograft studies have demonstrated that LFABP expression is not solely dependent on signals related to lipid flux. Rubin et al.[95] implanted fetal proximal small intestinal isografts into the subcutaneous tissues of adult mice, where luminal signals are absent, and found appropriate proximal-distal and crypt-villus positional expression of the LFABP gene. In addition, the proximal-to-distal gradients for LFABP and IFABP were seen at day 17 of gestation in the mouse, a time when exposure of the intestinal mucosa to luminal fat is quite low.[96]

6.4.2.2   Intestinal FABP

The correlation of intestinal IFABP expression with the anatomical localization of dietary lipid absorption,[97] the higher expression of IFABP in villus compared to crypt cells,[60] and the increased accumulation of IFABP mRNA at the onset of the suckling period,[87] all support a causal relationship between dietary fat and IFABP expression. Early studies of intestinal FABP showed no effect of high fat feeding on jejunal levels and a 40% increase in ileal levels in rats fed a high fat diet, with little effect or even a decrease in intestinal FABP levels in animals fed a high sucrose diet.[36] Fasted rats were found to have a sparing of intestinal FABP levels relative to total intestinal protein,[36] perhaps indicative of the need for maintaining maximal absorptive capacity. In contrast, a 16% fat diet, relative to an 8% diet, had no effect on IFABP mRNA levels in any segment of mouse small intestine.[86] Thus, there is a somewhat uncertain relationship between IFABP expression and luminal fat. Studies of the IFABP gene in intestinal isografts demonstrated the establishment of positional expression in the absence of exposure to luminal contents,[95] indicating that for IFABP, as for LFABP, expression is regulated by both nutritional and non-nutrient-related means.

Unlike the 2- to 3-fold increases of liver and intestinal LFABP expression in clofibrate-treated rats,[73,77] intestinal IFABP levels were increased by only 25%,[77] and no peroxisome proliferator-responsive element (PPRE) has been reported in the promoter region of the IFABP gene. Thus, for IFABP, the molecular mechanisms of dietary lipid modulation, if indeed present, are not known.

6.4.2.3   Adipocyte FABP

Our understanding of the nutritional regulation of AFABP expression has come mostly from studies using cultured adipocyte cell lines, with only a modest amount of information available about the dietary regulation of AFABP expression in animal models. Rats fed a high fat diet had a 50% increase in adipose tissue AFABP content,[84] a robust effect given existing high levels of AFABP expression. The involvement of insulin was first shown by studies in streptozotocin-diabetic rats, where AFABP protein and mRNA levels were decreased, and the changes reversed by insulin administration.[98]

Analysis of the promoter region of the AFABP gene in cultured cells has shown that the activation of expression by insulin is likely to occur indirectly, via CCAAT/enhancer-binding protein (C/EBPα)-stimulated transcription.[99,100] Insulin-like growth factor I, glucocorticoid, fatty acids, and agents that increase intracellular cAMP levels also increase AFABP expression.[101–105] Addition of oleic acid to confluent preadipocytes treated with the glucocorticoid analogue dexamethasone was shown to potentiate the increase in AFABP mRNA levels.[101] Treatment of preadipocytes with long-chain FA results in a dramatic (>20-fold) increase in AFABP mRNA levels.[106] As will be discussed further, AFABP expression is also regulated by the transcription factors peroxisomal proliferator activated receptor γ (PPARγ) and fatty acid activated receptor (FAAR, also termed PPARδ). Thus, the lipid effects noted above are likely mediated via these nuclear receptors.

6.4.2.4   Heart FABP

Heart and skeletal muscle utilize long-chain fatty acids to provide a majority of their oxidative requirements. Studies of the regulation of HFABP expression have, therefore, focused on conditions under which mitochondrial β-oxidation is modified.[84] For instance, higher levels of HFABP are expressed in red gastrocnemius muscle than white, and expression increases following endurance training, both situations that parallel the relative mitochondrial β-oxidation levels.[84,107–109] In a murine muscle cell line, HFABP content was increased in differentiated relative to undifferentiated cells, in parallel with the expression of creatine kinase activity and fatty acid β-oxidation.[110]

Little information is available about the regulation of HFABP expression by diet, and the available data are somewhat contradictory. Early studies by

Fournier and Rahim showed a 30% increase in heart HFABP levels following a high fat diet,[111] whereas more recently others found no change in HFABP levels in rats fed diets ranging from 5 to 40% fat.[84] It has also been reported that HFABP expression in mammary gland is increased upon feeding a high fat diet.[112] In contrast to results for LFABP and IFABP, fasting was reported to result in an increase in the level of HFABP expression in heart, via an increase in gene transcription rate.[113]

The developmental expression of HFABP may also offer some insight into its potential for nutritional regulation. HFABP mRNA levels rise rapidly in rat heart 2 days prior to birth, and continue to rise during the high-fat diet suckling period. They reach a peak at the initiation of weaning, upon transition from the maternal high fat diet, and then decline slightly into adulthood. It was noted that these changes parallel those in cardiac mitochondrial β-oxidative capacity and mitochondrial abundance.[114]

A number of investigators have reported that heart HFABP levels increase during experimental diabetes mellitus.[113,115,116] Although it would appear that the mechanism of this increase might be the same as that observed in starvation, the increase appears to be secondary to an increase in mRNA turnover time rather than to increased transcription rate.[113] Unlike HFABP expression in the heart, HFABP expression in the aorta was found to be decreased in streptozotocin-diabetic rats, and this was reversed upon insulin treatment.[117]

The mechanism(s) of nutritional regulation of HFABP expression are unknown at present. Peroxisome proliferators have little or no effect on the levels of HFABP in heart and skeletal muscles, and little information is available about the promoter region of the HFABP gene.[84,118] The existing literature supports the suggestion that the modulation of HFABP abundance is consistent with a role in fatty acid metabolism, particularly with the capacity of tissues to oxidize fatty acids for energy. The signals that affect this regulation remain to be revealed.

6.4.2.5   Other FABPs

Minimal information is available about the nutritional regulation of other members of the FABP family. Ibrahimi et al. reported an increase in the expression of KFABP (skin type) in Ob1771 adipocytes incubated with fatty acids or thiazolidinedione antidiabetic agents,[119] and it is thus likely that the KFABP promoter region will be found to contain a PPRE. Studies relevant to the nutritional regulation of myelin P2 protein (MFABP) and BFABP are not available at present. Of interest, however, is that these two proteins are maximally expressed during cellular growth and differentiation, when neuronal cells undergo abundant membrane biogenesis, rather than in fully mature cells, so signals regulating their expression are likely to be different than those regulating expression of other FABPs that are more highly expressed in differentiated cells.

6.5 Molecular Mechanism of Fatty Acid Regulation of Transport Proteins

The gross nutritional regulation of fatty acid transport proteins discussed above is likely facilitated in large part by a nuclear phenomenon whereby dietary ligands affect gene transcription through binding to a class of nuclear receptors. The role that fatty acids may play in nuclear transcriptional events and, in turn, in overall cellular homeostasis is summarized schematically in Fig. 6.1.

6.5.1 Peroxisome Proliferator-Activated Receptors

Peroxisome proliferation is a complex cellular phenomenon initiated by a class of structurally diverse compounds such as fibrates, herbicides, and pthalate plasticizers that increase peroxisomal β-oxidation of fatty acids. In 1990 the effects of these peroxisomal proliferating agents was shown to be mediated via a nuclear receptor.[120] Based on sequence homologies, this receptor was concluded to belong to the steroid–hormone superfamily of nuclear receptors and was named the peroxisome proliferator-activated receptor (PPAR). Thus far, three major PPARs, α, δ (also referred to as β, NUC-1, or FAAR) and γ have been cloned from multiple species, including *Xenopus*, rodents, and humans.[121–123] Each of the PPAR forms is coded by a separate gene and has a distinct tissue distribution. The PPAR receptors have retained the main functional domains of the other members of the steroid–hormone superfamily of receptors. Of note, they have a highly conserved DNA-binding domain and a multifunctional ligand-binding domain, which is responsible for ligand binding, dimerization with other receptors, and nuclear localization. Like other members of this superfamily, PPARs act at the nuclear level via ligand-induced binding to cognate DNA sequences on particular genes. These highly conserved DNA sequences on the target genes are referred to as peroxisome proliferator responsive elements (PPREs).[121–123]

PPARα was the first member of the subfamily to be cloned and is expressed mainly in tissues with high catabolic rates for fatty acid and peroxisomal metabolism (liver, kidney, heart, intestinal mucosa, and brown adipose tissue). PPARδ is also an abundant and widely distributed protein whereas PPARγ displays a distribution limited primarily to white adipose tissue and immune cells. The role of PPARδ is not as well understood as the other two. The discussion here will focus on the role of PPARs in the regulation of fatty acid transport proteins and thus will concentrate on known functions of PPARα and PPARγ.[121–125]

PPAR ligands include a broad array of both natural and pharmacological compounds. PPARα binds a variety of endogenous fatty acids,

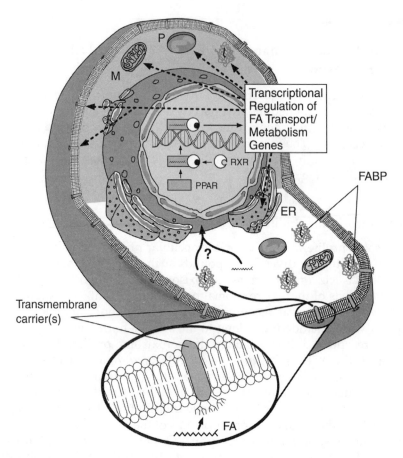

FIGURE 6.1

Fatty acid transport and fatty acid-induced nuclear regulation of transport protein genes. Schematic diagram of a fatty acid (FA) entering a mammalian cell through a putative transmembrane carrier, binding to the intracellular fatty acid binding proteins (FABPs) and moving to the nucleus. The mechanism(s) by which fatty acid enters the nucleus is unknown at this time. Upon entering the nucleus, the FA binds to a peroxisome proliferator-activated receptor (PPAR) that dimerizes with holo-retinioc acid X receptor (RXR). This heterodimer recognizes and binds to a peroxisome proliferator-responsive element (PPRE) on target DNA, thereby effecting transcription of a downstream coding region. In particular, the expression of membrane fatty acid transporters and FABPs as well as many genes involved in both mitochondiral (M) fatty acid metabolism and peroxisomal (P) fatty acid oxidation are mediated via PPRE elements.

although it demonstrates a preference for the C18 unsaturated fatty acids such as oleic (18:1) and α-linoleic acid (18:3), with binding affinities of approximately 5 nM, thought to be well within the physiological range.[126,127] PPARα is also activated by naturally occurring eicosanoids, such as leukotriene B4, a mediator of the inflammatory response, and by 8-hydroxyeicosoatetraenoic acid, a product of the lipoxygenase pathway. Synthetic ligands for PPARα include the fibrates, a class of hypolipidemic drugs widely prescribed for the treatment of hypertriglyceridemia. Recent competitive binding studies have demonstrated that naturally occurring fatty acids were actually more potent ligands for human PPARα than the synthetic fibrate WY-14,643, previously thought to be the highest-affinity ligand for PPARα.[126,127]

As with PPARα, PPARγ demonstrates broad ligand specificity. Natural ligands for PPARγ include prostaglandins A, D, and J, and certain mono- and polyunsaturated FAs, in particular, linolenic (18:2), linoleic (18:3), and arachidonic acid (20:4).[128] Synthetic activators of PPARγ include the insulin-sensitizing thiazolidinedione drugs used as oral antidiabetic agents.

6.5.2 Mode of Action — Ligand Binding and Cofactor Proteins

In order to affect the expression of target genes, ligand bound forms of both PPARα and PPARγ dimerize with the 9-*cis*-retinoic acid receptor, RXR, when it is also bound by ligand. This receptor dimer is the functional unit that recognizes and binds the PPRE on target DNA, thereby affecting transcriptional activity. RXR heterodimers are required for other members of the steroid hormone superfamily to modulate gene expression (i.e., other retinoic acid receptors, the thyroid hormone receptor, and the vitamin D receptor), and these dimers represent convergence in the signaling pathways of these hormone systems.[121–123] In addition to receptor dimerization, a series of cofactor proteins have also been shown to adjust the transcriptional activity of PPARs by interacting directly with the receptors, to either repress (corepressors) or enhance (coactivators) their activities. For example, p300, a component of the TATA-binding protein complex, has been shown to stimulate transcriptional activity of PPARα.[129] The number of identified protein cofactors for the PPARs is growing and reflects the complexity by which this nuclear receptor system regulates transcriptional activity.

The diversity of ligands that individual PPARs are capable of binding is unlike the strict ligand specificity observed for other members of the steroid–receptor superfamily, for example, RXR, which is thought to bind only the 9-*cis* form of retinoic acid. Recent crystallographic data on the ligand binding domain of PPARδ demonstrate that the carboxylic acid moieties of two structurally different classes of ligands for PPARδ, an eicosenoid and a fibrate, are both oriented toward a particular region of the receptor, and this orientation stabilizes a helical conformation via a series of highly conserved hydrogen bonds.[130] This stable helix within the holo-receptor, then, is thought to allow for dimerization and/or interaction with cofactor proteins. In addition, the X-ray data show that the binding pocket of PPARδ is relatively large and allows for binding of ligands in multiple configurations. The overall size of the binding pocket and its use of a number of stabilizing hydrophobic interactions help explain the structural diversity of PPAR ligands, as well as why PPARδ bind FA of only certain chain lengths ($14 \leq C \leq 20$).[130]

6.5.3   The Effect of PPARs on Fatty Acid Transport Proteins

6.5.3.1   *Membrane Fatty Acid Transport Proteins*

In general, PPARα and its concomitant ligands have been implicated in the regulation of many genes involved in hepatic lipid metabolism and energy homeostasis.[122,124,131] These include both mitochondrial and peroxisomal β-oxidative enzymes as well as fatty acid synthetase and lipoprotein assembly and transport proteins.[124,132] PPARγ has been associated primarily with lipolytic effects and is known to regulate enzymes involved in adipocyte differentiation and lipid storage and metabolism, for example, LPL and acyl-CoA synthetase, as well as the hormone leptin.[122,124,133]

Recent molecular evidence has shown that certain putative membrane fatty acid transport proteins are also modulated in a tissue specific manner via PPARs (Table 6.2). In mice, treatment with the synthetic fibrate WY-14,643 and other PPARα ligands resulted in increased mRNA levels of two of the three major membrane carrier proteins. FAT mRNA levels were increased in both liver and intestinal tissue by treatment with a fibrate,[71] whereas FATP mRNA increased primarily in liver only.[71,72] The observed increase in both FAT and FATP mRNA in liver was not observed in PPARα-null mice, demonstrating that PPARα was obligatory for the hepatic transcriptional effect.[71] FABPpm mRNA levels increased only slightly in liver following treatment with the fibrate and were unaffected by treatment with any other PPARα ligands. Transcription of FAT and FATP mRNA also increased in white adipose tissue of mice and in preadipocyte cell lines by treatment with PPARγ ligands, but again transcription of FABPpm was unaffected.[71,72] Thus, tissue-specific regulation of FAT and FATP expression has been demonstrated, with hepatic expression of FAT and FATP under the control of PPARα and adipocyte expression under the control of PPARγ.[71,72] In contrast, it appears that FABPpm expression is not under the control of PPARα or PPARγ.

Cloning and sequence analysis of the murine FATP gene identified a putative PPRE in its 5′ untranslated region.[68] A recent study further characterized

TABLE 6.2

Identified PPRE Sequences in Fatty Acid Transport Proteins

Protein	Species	Sequence	Proposed Function	Ref.
CONSENSUS PPRE SEQUENCE		AACT AGGTCA A AGGTCA T		121
AFABP	Mouse	CTCT GGGTGA A ATGTGC	Intracellular fatty acid binding/transport	159
LFABP	Rat	ATAT AGGCCA T AGGTCA	Intracellular fatty acid binding/transport	137
FATP	Mouse	AAGT GGGGCA A AGGGCA	Transmembrane fatty acid transport	134
FAT	Mouse	TGGCCT C TGACTT	Transmembrane fatty acid transport	a

ª P. Grimaldi and L. Teboul, personal communication.

the PPRE on FATP and found that this sequence is very similar to the consensus sequence for other identified PPREs (Table 6.2), and that it does confer transcriptional regulation of FATP mRNA by PPARs. Transient transfection of an FATP–luciferase reporter construct into CV-1 cells resulted in ligand-dependent upregulation of the reporter activity by both PPARα and PPARγ in a PPRE-mediated manner.[134] In 3T3-L1 adipocyte cells, luciferase reporter activity was increased by ligand bound PPARγ but not by PPARα. Further, in the 3T3-L1 cells activation of FATP expression with bound PPARγ correlated with an increased uptake of oleate into the cells; the physiological ligand, linoleic acid, was also shown to activate FATP transcription in a PPRE-dependent manner.[134] A functional PPRE has also been identified recently in the mouse FAT promoter (P. Grimaldi and L. Teboul, personal communication).

6.5.3.2   *Intracellular FABPs*

It has been known for some time that the expression of LFABP was increased by a seemingly heterogeneous group of compounds that caused the proliferation of peroxisomes,[124,135–138] and that induction of hepatic peroxisomal β-oxidation capacity correlates strongly with the increase in LFABP levels.[139] Indeed, when ethanol, which impairs mitochondrial β-oxidation and stimulates peroxisomal β-oxidation, was added to a high fat diet, LFABP was found to be expressed at levels up to 20% of soluble protein.[140] Dicarboxylic acids, FA metabolites that are found under conditions of impaired mitochondrial β-oxidation or with high levels of FA flux, have also been shown to increase LFABP mRNA levels in cultured hepatocytes.[135,141] It is now known that these compounds, which include long-chain FA, bind to and activate PPARs. In mice null for PPARα, fasting induced a fatty liver accompanied by severe impairment of fatty acid oxidation, and LFABP expression was dramatically decreased in the the PPARα$^{-/-}$ fasted rats.[142] The relationship between LFABP expression and peroxisome proliferation is not absolute, however, as normal LFABP levels are present in infants with Zellweger's syndrome, who have a complete absence of peroxisomal biogenesis.[73] Thus, LFABP expression appears to be coordinated with, but not dependent on, peroxisomal oxidative capacity.

Studies in cultured cell lin es are consistent with PPRE-mediated regulation of LFABP expression. Besnard and colleagues demonstrated that long-chain FA increases the transcription rate of the LFABP gene in rat hepatoma cells, and that 9-*cis*-retionoic acid enhances this induction.[143–145] Increased LFABP synthesis following incubation with linoleic acid was also reported,[146] although others have found that oleate was effective only under conditions where β-oxidation was inhibited.[135,141]

It is likely that the effects of long-chain fatty acids on AFABP expression are also mediated via interactions with PPAR transcription factors. PPARγ was shown to bind the arachidonate metabolite 15-deoxy $\Delta^{12,14}$ prostaglandin J$_2$,[147,136] forming a heterodimer with RXRα and thereby activating

AFABP transcription.[148] Indeed, both LFABP and AFABP contain functional PPRE homolog sequences in the promoter region of their genes (Table 6.2) and are upregulated by PPARα and PPARγ, respectively.[137,141,148] Antidiabetic agents such as the thiazolidinediones increase AFABP mRNA levels presumably by increasing insulin sensitivity, and appear to be operating via the same mechanism of activation of nuclear hormone receptors as do long-chain fatty acids.[119]

6.6   Concluding remarks

Nutritional regulation of FA transport protein gene expression, in particular by FA itself, highlights the potential for a direct effect of diet on transcription, and demonstrates at the molecular level how diet can directly influence gene transcription, even in the absence of metabolic transformation.

The effects of the PPARs on expression of numerous fatty acid metabolizing enzymes, and on particular fatty acid transport proteins (Fig. 6.1), demonstrate how PPARs and their associated ligands are capable of coordinate regulation of FA flux and metabolism at the nuclear level. Thus, the participation of intracellular FA in their pleiotropic functions requires regulation by a complex sequence of ligand–receptor–DNA interactions which, in turn, requires not only other hormone-signaling pathways but also a series of co-repressor/activator proteins. The result of these multiple regulatory events leads, ultimately, to a particular FA availability within the cell. The coordinated regulation of the transmembrane FA transporters and the intracellular FABPs, as well as particular enzymes of FA metabolism, supports the hypothesis that cellular FA trafficking is vectorial rather than simply random or diffusion controlled, and occurs via a series of specific protein–protein and/or protein–membrane interactions.[47,149]

The role of PPARα in hepatocyte lipid metabolism, and the role of PPARγ in adipocyte lipid metabolism, suggest that significant pathological conditions may be associated with aberrant function of these FA-activated transcription factors. For example, alterations in PPARα function may play a role in hyperlipoproteinemia and alterations in PPARγ may play a role in insulin resistance and diabetes. Therefore, the dietary availability, intracellular transport, and trafficking of their respective ligands may, by association, also play a significant role in certain pathological states. However, that both the intracellular and membrane transport proteins for FA are themselves regulated by PPARs (Fig. 6.1) and are, therefore, regulated by the availability of their FA ligands, highlights the complicated feedback regulation between dietary fats and nuclear events which may influence many metabolic conditions such as obesity and diabetes. Clearly, the involvement of fatty acids as transcriptional regulatory factors in their own homeostasis is complex, and to date may present more questions than answers. These questions include the complete identification of regulatory proteins, protein cofactors, and the cognate DNA sequences recognized by the various effectors, as well as the role of fatty acid specificity, and potential intracellular compartmentalization of different FA. The potential functional redundancies in both intracellular and transmembrane FA transport proteins, with two or three of each type expressed simultaneously in particular cell types, respectively, must also be clearly defined.

Abbreviations

AFABP adipocyte FABP
BFABP brain FABP
cAMP cyclic adenosine monophosphate
C/EBP-α CCAAT-enhancer binding protein α
FA fatty acid
FABP fatty acid binding protein
FABPpm plasma membrane fatty acid binding protein
FAT fatty acid translocase (CD36)
FATP fatty acid transport protein
HFABP heart FABP
IFABP intestinal FABP
KFABP keratinocyte FABP
LFABP liver FABP
MFABP myelin FABP (myelin P2)
mRNA messenger RNA
NMR nuclear magnetic resonance
PPAR peroxisome proliferator-activated receptor
PPRE peroxisome proliferator response element
PUFA polyunsaturated fatty acid
RXR retinoid X receptor
SFA saturated fatty acid
TG triacylglycerol

References

1. Carey, M. C. and Hernell, O., Digestion and absorption of fat, *Sem. Gastroint. Dis.*, 3, 189, 1992.
2. Noy, N., Donnelly, T. M., and Zakim, D., Physical-chemical model for the entry of water-soluble compounds into cells: Studies of fatty acid uptake by the liver, *Biochemistry*, 25, 2013, 1986.
3. Hamilton, J. A., Fatty acid transport: difficult or easy, *J. Lipid Res.*, 39, 467, 1998.
4. Kleinfeld, A. M. and Storch, J., Transfer of long-chain fluorescent fatty acids between small and large unilamellar vesicles, *Biochemistry*, 32, 2053, 1993.
5. Abumrad, N. A., Harmon, C. M., and Ibrahimi, A., Membrane transport of long-chain fatty acids: evidence for a facilitated process, *J. Lipid Res.*, 39, 2309, 1998.
6. Stremmel, W., Strohmeyer, G., Borchard, F., Kochwa, S., and Berk, P. D., Isolation and partial characterization of a fatty acid binding protein in rat liver plasma membranes, *Proc. Natl. Acad. Sci. USA*, 82, 4, 1985.
7. Trigatti, B. L., Mangroo, D., and Gerber, G. E., Photoaffinity labeling and fatty acid permeation in 3T3-L1 adipocytes, *J. Biol. Chem.*, 266, 22621, 1991.
8. Harmon, C. M., Luce, P., Beth, A. H., and Abumrad, N. A., Labeling of adipocyte membranes by sulfo-N-succinimidyl derivatives of long-chain fatty acids: inhibition of fatty acid transport, *J. Membrane Biol.*, 121, 261, 1991.
9. Schaffer, J. E. and Lodish, H. F., Expression cloning and characterization of a novel adipocyte long chain fatty acid transport protein, *Cell*, 79, 427, 1994.
10. Berk, P. D., Wada, H., Horio, Y., Potter, B. J., Sorrentino, D., Zhou, S., Isola, L. M., Stump, D., Kiang, C., and Thung, S., Plasma membrane fatty acid-binding protein and mitochondrial glutamic-oxaloacetic transaminase of rat liver are related, *Proc. Natl. Acad. Sci. USA*, 87, 3484, 1990.
11. Zhou, S., Stump, D., Sorrentino, D., Potter, B. J., and Berk, P. D., Adipocyte differentiation of 3T3-L1 cells involves augmented expression of a 43-kDa plasma membrane fatty acid-binding protein, *J. Biol. Chem.*, 267, 14456, 1992.
12. Luiken, J., Turcotte, L., and Bonen, A., Protein-mediated palmitate uptake and expression of fatty acid transport proteins in heart giant vesicles, *J. Lipid Res.*, 40, 1007, 1999.
13. Zhou, S. L., Stump, D., Isola, L. M., and Berk, P. D., Constitutive expression of a saturable transport system for non-esterified fatty acids in *Xenopus laevis* oocytes, *J. Biochem.*, 297, 315, 1994.
14. Isola, L. M., Zhou, S. L., Kiang, C. L., Stump, D. D., Bradbury, M. W., and Berk, P. D., 3T3 fibroblasts transfected with a cDNA for mitochondrial aspartate aminotransferase express plasma membrane fatty acid-binding protein and saturable fatty acid uptake, *Proc. Natl. Acad. Sci. USA*, 92, 9866, 1995.
15. Abumrad, N. A., El-Maghrabi, M. R., Amri, E., Lopez, E., and Grimaldi, P. A., Cloning of a rat adipocyte membrane protein implicated in binding or transport of long-chain fatty acids that is induced during preadipocyte differentiation: Homology with human CD36, *J. Biol. Chem.*, 268, 17665, 1993.
16. Baillie, A. G. S., Coburn, C. T., and Abumrad, N. A., Reversible binding of long-chain fatty acids to purified FAT, the adipose CD36 homolog, *J. Membrane Biol.*, 153, 75, 1996.

17. Abumrad, N. A., Perkins, R. C., Park, J. H., and Park, C. R., Mechanism of long chain fatty acid permeation in the isolated adipocyte, *J. Biol. Chem.*, 256, 9183, 1981.

18. Banaszak, L., Winter, N., Xu, Z., Bernlohr, D. A., Cowan, S., and Jones, T. A., Lipid-binding proteins: A family of fatty acid and retinoid transport proteins, *Adv. Prot. Chem.*, 45, 89, 1994.

19. Abumrad, N. A., Coburn, C., and Ibrahimi, A., Membrane proteins implicated in long-chain fatty acid uptake by mammalian cells: CD36, FATP and FABPpm, *Biochim. Biophys. Acta*, 1441, 4, 1999.

20. Dutta-Roy, A. K., Crosbie, L. C., Gordon, M. J., and Campbell, F. M., Platelet membrane glycoprotein IV (CD36) is involved in arachidonic acid induced-platelet aggregation, *Biochem. Soc. Trans.*, 24, 167S, 1996.

21. Ibrahimi, A., Sfeir, Z., Magharaie, H., Amri, E. Z., and Grimaldi, P., Expression of the CD36 homolog (FAT) in fibroblast cells: Effects on fatty acid transport, *Proc. Natl. Acad. Sci. USA*, 93, 2646, 1996.

22. Sfeir, Z., Ibrahimi, A., Ez-zoubir, A., Grimaldi, P., and Abumrad, N., CD36 antisense expression in 3T3-F442A preadipocytes, *Mol. Cell. Biochem.*, 192, 3, 1999.

23. Nozaki, S., Tanaka, T., Yamashita, S., Sohmiya, K., Yoshizumi, T., Okamoto, F., Kitaura, Y., Kotake, C., Nishida, H., Nakata, A., Nakagawa, T., Matsumoto, K., Kameda-Takemura, K., Tadokoro, S., Kurata, Y., Tomiyama, Y., Kawamura, K., and Matsuzawa, Y., CD36 mediates long-chain fatty acid transport in human myocardium: Complete myocardial accumulation defect of radiolabeled long-chain fatty acid analog in subjects with CD36 deficiency, *Mol. Cell. Biochem.*, 192, 129, 1999.

24. Febbraio, M., Abumrad, N., Hajjar, D. P., Sharma, K., Cheng, W., Pearce, S. F. A., and Silverstein, R. L., A null mutation in murine CD36 reveals an important role in fatty acid and lipoprotein metabolism, *J. Biol. Chem.*, 274, 19055, 1999.

25. Gargiulo, C., Stuhlsatz-Krouper, S., and Schaffer, J. E., Localization of adipocyte long-chain fatty acyl CoA synthetase at the plasma membrane, *J. Lipid Res.*, 40, 881, 1999.

26. Hirsch, D., Stahl, A., and Lodish, H. F., A family of fatty acid transporters conserved from mycobacterium to man, *Proc. Natl. Acad. Sci. USA*, 95, 8625, 1998.

27. Stuhlsatz-Krouper, S. M., Bennett, N., and Schaffer, J. E., Substitution of alanine for serine 250 in the murine fatty acid transport protein inhibits long chain fatty acid transport, *J. Biol. Chem.*, 273, 28642, 1998.

28. Watkins, P. A., Lu, J. F., Steinberg, S. J., Gould, S. J., Smith, K. D., and Braiterman, L. T., Disruption of the *Saccharomyces cerevisiae* FAT1 gene decreases very long-chain fatty acyl-CoA synthetase activity and elevates intracellular very long-chain fatty acid concentrations, *J. Biol. Chem.*, 273, 18210, 1998.

29. Gerber, G. E., Mangroo, D., and Trigatti, B. L., Identification of high affinity membrane-bound fatty acid-binding proteins using a photoreactive fatty acid, *Mol. Cell Biochem.*, 39, 1993.

30. Trigatti, B. L., Anderson, R. G. W., and Gerber, G. E., Identification of caveolin-1 as a fatty acid binding protein, *Biochem. Biophys. Res. Commun.*, 255, 34, 1999.

31. Smart, E. J., Graf, G. A., McNiven, M. A., Sessa, W. C., Engelman, J. A., Scherer, P. E., Okamoto, T., and Lisanti, M. P., Caveolins, liquid-ordered domains, and signal transduction, *Mol. Cell. Biol.*, 7289, 1999.

32. Fujii, S., Kawaguchi, H., and Yasuda, H., Purification of high affinity fatty acid receptors in rat myocardial sarcolemmal membranes, *Lipids*, 22, 544, 1987.

33. Fujii, S., Kawaguchi, H., and Yasuda, H., Purification and characterization of fatty acid-binding protein from rat kidney, *Arch. Biochem. Biophys.*, 254, 552, 1987.

34. Ockner, R. K., Manning, J. A., Poppenhausen, R. B., and Ho, W. K. L., A binding protein for fatty acids in cytosol of intestinal mucosa, liver, myocardium, and other tissues, *Science*, 177, 56, 1972.

35. Mishkin, S., Stein, L., Gatmaitan, Z., and Arias, I. M., The binding of fatty acids to cytoplasmic proteins: Binding to Z-protein in liver and other tissues of the rat, *Biochem. Biophys. Res. Comm.*, 47, 997, 1972.

36. Ockner, R. K. and Manning, J. A., Fatty acid-binding protein in small intestine: Identification, isolation, and evidence for its role in cellular fatty acid transport, *J. Clin. Invest.*, 54, 326, 1974.

37. Fournier, N. C., Geoffrey, M., and Deshusses, J., Purification and characterization of a long-chain fatty acid binding protein supplying the mitochondrial β-oxidation system in the heart, *Biochim. Biophys. Acta*, 533, 457, 1978.

38. Matarese, V. and Bernlohr, D. A., Purification of murine adipocyte lipid-binding protein: Characterization as a fatty acid- and retinoic acid-binding protein, *J. Biol. Chem.*, 263, 14544, 1988.

39. Narayanan, V., Barbosa, E., Reed, R. G., and Tennekoon, G., Characterization of a cloned cDNA encoding rabbit myelin P2 protein, *J. Biol. Chem.*, 263, 8332, 1988.

40. Feng, L., Hatten, M. E., and Heintz, N., Brain lipid-binding protein (BLBP): A novel signaling system in the developing mammalian CNS, *Neuron*, 12, 895, 1994.

41. Krieg, P., Feil, S., Fürstenberger, G., and Bowden, G. T., Tumor-specific overexpression of a novel keratinocyte lipid-binding protein: Identification and characterization of a cloned sequence activated during multistage carcinogenesis in mouse skin, *J. Biol. Chem.*, 268, 17362, 1993.

42. Kaikaus, R. M., Bass, N. M., and Ockner, R. K., Functions of fatty acid binding proteins, *Experientia*, 46, 617, 1990.

43. Li, E. and Norris, A. W., Structure/function of cytoplasmic vitamin A-binding proteins, *Annu. Rev. Nutr.*, 16, 205, 1996.

44. Napoli, J. L., Biosynthesis and metabolism of retinoic acid: roles of CRBP and CRABP in retinoic acid homeostasis, *J. Nutr.*, 123, 362, 1993.

45. Glatz, J. F. C., Börchers, T., Spener, F., and Van der Vusse, G. J., Fatty acids in cell signaling: Modulation by lipid binding proteins, *Prostaglandins Leukotrienes Essen. Fatty Acids*, 52, 121, 1995.

46. Glatz, J. F. C. and Van der Vusse, G. J., Cellular fatty acid-binding proteins: Their function and physiological significance, *Prog. Lipid Res.*, 35, 243, 1996.

47. Storch, J. and Thumser, A. E. A., The fatty acid transport function of fatty acid-binding proteins, *Biochim. Biophys. Acta*, 1486, 28, 2000.

48. Sacchettini, J. C., Gordon, J. I., and Banaszak, L. J., Crystal structure of rat intestinal fatty-acid-binding protein: Refinement and analysis of the Escherichia coli-derived protein with bound palmitate, *J. Mol. Biol.*, 208, 327, 1989.

49. Sacchettini, J. C., Scapin, G., Gopaul, D., and Gordon, J. I., Refinement of the structure of Escherichia coli-derived rat intestinal fatty acid binding protein with bound oleate to 1.75 Å resolution: Correlation with the structures of the apoprotein and the protein with bound palmitate, *J. Biol. Chem.*, 267, 23534, 1992.

50. Cistola, D. P., Sacchettini, J. C., Banaszak, L. J., Walsh, M. T., and Gordon, J. I., Fatty acid interactions with rat intestinal and liver fatty acid-binding proteins expressed in Escherichia coli: A comparative ^{13}C NMR study, *J. Biol. Chem.*, 264, 2700, 1989.

51. Jakoby, M. G., Miller, K. R., Toner, J. J., Bauman, A., Cheng, L., Li, E., and Cistola, D. P., Ligand-protein electrostatic interactions govern the specificity of retinol- and fatty acid-binding proteins, *Biochemistry*, 32, 872, 1993.

52. Richieri, G. V., Ogata, R. T., and Kleinfeld, A. M., Thermodynamic and kinetic properties of fatty acid interactions with rat liver fatty acid-binding protein, *J. Biol. Chem.*, 271, 31068, 1996.

53. Wilkinson, T. C. I. and Wilton, D. C., Studies on fatty acid-binding proteins: The binding properties of rat liver fatty acid-binding protein, *Biochem. J.*, 247, 485, 1987.

54. Burrier, R. E., Manson, C. R., and Brecher, P., Binding of acyl-CoA to liver fatty acid binding protein: Effect on acyl-CoA synthesis, *Biochim. Biophys. Acta*, 919, 221, 1987.

55. Takikawa, H. and Kaplowitz, N., Binding of bile acids, oleic acid, and organic anions by rat and human hepatic Z protein, *Arch. Biochem. Biophys.*, 251, 385, 1986.

56. Thumser, A. E. A., Voysey, J. E., and Wilton, D. C., The binding of lysophospholipids to rat liver fatty acid-binding protein and albumin, *Biochem. J.*, 301, 801, 1994.

57. Vincent, S. H. and Muller-Eberhard, U., A protein of the Z class of liver cytosolic proteins in the rat that preferentially binds heme, *J. Biol. Chem.*, 260, 14521, 1985.

58. Richieri, G. V., Ogata, R. T., and Kleinfeld, A. M., Equilibrium constants for the binding of fatty acids with fatty acid-binding proteins from adipocyte, intestine, heart, and liver measured with the flourescent probe ADIFAB, *J. Biol. Chem.*, 269, 23918, 1994.

59. Richieri, G. V., Ogata, R. T., Zimmerman, A. W., Veerkamp, J. H., and Kleinfeld, A. M., Fatty acid binding proteins from different tissues show distinct patterns of fatty acid interactions, *Biochemistry*, 39, 7197, 2000.

60. Shields, H. M., Bates, M. L., Bass, N. M., Best, C. J., Alpers, D. H., and Ockner, R. K., Light microscopic immunocytochemical localization of hepatic and intestinal types of fatty acid-binding proteins in rat small intestine, *J. Lipid Res.*, 27, 549, 1986.

61. Glatz, J.F.C. and van der Vusse, G. J., Cellular fatty acid-binding proteins: their function and physiological significance, *Prog. Lipid Res.*, 35, 243, 1996.

62. Berk, P. D., Zhou, S. L., Kiang, C. L., Stump, D., Bradbury, M. W., and Isola, L. M., Uptake of long chain free fatty acids is selectively up-regulated in adipocytes of Zucker rats with genetic obesity and non-insulin-dependent diabetes mellitus, *J. Biol. Chem.*, 272, 8830, 1997.

63. Turcotte, L., Srivastava, A. K., and Chiasson, J. L., Fasting increases plasma membrane fatty acid-binding protein (FABP(PM)) in red skeletal muscle, *Mol. Cell. Biochem.*, 166, 153, 1997.

64. Kiens, B., Kristiansen, S., Jensen, P., Richter, E., and Turcotte, L., Membrane associated fatty acid binding protein (FABPpm) in human skeletal muscle is increased by endurance training, *Biochem. Biophys. Res. Comm.*, 231, 463, 1997.

65. Turcotte, L., Richter, E., and Kiens, B., Increased plasma FFA uptake and oxidation during prolonged exercise in trained vs. untrained humans, *Am. J. Physiol.*, 262, E791, 1992.

66. Turcotte, L. P., Swenberger, J. R., Tucker, M. Z., and Yee, A. J., Training-induced elevation in FABP(PM) is associated with increased palmitate use in contracting muscle, *J. Applied Physiol.*, 87, 285, 1999.
67. Man, M. Z., Hui, T. Y., Schaffer, J. E., Lodish, H. F., and Bernlohr, D. A., Regulation of the murine adipocyte fatty acid transporter gene by insulin, *Mol. Endocrinol.*, 10, 1021, 1996.
68. Hui, T. Y., Frohnert, B. I., Smith, A. J., Schaffer, J. E., and Bernlohr, D. A., Characterization of the murine fatty acid transport protein gene and its insulin response sequence, *J. Biol. Chem.*, 273, 27420, 1998.
69. Greenwalt, D. E., Scheck, S. H., and Rhinehart-Jones, T., Heart CD36 expression is increased in murine models of diabetes and in mice fed a high fat diet, *J. Clin. Invest.*, 96, 1382, 1995.
70. Poirier, H., Degrace, P., Niot, I., Bernard, A., and Besnard, P., Localization and regulation of the putative membrane fatty-acid transporter (FAT) in the small intestine. Comparison with fatty acid-binding proteins (FABP), *Eur. J. Biochem.*, 238, 368, 1996.
71. Motojima, K., Passilly, P., Peters, J., Gonzalez, F. J., and Latruffe, N., Expression of putative fatty acid transporter genes are regulated by peroxisome proliferator-activated receptor α and γ activators in a tissue- and inducer-specific manner, *J. Biol. Chem.*, 273, 16710, 1998.
72. Martin, G., Schoonjans, K., Lefebvre, A., Staels, B., and Auwerx, J., Coordinate regulation of the expression of the fatty acid transport protein and acyl-CoA synthetase genes by PPAR α and PPAR γ activators, *J. Biol. Chem.*, 272, 28210, 1997.
73. Bass, N. M., The cellular fatty acid binding proteins: Aspects of structure, regulation, and function, *Intl. Rev. Cytol.*, 3, 143, 1988.
74. Cohn, S. M., Simon, T. C., Roth, K. A., Birkenmeier, E. H., and Gordon, J. I., Use of transgenic mice to map cis-acting elements in the intestinal fatty acid binding protein gene (Fabpi) that control its cell lineage-specific and regional patterns of expression along the duodenal-colonic and crypt-villus axes of the gut epithelium, *J. Cell. Biol.*, 119, 27, 1992.
75. Suzuki, T., Hitomi, M., and Ono, T., Immunohistochemical distribution of hepatic fatty acid-binding protein in rat and human alimentary tract, *J. Histochem. Cytochem.*, 36, 349, 1988.
76. Iseki, S., Hitomi, M., Ono, T., and Kondo, H., Immunocytochemical localization of hepatic fatty acid binding protein in the rat intestine: Effect of fasting, *Anat. Rec.*, 223, 283, 1989.
77. Bass, N. M., Manning, J. A., Ockner, R. K., Gordon, J. I., Seetharam, S., and Alpers, D. H., Regulation of the biosynthesis of two distinct fatty acid-binding proteins in rat liver and intestine: Influences of sex difference and clofibrate, *J. Biol. Chem.*, 260, 1432, 1985.
78. Gordon, J. I., Smith, D. P., Alpers, D. H., and Strauss, A. W., Cloning of a complementary deoxyribonucleic acid encoding a portion of rat intestinal preapolipoprotein AIV messenger ribonucleic acid, *Biochemistry*, 21, 5424, 1982.
79. Bass, N. M. and Manning, J. A., Tissue expression of three structurally different fatty acid binding proteins from rat heart muscle, liver, and intestine, *Biochem. Biophys. Res. Comm.*, 137, 929, 1986.
80. Spiegelman, B. M. and Green, H., Control of specific protein biosynthesis during the adipose conversion of 3T3 cells, *J. Biol. Chem.*, 255, 8811, 1980.

81. Bass, N. M., Manning, J. A., and Ockner, R. K., Turnover and short-term regulation of fatty acid binding protein in liver, *J. Biol. Chem.,* 260, 9603, 1985.

82. Malewiak, M.-I., Bass, N. M., Griglio, S., and Ockner, R. K., Influence of genetic obesity and of fat-feeding on hepatic FABP concentration and activity, *Intl. J. Obesity,* 12, 543, 1988.

83. St. John, L. C., Rule, D. C., Knabe, D. A., Mersmann, H. J., and Smith, S. B., Fatty acid-binding protein activity in tissues from pigs fed diets containing 0 and 20% high oleate oil, *J. Nutr.,* 117, 2021, 1987.

84. Veerkamp, J. H. and van Moerkerk, H. T. B., Fatty acid-binding protein and its relation to fatty acid oxidation, *Mol. Cell. Biochem.,* 123, 101, 1993.

85. Lin, M. C., Arbeeny, C., Bergquist, K., Kienzle, B., Gordon, D. A., and Wetterau, J. R., Cloning and regulation of hamster microsomal triglyceride transfer protein. The regulation is independent from that of other hepatic and intestinal proteins which participate in the transport of fatty acids and triglycerides, *J. Biol. Chem.,* 269, 29138, 1994.

86. Poirier, H., Niot, I., Degrace, P., Monnot, M., Bernard, A., and Besnard, P., Fatty acid regulation of fatty acid-binding protein expression in the small intestine, *Am. J. Physiol.,* 273, G289, 1997.

87. Gordon, J. I., Elshourbagy, N., Lowe, J. B., Liao, W. S., Alpers, D. H., and Taylor, J. M., Tissue specific expression and developmental regulation of two genes coding for rat fatty acid binding proteins, *J. Biol. Chem.,* 260, 1995, 1985.

88. Sheridan, M., Wilkinson, T. C. I., and Wilton, D. C., Studies on fatty acid-binding proteins: Changes in the concentration of hepatic fatty acid-binding protein during development in the rat, *Biochem. J.,* 242, 919, 1987.

89. Stein, L. B., Mishkin, S., Fleischner, G. M., Gatmaitan, Z., and Arias, I. M., Effect of fasting on hepatic ligandin, Z protein, and organic anion transfer, *Am. J. Physiol.,* 231, 1371, 1976.

90. Iseki, S., Kondo, H., Hitomi, M., and Ono, T., Localization of liver fatty acid-binding protein and its mRNA in the liver and jejunum of rats; an immuno-histochemical and in situ hybridization study, *Mol. Cell. Biochem.,* 98, 27, 1990.

91. Iseki, S. and Kondo, H., Light microscopic localization of hepatic fatty acid binding protein mRNA in jejunal epithelia of rats using in situ hybridization, immunohistochemical, and autoradiographic techniques, *J. Histochem. Cytochem.,* 38, 111, 1990.

92. Bass, N.M., Kaikaus, R. M., and Ockner, R. K., Physiology and molecular biology of hepatic cytosolic fatty acid-binding protein, in *Hepatic Transport and Bile Secretion: Physiology and Pathophysiology,* N. Tavolini and P.D. Berk, Eds., Raven Press, New York, 1993, 421.

93. Brandes, R. and Arad, R., Liver cytosolic fatty acid-binding proteins. Effect of diabetes and starvation, *Biochim. Biophys. Acta,* 750, 334, 1983.

94. Nakagawa, S., Kawashima, Y., Hirose, A., and Kozuka, H., Regulation of hepatic level of fatty-acid-binding protein by hormones and clofibric acid in the rat, *Biochem. J.,* 297, 581, 1994.

95. Rubin, D. C., Swietlicki, E., Roth, K. A., and Gordon, J. I., Use of fetal intestinal isografts from normal and transgenic mice to study the programming of positional information along the duodenal-to-colonic-axis, *J. Biol. Chem.,* 267, 15122, 1992.

96. Hauft, S. M., Sweetser, D. A., Rotwein, P. S., Lajara, R., Hoppe, P. C., Birkenmeier, E. H., and Gordon, J. I., A transgenic mouse model that is useful for analyzing cellular and geographic differentiation of the intestine during fetal development, *J. Biol. Chem.,* 264, 8419, 1989.

97. Sweetser, D. A., Hauft, S. M., Hoppe, P. C., Birkenmeier, E. H., and Gordon, J. I., Transgenic mice containing intestinal fatty acid-binding protein-human growth hormone fusion genes exhibit correct regional and cell-specific expression of the reporter gene in their small intestine, *Proc. Natl. Acad. Sci. USA*, 85, 9611, 1988.

98. Melki, S. A. and Abumrad, N. A., Expression of the adipocyte fatty acid-binding protein in streptozotocin-diabetes: Effects of insulin deficiency and supplementation, *J. Lipid Res.*, 34, 1527, 1993.

99. Smas, C. M. and Sul, H. S., Control of adipocyte differentiation, *Biochem. J.*, 309, 697, 1995.

100. Sul, H. S., Smas, C. M., and Moustaïd, N., Positive and negative regulators of adipocyte differentiation, *J. Nutr. Biochem.*, 4, 554, 1993.

101. Amri, E., Bertrand, B., and Grimaldi, P., Regulation of adipose cell differentiation: I. Fatty acids are inducers of the aP2 gene expression, *J. Lipid Res.*, 32, 1449, 1991.

102. Cook, J. S., Lucas, J. J., Sibley, E., Bolanowski, M. A., Christy, R. J., Kelly, T. J., and Lane, M. D., Expression of the differentiation-induced gene for fatty acid-binding protein is activated by glucocorticoid and cAMP, *Proc. Natl. Acad. Sci. USA*, 85, 2949, 1988.

103. Blake, W. L. and Clarke, S. D., Induction of adipose fatty acid binding protein (a-FABP) by insulin-like growth factor-1 (IGF-1) in 3T3-L1 preadipocytes, *Biochem. Biophys. Res. Comm.*, 173, 87, 1990.

104. MacDougald, O. A. and Lane, M. D., Transcriptional regulation of gene expression during adipocyte differentiation, *Annu. Rev. Biochem.*, 64, 345, 1995.

105. Grimaldi, P. A., Knobel, S. M., Whitesell, R. R., and Abumrad, N. A., Induction of aP2 gene expression by nonmetabolized long-chain fatty acids, *Proc. Natl. Acad. Sci. USA*, 89, 10930, 1992.

106. Distel, R. J., Robinson, G. S., and Spiegelman, B. M., Fatty acid regulation of gene expression: Transcriptional and post-transcriptional mechanisms, *J. Biol. Chem.*, 267, 5937, 1992.

107. van Breda, E., Keizer, H. A., Vork, M. M., Surtel, D. A., de Jong, Y. F., Van der Vusse, G. J., and Glatz, J. F., Modulation of fatty-acid-binding protein content of rat heart and skeletal muscle by endurance training and testosterone treatment, *Euro. J. Physiol.*, 421, 274, 1992.

108. Claffey, K. P., Herrera, V. L., Brecher, P., and Ruiz-Opazo, N., Cloning and tissue distribution of rat heart fatty acid binding protein mRNA: Identical forms in heart and skeletal muscle, *Biochemistry*, 26, 7900, 1987.

109. Bonen, A., Luiken, J. J. F. P., Liu, S., Dyck, D., Kiens, B., Kristiansen, S., Turcotte, L., Van der Vusse, G. J., and Glatz, J. F. C., Palmitate transport and fatty acid transporters in red and white muscles, *Am. Physiol. Soc.*, 193, 1849, 1998.

110. Rump, R., Buhlmann, C., Borchers, T., and Spener, F., Differentiation-dependent expression of heart type fatty acid-binding protein in C2C12 muscle cells, *Eur. J. Cell. Biol.*, 69, 135, 1996.

111. Fournier, N. C. and Rahim, M., Control of energy production in the heart: A new function for fatty acid binding protein, *Biochemistry*, 24, 2387, 1985.

112. Jones, P. D., Carne, A., Bass, N. M., and Grigor, M. R., Isolation and characterization of fatty acid binding proteins from mammary tissue of lactating rats, *Biochem. J.*, 251, 919, 1988.

113. Carey, J. O., Neufer, P. D., Farrar, R. P., Veerkamp, J. H., and Dohm, G. L., Transcriptional regulation of muscle fatty acid-binding protein, *Biochem. J.*, 298, 613, 1994.
114. Heuckeroth, R. O., Birkenmeier, E. H., Levin, M. S., and Gordon, J. I., Analysis of the tissue-specific expression, developmental regulation, and linkage relationships of a rodent gene encoding heart fatty acid binding protein, *J. Biol. Chem.*, 262, 9709, 1987.
115. Veerkamp, J. H., van Moerkerk, H. T. B., and Van den Born, J., No correlation between changes in fatty acid-binding protein content and fatty acid oxidation capacity of rat tissues in experimental diabetes, *Int. J. Biochem. Cell. Biol.*, 28, 473, 1996.
116. Glatz, J. F. C., van Breda, E., Keizer, H. A., de Jong, Y. F., Lakey, J. R. T., Rajotte, R. V., Thompson, A., Van der Vusse, G. J., and Lopaschuk, G. D., Rat heart fatty acid-binding protein content is increased in experimental diabetes, *Biochem. Biophys. Res. Comm.*, 199, 639, 1994.
117. Sakai, K., Fujii, H., Yamamoto, T., Sakakibara, J., Izumi, T., Shibata, A., and Ono, T., Tissue-specific suppression of aortic faty-acid-binding protein in streptozotocin-induced diabetic rats, *Eur. J. Biochem.*, 229, 201, 1995.
118. Veerkamp, J. H. and Maatman, R. G. H. J., Cytoplasmic fatty acid-binding proteins: Their structure and genes, *Prog. Lipid Res.*, 34, 17, 1995.
119. Ibrahimi, A., Teboul, L., Gaillard, D., Amri, E. Z., Ailhaud, G. P., Young, P., Cawthorne, M. A., and Grimaldi, P. A., Evidence for a common mechanism of action for fatty acids and thiazolidinedione antidiabetic agents on gene expression in preadipose cells, *Mol. Pharmacol.*, 46, 1070, 1994.
120. Issemann, I. and Green, S., Activation of a member of the steroid hormone receptor superfamily by peroxisome proliferators, *Nature*, 347, 645, 1990.
121. Desvergne, B., IJpenberg, A., Devchand, P. R., and Wahli, W., The peroxisome proliferator-activated receptors at the cross-road of diet and hormonal signalling, *J. Steroid Biochem. Molec. Biol.*, 65, 65, 1998.
122. Vamecq, J. and Latruffe, N., Medical significance of peroxisome proliferator-activated receptors, *Lancet*, 354, 141, 1999.
123. Vanden Heuvel, J. P., Peroxisome proliferator-activated receptors: a critical link among fatty acids, gene expression and carcinogenesis, *J. Nutr.*, 129, 575S, 1999.
124. Schoonjans, K., Staels, B., and Auwerx, J., Role of the peroxisome proliferator-activated receptor (PPAR) in mediating the effects of fibrates and fatty acids on gene expression, *J. Lipid Res.*, 37, 907, 1996.
125. Latruffe, N. and Vamecq, J., Peroxisome proliferators and peroxisome proliferator activated receptors (PPARs) as regulators of lipid metabolism, *Biochimie*, 79, 81, 1997.
126. Murakami, K., Ide, T., Suzuki, M., Mochizuki, T., and Kadowaki, T., Evidence for direct binding of fatty acids and eicosenoids to human peroxisome proliferators-activated receptor alpha, *Biochem. Biophys. Res. Comm.*, 260, 609, 1999.
127. Lin, Q., Ruuska, S. E., Shaw, N. S., Dong, D., and Noy, N., Ligand selectivity of the peroxisome proliferator-activated receptor α, *Biochemistry*, 38, 185, 1999.
128. Kliewer, S. A., Sundseth, S. S., Jones, S. A., Brown, P. J., Wisely, G. B., Koble, C. S., Devchand, P., Wahli, W., Willson, T. M., Lenhard, J. M., and Lehmann, J. M., Fatty acids and eicosanoids regulate gene expression through direct interactions with peroxisome proliferator-activated receptors α and γ, *Proc. Natl. Acad. Sci. USA*, 94, 4318, 1997.

129. Dowell, P., Ishmael, J. E., Avram, D., Peterson, V. J., Nevrivy, D. J., and Leid, M., p300 functions as a coactivator for the peroxisome proliferator-activated receptor alpha, *J. Biol. Chem.*, 272, 33435, 1997.

130. Xu, H. E., Lambert, M. H., Montana, V. G., Parks, D. J., Blanchard, S. G., Brown, P. J., Sternbach, D. D., Lehmann, J. M., Wisely, G. B., Willson, T. M., Kliewer, S. A., and Milburn, M. V., Molecular recognition of fatty acids by peroxisome proliferator-activated receptors, *Mol. Cell*, 3, 397, 1999.

131. Pineda Torra, I., Gervois, P., and Staels, B., Peroxisome proliferator-activated receptor alpha in metabolic disease, inflammation, atherosclerosis and aging, *Curr. Opin. Lipidol.*, 10, 151, 1999.

132. Aoyama, T., Peters, J., Iritani, N., Nakajima, T., Furihata, K., Hashimoto, T., and Gonzalez, F. J., Altered constitutive expression of fatty acid-metabolizing enzymes in mice lacking the peroxisome proliferator-activated receptor α (PPARα), *J. Biol. Chem.*, 273, 5678, 1998.

133. Schoonjans, K., Peinado-Onsurbe, J., Lefebvre, A., Heyman, R. A., Briggs, M., Deeb, S., Staels, B., and Auwerx, J., PPARα and PPARγ activators direct a distinct tissue-specific transcriptional response via a PPRE in the lipoprotein lipase gene, *EMBO J.*, 15, 5336, 1996.

134. Frohnert, B. I., Hui, T. Y., and Bernlohr, D. A., Identification of a functional peroxisome proliferator-responsive element in the murine fatty acid transport protein gene, *J. Biol. Chem.*, 274, 3970, 1999.

135. Kaikaus, R. M., Sui, Z., Lysenko, N., Wu, N. Y., Ortiz de Montellano, P. R., Ockner, R. K., and Bass, N. M., Regulation of pathways of extramitochondrial fatty acid oxidation and liver fatty acid-binding protein by long-chain monocarboxylic fatty acids in hepatocytes: Effect of inhibition of carnitine palmitoyltransferase I, *J. Biol. Chem.*, 268, 26866, 1993.

136. Forman, B. M., Chen, J., and Evans, R. M., Hypolipidemic drugs, polyunsaturated fatty acids, and eicosanoids are ligands for peroxisome proliferator-activated receptors α and δ, *Proc. Natl. Acad. Sci. USA*, 94, 4312, 1997.

137. Issemann, I., Prince, R. A., Tugwood, J. D., and Green, S., A role for fatty acids and liver fatty acid binding protein in peroxisome proliferation?, *Biochem. Soc. Trans.*, 20, 824, 1992.

138. Kaikaus, R. M., Chan, W. K., Ortiz de Montellano, P. R., and Bass, N. M., Mechanisms of regulation of liver fatty acid-binding protein, *Mol. Cell. Biochem.*, 123, 93, 1993.

139. Kawashima, Y., Nakagawa, S., Tachibana, Y., and Kozuka, H., Effects of peroxisome proliferators on fatty acid-binding protein in rat liver, *Biochim. Biophys. Acta*, 754, 21, 1983.

140. Pignon, J. P., Bailey, N. C., Baraona, E., and Lieber, C. S., Fatty acid-binding protein: a major contributor to the ethanol-induced increase in liver cytosolic proteins in the rat, *Hepatology*, 7, 865, 1987.

141. Kaikaus, R. M., Chan, W. K., Lysenko, N., Ray, R., Ortiz de Montellano, P. R., and Bass, N. M., Induction of peroxisomal fatty acid β-oxidation and liver fatty acid-binding protein by peroxisome proliferators: Mediation via the cytochrome P-450IVA1 ω-hydroxylase pathway, *J. Biol. Chem.*, 268, 9593, 1993.

142. Kersten, S., Seydoux, J., Peters, J. M., Gonzalez, F. J., Desvergne, B., and Wahli, W., Peroxisome proliferator-activated receptor alpha mediates the adaptive response to fasting, *J. Clin. Invest.*, 103, 1489, 1999.

143. Besnard, P., Mallordy, A., and Carlier, H., Transcriptional induction of the fatty acid binding protein gene in mouse liver by bezafibrate, *FEBS Lett.*, 327, 219, 1993.

144. Poirier, H., Braissant, O., Niot, I., Wahli, W., and Besnard, P., 9-*cis*-retinoic acid enhances fatty acid-induced expression of the liver fatty acid-binding protein gene, *FEBS Lett.*, 412, 480, 1997.

145. Meunier-Durmort, C., Poirier, N., Noit, I., Forest, C., and Besnard, P., Up-regulation of the expression of the gene for liver fatty acid-binding protein by long-chain fatty acids, *Biochem. J.*, 319, 483, 1996.

146. Clarke, S. D. and Armstrong, M. K., Cellular lipid binding proteins: expression, function, and nutritional regulation, *FASEB J.*, 3, 2480, 1989.

147. Teboul, L., Gaillard, D., Staccini, L., Inadera, H., Amri, E. Z., and Grimaldi, P. A., Thiazolidinediones and fatty acids convert myogenic cells into adipose-like cells, *J. Biol. Chem.*, 270, 28183, 1995.

148. Tontonoz, P., Hu, E., and Spiegelman, B. M., Regulation of adipocyte gene expression and differentiation by peroxisome proliferator activated receptor γ, *Curr. Opin. Genet. Develop.*, 5, 571, 1995.

149. Spitsberg, V. L., Matitashvili, E., and Gorewit, R. C., Association and coexpression of fatty-acid-binding protein and glycoprotein CD36 in the bovine mammary gland, *Eur. J. Biochem.*, 230, 872, 1995.

150. Gordon, J. I., Alpers, D. H., Ockner, R. K., and Strauss, A. W., The nucleotide sequence of rat liver fatty acid binding protein mRNA, *J. Biol. Chem.*, 258, 3356, 1983.

151. Takahashi, K., Odani, S., and Ono, T., A close structural relationship of rat liver Z-protein to cellular retinoid binding proteins and peripheral nerve myelin p2 protein, *Biochem. Biophys. Res. Comm.*, 106, 1099, 1982.

152. Alpers, D. H., Strauss, A. W., Ockner, R. K., Bass, N. M., and Gordon, J. I., Cloning of a cDNA encoding rat intestinal fatty acid binding protein, *Proc. Natl. Acad. Sci. USA*, 81, 313, 1984.

153. Sacchettini, J. C., Said, B., Schulz, H., and Gordon, J. I., Rat heart fatty acid-binding protein is highly homologous to the murine adipocyte 422 protein and the P2 protein of peripheral nerve myelin, *J. Biol. Chem.*, 261, 8218, 1986.

154. Spiegelman, B. M., Frank, M., and Green, H., Molecular cloning of mRNA from 3T3 adipocytes: Regulation of mRNA content for glycerophosphate dehydrogenase and other differentiation-dependent proteins during adipocyte development, *J. Biol. Chem.*, 258, 10083, 1983.

155. Bernlohr, D. A., Angus, C. W., Lane, M. D., Bolanowski, M. A., and Kelly, Jr., T. J., Expression of specific mRNAs during adipose differentiation: Identification of an mRNA encoding a homologue of myelin P2 protein, *Proc. Natl. Acad. Sci. USA*, 81, 5468, 1984.

156. Kurtz, A., Zimmer, A., Schnutgen, F., Bruning, G., Spener, F., and Muller, T., The expression pattern of a novel gene encoding brain-fatty acid binding protein correlates with neuronal and glial cell development, *Development*, 120, 2637, 1994.

157. Madsen, P., Rasmussen, H. H., Leffers, H., Honore, B., and Celis, J. E., Molecular cloning and expression of a novel keratinocyte protein (psoriasis-associated fatty acid-binding protein [PA-FABP]) that is highly up-regulated in psoriatic skin and that shares similarity to fatty acid-binding proteins, *J. Invest. Dermatol.*, 99, 299, 1992.

158. Narayanan V., Barbosa E., Reed R., and Tennekoon G., Characterization of a cloned cDNA encoding rabbit myelin P2 protein, *J. Biol. Chem.*, 263, 8332, 1988.
159. Tontonoz, P., Hu, E., Graves, R. A., Budavari, A. I., and Spiegelman, B. M., mPPAR gamma 2: tissue-specific regulator of an adipocyte enhancer, *Genes Dev.*, 8, 1224, 1994.

7

Alcohol and Gene Expression in the Central Nervous System

Matthew T. Reilly, Christoph Fehr, and Kari J. Buck

CONTENTS

7.1 Introduction 132
7.2 Ligand-Gated Receptors 132
    7.2.1 NMDA Receptors 132
    7.2.2 GABA$_A$ Receptors... 137
    7.2.3 Glycine Receptors 139
7.3 Voltage-Operated Channels... 140
    7.3.1 L-Type Calcium Channels... 140
7.4 G-Protein Coupled Receptors 141
    7.4.1 Dopamine Receptors 141
    7.4.2 Serotonin Receptors... 143
    7.4.3 Noradrenergic Receptors 144
    7.4.4 Opioid Receptors.. 145
    7.4.5 Other G-Protein Coupled Receptors 145
7.5 Neurotransmitter Transporters 146
    7.5.1 Dopamine Transporter 146
    7.5.2 Serotonin Transporter.. 146
7.6 Second Messenger Systems 147
    7.6.1 G-Proteins.. 147
    7.6.2 Adenylyl Cyclase 147
7.7 Transcription Factors 147
    7.7.1 cAMP Responsive Element-Binding Protein (CREBP)............. 147
    7.7.2 Immediate Early Genes (IEGs)... 148
    7.7.3 Retinoic Acid Receptors (RARs) 148
7.8 Growth Factors... 150
7.9 Summary 150
References 152

0-8493-2216-2/01/$0.00+$1.50
© 2001 by CRC Press LLC

7.1   Introduction

Alcohol is one of the most widely used chemical substances in our society. Nearly 75% of American adults use alcohol, and 15% of these adults develop life-long health problems associated with its abuse. Alcohol dependence (alcoholism) is characterized by the development of tolerance (a reduction in the effect of alcohol after single or repeated administration), withdrawal (a state of central nervous system hyperexcitability once alcohol is removed), and a maladaptive pattern of use (loss of control).[1] Why some individuals become alcoholics and others do not has been a question under active investigation by researchers for a number of years. There are clear genetic components to the multidimensional disorder of alcoholism supported by half-sibling and adoption studies.[2-5]

Animal models also provide evidence for the role that genetics plays in the development of alcohol dependence and other drug-related disorders.[6] However, no one animal model of alcoholism encompasses every aspect involved with the disorder, but some key advantages of using animal models are (1) the experimenter controls the genotype, i.e., reduced heterogeneity; (2) a plethora of inbred strains are available in both rats and mice for testing; and (3) the use of forward and reverse genetic techniques can be utilized.[6] Even though these studies indicate that genetics are an important factor in determining susceptibility for the development of alcoholism, the specific genes involved and their mode of regulation have yet to be identified.

Alcohol affects a wide range of activities in the central nervous system including the activity of numerous genes expressed within this system (Fig. 7.1). Thus, understanding the genetics underlying the development of alcoholism will require not only the identification of the genes involved but also how alcohol regulates their expression. The aim of this chapter is to present and discuss findings on how alcohol (ethanol) affects the expression of genes in the central nervous system (CNS), and how this might result in the development of alcoholism. Our review will focus on ethanol's effects on gene expression *in vivo* within the central nervous system. Other reviews have recently focused on the effects of ethanol on expression in cultured cells, and the effects of ethanol outside the central nervous system. These data are reviewed elsewhere in several excellent reviews.[7-9]

7.2   Ligand-Gated Receptors

7.2.1   NMDA Receptors

Glutamate is the primary mediator of excitatory neurotransmission in the mammalian brain, and studies have suggested a role for glutamate in ethanol

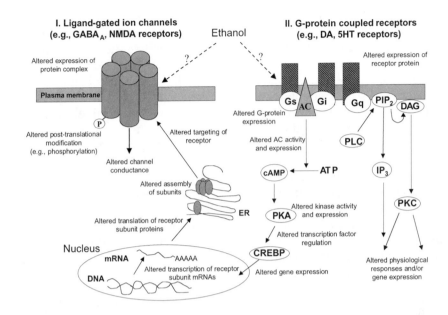

FIGURE 7.1

Potential adaptations of neurotransmitter receptors after chronic ethanol exposure in animal models of ethanol physical dependence. (I) Ligand-gated ion channels. GABA$_A$ and NMDA receptors are two examples of ligand-gated ion channels that are affected by chronic ethanol exposure. GABA$_A$ receptors are the primary sites of inhibitory neurotransmission, while NMDA receptors mediate excitatory neurotransmission in the mammalian brain. These receptors are thought to be constructed from four to five subunits, and modulate neuronal activity by changes in channel conductance. GABA$_A$ receptors are permeable to Cl$^-$ ions, while NMDA receptors are permeable to Ca^{2+} and monovalent cations. There is evidence to suggest several mechanisms by which chronic ethanol exposure alters these ion channels including functional alterations in channel conductance, altered transcription of receptor subunit mRNAs, altered translation of receptor subunit proteins, altered assembly of receptor subunits, altered targeting of receptor to plasma membrane, altered post-translational modifications, and altered expression of the protein complex. (II) G-protein coupled receptors. DA and 5HT receptors are two examples of G-protein coupled receptors affected by chronic ethanol exposure. There are multiple subclasses of DA receptors (e.g., D1 and D2) that are either positively or negatively coupled to AC. There also exist several subclasses of 5HT receptors (e.g., 5HT-2A and 5HT-2C) that are coupled to the phosphoinositol second messenger pathway. Chronic ethanol exposure may alter G-protein coupled receptors and their associated second messenger pathways through several mechanisms, including altered expression of G-proteins, altered AC activity and expression, altered protein kinase activity and expression (e.g., PKA and PKC), altered transcription factor regulation (e.g., CREBP), and altered expression of receptor proteins. Any of these alterations may affect a host of other physiological responses downstream of the receptor (e.g., gene expression, phosphorylation of ion channels, general metabolism, and neurotransmitter synthesis). It is not known if ethanol interacts directly or indirectly to produce these effects.

Abbreviations: γ-aminobutyric acid type A receptor (GABA$_A$), N-methyl-D-asparate receptor (NMDA), dopamine (DA), 5-hydroxytryptamine (5-HT), adenylyl cyclase (AC), protein kinase A (PKA), protein kinase C (PKC), phospholipase C (PLC), phosphoinositolbishophate (PIP$_2$), inositoltriphosphate (IP$_3$), cAMP responsive element-binding protein (CREBP), diacylglycerol (DAG).

dependence.[10] Glutamate-N-methyl-D-aspartic acid (NMDA) receptors are linked to a voltage-sensitive ion channel permeable to calcium and monovalent cations (e.g., Na[+], K[+]). This receptor contains binding sites for a number of amino acids including glutamate, glycine (a co-agonist required for activation), D-serine, and L-aspartate. In addition, the NMDA receptor contains binding sites for the dissociative anesthetic phencyclidine (PCP), and dizcolipine (MK-801), which work as noncompetitive antagonists. The NMDA receptor is thought to be constructed of five subunits. There are two major classes of NMDA subunits: NR1 (ζ1 in the mouse) with eight possible splice variants, and NR2 of which there are four distinct subtypes (NR2A, -2B, -2C, and -2D; ε1 to 4 in the mouse, respectively). Both classes of NMDA receptor subunits show distinct brain regional distributions, which provide for a great degree of receptor heterogeneity and suggest functionally distinct isoforms of the receptor. Along these lines, acute ethanol has been found to inhibit NMDA receptor responses in certain brain regions (e.g., inferior colliculus and hippocampus), while having no effect in others (lateral septum).[11]

Receptor binding studies of NMDA receptors after chronic ethanol have produced somewhat contradictory results (Table 7.1). Early studies reported both increases and decreases in the density of [3H]glutamate-binding sites after acute and chronic ethanol.[12,13] Chronic ethanol also increases the binding density of [3H]MK-801 in certain brain regions,[14–16] but some studies have reported no change with 4 to 8 months of ethanol exposure.[17] Thus, it is unclear whether the effects of chronic ethanol are reflected consistently in changes in binding site densities of the NMDA receptor. These contradictory results have forced researchers to investigate more specific molecular mechanisms resulting from chronic ethanol exposure. Specifically, researchers have begun to focus on the effects of chronic ethanol on the expression of NMDA receptor subunits.

TABLE 7.1

Effect of Chronic *in Vivo* Ethanol Administration on Ligand and Voltage-Operated Ion Channels, Receptor Recognition Sites, and mRNA and Peptide Expression in the Brain

Receptor /Property	Alteration	Refs.
Ligand-Gated Ion Channels		
NMDA Receptor		
[3H]glutamate binding [c]	Increased	12
	Decreased	13
[3H]MK-801 binding [a, c]	Increased	14
		15, 16
	No change	17
NR2A mRNA and peptides [a, b, c, e]	Increased	18–20, 23
	No change	18, 21
NR2B mRNA and peptides [a, b, c]	Increased	18, 19, 21–23
	No change	18

TABLE 7.1 (CONTINUED)

Effect of Chronic *in Vivo* Ethanol Administration on Ligand and Voltage-Operated Ion Channels, Receptor Recognition Sites, and mRNA and Peptide Expression in the Brain

Receptor /Property	Alteration	Refs.
NR2C mRNA [a, b]	No change	18, 21
NR1 mRNA and peptides [a, b, c, e]	Increased	19, 20, 23
	No change	18, 20, 21
NR1 (5′ insert) mRNA [a]	Decreased	21
NR1 (3′ insert) mRNA [a]	No change	21
GABA$_A$ Receptor		
GABA-mediated Cl⁻ flux [a, b]	Decreased	28, 29, 40, 46
	No change	30, 33
Pentobarbital-enhanced Cl⁻ flux [a]	Decreased	28
	No change	30
Benzodiazepine-enhanced Cl⁻ flux [a]	Decreased	30
Inverse agonist-inhibition of Cl⁻ flux [a]	Increased	30
Low affinity [³H]GABA binding [d]	Decreased	35
[³H]Flunitrazepam binding [a, b]	No change	37–39
[³H]zolpidem binding [a, b]	Increased	48
	No change	49
[³H]Ro 15-4513 binding [a, b]	Increased	54, 55
α_1 subunit mRNA and peptides [a-d]	Decreased	41–45, 47, 51, 61, 65
α_2 subunit mRNA and peptides [a]	Decreased	42–44
α_3 subunit mRNA [a]	No change	42, 44
α_4 subunit mRNA and peptides [a, c]	Increased	45, 47, 63
	No change	62
α_5 subunit mRNA [a, c]	Increased	45
	No change	61
α_6 subunit mRNA and peptides [b]	Increased	43, 51, 52
β_1 subunit mRNA [a]	Increased	57
β_1 subunit mRNA [a]	No change	45
β_2 subunit mRNA and peptides [c, d]	Increased	47, 57
β_2 subunit mRNA and peptides [a, b, c]	Increased	58, 59
	No change	45, 58, 62
β_3 subunit mRNA and peptides [a, c]	Increased	47, 57
	No change	45, 62
γ_1 subunit mRNA and peptides [a]	Increased	45, 47
γ_{2S} subunit mRNA [a]	Increased	45
γ_{2L} subunit mRNA [a]	No change	45
γ_2 subunit peptides [a, c]	No change	47, 62
γ_3 subunit mRNA [a]	No change	45
δ subunit mRNA [a]	No change	45
Glycine Receptor		
[³H]glycine binding [c]	No change	15
Voltage-Operated Channels		
L-Type Calcium Channel		
[³H]nitrendipine binding [a, d]	Increased	69, 70

[a] Cerebral cortex, [b]cerebellum, [c]hippocampus, [d]whole brain, [e]hypothalamus

Several studies have shown that chronic ethanol exposure alters the expression of both NR1 and NR2 subunits (Table 7.1). The hippocampus seems to be a brain region where most of the changes in NMDA receptor subunit messenger RNA (mRNA) and protein are observed, probably due to the high abundance of NMDA receptors in this region. Follesa and Ticku[18] found a 30% increase in both the NR2A and NR2B subunit mRNAs in rat hippocampus, but only in rats withdrawing from chronic ethanol. In addition, they also found similar increases in these subunit mRNAs in the cerebral cortex from the same rats, but found no changes in NR1 subunit mRNA at any time point or in any brain region tested (e.g., cerebral cortex, cerebellum, and hippocampus). This same group also found an upregulation of the NR1, NR2A, and NR2B subunit proteins by approximately 35% compared to both the hippocampus and cerebral cortex in ethanol-naive rats.[19] These observed increases in NMDA receptor subunit proteins returned to control values by 48 h, which parallels the disappearance of behavioral signs of withdrawal. Thus, these results suggest that alterations in NMDA receptor subunit expression following chronic ethanol could contribute to CNS hyperexcitability observed during ethanol withdrawal. Another group has reported increases compared to control values in NR1 subunit protein in the hippocampus and cerebellum (50 and 95%, respectively) as well as an upregulation of NR2A subunit protein in the hippocampus and cerebral cortex of mice (25 and 40%, respectively) with no alterations in these subunit mRNAs.[20] As mentioned previously the NR1 subunit may be expressed as one of eight possible alternatively spliced variants. In an attempt to delineate a role of individual NR1 splice variants, Hardy et al.[21] reported a decrease in mRNA encoding the NR1 subunit containing a 5′ insert compared to those lacking it in ethanol-dependent rats. This change persisted through 48 h of ethanol withdrawal. This 5′ NR1 subunit insert is located in the N-terminal domain of the protein. The authors suggest that reduced expression of the N-terminal domain insert may result in NMDA receptors that have a greater likelihood of agonist activation, and thus increased NMDA receptor function.[21] This result further supports the hypothesis that NMDA receptor function is increased as a consequence of chronic ethanol exposure.

Another report of mice made physically dependent on ethanol using a multiple withdrawal paradigm, which results in an exacerbation of seizure severity following repeated episodes of intoxication and withdrawal, has shown an increase in the ε2 subunit mRNA in the hippocampus which was greater than that in mice continuously exposed to ethanol (i.e., uninterrupted chronic ethanol exposure).[22] In contrast, this same treatment paradigm resulted in a greater increase in ε2 subunit mRNA in the cerebral cortex of continuously exposed mice compared to mice undergoing multiple ethanol withdrawals.[22] Thus, these results indicate that the type of ethanol treatment paradigm used differentially alters NMDA receptor subunits, and a previous withdrawal history influences NMDA receptor subunit gene expression. Gender is another important variable which may affect the expression of NMDA receptor subunits following chronic ethanol. Devaud and Morrow[23] reported gender-specific effects of chronic ethanol on the expression of NMDA receptor subunits in rats. They found that males showed increases in NR1 protein in the hippocampus, whereas females showed increases in the cerebral cortex and hypothalamus. In addition, hippocampal NR2A subunit protein was only increased in males, with no changes observed in females, while NR2B subunit protein was increased similarly in the cerebral cortex of both males and females.[23]

Taken together, these results suggest that ethanol regulates the expression of NMDA receptor subunit genes which may contribute to ethanol withdrawal-related CNS hyperexcitability. The majority of evidence points to an augmentation of NMDA receptor function following chronic ethanol as shown by upregulation of both NR1 and NR2 subunits in specific brain regions. This overexpression of NMDA receptor subunits might be a neuroadaptive mechanism by which the central nervous system compensates for the chronic inhibitory effects of ethanol.

7.2.2   GABA$_A$ Receptors

γ-Aminobutyric acid (GABA) is the major inhibitory neurotransmitter in the mammalian brain, and thus plays an important role in regulating neuronal excitability. GABA$_A$ receptors consist of a heterologous combination of subunits that are assembled as a pentamer and form a Cl$^-$ channel. The majority of these subunits exist in variant forms (e.g., α_{1-6}, β_{1-3}, γ_{1-3}, δ, and ε) which adds another degree of complexity to the structure of the GABA$_A$ receptor.[24-26] GABA$_A$ receptors are members of the ligand-gated ion channel superfamily of neurotransmitter receptors. The GABA$_A$ receptor contains several recognition sites for various sedative (e.g., benzodiazepines, barbiturates, neurosteroids) and convulsant agents (e.g., β-carbolines, picrotoxin) which are allosterically coupled to a Cl$^-$ channel. These agents work by allosterically modulating the actions of GABA at the GABA$_A$ receptor.

There is a substantial amount of evidence suggesting that both acute and chronic ethanol affect the GABA$_A$ receptor system.[27] It is widely established that GABA$_A$ receptor subunit genes are sensitive to ethanol manipulations (Table 7.1). These effects on gene expression have been demonstrated at the level of both mRNA and protein regulation after chronic ethanol. Alterations in GABA$_A$ receptor subunit expression following chronic ethanol could result in receptors with different functional and pharmacological properties from the native receptor. This hypothesis is supported by numerous functional studies of GABA$_A$ receptor activity following chronic ethanol treatment along with studies of recombinant GABA$_A$ receptors expressed in *Xenopus* oocytes or other expression systems.[28-32] Functional studies show that after chronic ethanol the ability of GABA to gate the associated Cl$^-$ channel is reduced, although some studies show no change.[28-30,33] In addition, while pentobarbital- and benzodiazepine-mediated ^{36}Cl$^-$ flux is also reduced, the ability of benzodiazepine inverse agonists (e.g., Ro 15-4513, DMCM) to inhibit ^{36}Cl$^-$ flux is enhanced.[28,30] Recombinant expression studies of GABA$_A$

receptors, which examine the relationships between subunit composition and receptor function show that different combinations of subunits confer different functional and pharmacological properties to the receptor.[24,34] These studies have also identified combinations of subunits that show differential responses to ethanol.[31,32] In light of this evidence, changes in $GABA_A$ receptor densities at various modulatory sites after chronic ethanol have not correlated well with measures of subunit expression and function.[35-40] Thus, it appears that altered expression of $GABA_A$ subunits is most likely reflected in the functional status of the receptor rather than in the total density of its modulatory binding sites. Therefore, understanding the underlying mechanisms of functional alterations will require a thorough understanding of how ethanol regulates $GABA_A$ receptor subunit gene expression.

$GABA_A$ receptor subunit expression is affected by chronic ethanol in several brain regions including the cerebral cortex, cerebellum, and hippocampus. In addition, subunit gene expression has been shown to be bi-directionally altered. Bi-directional expression patterns of $GABA_A$ receptor subunits might be a unique neuroadaptive mechanism by which the central nervous system compensates for the continued presence of ethanol without affecting receptor density. In the cerebral cortex the α subunit genes appear to show the most consistent changes with chronic ethanol. The α_1 and α_2 subunit mRNAs and peptides are decreased, while α_4 subunit mRNA and peptides are increased.[41-47] However, binding-site densities are slightly increased or unchanged for the selective α_1 subunit ligand, [³H]zolpidem, following chronic ethanol exposure in the cerebral cortex and cerebellum.[48-50] In contrast, α_3 and α_5 subunit mRNAs show no change.[41,42] In the cerebellum, the α_1 subunit mRNA and peptide are decreased, while the α_6 subunit mRNA peptide is increased.[43,44,51,52] The α_6 subunit is only found in the cerebellum and is thought to confer binding to a diazepam-insensitive site labeled by [³H]Ro 15-4513, a partial inverse agonist.[53] Thus, an increase in the α_6 with a concomitant decrease in the α_1 subunit might explain the upregulation of diazpam-insensitive [³H]Ro 15-4513 binding-site densities in the cerebellum,[54,55] and behavioral sensitization to benzodiazepine inverse agonist following chronic ethanol.[56]

After chronic ethanol the β subunits appear to show increases in expression in the cerebral cortex and cerebellum, but some studies have reported no change. For example, in a study conducted by Mhatre and Ticku[57] they found increases in all three β subunit mRNAs (i.e., β_1, β_2, and β_3) in rats chronically exposed to ethanol within the cerebral cortex. In contrast, Devaud et al.[45] found no changes in any of the β subunit mRNAs following ethanol treatment. We also found no consistent changes in the cerebral cortex for β_2 subunit mRNA in C57BL/6J (B6) or DBA/2J (D2) mice chronically exposed to ethanol for a period of 72 h.[58] Although in all these studies rodents were ethanol-dependent, there were variations in blood ethanol concentrations (BECs) maintained among the animals which might explain the discrepancies. For example, in the study by Mhatre and Ticku[57] rats had BECs of about 4.0 mg/ml, whereas in our study, Reilly and Buck,[58] and the study conducted by Devaud et al.[45] rodents had BECs between 1.0 and 2.0 mg/ml. These results suggest that the β subunit mRNAs might only be sensitive to ethanol regulation in the cerebral cortex at higher BECs, which may or may not reflect direct effects of chronic ethanol exposure. In contrast, we and others have reported increases in the β_2 subunit mRNA following chronic ethanol treatment in the cerebellum.[58,59] Using RNase protection analysis we found a differential regulation of β_2 subunit mRNA content in the cerebellum of B6 and D2 mice. The D2 strain was more sensitive to ethanol-induced increases in β_2 subunit mRNA content in the cerebellum, showing significant increases at lower blood ethanol concentrations than B6 mice. The ethanol-induced regulation in B6 mice appeared to be more complex, with decreases in β_2 subunit mRNA content at low blood ethanol concentrations, and increases at higher concentrations. These data suggest that differences between B6 and D2 mice in the degree of physical dependence (withdrawal) on ethanol may be related to differential sensitivity to ethanol regulation of β_2 subunit expression.

The hippocampus is another region that shows changes in GABA$_A$ receptor subunit expression after chronic ethanol, but in this region the changes observed seem to depend on duration of ethanol exposure. Decreases in subunit gene expression have been noted for the α_1 subunit mRNA and peptide after 12 weeks of chronic ethanol in rats,[61] while longer durations of exposure (e.g., 40 days) produce no change in α_1 peptide content.[62] In contrast, the α_4 subunit mRNA and peptides are found to be increased after either 40 days of continuous ethanol exposure, or after using a 60-day, chronic, intermittent ethanol exposure paradigm.[62,63] The hippocampus has not been found to show changes in $\beta_{2/3}$ peptide content.[62] In addition, γ_2 subunit peptide content shows no change after chronic ethanol exposure in this region.[62]

In summary, it is clear that GABA$_A$ receptor subunit gene expression is sensitive to ethanol manipulations. Alterations in subunit gene expression may alter the functional properties of the GABA$_A$ receptor, which seems to be a likely mechanism by which the central nervous system adapts to the continued presence of ethanol. Further studies will be needed to determine how altered subunit gene expression affects receptor assembly, post-translational modifications, and interactions with second messenger systems.

7.2.3   Glycine Receptors

Glycine, like GABA, is an inhibitory neurotransmitter that is primarily localized in the brain stem and spinal cord where it acts on strychnine-sensitive receptors.[65] Two types of subunits have been identified for the glycine receptor: an α subunit which has three isoforms denoted (α_{1-3}) and a β subunit. Despite low levels of strychnine binding in the forebrain, more specific molecular biological techniques have shown the presence of glycine receptor α subunits in the cerebral cortex,[66] and have provided evidence for a widespread distribution of the β subunit throughout the brain.[67] Receptor-binding studies have not shown changes in glycine receptor densities in the hippocampus of ethanol-dependent mice,[15] but as we have seen for $GABA_A$ and NMDA receptors a more specific analysis of subunit expression might indicate that the glycine receptor does contribute to ethanol withdrawal severity.

7.3   Voltage-Operated Channels

7.3.1   L-Type Calcium Channels

The L-type calcium channel is a member of the voltage-operated calcium channel family which also includes N, P, T, and Q-type channels. It is distinguished from the other voltage-operated calcium channels based on both electrophysiological and pharmacological properties. The L-type channel is activated under high voltage, and is blocked by dihydropyridines. The L-type channel consists of five subunit proteins (α_{1-2}, β, γ, and δ) of which the α_1 subunit is thought to be the major voltage sensor and pore-forming protein,[68] but the native subunit composition of the L-type channel is not known. In addition, how each subunit contributes to the functional properties of the channel has not been completely determined. However, the L-type calcium channel may represent an important target for regulation by chronic ethanol due to its effects on neurotransmitter release and second-messenger mediating functions in neurons.

Several studies have noted an upregulation of the L-type calcium channel following chronic ethanol exposure as determined by [³H]nitrendipine-binding-site densities.[69,70] For example, Guppy and Littleton[69] found a 40% increase in [³H]nitrendipine-binding sites in ethanol-dependent rats. To further examine the time course of changes in L-type calcium channel regulation by chronic ethanol, Guppy et al.[70] measured [³H]nitrendipine-binding-site densities in mice during (i.e., up to ten days) and after the induction of ethanol physical dependence (i.e., 8 and 24 h of withdrawal). In the cerebral cortex, [³H]nitrendipine-binding site densities show a sharp increase between days 3 and 4 and remain at this level throughout the 10-day ethanol exposure. This change in receptor density is preceded by a decrease in receptor affinity, which returns to control values by 6 days of exposure.[70] In contrast, [³H]nitrendipine-binding-site densities are reduced at 8 h of withdrawal compared to ethanol-dependent mice, and return to control values by 24 h of withdrawal.[70] These observed time-dependent changes in the regulation of L-type calcium channels by chronic ethanol correlate well with the time course of the appearance of ethanol withdrawal signs in mice.

This evidence suggests that the L-type calcium channels are potential targets of ethanol regulation which may contribute to ethanol withdrawal severity. Further studies will be needed to determine how this ethanol-induced upregulation of the L-type calcium channels occurs on a molecular level in terms of specific subunits.

7.4 G-Protein Coupled Receptors

7.4.1 Dopamine Receptors

Special interest has been raised on alterations in the dopaminergic system, since it is believed to be an important interface for multiple substances of abuse.[71] Behavioral studies of rodents administered electric currents intracranially have shown that electrical stimulation in the ventral tegmental area triggers repetitive self-stimulating behavior and a dopaminergic efflux in the nucleus accumbens core and shell.[72,73] Lesions of the pathway abolish the rewarding efficacy of multiple substances of abuse, e.g., ethanol, cocaine, and amphetamine.[74] Moreover, chronic intake of multiple substances of abuse like ethanol, cocaine, amphetamine, or opioids induces a dopamine efflux in the nucleus accumbens, which is important for the rewarding efficacy of these drugs.[71,75–78] These findings have initiated a number of investigations on the interactions between ethanol administration or withdrawal and the activity of the limbic and forebrain dopaminergic system.[79] Molecular-cloning studies have revealed at least five distinct dopaminergic receptors. The D_1 and the D_5 receptor subtypes belong to the D_1 family, while the D_2, D_3, and D_4 subtypes belong to the D_2-like group.[80]

Chronic ethanol treatment alters the expression of a number of dopaminergic receptors in a complex manner (see Table 7.2).[81] Two studies showed an increase in D_1-receptor binding sites in the striatum,[82–83] whereas three other groups failed to confirm this finding (see Table 7.2).[84–86] In the case of D_2 receptors three studies reported a strong increase in receptor binding or D_2 mRNA expression after chronic ethanol ingestion,[83,86,87] but these results were not replicated in independent studies (see Table 7.2).[84,85,88] There are several differences in ethanol treatment (injection vs. free choice two-bottle regimen) and duration (7 days vs. e.g., 7 months) among the investigations that strongly affect blood ethanol levels and subsequent gene expression. The expression of important target genes also varies on the genetic background of the animals. The ethanol-preferring C57BL/6J mice displayed higher D_1 and D_2 receptor mRNA content and higher D_1 and D_2 receptor densities in the limbic forebrain than the ethanol-avoiding DBA/2J strain under non-ethanol conditions.[89] Controversial findings might also result from an age dependent decline in receptor density, especially of D_2 receptors in the forebrain regions beginning at the age of 5 months as well in ethanol-treated animals as in the controls.[87] Fewer studies have been performed for the D_3, D_4, or the D_5 dopaminergic receptors. Eravci et al.[85] reported a decrease in dopamine D_3

TABLE 7.2

Expression of G-Protein Coupled Receptors and Related Peptides in the CNS after Chronic Ethanol Treatment

Receptor/Property	Alteration	Refs.
G-protein Coupled Receptors		
Dopamine Receptor		
[3H]SCH 23390 binding[a,e]	Increased	82, 83
	No change	84
D_1 mRNA[a,c,e]	No change	85
D_2 mRNA[c,e]	No change	85
	Increased	86
[3H]spiperone binding[a,c,e]	Increased	83, 87
	No change	84
[3H]YM09151 binding[e]	Decreased	88
	Increased[o]	
D_3 mRNA[c,e]	Decreased	85
D_4 mRNA[c,e]	No change	85
D_5 mRNA[c,e]	No change	85
Serotonin Receptors		
5-HT_{1A} mRNA[a,b,h]	Increased	100
	Decreased	100
[3H]8-OH-(DPAT) binding[a,b,h]	Increased	100
	Decreased	100–102
5-HT_{1B} mRNA[e,g]	Increased	100
	No change	100
[125I]GTI- binding[f]	Increased	100
[3H]ketanserin binding[a,b,e,h]	No change	102, 104
5-HT stimulated phosphoinositide hydrolysis[a]	No change	105
Noradrenergic Receptors		
[125I]pindolol binding[a]	No change[p]	118, 119
Opioid Receptors		
δ-opioid receptor mRNA[d,e]	No change	127, 128
[3H]H-Tyr-Tic psi[CH2-NH] Phe-Phe-OH binding[e]	No change	129
μ-opioid receptor mRNA[d,e]	No change	127
[3H]Tyr-D-Ala-Gly-MePhe-Gly-binding[c]	Decreased	129
prodynorphin, mRNA[d]	Increased	130
vasopressin, mRNA[d]	Decreased	130
Other G-Protein Coupled Receptors		
mACh-receptor [3H]quinuclidinylbenzilate binding[a,b,e]	No change	132
	Decreased	131
Adenosine A_1 receptor mRNA and [3H]DPCPX binding[e]	No change	135
Adenosine A_2 receptor mRNA and [3H]CGS 21680 binding[e]	No change	135
neurotensin receptor [3H]SCH23390 binding	Decreased	133
Neurotransmitter Transporters		
5-HT transporter [3H]serotonin binding[a]	Increased	140, 141
[3H]citalopram binding[a,b,h,e]	No change	102

TABLE 7.2 (CONTINUED)

Expression of G-Protein Coupled Receptors and Related Peptides in the CNS after Chronic Ethanol Treatment

Receptor/Property	Alteration	Refs.
Second Messenger Systems		
G-Proteins		
G_s mRNA and protein[a,b,c,e,j]	No change	144, 145
G_0 mRNA and protein[a,b,g,j]	Decreased	144
	No change	145
G_{i1} mRNA and protein[a,b,c,e]	No change	144, 145
	Increased	145
G_{i2} mRNA and protein[a,b,c,e,j]	No change	144, 145
G_{i3} mRNA and protein[a,b,e,f,j,k]	Increased	144
	No change	145
Adenylyl Cyclase System		
protein kinase A (PKA) protein[j]	Decreased	149
CAM-kinase protein[j]	Decreased	149

[a]cortex; [b]hippocampus; [c]nucleus accumbens; [d]hypothalamus; [e]striatum; [f]globus pallidum; [g]substantia nigra; [h]dorsal raphe; [i]cerebellum; [k]ventral tegmental area; [l]whole brain; [m]amygdala; [n]parvoventricular nucleus; [o]stimulation 2 weeks, decrease after 10 weeks; [p]K_d decrease

mRNA expression whereas D_4 and D_5 receptor densities remain unaltered (see Table 7.2). There is special interest on ethanol's effects on the gene expression of the D_3 and D_4 receptors since they are preferentially expressed in the mesofrontal/mesolimbic dopaminergic system.[80] These receptors display a high affinity to several clinically used atypical antipsychotic agents like clozapine or olanzapine. Clozapine administration has been shown to reduce stimulant and ethanol abuse in patients with a double diagnosis of psychotic and substance abuse disorder.[90,91]

Overall, a significant number of studies have shown an increase in D_1 or D_2 receptors in the nucleus accumbens and cortex of rodents. Increased numbers of D_1 and D_2 receptors might also induce ethanol-seeking behavior or a relapse in humans. The behavioral relevance is supported by studies on knockout animals. Animals lacking the D_1 receptor gene consumed significantly lower amounts of ethanol than the control mice.[92] Taken together, these studies argue for a sensitization of the dopaminergic system after chronic alcohol intake that might be important for the reinforcing properties of the drug.

7.4.2 Serotonin Receptors

Studies using knockout and transgenic animals indicate that the intake of ethanol is dramatically influenced by functional alterations in the serotonergic system.[93] Moreover, a number of human serotonergic genes may be associated with subtypes of alcohol dependence.[94–96] Molecular-cloning studies have yielded at least fourteen subtypes of serotonergic receptors.[97] The serotonergic receptors are widely expressed in the CNS on non-serotonergic and serotonergic neurons thereby influencing the activity of several other neurotransmitter systems, including the dopaminergic system.[97] There is some evidence for decreased function of the serotonergic system by ethanol.[81,98] Chronic ethanol treatment induced a strong decrease in the density of postsynaptic 5-HT_{1A} receptors in cortex and hippocampus (see Table 7.2).[99–102] In contrast, the number of presynaptic auto-inhibiting 5-HT_{1A} and 5-HT_{1B} receptors in the dorsal raphe was markedly increased (see Table 7.2).[100]

Interestingly, the 5-HT_{1B} knockout mice consume greater amounts of ethanol (10% unsweetened solution) in a two-bottle choice paradigm.[93] Using an operant ethanol self-administration procedure the differences between the 5-HT_{1B} knockout animals and controls were only statistically significant for the groups consuming the unsweetened 10% ethanol solutions, but not for the either unsweetened or sweetened 5%, 10%, 20%, solutions.[103] In contrast to the alterations in the densities of the 5-HT_{1A} or 5-HT_{1B} receptors, the number of 5-HT_{2A} or 5-HT_{2C} receptors in the cortex or hippocampus remains unaltered after chronic ethanol treatment (see Table 7.2).[102,104,105] Overall, these studies argue for different ethanol-induced changes in the serotonergic neurotransmission: enhanced 5-HT_{1A}- or 5-HT_{1B}-mediated inhibition of serotonergic neurons in the dorsal raphe nuclei, impaired 5-HT_{1A} postsynaptic transmission in the hippocampus and the cortex, but unaltered 5-HT_{2A} expression in all areas investigated. A gain in 5-HT_3 receptor function is also evident in *in vitro* studies,[106–109] but no studies regarding direct effects of ethanol on 5-HT_3 receptor expression have been carried out. These alterations do not fit into a simple model of reinforcement or impairment of serotonergic neurotransmission and may be related to the inconclusive findings of treatment trials using selective serotonin reuptake inhibitors (SSRIs) for relapse prevention in alcohol-dependent patients.[110–112]

7.4.3 Noradrenergic Receptors

In comparison to studies on the serotonergic and dopaminergic systems fewer studies have been reported on ethanol's effects on the noradrenergic system. Ethanol withdrawal induces a strong increase in the activity of the brainstem noradrenergic system[113] that can be abolished by bilateral lesions of the locus coeruleus area.[114] Moreover, α_2-adrenergic receptor agonists like clonidine are commonly used drugs in the treatment of ethanol withdrawal symptoms[115,116] In vitro ethanol administration in NG108-15 cells induced a strong induction of α_{2B}-adrenergic receptors over 48 h and α_{2C}-adrenergic receptor expression over a 5-day treatment period.[117] Unfortunately, no comparable *in vivo* studies on α_2-adrenergic receptor expression have been reported. Studies on ethanol's effects on the densities of β-adrenergic receptors have shown controversial results (see Table 7.2), but a decrease of high affinity β-adrenergic binding sites is evident in some investigations.[118,119] These data also correspond to a recently reported finding that chronic ethanol intake reduces adenylyl cyclase activity only in intoxicated alcohol dependent patients.[120,121] Taken together, these studies provide evidence that ethanol intoxication impairs noradrenergic neurotransmission, as indicated by reduced high affinity adrenoceptor binding sites.

7.4.4 Opioid Receptors

The endogenous opioid system has been implicated in mediating the effects of ethanol and other drugs of abuse. Ethanol withdrawal is associated with an increased endorphin release in the nucleus accumbens.[122] Special interest has been raised on the µ-opioid receptor function, since animals lacking the µ-opioid receptor lose almost all the rewarding efficacy of morphine.[123,124] Two clinical treatment trials with the µ-opioid receptor antagonist naltrexone have reported reduced relapses in ethanol-dependent patients.[125,126] The expression studies provide preliminary evidence of specific alterations in the opioid system by ethanol. Chronic ethanol treatment induced a decrease of µ-opioid receptor expression in the hypothalamus,[127] the nucleus accumbens, but not in the striatum of mice (see Table 7.2). In contrast, the density and mRNA expression of the δ-opioid receptors remain unaltered after continuous ethanol administration in all brain regions investigated (see Table 7.2).[127–129] The expression of opioid ligands is also altered by chronic ethanol administration. One week of ethanol treatment induced a 50 to 60% increase in prodynorphin mRNA expression and 60% decrease in vasopressin mRNA expression (see Table 7.2).[130]

In conclusion, ethanol and ethanol withdrawal alter the expression of opioid genes, particularly the µ-opioid receptor. This might have relevance to drug-seeking behavior in animals and in humans.

7.4.5 Other G-Protein Coupled Receptors

Chronic ethanol treatment has been shown to affect a number of other G-protein receptors. Syvalahti et al.[131] reported a 30% downregulation in the density of the muscarinergic acetylcholine receptor (mAChR) after chronic ethanol treatment, but Rothberg et al.[132] found no change (see Table 7.2). Special interest has focused on receptors that are colocalized with dopamine or opioid receptors, e.g., neurotensin receptors and adenosine receptors. The results of these studies are shown in Table 7.2. Chronic ethanol administration induced a significant reduction in neurotensin receptor density and binding affinity in the striatum of different mice lines.[133,134] Adenosine receptor densities were measured in brains of rats who had lifelong access to ethanol solutions as well as in rats who had no access to alcohol.[135] This study reported an age-dependent decline in the number of adenosine A_1 and adenosine A_2 receptors in striatopallidal cells that was observed in both the drug naive and in ethanol-consuming groups.[135] In contrast, ethanol withdrawal (either single or multiple episodes) was able to induce a 20 to 50% increase in adenosine A_1 receptor densities in the cerebral cortex of standard laboratory mice.[136] Clearly, more work is needed examining ethanol's effects on gene expression of neurotensin and adenosine receptors before conclusions can be drawn about their roles in ethanol dependence.

7.5 Neurotransmitter Transporters

7.5.1 Dopamine Transporter

The dopamine transporter (DAT) is an important molecule for controlling dopaminergic turnover in the brain. Moreover, it is an important initial site of action for psychostimulants such as amphetamine and cocaine. Chronic ethanol treatment affects the function of the DAT: A single photon emission computer tomography (SPECT) study on Finish alcohol-dependent patients found a 30% decrease in the DAT while these patients were intoxicated.[137] However, another human positron emission tomography (PET) study with the radioligand 11C d-threo-methylphenidate showed no significant difference in DAT densities between alcohol-dependent patients and normal healthy volunteers.[138] The divergence among the data might be related to different blood ethanol levels that were not controlled in these studies. Further investigations will help to clarify the functional meaning of this molecule.

7.5.2 Serotonin Transporter

The serotonin transporter (5-HTT) has received attention in alcohol research since human studies have identified a promotor polymorphism in the gene that encodes this transporter.[139] This polymorphism is associated with several subtypes of alcoholism.[94,95] Initial animal studies have indicated that chronic ethanol treatment increases [³H]serotonin uptake after chronic ethanol ingestion.[140,141] However, human studies on ethanol's effects on 5-HTT expression have shown controversial results. A PET study with the radioligand [125I]-citalopram showed a 30% decrease in density of 5-HTT sites in the dorsal raphe region of ethanol-dependent patients.[142] Another post-mortem study in humans reported an overall increase in 5-HTT sites in the dorsal raphe region of alcohol-dependent patients as well as increased ligand binding with [125I]-citalopram.[143] Interestingly, the binding intensity was largely influenced by the 5-HTT genotype.[143] Further imaging studies on a larger number of subjects are needed to confirm the 5-HTT as a trait marker for alcoholism.

7.6   Second Messenger Systems

7.6.1   G-Proteins

The observed changes in radioligand binding studies for several neurocep-
tors after chronic ethanol administration raise the question whether these
alterations might be accompanied by changes in second messenger function
or gene expression. Interest has focused on G-protein subunits, adenylyl
cyclases, and components of the phosphoinositoldiphosphate signaling system (see Table 7.2). Two investigations argue for a shift of G-protein function
toward an increased expression of several inhibitory G-protein subunits after
chronic ethanol exposure (see Table 7.2).[144,145] However, the study of Wenrich
et al.[146] emphasizes that these alterations in G-protein subunit expression
depend dramatically on the duration of ethanol treatment and the method of
ethanol administration. Further investigations using more standardized ethanol treatment protocols and behavioral analyses will help to elucidate the
functional meaning of these findings.

7.6.2   Adenylyl Cyclase

Interest has focused on adenylyl cyclase (AC) activity, since this enzyme can
easily be measured in human platelets. One clinical study reported a significant decrease in adenylyl cyclase activity in platelets of alcohol-dependent
patients after stimulation with guanine nucleotide or prostaglandinE (PGE) as
compared to normal healthy volunteers, even if they were abstinent for more
than a year.[147] The same group showed that basal activity of adenylyl cyclase
was reduced in platelets of male alcohol-dependent patients.[148] Data on animal
models support these findings. Seven days of oral ethanol administration
reduced forskolin-stimulated AC activity in the cerebral cortex of mice by
about 20%.[145] However, more recent clinical investigations show that the
reduced activity of platelet adenylyl cyclase might be due to elevated blood
ethanol levels, which was not controlled for in previous investigations.[120,121]

7.7   Transcription Factors

7.7.1   cAMP Responsive Element-Binding Protein (CREBP)

The induction of different transcription factors is believed to play an important role in mediating the effects of long-term ethanol exposure. Pandey et
al.[150] investigated the effects of ethanol on the expression of the cAMP-
responsive element-binding protein (CREBP). Acute ethanol administration

or withdrawal did not alter CREBP-binding activity,[150] but did stimulate CREBP phosphorylation in granular cells of the cerebellum in rats.[151] In contrast, withdrawal after chronic ethanol treatment induced a strong expression of CREBP-binding in the rat cortex.[150] Interestingly, the expression of the brain-derived neurotrophic factor (BDNF) was increased in a similar manner.[150] Since the observed changes in CREBP expression occur nearly in the same time window as withdrawal induced anxiety syndromes,[150] these alterations may contribute to drug-seeking behavior and ethanol craving.

7.7.2 Immediate Early Genes (IEGs)

Investigation of IEG expression has been an interesting research field, since IEGs are believed to represent neuronal activity after different tasks, e.g., after seizures or other stress related behavioral events.[152] In addition, long-term changes in gene expression are often preceded by the activation of genes of the IEG group. The *c-fos* gene is one well-characterized IEG member. The activator protein 1 (AP-1) complex is formed from hetero- and homodimers of the c-fos protein.[153] Early studies indicated that acute ethanol administration strongly suppresses pentylentetrazole-induced *c-fos* mRNA expression, whereas the noncompetitive NMDA receptor antagonist dizocilpine (MK-801) suppresses ethanol withdrawal-induced *c-fos* mRNA expression in rat hippocampus and cortex.[154,155] In addition, an acute ethanol administration (2 g/kg i.p.) was able to suppress stress-induced *c-fos* mRNA expression and immunoreactivity in the hippocampus and piriform cortex of the rat (see Table 7.3).[156] Moreover, low doses of acute ethanol reduced some enviromental induced *c-fos* expression in the cortex, the hippocampus, and hypothalamus, but also induced expression in the central nucleus of amygdala of mice, which may represent GABA ergic activity (see Table 7.3).[157] Interestingly, the ethanol-specific induction of *c-fos* mRNA expression was 2-fold greater in the DBA/2J mouse strain, as compared to the C57BL/6 strain, which may underlie genetic differences in ethanol withdrawal severity.[158] Other IEGs have not been extensively studied for alterations in gene expression following ethanol exposure. Some interest has focused on the expression of a zinc finger protein termed zif268 (also termed egr-1, NGFI-A)[159] and the *c-fos*-related gene fosB. Acute ethanol strongly suppressed the expression of zif268 and fosB after a stress paradigm (see also, Table 7.3),[160] whereas ethanol withdrawal is able to induce an increase in expression.[161] The IEG activation during ethanol withdrawal induces the expression of a variety of other genes like neuroreceptors and other transcription factors, which might be responsible for prolonged withdrawal syndromes or relapse.

7.7.3 Retinoic Acid Receptors (RARs)

Prenatal vitamin A-deficiency syndrome has been viewed under certain aspects as a model disease for the fetal alcohol syndrome.[164–166] Although

TABLE 7.3

Ethanol-Induced Changes in Transcription Factors or Growth Factors Gene Expression

Gene	Alteration	Refs.
Transcription Factors		
CREB		
CREB protein[a]	No change	150
Immediate Early Genes (IEGs)		
c-fos[q] mRNA and protein[a,b,e,m,n]	Decreased	156
	Increased	157, 158, 163
NGFI-A[q] mRNA and protein[a,b]	Decreased	160, 162
fosB[q] protein[b]	Decreased	160
Growth Factors		
NGF mRNA and protein[b]	No change	175
	Decreased	174
p75 protein[j]	Decreased	176
trkA protein[j]	Decreased	176
BDNF mRNA[b]	Decreased	171
trkB mRNA[b]	Increased	172
b-FGF mRNA[b]	No change	171
neutrotrophin3 mRNA[b]	No change	171

[a]cortex; [b]hippocampus; [c]nucleus accumbens; [d]hypothalamus; [e]striatum; [f]globus pallidum; [g]substantia nigra; [h]dorsal raphe; [i]cerebellum; [k]ventral tegmental area; [l]whole brain; [m]amygdala; [n]parvoventricular nucleus; [o]stimulation 2 weeks, decrease after 10 weeks; [p]K_d decrease; [q]acute high-dose ethanol administration.

ethanol treatment did not alter brain vitamin A levels, the embryos of the ethanol-fed mothers displayed a 70% decreased concentration of RAR_β mRNA in the fetal brain on gestation day 12, which returned to control values by day 20 of gestation.[165] Moreover, maternal ethanol treatment resulted in increased RAR_α mRNA expression in the fetal brain at gestation day 20, which was accompanied by normal RAR_β and RAR_γ mRNA levels. The availability of free vitamin A was reduced via increased levels of cellular retinol-binding protein (CRBP) on both dates investigated.[165] However, only one study regarding ethanol's effects on the retinoic acid system in adult animals has been reported. Chronic ethanol intake in the ethanol-tolerant C57BL/6J mice induced an 80 to 90% increase in RAR_β receptor mRNA expression in whole brain homogenates, which was reversed 4 months after ethanol withdrawal.[167] Interestingly, chronic ethanol exposure induced the expression of the enzyme transglutaminase (tTG) by 40 to 50%,[167] an enzyme, which is involved in RAR-dependent apoptotic processes.[168] These data support the hypothesis that interactions between ethanol and the retinol system are partially responsible for fetal alcohol syndrome abnormalities,[169] but further studies are needed to clarify the role of the retinoic acid receptor system in adult animals.

7.8   Growth Factors

Interest in growth factors has risen since neurodevelopmental abnormalities are observed in fetal alcohol syndrome. The findings on the expression of the nerve growth factor (NGF) have remained controversial. Angelucci et al.[170] demonstrated that a single intraperitoneal ethanol injection at gestation day 15 reduced the expression of NGF and the NGF receptor (p75NGFR) in the hippocampus of a developing rat at various time points. Chronic ethanol treatment alters the expression of various growth factors and their receptors (see Table 7.3). These data suggest that chronic ethanol exposure during pregnancy, in particular, alters the expression of brain-derived neurotrophic factor (BDNF) and its receptor trkB in the rat hippocampus.[171,172] However, studies on the expression of NGF, basic-fibroblast-growth-factor (bFGF) and neurotrophin-3 have shown unaltered expression or controversial results.[171,173–175] Interestingly, chronic ethanol treatment in adult animals induced the expression of the NGF receptor p75 and trkA in the hippocampus.[176] Studies on adult animals will help to understand the relationship between altered growth factor expression and neurotransmitter function. Taken together, the changes in expression of several growth factors and their receptors might partially explain long-lasting cognitive impairments observed after fetal chronic ethanol intake.

7.9   Summary

Alcohol clearly affects the expression of numerous genes within the central nervous system. Within the last 10 years knowledge about which genes are regulated by alcohol has increased rapidly, and with the advent of gene expression micro arrays (gene chips) the next 10 years should expand this knowledge at an even greater speed by enabling the researcher to examine simultaneously the regulation of thousands of genes. For example, a recent study using microarray analysis to examine gene expression changes in the frontal cerebral cortex of human alcoholics found selective reprogramming of myelin-related genes as well as changes in cell cycle genes and several neuronal genes.[177] Animal models for specific alcohol responses have been an important tool of researchers for identifying which genes are regulated by alcohol in the mammalian brain. However, it remains to be determined to what extent genetic variation in the expression of these genes contributes to a predisposition to alcoholism. This will be an important area of investigation, and should provide exciting new insights into the genetic basis of alcoholism.

Acknowledgments: This work was supported by the Department of Veterans Affairs, PHS grants AA11114 (K.J.B.), AA07468 (M.T.R.), AA10760 (Alcohol Research Center), and Fe 524/1-1 from the Deutsche Forschungsgemeinschaft (C.F.).

Abbreviations

AP-1   activator protein 1

AC   adenylyl cyclase

bFGF   basic-fibroblast-growth-factor

BDNF   brain-derived neurotrophic factor

CAM-kinase calmodulin dependent kinase

CREBP cAMP responsive element binding protein

CRBP   cellular retinol binding protein

CNS   central nervous system

MK-801 dizocilpine

DA   dopamine

DAT   dopamine transporter

GABA$_A$ γ-aminobutyric acid type A receptor

5-HT   5-hydroxytryptamin

5-HTT 5-hydroxytryptamin transporter

IEG   immediate early gene

G$_i$ inhibitory G-protein

G$_0$ modulatory G-protein subunit

mAChR muscarinergic acetylcholine receptor

NGF   nerve growth factor

NGFI-A nerve growth factor inducible gene A

NMDA   *N*-methyl-D-aspartate receptor

PET   positron emission tomography

PGE   prostaglandin$_E$

PKA   protein kinase A

RAR   retinoic acid receptor

SSRI   selective serotonin reuptake inhibitor

SPECT single photon emission tomography

G$_s$ stimulatory G-protein

tTG   transglutaminase

trkA   tyrosin kinase A

trkB   tyrosine kinase B

VOCC   voltage-operated calcium channel

References

1. DSM-IV *Diagnostic and Statistical Manual of Mental Disorders*, 4th ed. American Psychiatric Assoc. Washington, D.C., 1994, 175.
2. Schuckit, M. A., Goodwin, D. A., and Winokur, G. A., A study of alcoholism in half siblings, *Am. J. Psychiatr.*, 128, 1132, 1972.
3. Goodwin, D. W., Schulsinger, F., Moller, N., Hermansen, L., Winokur, G., and Guze, S.B., Drinking problems in adopted and nonadopted sons of alcoholics, *Arch. Gen. Psychiatr.*, 31, 164, 1974.
4. Bohman, M., Some genetic aspects of alcoholism and criminality: a population of adoptees, *Arch. Gen. Psychiatr.*, 35, 269, 1978.
5. Cadoret, R. J., Cain, C. A., and Grove, W. M., Development of alcoholism in adoptees raised apart from alcoholic biologic relatives, *Arch. Gen. Psychiatr.*, 37, 56, 1980.
6. Crabbe, J. C., Belknap, J. K., and Buck, K. J., Genetic animal models of alcohol and drug abuse, *Science,* 264, 1715, 1994.
7. Miles, F. M., Alcohol's effects on gene expression, *Alcohol Hlth Res. World*, 19(3), 237, 1995.
8. Diamond, I. and Gordon, A. S., Cellular and molecular neuroscience of alcoholism, *Physiol. Rev.*, 77, 1, 1997.
9. Harris, R. A., Mihic, S. J., and Valenzuela, C. F., Alcohol and benzodiazepines: recent mechanistic studies, *Drug Alcohol Depend.*, 51, 155, 1998.
10. Woodward, J. J., Ionotrophic glutamate receptors as sites of action for ethanol in the brain, *Neurochem. Int.*, 35, 107, 1999.
11. Simson, P. E., Criswell, H. E., and Breese, G. R., Inhibition of NMDA-evoked electrophysiological activity by ethanol in selected brain regions: evidence for ethanol-sensitive NMDA-evoked responses, *Brain Res.*, 607, 9, 1993.
12. Michaelis, E. K., Mulvaney, M. J., and Freed, W. J., Effects of acute and chronic ethanol intake on synaptosomal glutamate binding activity, *Biochem. Pharmacol.*, 27, 1685, 1978.
13. Savage, D. D., Queen, S. A., Sanchez, C. F., Paxton, L. L., Mahoney, J. C., Goodlett, C. R., and West, J. R., Prenatal ethanol exposure during the last third of gestation in rats reduces hippocampal NMDA agonist binding site density in 45-day old offspring, *Alcohol*, 9, 37, 1992.
14. Gulya, K., Grant, K. A., Valverius, R., Hoffman, P. L., and Tabakoff, B., Brain regional specificity and time-course of changes in NMDA receptor-ionophore complex during ethanol withdrawal, *Brain Res.*, 547, 129, 1991.
15. Snell, L. D., Tabakoff, B., and Hoffman, P. L., The density of NMDA but not glycine binding sites is increased in ethanol-dependent mice, *Alcohol Clin. Exp. Res.*, 15, 333, 1991.
16. Snell, L. D., Tabakoff, B., and Hoffman, P. L., Radioligand binding to the N-methyl-D-aspartate receptor/ionophore complex: alterations by ethanol *in vitro* and by chronic *in vivo* ethanol ingestion, *Brain Res.*, 602, 91, 1993.
17. Tremwel, M. F., Anderson, K. J., and Hunter, B. E., Stability of [³H]MK-801 binding sites following chronic ethanol consumption, *Alcohol Clin. Exp. Res.*, 18, 1004, 1994.

18. Follesa, P. and Ticku, M. K., Chronic ethanol treatment differentially regulates NMDA receptor subunit mRNA expression in rat brain, *Molec. Brain Res.*, 29, 99, 1995.
19. Kalluri, H. S. G., Mehta, A. K., and Ticku, M. K., Up-regulation of NMDA receptor subunits in rat brain following chronic ethanol treatment, *Molec. Res.*, 58, 221, 1998.
20. Snell, L. D., Nunley, K. R., Lickteig, R. L., Browning, M. D., Tabakoff, B., and Hoffman, P. L., Regional and subunit specific changes in NMDA receptor mRNA and immunoreactivity in mouse brain following chronic ethanol ingestion, *Molec. Brain Res.*, 40, 71, 1996.
21. Hardy, P. A., Chen, W., and Wilce, P. A., Chronic ethanol exposure and withdrawal influence NMDA receptor subunit and splice variant mRNA expression in the rat cerebral cortex, *Brain Res.*, 8198, 33, 1999.
22. Nowak, M. W., Redmond, D., Sullivan, M., Fidan-Nowak, M., Fernandez, K., Hoffman, P. L., and Becker, H. C., Effect of repeated chronic ethanol exposure and withdrawal on NMDAR subunit mRNA levels in mouse brain, *Alcohol Clin. Exp. Res.*, 23, 29, 1999.
23. Devaud, L. L. and Morrow, A. L., Gender-selective effects of ethanol dependence on NMDA receptor subunit expression in cerebral cortex, hippocampus, and hypothalamus, *Eur. J. Pharmacol.*, 369, 331, 1999.
24. Sieghart, W., Structure and pharmacology of γ-aminobutyric acidA receptor subtypes, *Pharmacol. Rev.*, 47, 182, 1995.
25. Smith, G. B. and Olsen, R. W., Functional domains of GABA$_A$ receptors, *Trends Pharmacol. Sci.*, 16, 162, 1995.
26. McKernan, R. M. and Withing, P. J., Which GABA$_A$ receptors really occur in the brain?, *Trends Neurosci.*, 19, 139, 1996.
27. Grobin, A. C., Matthews, D. B., Devaud, L. L., and Morrow, A. L., The role of GABA$_A$ receptors in the acute and chronic effects of ethanol, *Psychopharmacol.* 139, 2, 1998.
28. Morrow, A. L., Suzdak, P. D., Karanian, J. W., and Paul, S. M., Chronic ethanol adminstration alters γ-aminobutyric acid, pentobarbital and ethanol-mediated ^{36}Cl$^-$ uptake in cerebral cortical synaptoneurosomes, *J. Pharmacol. Exp. Ther.*, 246, 158, 1988.
29. Criswell, H. E., Simson, P. E., Johnson, K. B., and Breese, G. R., Chronic ethanol decreases the ability of GABA to inhibit ethanol-sensitive neurons in the medial septum, *Alcohol Clin. Exp. Res.*, 17, 477, 1993.
30. Buck, K. J. and Harris, R. A., Benzodiazepine agonist and inverse agonist actions on GABA$_A$ receptor-operated chloride channels. II. chronic effects of ethanol, *J. Pharmacol. Exp. Ther.*, 253, 713, 1990.
31. Witten, R. J., Maitra, R., and Reynolds, J. N., Modulation of GABA$_A$ receptor function by alcohols: effects of subunit composition and differential effects of ethanol, *Alcohol Clin. Exp. Res.*, 20(7), 1313, 1996.
32. Harris, R. A., Mihic, S. J., Brozowski, S., and Hadingham, K., Ethanol, flunitrazepam, and pentobarbital modulation of GABA$_A$ receptors expressed in mammalian cells and *Xenopus* oocytes, *Alcohol Clin. Exp. Res.*, 21, 444, 1997.
33. Allan, A. M. and Harris, R. A., Acute and chronic ethanol treatments alter GABA receptor-operated chloride channels, *Pharmacol. Biochem. Behav.*, 27, 665, 1987.

34. Verdoorn, T. A., Draguhn, A., Umer, S., Seeburg, P. H., and Sakmann, B., Functional properties of recombinant rat GABA$_A$ receptors depend upon subunit composition, *Neuron*, 4, 919, 1990.

35. Ticku, M. K. and Burch, T., Alterations in γ-aminobutyric acid receptor sensitivity following acute and chronic ethanol treatment, *J. Neurochem.*, 34(2), 417, 1980.

36. Unwin, J. W. and Taberner, P. V., Sex and strain differences in GABA receptor binding after chronic ethanol drinking in mice, *Neuropharmacology*, 19, 1257, 1980.

37. Karobath, M., Rogers, J., and Bloom, F. E., Benzodiazepine receptors remain unchanged after chronic ethanol adminstration, *Neuropharmacology*, 19, 125, 1980.

38. Volicer, L. and Biagioni, T. M., Effect of ethanol adminstration and withdrawal on benzodiazepine receptor binding in rat brain, *Neuropharmacology*, 21, 283, 1982.

39. Rastogi, S. K., Thyagarajan, R., Clothier, J., and Ticku, M. K., Effect of chronic treatment of ethanol on benzodiazepine and picrotoxin sites on the GABA receptor complex in regions of the brain of the rat, *Neuropharmacology*, 25, 1179, 1986.

40. Sanna, E., Serra, M., Cossu, A., Colombo, G., Follesa, P., Cuccheddu, T., Concas, A., and Biggio, G., Chronic ethanol intoxication induces differential effects on GABA$_A$ and NMDA receptor function in the rat brain, *Alcoholism Clin. Exp. Res.*, 17(1), 115, 1993.

41. Morrow, A. L., Montpied, P., Lingford-Hughes, A., and Paul, S. M., Chronic ethanol and pentobarbital administration in the rat: effects on GABA$_A$ receptor function and expression in brain, *Alcohol* , 7, 237, 1990.

42. Montpied, P., Morrow, A. L., Karanian, J. W., Ginns, E. I., Martin, B. M., and Paul, S. M., Prolonged ethanol inhalation decreases gamma-aminobutyric acidA receptor α subunit mRNAs in the rat cerebral cortex, *Molec. Pharmacol.*, 39, 157, 1991.

43. Mhatre, M. C. and Ticku, M. K., Chronic ethanol administration alters γ-aminobutyric acid$_A$ receptor gene expression, *Molec. Pharmacol.*, 42, 415, 1992.

44. Mhatre, M. C., Pena, G., Sieghart, W., and Ticku, M. K., Antibodies specific for GABA$_A$ receptor α subunits reveal that chronic alcohol treatment down-regulates α-subunit expression in rat brain regions, *J. Neurochem.*, 61(5), 1620, 1993.

45. Devaud, L. L., Smith, F. D., Grayson, D. R., and Morrow, A. L., Chronic ethanol consumption differentially alters the expression of γ-aminobutyric acidA receptor subunit mRNAs in rat cerebral cortex: competitive quantitative reverse transcriptase polymerase chain reaction analysis, *Molec. Pharmacol.*, 48, 861, 1995.

46. Devaud, L. L., Purdy, R. H., Finn, D. A., and Morrow, A. L., Sensitization of γ-aminobutryric acidA receptors to neuroactive steroids in rats during ethanol withdrawal, *J. Pharmacol. Exp. Ther.*, 278, 510, 1996.

47. Devaud, L. L., Fritschy, J. M., Sieghart, W., and Morrow, A. L., Bi-directional alterations of GABA$_A$ receptor subunit peptide levels in rat cortex during chronic ethanol consumption and withdrawal, *J. Neurochem.*, 69, 126, 1997.

48. Devaud, L. L. and Morrow, A. L., Effects of chronic ethanol adminstration on [^{3}H]zolpidem binding in the rat brain, *Eur. J. Pharmacol.*, 267, 243, 1994.

49. Devaud, L. L., Morrow, A. L., Criswell, H. E., Breese, G. R., and Duncan, G. E., Regional differences in the effects of chronic ethanol adminstration on [³H]zolpidem binding in the rat brain, *Alcoholism Clin. Exp. Res.*, 19(4), 910, 1995.

50. Depoortere, H. B., Zivkovic, B., Lloyd, K. G., Sanger, D., Perrault, G., Langer, S. Z., and Bartholini, G., Zolpidem, a novel non-benzodiazepine hypnotic. I. Neuropharmacological and behavioral effects, *J. Pharmacol. Exp. Ther.*, 237, 649, 1986.

51. Morrow, A. L., Herbert, J. S., and Montpied, P., Differential effects of chronic ethanol administration on GABA$_A$ receptor α_1 and α_6 subunit mRNA levels in rat cerebellum, *Molec. Cell. Neurosci.*, 3, 251, 1992.

52. Wu, C. H., Frostholm, A., DeBlas, A. L., and Rotter, A., Differential expression of GABA$_A$ benzodiazepine receptor subunit mRNAs and ligand binding sites in mouse cerebullar neurons following *in vivo* ethanol administration: an autoradiographic study, *J. Neurochem.*, 65, 1229, 1995.

53. Luddens, H., Pritchett, D. B., Koehler, M., Killisch, I., Keinaenen, K., Monyer, H., Sprengel, R., and Seeburg, P. H., Cerebellar GABA$_A$ receptor selective for a behavioral alcohol antagonist, *Nature*, 346, 648, 1990.

54. Mhatre, M. C., Mehta, A. K., and Ticku, M. K., Chronic ethanol adminstration increases the binding of the benzodiazepine inverse agonist and alcohol antagonist [³H]Ro 15-4513 in rat brain, *Eur. J. Pharmacol.*, 153, 141, 1988.

55. Becker, H. C. and Jarvis, M. F., Chronic ethanol selectively increases diazepam-insensitive [³H]Ro 15-4513 binding in mouse cerebellum, *Eur. J. Pharmacol.*, 296(1), 43, 1995.

56. Mehta, A. K. and Ticku, M. K., Chronic ethanol treatment alters the behavioral effects of Ro 15-4513, a partially negative ligand for benzodiazepine binding sites, *Brain Res.*, 489, 93, 1989.

57. Mhatre, M. and Ticku, M.K., Chronic ethanol treatment upregulates the GABA receptor β subunit expression, *Molec. Brain Res.*, 23, 246, 1994.

58. Reilly, M. T. and Buck, K. J., GABA$_A$ receptor β$_2$ subunit mRNA content is differentially regulated in ethanol-dependent DBA/2J and C57BL/6J mice, *Neurochem. Int.*, 37, 443, 2000.

59. Morrow, A. L., Herbert, J. S., Pritchett, D. B., Breese, G. R., Duncan, G. E., Simson, P. E., Criswell, H. E., and Keir, W. J., GABA$_A$ receptor subunit composition in animal models of alcoholism, *Alcohol Clin. Exp. Res.*, 16, 356, 1992.

60. Buck, K. J., Metten, P., Belknap, J. K., and Crabbe, J. C., Quantitative trait loci involved in genetic predisposition to acute alcohol withdrawal in mice, *J. Neurosci.*, 17, 3946, 1997.

61. Charlton, M. E., Sweetnam, P. M., Fitzgerald, L. W., Terwilliger, R. Z., Nestler, E. J., and Duman, R. S., Chronic ethanol adminstration regulates the expression of GABA$_A$ receptor α_1 and α_5 subunits in the ventral tegmental area and hippocampus, *J. Neurochem.*, 68, 121, 1997.

62. Matthews, D. B., Devaud, L. L., Fritschy, J. M., Sieghart, W., and Morrow, A. L., Differential regulation of GABA$_A$ receptor gene expression by ethanol in rat hippocampus versus cerebral cortex, *J. Neurochem.*, 70(3), 1160, 1998.

63. Mahmoudi, M., Kang, M. H., Tillakarartne, N., Tobin, A. J., and Olsen, R. W., Chronic intermittent ethanol treatment in rats increases GABA$_A$ receptor α_4-subunit expression: possible relevance to alcohol dependence, *J. Neurochem.*, 68, 2485, 1997.

64. Buck, K. J., Hahner, L., Sikela, J., and Harris, R. A., Chronic ethanol treatment alters brain levels of gamma-aminobutyric acidA receptor subunit mRNAs: relationship to genetic differences in ethanol withdrawal severity, *J. Neurochem.,* 57, 1452, 1991.

65. Aprison, M. H. and Daly, E. C., Biochemical aspects of transmission at inhibitory synapses: the role of glycine, *Adv. Neurochem.,* 3, 203, 1978.

66. Naas, E., Zilles, K., Gnahn, H., Betz, H., Becker, C. M., and Schroder, H., Glycine receptor immunoreactivity in rat and human cerebral cortex, *Brain Res.,* 561, 139, 1991.

67. Malosio, M., Marqueze-Pouey, B., Kuhse, J., and Betz, H., Widespread expression of glycine receptor subunit mRNAs in the adult and developing rat brain, *EMBO J.,* 10, 2401, 1991.

68. Ellinor, P. T., Zhang, J. F., Randall, A. D., Zhou, M., Schwarz, T. L., Tsien, R. W., and Horne, W. A., Functional expression of a novel neuronal voltage-dependent calcium channel, *Nature,* 363, 455, 1993.

69. Guppy, L. J. and Littleton, J. M., Binding characteristics of the calcium channel antagonist [³H]-nitrendipine in tissues from ethanol-dependent rats, *Alcohol Alcoholism,* 29, 283, 1994.

70. Guppy, L. J., Crabbe, J. C., and Littleton, J. M., Time course and genetic variation in the regulation of calcium channel antagonist binding sites in rodent tissues during the induction of ethanol-physical dependence and withdrawal, *Alcohol Alcoholism,* 30, 607, 1995.

71. Wise, R. A. and Rompre, P. P., Brain dopamine and reward, *Ann. Rev. Psychol.,* 1989, 40, 191–225.

72. Rompre, P. P. and Boye, S., Localization of reward-relevant neurons in the pontine tegmentum: a moveable electrode mapping study, *Brain Res.,* 496, 295, 1989.

73. Phillips, A. G., Coury, A., Fiorino, D., LePiane, F. G., Brown, E., and Fibiger, H. C., Self-stimulation of the ventral tegmental area enhances dopamine release in the nucleus accumbens: a microdialysis study, *Ann. NY Acad. Sci.,* 654, 199, 1992.

74. Koob, G. F., Maldonado, R., and Stinus, L., Neural substrates of opiate withdrawal, *Trends Neurosci.,* 15, 186, 1992.

75. Imperato, A. and Di Chiara, G., Preferential stimulation of dopamine release in the nucleus accumbens of freely moving rats by ethanol, Preferential stimulation of dopamine release in the nucleus accumbens of freely moving rats by ethanol, *J. Pharmacol. Exp. Ther.,* 239, 219, 1986.

76. Di Chiara, G. and Imperato, A., Drugs abused by humans preferentially increase synaptic dopamine concentrations in the mesolimbic system of freely moving rats, *Proc. Natl. Acad. Sci. USA,* 85, 5274, 1988.

77. Gonzales, R. A. and Weiss, F., Suppression of ethanol-reinforced behavior by naltrexone is associated with attenuation of the ethanol-induced increase in dialysate dopamine levels in the nucleus accumbens, *J. Neurosci.,* 18, 10663, 1998.

78. Nestby, P., Vanderschuren, L. J., De Vries, T. J., Mulder, A. H., Wardeh, G., Hogenboom, F., and Schoffelmeer, A. N., Unrestricted free-choice ethanol self-administration in rats causes long-term neuroadaptations in the nucleus accumbens and caudate putamen, *Psychopharmacology (Berlin),* 141, 307, 1999.

79. Diana, M., Drugs of abuse and dopamine cell activity, *Adv. Pharmacol.,* 42, 998, 1998.

80. Kuhar, M. J., Couceyro, P. R., and Lambert, P. D., Catecholamines, in *Basic Neurochemistry*, 6th ed., Siegel, G. J., Agranoff, B. W., Albers, R. W., Fisher, S. K., Uhler, M. D., Eds., Lippincott-Raven, Philadelphia, 1998.
81. Nevo, I. and Hamon, M., Neurotransmitter and neuromodulatory mechanisms involved in alcohol abuse and alcoholism, *Neurochem. Int.*, 26, 305, 1995.
82. Hruska, R. E., Effect of ethanol administration of striatal D1 and D2 dopamine receptors, *J. Neurochem.*, 50, 1929, 1988.
83. Lograno, D. E., Matteo, F., Trabucchi, M., Govini, I., Cagiano, R., Lacomba, C., and Cuomo, V., Effects of chronic ethanol intake at a low dose on the rat brain dopaminergic system, *Alcohol*, 10, 45, 1993.
84. Hietala, J., Salonen, I., Lappalainen, J., and Syvalahti, E., Ethanol administration does not alter dopamine D1 and D2 receptor characteristics in rat brain, *Neurosci. Lett.*, 108, 289, 1990.
85. Eravci, M., Grosspietsch, T., Pinna, G., Schulz, O., Kley, S., Bachmann, M., Wolffgramm, J., Gotz, E., Heyne, A., Meinhold, H., and Baumgartner, A., Dopamine receptor gene expression in an animal model of 'behavioral dependence' on ethanol, *Brain Res. Molec. Brain Res.*, 50, 221, 1997.
86. Kim, M. O., Lee, Y. K., Choi, W. S., Kim, J. H., Hwang, S. K., Lee, B. J., Kang, S. G., Kim, K., and Baik, S. H., Prolonged ethanol intake increases D2 dopamine receptor expression in the rat brain, *Mol. Cells*, 7, 682, 1997.
87. Tajuddin, N. F. and Druse, M. J., Effects of chronic alcohol consumption and aging on dopamine D2 receptors in Fischer 344 rats, *Alcohol Clin. Exp. Res.*, 20, 144, 1996.
88. Hamdi, A. and Prasad, C., Bidirectional changes in striatal D2-dopamine receptor density during chronic ethanol intake, *Alcohol*, 9, 133, 1992.
89. Ng, G. Y., O'Dowd, B. F., and George, S. R., Genotypic differences in brain dopamine receptor function in the DBA/2J and C57BL/6J inbred mouse strains, *Eur. J. Pharmacol.*, 269, 349, 1994.
90. Marcus, P. and Snyder, R., Reduction of comorbid substance abuse with clozapine, *Am. J. Psychiatr.*, 152, 959, 1995.
91. Tsuang, J. W., Eckman, T. E., Shaner, A., and Marder, S. R., Clozapine for substance-abusing schizophrenic patients., *Am. J. Psychiatr.*, 156, 1119, 1999.
92. El-Ghundi, M., George, S. R., Drago, J., Fletcher, P. J., Fan, T., Nguyen, T., Liu, C., Sibley, D. R., Westphal, H., and O'Dowd, B. F., Disruption of dopamine D1 receptor gene expression attenuates alcohol-seeking behavior, *Eur. J. Pharmacol.*, 353, 149, 1998.
93. Crabbe, J. C., Phillips, T. J., Feller, D. J., Hen, R., Wenger, C. D., Lessov, C. N., and Schafer, G. L., Elevated alcohol consumption in null mutant mice lacking 5-HT1B serotonin receptors, *Nature Genet.*, 14, 98, 1996.
94. Hill, E. M., Stoltenberg, S. F., Burmeister, M., Closser, M., and Zucker, R. A., Potential associations among genetic markers in the serotonergic system and the antisocial alcoholism subtype, *Exp. Clinical Psychopharmacol.*, 7, 103, 1999.
95. Hammoumi, S., Payen, A., Favre, J. D., Balmes, J. L., Benard, J. Y., Husson, M., Ferrand, J. P., Martin, J. P., and Daoust, M., Does the short variant of the serotonin transporter linked polymorphic region constitute a marker of alcohol dependence?, *Alcohol*, 17, 107, 1999.
96. Lappalainen, J., Long, J. C., Eggert, M., Ozaki, N., Robin, R.W., Brown, G. L., Naukkarinen, H., Virkkunen, M., Linnoila, M., and Goldman, D., Linkage of antisocial alcoholism to the serotonin 5-HT1B receptor gene in 2 populations, *Arch. Gen. Psychiatr.*, 55, 989, 1998.

97. Frazer, A. and Hensler, J. G., Serotonin, in *Basic Neurochemistry, Molecular, Cellular and Medical Aspects*, Siegel, G. J., Agranoff, B. W., Albers, R. W., Fisher, S. K., and Uhler, M. D., Eds., Lippincott-Raven, Philadephia, 1998, 263–292.
98. McBride, W. J. and Li, T. K., Animal models of alcoholism: neurobiology of high alcohol-drinking behavior in rodents, *Crit. Rev. Neurobiol.*, 12, 339, 1998.
99. Druse, M. J., Kuo, A., and Tajuddin, N., Effects of in utero ethanol exposure on the developing serotonergic system, *Alcohol Clin. Exp. Res.*, 15, 678, 1991.
100. Nevo, I., Langlois, X., Laporte, A. M., Kleven, M., Koek, W., Lima, L., Maudhuit, C., Martres, M.P., and Hamon, M., Chronic alcoholization alters the expression of 5-HT1A and 5-HT1B receptor subtypes in rat brain, *Eur. J. Pharmacol.*, 281, 229, 1995.
101. Ulrichsen, J., Alterations in serotonin receptor subtypes in ethanol-dependent rats, *Alcohol Alcoholism*, 26, 567, 1991.
102. Kim, J. A., Gillespie, R. A., and Druse, M. J., Effects of maternal ethanol consumption and buspirone treatment on 5-HT1A and 5-HT2A receptors in offspring, *Alcohol Clin. Exp. Res.*, 21, 1169, 1997.
103. Risinger, F. O., Doan, A. M., and Vickrey, A. C., Oral operant ethanol self-administration in 5-HT1b knockout mice, *Behav. Brain Res.*, 102, 211, 1999.
104. Druse, M. J., Tajuddin, N. F., and Ricken, J.D., Effects of chronic ethanol consumption and aging on 5-HT2A receptors and 5-HT reuptake sites, *Alcohol Clin. Exp. Res.*, 21, 1157, 1997.
105. Pandey, S. C. and Pandey, G. N., Modulation of serotonin2A/2C receptors and these receptor-linked phosphoinositide system by ethanol, *Behav. Brain Res.*, 73, 235, 1996.
106. Grant, K. A., The role of 5-HT3 receptors in drug dependence, *Drug Alcohol Depend.*, 38, 155, 1995.
107. Zhou, Q., Verdoorn, T. A., and Lovinger, D. M., Alcohols potentiate the function of 5-HT3 receptor-channels on NCB-20 neuroblastoma cells by favouring and stabilizing the open channel state, *J. Physiol.*, 507, 335, 1998.
108. Lovinger, D. M., 5-HT3 receptors and the neural actions of alcohols: an increasingly exciting topic, *Neurochem. Int.*, 35, 125, 1999.
109. Lovinger, D. M. and Zhou, Q., Alcohol effects on the 5-HT3 ligand-gated ion channel, *Toxicol. Lett.*, 23, 239, 1998.
110. Naranjo, C. A., Poulos, C. X., Bremner, K. E., and Lanctot, K. L., Fluoxetine attenuates alcohol intake and desire to drink, *Int. Clin. Psychopharmacol.*, 9, 163, 1994.
111. Miller, N. S., Pharmacotherapy in alcoholism, *J. Addictive Dis.*, 14, 23, 1995.
112. Kranzler, H. R., Burleson, J. A., Brown, J., and Babor, T. F., Fluoxetine treatment seems to reduce the beneficial effects of cognitive-behavioral therapy in type B alcoholics, *Alcohol Clin. Exp. Res.*, 20, 1534, 1996.
113. Eisenhofer, G., Szabo, G., and Hoffman, P. L., Opposite changes in turnover of noradrenaline and dopamine in the CNS of ethanol-dependent mice, *Neuropharmacology*, 29, 37, 1990.
114. Clemmesen, L., Lindvall, O., Hemmingsen, R., Ingvar, M., and Bolwig, T. G., Convulsive and non-convulsive ethanol withdrawal behavior in rats with lesions of the noradrenergic locus coeruleus system, *Brain Res.*, 346, 164, 1985.
115. Baumgartner, G. R. and Rowen, R. C., Clonidine vs chlordiazepoxide in the management of acute alcohol withdrawal syndrome, *Arch. Intern. Med.*, 147, 1223, 1987.

116. Spies, C. D., Dubisz, N., Neumann, T., Blum, S., Muller, C., Rommelspacher, H., Brummer, G., Specht, M., Sanft, C., Hannemann, L., Striebel, H. W., and and Schaffartzik, W., Therapy of alcohol withdrawal syndrome in intensive care unit patients following trauma: results of a prospective, randomized trial, *Crit. Care Med.,* 24, 414, 1996.

117. Hu, G., Querimit, L. A., Downing, L. A., and Charness, M. E., Ethanol differentially increases alpha 2-adrenergic and muscarinic acetylcholine receptor gene expression in NG108-15 cells, *J. Biol. Chem.,* 268, 23441, 1993.

118. Valverius, P., Borg, S., Valverius, M. R., Hoffman, P. L., and Tabakoff, B., Beta-adrenergic receptor binding in brain of alcoholics, *Exp. Neurol.,* 105, 280, 1989.

119. Valverius, P., Hoffman, P. L., and Tabakoff, B., Effects of chronic ethanol ingestion on mouse brain beta-adrenergic receptors (BAR) and adenylate cyclase, *Adv. Alcohol Substance Abuse,* 7, 99, 1988.

120. Szegedi, A., Anghelescu, I., Pauly, T., Dahmen, N., Muller, M. J., Wetzel, H., and Hiemke, C., Activity of the adenylyl cyclase in lymphocytes of male alcoholic patients is state dependent, *Alcohol Clin. Exp. Res.,* 22, 2073, 1998.

121. Pauly, T., Dahmen, N., Szegedi, A., Wetzel, H., Bol, G. F., Ferdinand, K., and Hiemke, C., Blood ethanol levels and adenylyl cyclase activity in lymphocytes of alcoholic patients, *Biol. Psychiatr.,* 45, 489, 1999.

122. Przewlocka, B., Turchan, J., Lason, W., and Przewlocki, R., Ethanol withdrawal enhances the prodynorphin system activity in the rat nucleus accumbens, *Neurosci. Lett.,* 238, 13, 1997.

123. Sora, I., Takahashi, N., Funada, M., Ujike, H., Revay, R. S., Donovan, D. M., Miner, L. L., and Uhl, G. R., Opiate receptor knockout mice define mu receptor roles in endogenous nociceptive responses and morphine-induced analgesia, *Proc. Natl. Acad. Sci. USA,* 94, 1544, 1997.

124. Matthes, H. W., Maldonado, R., Simonin, F., Valverde, O., Slowe, S., Kitchen, I., Befort, K., Dierich, A., Le Meur, M., Dolle, P., Tzavara, E., Hanoune, J., Roques, B. P., and Kieffer, B. L., Loss of morphine-induced analgesia, reward effect and withdrawal symptoms in mice lacking the mu-opioid-receptor gene, *Nature,* 383, 819, 1996.

125. O'Malley, S. S., Jaffe, A. J., Chang, G., Schottenfeld, R. S., Meyer, R. E., and Rounsaville, B., Naltrexone and coping skills therapy for alcohol dependence. A controlled study, *Arch. Gen. Psychiatr.,* 49, 881, 1992.

126. Volpicelli, J. R., Alterman, A. I., Hayashida, M., and O'Brien, C. P., Naltrexone in the treatment of alcohol dependence, *Arch. Gen. Psychiatr.,* 49, 876, 1992.

127. Winkler, A., Buzas, B., Siems, W. E., Heder, G., and Cox, B. M., Effect of ethanol drinking on the gene expression of opioid receptors, enkephalinase, and angiotensin-converting enzyme in two inbred mice strains, *Alcohol Clin. Exp. Res.,* 22, 1262, 1998.

128. Shen, J., Chan, K. W., Chen, B. T., Philippe, J., Sehba, F., Duttaroy, A., Carroll, J., and Yoburn, B. C., The effect of *in vivo* ethanol consumption on cyclic AMP and delta-opioid receptors in mouse striatum, *Brain Res.,* 770, 65, 1997.

129. Turchan, J., Przewlocka, B., Toth, G., Lason, W., Borsodi, A., and Przewlocki, R., The effect of repeated administration of morphine, cocaine and ethanol on mu and delta opioid receptor density in the nucleus accumbens and striatum of the rat, *Neurosci.,* 91, 971, 1999.

130. Gulya, K., Orpana, A. K., Sikela, J. M., and Hoffman, P. L., Prodynorphin and vasopressin mRNA levels are differentially affected by chronic ethanol ingestion in the mouse, *Brain Res. Molec. Brain Res.,* 20, 1, 1993.

131. Syvalahti, E. K., Hietala, J., Roytta, M., and Gronroos, J., Decrease in the number of rat brain dopamine and muscarinic receptors after chronic alcohol intake, *Pharmacol. Toxicol.,* 62: 210, 1988.
132. Rothberg, B. S., Hunter, B. E., Walker, D. W., Anderson, J. F., and Anderson, K. J., Long-term effects of chronic ethanol on muscarinic receptor binding in rat brain, *Alcohol Clin. Exp. Res.,* 20, 1613, 1996.
133. Campbell, A. D. and Erwin, V. G., Chronic ethanol administration downregulates neurotensin receptors in long- and short-sleep mice, *Pharmacol. Biochem. Behav.,* 45, 95, 1993.
134. Erwin, V. G., Jones, B. C., and Myers, R., Effects of acute and chronic ethanol administration on neurotensinergic systems, *Ann. NY Acad. Sci.,* 739, 185, 1994
135. Fredholm, B. B., Johansson, B., Lindstrom, K., and Wahlstrom, G., Age-dependent changes in adenosine receptors are not modified by life-long intermittent alcohol administration, *Brain Res.,* 791, 177, 1998.
136. Jarvis M. F. and Becker, H. C., Single and repeated episodes of ethanol withdrawal increase adenosine A1, but not A2A, receptor density in mouse brain, *Brain Res.,* 786, 80, 1998.
137. Laine, T. P., Ahonen, A., Torniainen, P., Heikkila, J., Pyhtinen, J., Rasanen, P., Niemela, O., and Hillbom, M., Dopamine transporters increase in human brain after alcohol withdrawal, *Molec. Psychiatr.,* 4, 189, 104, 1999.
138. Volkow, N. D., Wang, G. J., Fowler, J. S., Logan, J., Hitzemann, R., Ding, Y. S., Pappas, N., Shea, C., and Piscani, K., Decreases in dopamine receptors but not in dopamine transporters in alcoholics, *Alcohol Clin. Exp. Res.,* 20, 1594, 1996.
139. Lesch, K. P., Bengel, D., Heils, A., Sabol, S. Z., Greenberg, B. D., Petri, S., Benjamin, J., Muller, C. R., Hamer, D. H., and Murphy, D. L., Association of anxiety-related traits with a polymorphism in the serotonin transporter gene regulatory region, *Science,* 274, 1527, 1996.
140. Daoust, M., Chretien, P., Moore, N., Saligaut, C., Lhuintre, J. P., and Boismare, F., Isolation and striatal (3H) serotonin uptake: role in the voluntary intake of ethanol by rats, *Pharmacol. Biochem. Behav.,* 22, 205, 1985.
141. Daoust, M., Compagnon, P., Legrand, E., and Boucly, P., Ethanol intake and 3H-serotonin uptake I: A study in Fawn-Hooded rats, *Life Sci.,* 48, 1969, 1991.
142. Heinz, A., Ragan, P., Jones, D. W., Hommer, D., Williams, W., Knable, M. B., Gorey, J. G., Doty, L., Geyer, C., Lee, K. S., Coppola, R., Weinberger, D. R., and Linnoila, M., Reduced central serotonin transporters in alcoholism, *Am. J. Psychiatr.,* 155, 1544, 1998.
143. Little, K. Y., McLaughlin, D. P., Zhang, L., Livermore, C. S., Dalack, G. W., McFinton, P. R., DelProposto, Z. S., Hill, E., Cassin, B. J., Watson, S. J., and Cook, E. H., Cocaine, ethanol, and genotype effects on human midbrain serotonin transporter binding sites and mRNA levels, *Am. J. Psychiatr.,* 155, 207, 1998.
144. Pellegrino, S. M., Woods, J. M., and Druse, M. J., Effects of chronic ethanol consumption on G proteins in brain areas associated with the nigrostriatal and mesolimbic dopamine systems, *Alcohol Clin. Exp. Res.,* 17, 1247, 1993.
145. Tabakoff, B., Whelan, J. P., Ovchinnikova, L., Nhamburo, P., Yoshimura, M., and Hoffman, P. L., Quantitative changes in G proteins do not mediate ethanol-induced downregulation of adenylyl cyclase in mouse cerebral cortex, *Alcohol Clin. Exp. Res.,* 19, 187, 1995.

146. Wenrich, D., Lichtenberg-Kraag, B., and Rommelspacher, H., G-protein pattern and adenylyl cyclase activity in the brain of rats after long-term ethanol, *Alcohol*, 16, 285, 1998.

147. Tabakoff, B., Hoffman, P. L., Lee, J. M., Saito, T., Willard, B., and De Leon-Jones, F., Differences in platelet enzyme activity between alcoholics and nonalcoholics, *N. Eng. J. Med.*, 318, 134, 1988.

148. Parsian, A., Todd, R. D., Cloninger, C. R., Hoffman, P. L., Ovchinnikova, L., Ikeda, H., and Tabakoff, B., Platelet adenylyl cyclase activity in alcoholics and subtypes of alcoholics. WHO/ISBRA Study Clinical Centers, *Alcohol Clin. Exp. Res.*, 20, 745, 1996.

149. Yang, X., Horn, K., Baraban, J. M., and Wand, G. S., Chronic ethanol administration decreases phosphorylation of cyclic AMP response element-binding protein in granule cells of rat cerebellum, *J. Neurochem.*, 70, 224, 1998.

150. Pandey, S. C., Zhang, D., Mittal, N., and Nayyar, D., Potential role of the gene transcription factor cyclic AMP-responsive element binding protein in ethanol withdrawal-related anxiety, *J. Pharmacol. Exp. Ther.*, 288, 866, 1999.

151. Yang, X., Diehl, A. M., and Wand, G. S., Ethanol exposure alters the phosphorylation of cyclic AMP responsive element binding protein and cyclic AMP responsive element binding activity in rat cerebellum, *J. Pharmacol. Exp. Ther.*, 278, 338, 1996.

152. Morgan, J. I. and Curran, T., Proto-oncogene transcription factors and epilepsy, *Trends Pharmacol. Sci.*, 12, 343, 1991.

153. Curran, T. and Franza, Jr., B. R., Fos and Jun: the AP-1 connection, *Cell*, 55, 395, 1988.

154. Le, F., Wilce, P. A., Cassady, I., Hume, D. A., and Shanley, B. C., Acute administration of ethanol suppresses pentylenetetrazole-induced c-fos expression in rat brain, *Alcohol Alcoholism Suppl.*, 1, 211, 1991.

155. Wilce, P. A., Le, F., Matsumoto, I., and Shanley, B. C., Ethanol inhibits NMDA-receptor mediated regulation of immediate early gene expression, *Alcohol Alcoholism Suppl.*, 2, 359, 1993.

156. Ryabinin, A. E., Melia, K. R., Cole, M., Bloom, F. E., and Wilson, M. C., Alcohol Selectively attenuates stress-induced c-fos expression in rat hippocampus, *J. Neurosci.*, 15, 721, 1995.

157. Ryabinin, A. E., Criado, J. R., Henriksen, S. J., Bloom, F. E., and Wilson, M. C., Differential sensitivity of c-Fos expression in hippocampus and other brain regions to moderate and low doses of alcohol, *Molec. Psychiatr.*, 2, 32, 1997.

158. Hitzemann, B. and Hitzemann, R., Genetics ethanol and the Fos response: a comparison of the C57BL/6J and DBA/2J inbred mouse strains, *Alcohol Clin. Exp. Res.*, 21, 1497, 1997.

159. Christy, B. and Nathans, D., DNA binding site of the growth factor-inducible protein Zif268. *Proc. Natl. Acad. Sci. USA*, 86, 8737, 1989.

160. Ryabinin, A. E., Wang, Y. M., Freeman, P., and Risinger, F. O., Selective effects of alcohol drinking on restraint-induced expression of immediate early genes in mouse brain, *Alcohol Clin. Exp. Res.*, 23, 1272, 1999.

161. Beckmann, A. M., Matsumoto, I., and Wilce, P. A., AP-1 and Egr DNA-binding activities are increased in rat brain during ethanol withdrawal, *J. Neurochem.*, 69, 306, 1997.

162. Ueyama, T., Ohya, H., Yoshimura, R., and Senba, E., Effects of ethanol on the stress-induced expression of NGFI-A mRNA in the rat brain, *Alcohol*, 18, 171, 1999.

163. Zoeller, R. T. and Fletcher, D. L., A single administration of ethanol simultaneously increases c-fos mRNA and reduces c-jun mRNA in the hypothalamus and hippocampus, *Brain Res. Molec. Brain Res.*, 24, 185, 1994.

164. Pullarkat, R. K., Hypothesis: prenatal ethanol-induced birth defects and retinoic acid, *Alcohol Clin. Exp. Res.*, 15, 565, 1991.

165. Grummer, M. A. and Zachman, R. D., Prenatal ethanol consumption alters the expression of cellular retinol binding protein and retinoic acid receptor mRNA in fetal rat embryo and brain, *Alcohol Clin. Exp. Res.*, 19, 1376, 1995.

166. Grummer, M. A., Langhough, R. E., and Zachman, R. D., Maternal ethanol ingestion effects on fetal rat brain vitamin A as a model for fetal alcohol syndrome, *Alcohol Clin. Exp. Res.*, 17, 592, 1993.

167. Alfos, S., Higueret, P., Pallet, V., Higueret, D., Garcin, H., and Jaffard, R., Chronic ethanol consumption increases the amount of mRNA for retinoic acid and triiodothyronine receptors in mouse brain, *Neurosci. Lett.*, 206, 73, 1996.

168. Piacentini, M., Annicchiarico-Petruzzelli, M., Oliverio, S., Piredda, L., Biedler, J. L., and Melino, E., Phenotype-specific "tissue" transglutaminase regulation in human neuroblastoma cells in response to retinoic acid: correlation with cell death by apoptosis, *Int. J. Cancer,* 52, 271, 1992.

169. Zachman, R. D. and Grummer, M. A., The interaction of ethanol and vitamin A as a potential mechanism for the pathogenesis of Fetal Alcohol syndrome, *Alcohol Clin. Exp. Res.*, 22, 1544, 1998.

170. Angelucci, F., Cimino, M., Balduini, W., Piltillo, L., and Aloe, L., Prenatal exposure to ethanol causes differential effects in nerve growth factor and its receptor in the basal forebrain of preweaning and adult rats, *J. Neural Transpl. Plastic.*, 6, 63, 1997.

171. MacLennan, A. J., Lee, N., and Walker, D. W., Chronic ethanol administration decreases brain-derived neurotrophic factor gene expression in the rat hippocampus, *Neurosci. Lett.*, 197, 105, 1995.

172. Baek, J. K., Heaton, M. B., and Walker, D. W., Up-regulation of high-affinity neurotrophin receptor, trk B-like protein on western blots of rat cortex after chronic ethanol treatment, *Brain Res. Molec. Brain Res.*, 40, 161, 1996.

173. Walker, D. W., Lee, N., Heaton, M. B., King, M. A., and Hunter, B. E., Chronic ethanol consumption reduces the neurotrophic activity in rat hippocampus, *Neurosci. Lett.*, 23, 147, 77, 1992.

174. Aloe, L., Bracci-Laudiero, L., and Tirassa, P., The effect of chronic ethanol intake on brain NGF level and on NGF-target tissues of adult mice, *Drug Alcohol Depend.,* 31, 159, 1993.

175. Baek, J. K., Heaton, M. B., and Walker, D. W., Chronic alcohol ingestion: nerve growth factor gene expression and neurotrophic activity in rat hippocampus, *Alcohol Clin. Exp. Res.*, 18, 1368, 1994.

176. Dohrman, D. P., West, J. R., and Pantazis, N. J., Ethanol reduces expression of the nerve growth factor receptor, but not nerve growth factor protein levels in the neonatal rat cerebellum, *Alcohol Clin. Exp. Res.*, 21, 882, 1997.

177. Lewohl, J. M., Wang, L., Miles, M. F., Zhang, L., Dodd, P. R., and Harris, R. A., Gene expression in human alcoholism: microarray analysis of frontal cortex, *Alcohol Clin. Exp. Res.*, 24, 1873, 2000.

8

Nutrient Control of Insulin-Stimulated Glucose Transport in 3T3-L1 Adipocytes

Joseph P. Hwang, Greg Marshall, Daniel Fallon, and Susan C. Frost

CONTENTS

8.1   Introduction 163
8.2   Facilitated Glucose Transporters 164
8.3   Alteration in Glucose Transporter Activity in Response
      to Glucose Stress in 3T3-L1 Adipocytes 164
8.4   Effect of Glucose Deprivation on GLUT4 mRNA Expression 166
8.5   Effect of Glucose Deprivation on GLUT4 Protein Expression 168
8.6   Effect of Glucose Deprivation on GLUT4 Translocation 170
8.7   Conclusions and Future Directions 170
References 171

8.1   Introduction

It has been known for many years that nutrients control the expression of genes in bacteria and lower eucaryotes, which control hexose transport.[1-3] It is only more recently that the effects of nutrient availability on mammalian transport systems have been examined. These studies have been aided by the development of cell lines and culture techniques which allow long-term exposure to nutrients under defined conditions. For lack of model systems much of the earlier work focused on the effect of glucose deprivation on insulin-insensitive transport activity.[4-10] Results showed that in every system glucose transport activity increased in response to glucose deprivation in a protein synthesis-dependent fashion. Conversely, raising glucose concentrations decreased transport activity in a protein synthesis-independent manner. With the development of insulin-sensitive cell lines like the murine 3T3-L1 adipocytes and rat L6 and L8 myocytes, experiments like these were repeated. For example, van Putten and Krans[11] showed in the mid-1980s that glucose deprivation of 3T3-L1 adipocytes resulted in an increase in the V_{max} of glucose transport activity similar to that seen in the non-insulin-dependent cells. Together these results suggested that either the number of transport molecules were increasing at the cell surface in response to glucose deprivation or that the transporter at the cell surface was activated in some fashion.

8.2 Facilitated Glucose Transporters

Mueckler et al.[12] cloned the first mammalian transporter from human hepatoma cells. The expression of this transporter was widespread and became known as the constitutive glucose transporter, GLUT1; cloning of the insulin-sensitive glucose transporter by a number of laboratories followed within a few years.[13–15] To date, a total of five* transporters have been cloned, one of which possesses significant fructose transport activity.[16] These transport proteins have in common a structure which includes a 12-membrane spanning domain and an N-linked glycosylation site within the first extracellular loop. Although mutant and chimeric transporters have been designed[17–23] these expression studies have revealed few clues in understanding the relationship of structure and function.

8.3 Alteration in Glucose Transporter Activity in Response to Glucose Stress in 3T3-L1 Adipocytes

Fig. 8.1 shows an experiment similar to that published by Van Putten and Krans[11] and later by others,[24] including our own laboratory.[25] In this experiment, fully differentiated 3T3-L1 adipocytes were incubated for up to 24 h in the presence of 25 mM glucose (A), the absence of glucose (B), or the absence of glucose but presence of 25 mM fructose (C). At specific times, transport activity was evaluated under both basal (open symbols) and insulin-stimulated (closed symbols) conditions. In glucose-fed cells, basal transport values remained fairly constant over the course of the experiment. Insulin stimulation was robust with a 6-fold increase in activity relative to basal values. This stimulation rate was also fairly constant over the course of the experiment. Glucose deprivation increased the basal activity and over time reduced the ability of insulin to further stimulate (see also Fig. 8.2). Interestingly, fructose when substituted for glucose resulted in the same changes (C) as did glucose deprivation.

---

* Three new members of the glucose transporter family have been identified since this manuscript was first submitted. These include GLUTXI,[54] GLUT8,[55,56] and GLUT9.[57]

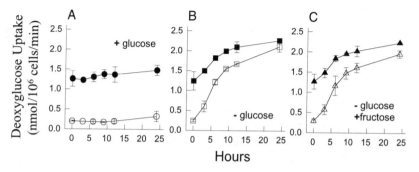

FIGURE 8.1

Effect of glucose deprivation on insulin-sensitive glucose transport activity. 3T3L1 cells were grown and differentiated according to Frost and Lane.[26] Cells were fed 24 h in advance of the experiment with complete medium to assure metabolic uniformity. At time 0, cells were exposed to medium that contained 25 mM glucose (+glucose), no glucose (–glucose), or no glucose but supplemented with 25 mM fructose (–glucose, +fructose). Transport activity was measured in the absence or presence of 1 µM insulin as previously described.[26] Data are expressed as the mean ± S.D. of three independent experiments with each time point run in duplicate.

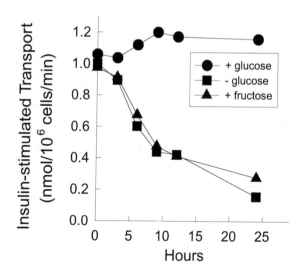

FIGURE 8.2

Change in insulin-sensitive transport activity in response to glucose deprivation. Basal transport values from Fig. 8.1 were subtracted from insulin-stimulated values and plotted against time of deprivation.

8.4 Effect of Glucose Deprivation on GLUT4 mRNA Expression

With the development of molecular probes for GLUT1 and GLUT4, a better understanding of the mechanism underlying the glucose-dependent changes in glucose transport activity has surfaced. First, it must be stated that regulation appears to be cell-type specific. In rat glial cells, Northern blot analysis revealed that glucose deprivation increases the expression of GLUT1 mRNA by 4 to 6-fold over glucose-fed controls.[27] This correlated with an increase in the expression of GLUT1 protein. While it was not established that the increase occurred in the plasma membrane, it is reasonable to assume such as transport activity increases coordinately with increased GLUT1. Similar results were observed in L6, L8, and BC₃H1 myocytes,[28,29] leading to the hypothesis that GLUT1 belongs to the stress-inducible, glucose-regulated protein family.[28] Other explanations have also been offered to explain the increase in transport activity. Ortiz et al.[30] have demonstrated that lysosomal degradation of GLUT1 in murine fibroblasts is blocked in the absence of glucose which allows the accumulation of GLUT1 protein in the face of constant synthesis. In these cells, GLUT1 mRNA was unchanged by glucose deprivation. We have shown that neither the expression of GLUT1 mRNA nor GLUT1 protein is affected in 3T3-L1 adipocytes during the early stages of glucose deprivation where much of the activation occurs. This suggests the synthesis of another transport protein or the synthesis of a transport activating protein. Several investigators have identified proteins which interact with GLUT1, but thus far none of these proteins have been shown to alter transport activity or are induced by glucose deprivation.[31–33]

In 3T3-L1 adipocytes and other insulin-sensitive cells, GLUT4 expression must be considered in addition to GLUT1 in order to understand the effects of glucose deprivation. Like GLUT1, the expression of GLUT4 appears to be regulated in a cell-specific fashion. Koivisto et al.[34] showed little effect of glucose deprivation on GLUT4 mRNA expression in L6 myocytes. Mayor et al.[29] were actually unable to detect GLUT4 in BC₃H1 cells in either the presence or absence of glucose. However, we have shown a significant decrease in GLUT4 mRNA in 3T3-L1 adipocytes in response to glucose deprivation such that by 48 h, no GLUT4 could be detected.[25] An experiment similar in design to this is shown in Fig. 8.3. The level of GLUT4 mRNA in glucose-fed cells was nearly constant over the course of 24 h (Fig. 8.3A). In glucose-deprived cells, we observed a decrease in GLUT4 mRNA at 15 h. By 24 h, there was little GLUT4 remaining. Note that actin mRNA expression was relatively constant over this timeframe. Fig. 8.3B shows a composite of three separate experiments, demonstrating that from 15 to 24 h there was a statistically significant decrease in GLUT4 mRNA expression. Despite the fact that glucose was removed from the cells at time zero, it is interesting that the level of GLUT4 mRNA remained stable over the first 12 h. We believe that this is

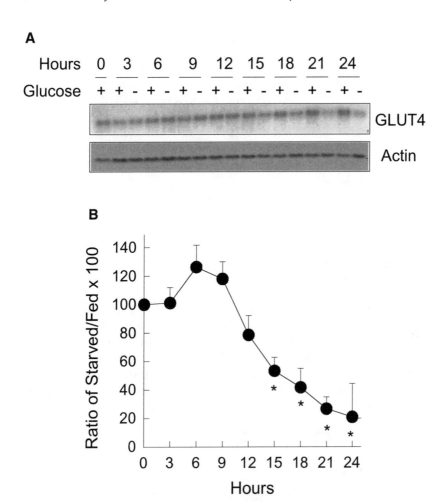

FIGURE 8.3

Time-dependent loss of GLUT4 mRNA in response to hexose deprivation. (A) Cells were treated for 24 h in advance of the start of the experiment. At time zero, cells were exposed to medium containing 25 mM glucose in the presence of 10% FBS or to glucose-free DMEM containing 10% dialyzed FBS. After the indicated time, tot.al RNA was isolated and separated by size on a horizontal polyacrylamide gel. After transfer to nylon overnight and UV cross-linking, the blot was probed with a GLUT4 cDNA (provided by Maureen Charron) or an actin cDNA (provided by Harry Nick).[25] (B) Three replicates of the experiment described in (A) were used to calculate the mean ± S.D. of the starved-to-fed ratios. *, $p < .05$.

related to the provision of intracellular glucose through an endogenous source, namely, glycogen.[35] Removal of glucose from the medium results in a time-dependent loss of glycogen. With a $t_{1/2}$ for glycogen loss of approximately 6 h, nearly 80% of the pool is gone by 12 h and greater than 90% at 24 h. We conclude from these combined studies that glucose regulates the expression of GLUT4 mRNA. Tordjman et al. reported similar results in this same cell line.[24]

We were intrigued by the similarity in the effect of glucose deprivation on insulin-sensitive transport activity in the presence or absence of fructose (see Fig. 8.1). Thus, we examined for the first time the effect of fructose, in a glucose-free background, on GLUT4 expression (Fig. 8.4). These results show that the presence of fructose prevents the loss of GLUT4, despite the lack of glucose. This suggests that a metabolite of glucose rather than glucose itself is responsible for regulating the expression of GLUT4. In this regard, both glucose 6-P[36,37] and xylulose 6-P[38] have been implicated as potential mediators of other glucose-dependent genes, although this has not been studied with respect to GLUT4.

8.5   Effect of Glucose Deprivation on GLUT4 Protein Expression

Changes in mRNA would only have significance if the level of protein expression were, in turn, affected. To determine whether glucose deprivation leads to changes in the expression and compartmentalization of GLUT4 protein, we fractionated cells which had been exposed or not to glucose for 24 h. Shown in Fig. 8.5 is the distribution of GLUT4 in the plasma membrane (PM), the high-density microsomal fraction (HDM), or the low-density membrane fraction (LDM). The PM fraction contains little

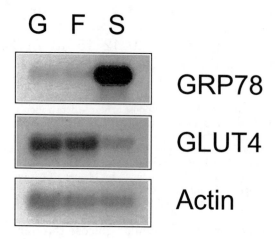

FIGURE 8.4

Effect of glucose deprivation on GLUT4 mRNA expression. Cells were fed 24 h in advance of the experiment and then 24 h in the presence of glucose (G), in the absence of glucose, but presence of 25 mM fructose (F), or in the complete absence of hexose (S). Total RNA was isolated using techniques described previously.[25] Northern blots were probed with cDNA for GLUT4, Actin, or GRP78 (provided by Amy Lee).

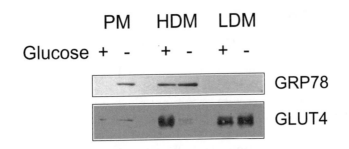

FIGURE 8.5
Distribution of GLUT4 in control and glucose-deprived cells. Cells were incubated in complete medium or glucose-free medium for 24 h. Membranes were isolated as described and characterized previously.[39] Proteins were separated by SDS-PAGE (7.5%) and transferred to nitrocellulose. Immunoblot analysis was performed using an antibody generated against a synthetic peptide analogous to the 12 N-terminal amino acids of GRP78 or an antibody generated against a synthetic peptide analogous to the 12 C-terminal amino acids of GLUT4. Enhanced chemiluminescence was used for final detection.

GLUT4 in control cells (glucose-fed), as noted previously.[39,40] Likewise, there is little GLUT4 in the glucose-deprived cells. This provides evidence that the increase in basal activity observed in the absence of glucose is not contributed to by an increase in GLUT4. The HDM fraction contains both endoplasmic reticulum (ER) and Golgi membranes and thus represents the biosynthetic compartment. This is illustrated here by the presence of GRP78. The amount of GLUT4 in glucose-deprived cells in the HDM fraction relative to the controls is significantly reduced. Interestingly, there appears to be little difference in the level of GLUT4 in the LDM fraction in glucose-deprived cells relative to the fed controls. This membrane fraction contains the pool of GLUT4 which we and others have shown translocates to the plasma membrane in response to insulin.[40] The reason for this protection is not completely clear. It is possible that insufficient time had passed for the storage compartment to reflect the decrease in the synthetic pool. However, we have also shown that protein degradation, specifically that of GLUT1, is inhibited with extended glucose deprivation.[41] As GLUT1 appears to resemble total protein in this instance, it is possible that GLUT4 degradation is blocked, as well. Regardless, our data show that GLUT4 protein is downregulated, which reflects the loss of GLUT4 mRNA. Tordjman et al.[24] came to a different conclusion in studies performed similarly. As mentioned above, these investigators showed that GLUT4 mRNA decreased over time in response to glucose deprivation. Yet, their data also suggested that GLUT4 protein did not reflect this decrease. However, these investigators examined only the PM and LDM fractions. It is thus easy to understand the reason for their conclusion. We would have concluded the same, had we not examined the biosynthetic pool, the HDM fraction, as well.

8.6   Effect of Glucose Deprivation on GLUT4 Translocation

To determine whether the lack of insulin-sensitive transport was due to a defect in translocation, we examined subcellular fractions isolated from cells exposed to medium with or without glucose for 24 h and then challenged acutely with insulin. Shown in Fig. 8.6 is the result of this experiment. As seen before in glucose-fed controls, insulin stimulated the recruitment of GLUT4 from the LDM fraction to the PM. Surprisingly, translocation of GLUT4 in the glucose-deprived cells was similar to that in control cells. Thus, despite the loss of insulin-sensitive glucose transport in glucose-deprived cells, the level of GLUT4 in the PM after exposure to insulin appears similar to glucose-fed cells. This may suggest that the transporter is not correctly inserted in the PM for functional expression. One way to test this is to label the transporter at the exofacial glucose-binding site. Experiments like this were done in the early 1990s by Kozka et al.[42] using cell the impermeant bis-mannose photolabel, 2-*N*-(4-(1-azi-2, 2, 2-trifluoroethyl)benzoyl-1,3-bis(D-mannos-4-yloxy)-2-propylamine (ATB-BMPA). In fact, these investigators showed essentially the same level of GLUT4 on the cell surface in response to insulin in glucose-fed vs. glucose-deprived cells. Thus arises a dilemma. Not only is there an increase in the amount of GLUT4 on the cell surface in glucose-deprived cells in response to insulin, but also, the transporter is inserted such that the exofacial glucose-binding site is accessible to extracellular glucose. Why there is no insulin-stimulated glucose transport activity remains a mystery.

8.7   Conclusions and Future Directions

In recent reviews of this topic, questions were raised for future investigation.[43,44] Among these were questions regarding how glucose affects transport distribution and gene expression. It seems little information has been gained in the intervening years despite solid evidence that such regulation must exist. Thus, we still have many challenges ahead. For example, is it possible that the activity of GLUT4 is regulated by a protein which does not exist in glucose-deprived cells? Or is the activity associated with transport activation in glucose-deprived cells a function which is distributed between that process and the GLUT4 transporter? Or perhaps GLUT4 substitutes for the activation process which might mean that the PM can accommodate only a limited number of transport proteins.

At the transcriptional level, one possible avenue of investigation may lie in the identification of regulatory elements in the promoter regions of GLUT4, in particular, and identification of proteins that interact with those

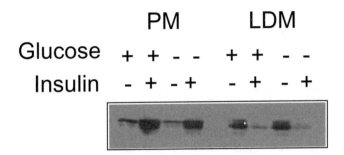

FIGURE 8.6

Translocation of GLUT4 in response to insulin. 3T3-L1 Adipocytes were incubated in Dulbecco's modified Eagle's medium (DMEM) in the presence or absence of 25 mM glucose. Cells were then washed and treated with 1 μM insulin for 10 min in KRP. Membrane fractions were collected and proteins separated by SDS-PAGE (10%). After transfer, GLUT4 was identified by immunoblotting.

elements. Other genes like those which encode pyruvate kinase,[45] fatty acid synthase,[46] and spot14[47] appear to be controlled by glucose availability through regions, known as E-boxes, which have the canonical sequence CANNTG.[48] This motif is recognized by the transcription factors USF1 or USF2 (upstream stimulatory factors).[49–51] These proteins are members of the basic helix-loop-helix leucine zipper family of transcription factors, characterized by a highly conserved C-terminal domain responsible for their dimerization and DNA binding.[52] Evaluation of the 5' promoter region of GLUT4 [see Reference 53] reveals the presence of a single non-palindromic E-box CACGTG upstream from the typical AP2 and SP1 binding sites. Studies investigating the regulatory potential of this site would be of significant interest.

Acknowledgments: The authors would like to thank previous members of the laboratory who contributed to the body of information presented, including Harvey Kitzman, Martin Williams, Bob McMahon, Maxine Fisher, Mike Thomson, and Payal Fadia. This work was funded in part by grant DK 45035 to S. C. Frost.

References

1. Celenza, J. L. and Carlson, M., Structure and expression of the *SNF1* gene of *Saccharomyces cerevisiae, Molec. Cell. Biol.,* 4, 54, 1984.
2. Celenza, J. L., Marshall-Carlson, L., and Carlson, M., The yeast SNF32 gene encodes a glucose transporter homologous to the mammalian protein, *Biochemistry,* 85, 2130, 1988.
3. Sarier, M. H., Protein phosphorylation and allosteric control of inducer exclusion and catabolite repression by the bacterial phosphoenolpyruvate: Sugar phosphotransferase system, *Microbiol. Rev.,* 53, 109, 1989.

4. Fung, K. P., Choy, Y. M., Chan, T. W., Lam, W. P., and Lee, C. Y., Glucose regulates its own transport in Ehrlich ascites tumour cells, *Biochem. Biophys. Res. Comm.*, 134, 1231, 1986.

5. Yamada, K., Tillotson, L. G., and Isselbacher, K. J., Regulation of hexose carriers in chicken embryo fibroblasts: Effect of glucose starvation and role of protein synthesis, *J. Biol. Chem.*, 258, 9786, 1983.

6. Pessin, J. E., Tillotson, L. G., Yamada, K., Gitomer, W., Carter-Su, C., Mora, R., Isselbacher, K. J., and Czech, M. P., Identification of the stereospecific hexose transporter from starved and fed chicken embryo fibroblasts, *Proc. Natl. Acad. Sci. USA*, 79, 2286, 1982.

7. Ullrey, D. B. and Kalckar, H. M., The nature of regulation of hexose transport in cultured mammalian fibroblasts: Aerobic "repressive" control by D-glucosamine, *Arch. Biochem. Biophys.*, 209, 168, 1981.

8. O'Brien, T. G. and Saladik, D., Regulation of hexose transport in BALB/c 3T3 preadipose cells: Effect of glucose concentration and 12-O-tetradecanoylphorbol-13-acetate, *J. Cell. Physiol.*, 112, 376, 1982.

9. Germinario, R. J., Ozaki, S., and Kalant, N., Regulation of insulin binding and stimulation of sugar transport in cultured human fibroblasts by sugar levels in the culture medium, *Arch. Biochem. Biophys.*, 234, 559, 1984.

10. Germinario, R. J., Rockman, H., Oliveira, M., Manuel, S., and Taylor, M., Regulation of sugar transport in cultured diploid human skin fibroblasts, *J. Cell. Physiol.*, 112, 367, 1982.

11. VanPutten, J. P. M. and Krans, H. M. J., Glucose as a regulator of insulin-sensitive hexose uptake in 3T3 adipocytes, *J. Biol. Chem.*, 260, 7996, 1985.

12. Mueckler, M., Caruso, C., Baldwin, S. A., Panico, M., Blench, I., Morris, H. R., Allard, W. J., Lienhard, G. E., and Lodish, H., Sequence and structure of a human glucose transporter, *Science*, 229, 941, 1985.

13. James, D. E., Strube, M., and Mueckler, M., Molecular cloning and characterization of an insulin-regulatable glucose transporter, *Nature*, 338, 83, 1989.

14. Birnbaum, M. J., Identification of a novel gene encoding an insulin-responsive glucose transporter protein, *Cell*, 57, 305, 1989.

15. Fukumoto, J., Kayano, T., Buse, J. B., Edwards, Y., Pilch, P. F., Bell, G. I., and Seino, S., Cloning and characterization of the major insulin-responsive glucose transporter expressed in human skeletal muscle and other insulin-responsive tissues, *J. Biol. Chem.*, 264, 7776, 1989.

16. Kayano, T., Burant, C. F., Fukumoto, H., Gould, G. W., Fan, Y., Eddy, R. L., Byers, M. G., Shows, T. B., Seino, S., and Bell, G. I., Human facilitative glucose transporters: Isolation, functional characterization, and gene localization of cDNA's encoding an isoform (GLUT5) expresssed in small intestine, kidney, muscle, and adipose tissue and an unusual glucose transporter pseudogene-like sequence (GLUT6), *J. Biol. Chem.*, 265, 13276, 1990.

17. Hresko, R. C., Kruse, M., Strube, M., and Mueckler, M., Topology of the GLUT1 glucose transporter deduced from glycosylation scanning mutagenesis, *J. Biol. Chem.*, 269, 20482, 1994.

18. Tamori, Y., Hashiramoto, M., Clark, A. E., Mori, H., Muraoka, A., Kadowaki, T., Holman, G. D., and Kasuga, M., Substitution at pro[385] of GLUT1 perturbs the glucose transport function by reducing conformational flexibility, *J. Biol. Chem.*, 269, 2982, 1994.

19. Williams, K. A. and Deber, C. M., Proline residues in transmembrane helices: structural or dynamic role, *Biochemistry*, 30, 8919, 1991.

20. Lin, J.-L., Asano, T., Katagiri, H., Tsukuda, K., Ishihara, H., Inukai, K., Yazaki, Y., and Oka, Y., Deletion of C-terminal 12 amino acids of GLUT1 protein does not abolish the transport activity, *Biochem. Biophys. Res. Comm.*, 184, 865, 1992.
21. Schurmann, A., Keller, K., Monden, I., Brown, F. M., Wandel, S., Shanahan, M. F., and Joost, H. G., Glucose transport activity and photolabelling with 3-[¹²⁵I]iodo-4-azidophenethylamido-7-O-succinyldeacetyl (IAPS)-forskolin of two mutants at tryptophan-388 and -412 of the glucose transporter GLUT1: dissociation of the binding domains of forskolin and glucose, *Biochem. J.*, 290, 497, 1993.
22. Mori, H., Hashiramoto, M., Clark, A. E., Yang, J., Muraoka, A., Tamori, Y., Kasuga, M., and Holman, G. D., Substitution of tyrosine 293 of GLUT1 locks the transporter into an outward facing conformation, *J. Biol. Chem.*, 269, 11578, 1994.
23. Piper, R. C., Tai, C., Slot, J. W., Chang, C. S., Rice, C. M., Huang, H., and James, D. E., The efficient intracellular sequestration of the insulin-regulatable glucose transporter (GLUT-4) is conferred by the NH₂ terminus, *J. Cell Biol.*, 117, 729, 1992.
24. Tordjman, K. M., Leingang, K. A., and Mueckler, M., Differential regulation of the HepG2 and adipocyte/muscle glucose transporters in 3T3-L1 adipocytes: effect of chronic glucose deprivation, *Biochem. J.*, 271, 201, 1990.
25. Kitzman, Jr., H. H., McMahon, R. J., Williams, M. G., and Frost, S. C., Effect of glucose deprivation on GLUT1 expression in 3T3-L1 adipocytes, *J. Biol. Chem.*, 268, 1320, 1993.
26. Frost, S. C. and Lane, M. D., Evidence for the involvement of vicinal sulfhydryl groups in insulin-activated hexose transport by 3T3-L1 adipocytes, *J. Biol. Chem.*, 260, 2646, 1985.
27. Walker, P. S., Donovan, J. A., VanNess, B. G., Fellows, R. E., and Pessin, J. E., Glucose-dependent regulation of glucose transport activity, protein, and mRNA in primary cultures of rat brain glial cells, *J. Biol. Chem.*, 263, 15594, 1988.
28. Wertheimer, E., Sasson, S., Cerasi, E., and Ben-Neriah, Y., The ubiquitous glucose transporter GLUT-1 belongs to the glucose-regulated protein family of stress-inducible proteins, *Proc. Natl. Acad. Sci. USA*, 88, 2525, 1991.
29. Mayor, P., Maianu, L., and Garvey, W. T., Glucose and insulin chronically regulate insulin action via different mechanisms in BC₃H1 myocytes, *Diabetes*, 41, 274, 1992.
30. Ortiz, P. A., Honkanen, R. A., Klingman, D. E., and Haspel, H. C., Regulation of the functional expression of hexose transporter GLUT-1 by glucose in murine fibroblasts: role of lysosomal degradation, *Biochemistry*, 31, 5386, 1992.
31. De Vries, L., Lou, X., Zhao, G., Zheng, B., and Faruhar, M. G., GIPC, a PDZ domain containing protein, interacts specifically with the C terminus of RGS-GAIP, *Proc. Natl. Acad. Sci. USA*, 95, 12340, 1998.
32. Liu, H., Xiong, S., Shi, Y., Samuel, S. J., Lachaal, M., and Jung, C. Y., ATP-sensitive binding of a 70-kDa cytosolic protein to the glucose transporter in rat adipocytes, *J. Biol. Chem.*, 270, 7869, 1995.
33. Lachaal, M., Berenski, C. J., Kim, J., and Jung, C. Y., An ATP-modulated specific association of glyceraldehyde-3-phosphate dehydrogenase with human erythrocytes glucose transporter, *J. Biol. Chem.*, 265, 15449, 1990.
34. Koivisto, U.-M., Martinex-Valdez, H., Bilan, P. J., Burdett, E., Ramlal, T., and Klip, A., Differential regulation of the GLUT-1 and GLUT-4 glucose transport systems by glucose and insulin in L6 muscle cells in culture, *J. Biol. Chem.*, 266, 2615, 1991.

35. McMahon, R. J. and Frost, S. C., Glycogen serves as a carbohydrate source for GLUT1 glycosylation during glucose deprivation in 3T3-L1 adipocytes, *Am. J. Physiol.*, 270, E640, 1996.

36. Foufelle, F., Gouhot, B., Pegorier, J.-P., Perdereau, D., Girard, J., and Ferre, P., Glucose stimulation of lipogenic enzyme gene expression in cultured white adipose tissue: A role for glucose 6-phosphate, *J. Biol. Chem.*, 267, 20543, 1992.

37. Mourrieras, F., Foufelle, F., Foretz, M., Morin, J., Bouche, S., and Ferre, P., Induction of fatty synthase and S14 gene expression by glucose, xylitol and dihydroxyacetone in cultured rat hepatocytes is closely correlated with glucose 6-phosphate concentrations, *Biochem. J.*, 326, 345, 1997.

38. Doiron, B., Cuif, M.-H., Chen, R., and Kahn, A., Transcriptional glucose signaling through the glucose response element is mediated by the pentose phosphate pathway, *J. Biol. Chem.*, 271, 5321, 1997.

39. Fisher, M. D. and Frost, S. C., Translocation of GLUT1 does not account for elevated glucose transport in glucose-deprived 3T3-L1 adipocytes, *J. Biol. Chem.*, 271, 11806, 1996.

40. Thomson, M. J., Williams, M. G., and Frost, S. C., Development of insulin resistance in 3T3-L1 adipocytes, *J. Biol. Chem.*, 272, 7759, 1997.

41. McMahon, R. J. and Frost, S. C., Nutrient control of GLUT1 processing and turnover in 3T3-L1 adipocytes, *J. Biol. Chem.*, 270, 12094, 1995.

42. Kozka, I. J., Clark, A. E., and Holman, G. D., Chronic treatment with insulin selectively down-regulates cell-surface GLUT4 glucose transporters in 3T3-L1 adipocytes, *J. Biol. Chem.*, 266, 11726, 1991.

43. Klip, A. and Marette, A., Acute and chronic signals controlling glucose transport in skeletal muscle, *J. Cell. Biochem.*, 48, 51, 1992.

44. Klip, A., Tsakiridis, T., Marette, A., and Ortiz, P. A., Regulation of expression of glucose transporters by glucose: A review of studies in vivo and in cell cultures, *FASEB J.*, 8, 43, 1994.

45. Moriizumi, S., Gourdon, L., Lefrancois-Martinez, A., Kahn, A., and Raymond-jean, M., Effect of different basic helix-loop-helix leucine zipper factors on the glucose response unit of the L-type pyruvate kinase gene, *Gene Expression*, 7, 103, 1998.

46. Casado, M., Vallet, V. S., Kahn, A., and Vaulont, S., Essential role in vivo of upstream stimulatory factors for a normal dietary response to the fatty acid synthase gene in the liver, *J. Biol. Chem.*, 274, 2009, 1999.

47. Harmon, J. S. and Mariash, C. N., Identification of a carbohydrate response element in rat S14, *Molec. Cell. Endocrin.*, 123, 37, 1996.

48. Sawadogo, M., Multiple forms of the human gene-specific transcription factor USF: II DNA binding properties and transcriptional activity of the purified HeLa USF, *J. Biol. Chem.*, 263, 11994, 1988.

49. Henrion, A. A., Marinez, A., Mattei, M. G., Kahn, A., and Raymoondjean, M., Structure, sequence, and chromosomal location of the gene for USF2 transcription factors in mouse, *Genomics*, 25, 36, 1995.

50. Aperlo, C., Boulukos, K. E., Sage, J., Cuzin, F., and Pognonec, P., Complete sequencing of the murine USF gene and comparison of its genomic organization to that of mFIP/USF2, *Genomics*, 37, 337, 1996.

51. Lin, Q., Luo, X., and Sawadogo, M., Archaic structure of the gene encoding transcription factor USF, *J. Biol. Chem.*, 269, 23894, 1994.

52. Littlewood, T. D. and Evan, G. I., Transcription factors 2: Helix-loop-helix, *Protein Profile*, 2, 621, 1995.

53. Buse, J. B., Yasuda, K., Lay, T. P., Seo, T. S., Olson, A. L., Pessin, J. E., Karam, J. H., Seino, S., and Bell, G. I., Human GLUT4/muscle-fat glucose-transporter gene: characterization and genetic variation, *Diabetes,* 41, 1436, 1992.
54. Ibberson, M., Uldry, M., and Thorens, B., GLUTX1, a novel mammalian glucose transporter expressed in the central nervous system and insulin-sensitive tissues, *J. Biol. Chem.,* 275, 4607, 2000.
55. Carayannopoulos, M. O., Chi, M. M. Y., Cui, Y., Pingsterhaus, J. M., McKnight, R. A., Mueckler, M., Devaskar, S. U., and Moley, K. H., GLUT8 is a glucose transporter responsible for insulin-stimulated glucose uptake in the blastocyst, *Proc. Natl. Acad. Sci. U.S.A.,* 97, 7313, 2000.
56. Doege, H., Schurmann, A., Bahrenberg, G., Brauers, A., and Joost, H. G., GLUT8, a novel member of the sugar transport facilitator family with glucose transport activity, *J. Biol. Chem.,* 275, 16275, 2000.
57. Phay, J. E., Hussain, H. B., and Moley, J. F., Cloning and expression analysis of a novel member of the facilitative glucose transporter family, SLC2A9 (GLUT9), *Genomics,* 66, 217, 2000.

9

Prohormone Processing and Disorders of Energy Homeostasis

Jung Han Kim and Jürgen K. Naggert

CONTENTS

9.1 Introduction 178
9.2 Processing of Neuro-Endocrine Peptides...179
    9.2.1 The Prohormone Processing Pathway 181
    9.2.2 Proopiomelanocortin, an Example
          of Prohormone Processing..182
    9.2.3 The Major Processing Enzymes 183
          9.2.3.1 Endoproteases 183
          9.2.3.2 Carboxypeptidases 184
    9.2.4 Regulation of Prohormone Processing.......................................184
    9.2.5 Precursor Molecules and Peptides Important
          in Energy Homeostasis...185
9.3 Animal Models with Defects in the Processing Pathway 185
    9.3.1 Cpe^{fat}...186
    9.3.2 PC2 Null Mutant...188
    9.3.3 7B2 Null Mutant...189
    9.3.4 The Murine Anorexia Mutation...190
9.4 Human Disease Associated with Processing Defects 190
    9.4.1 PC1 Mutations...191
    9.4.2 POMC Mutations..192
    9.4.3 Processing Defects in the Human Population 193
9.5 A Genetic Approach for Identifying Distal Effects on Energy
    Homeostasis...193
9.6 Conclusion 195
References 195

9.1   Introduction

Research into the molecular causes of obesity and diabetes has grown significantly in recent years. This is due in part to the rapid increase in the prevalence of obesity and related morbidities, and most importantly because the molecular genetic tools to identify underlying causes for these diseases have now become available. The identification of the five single-gene obesity mutations in the mouse has, in particular, changed the field of obesity. Whereas in the past, obesity was perceived predominantly as a metabolic disease, the notion that obesity is a disease of the central nervous system (CNS) has now gained wide acceptance. A striking feature of the genes underlying the "big" five spontaneous single-gene mutations in mouse, *ob*, *db* (encoding leptin and leptin receptor, respectively), *A^y* (encoding agouti — antagonist for melanocortin receptors), *fat* (encoding carboxypeptidase E), and *tub* (encoding a novel neuronal protein) is that they all act in the hypothalamus and affect neuro/endocrine signaling.[1] This suggests that, at the least, a significant subgroup of obesities arises from defects in the central regulation of energy homeostasis, and not simply from defects in metabolic pathways.

Food intake behavior is controlled primarily by inhibitory neural and humoral signals (e.g., melanin stimulating hormone (MSH), leptin, or insulin) that lead to cessation of ongoing ingestion; a new meal is initiated when these signals diminish in the post-absorptive state. However, this apparently simple behavior is modulated by a multitude of internal and external stimuli whose modes of action are not well understood. Control over feeding behavior rests within the CNS. For example, the spinal cord and brainstem affect energy homeostasis via the autonomic nervous system. The hypothalamus and the limbic system receive signals indicating the metabolic state of the body (quality of ingested food, gastric extension, etc.) and integrate this information with cortical information about factors such as taste, memory, and competing desires.[2,3]

Important neuro/endocrine signals that govern energy homeostasis involve the neuropeptides. Although these neuropeptides were originally thought only to function as hormones, it has become clear that they possess hormonal as well as neuromodulator and neurotransmitter activities.[4] Often the same peptide can carry out several of these functions, depending upon the cell type in which it is expressed. The insights gained from the obesity mutations are, in part, responsible for the expanded research interest into the action, biosynthesis, and regulation of neuro/endocrine peptides. This renewed interest builds upon a successful half a century of research, primarily at the biochemical level, which has shown that neuro/endocrine peptides are synthesized as precursor proteins and undergo extensive processing before they are released as mature peptides upon stimulation.[5-7] Many of the mechanisms and enzymes involved in prohormone processing have been identified and it has recently been shown that rare mutations in the genes of processing enzymes can lead to syndromes of obesity in animals and humans.[8-9]

Interest in novel neuropeptides and peptide hormones has also increased because their receptors are attractive drug targets. In the course of the genome project, a large number of orphan receptors, particularly the G-coupled seven transmembrane spanning receptors, were discovered, suggesting the existence of currently unknown peptides. Indeed, the search for endogenous agonists for these orphan receptors has become a new paradigm for the identification of novel bioactive peptides.[10,11]

In this brief overview, we will outline the prohormone processing pathway as it acts in most neuro/endocrine tissues and describe the major enzymes constituting this pathway. We will introduce mouse models with defects in prohormone processing and describe two human conditions in which processing defects lead to obesity syndromes. Finally, we will discuss a genetic approach for identifying factors that act downstream of the processing pathway in mediating the effects of prohormone maturation on energy homeostasis.

9.2 Processing of Neuro-Endocrine Peptides

Even with our currently limited knowledge, we are faced with a bewildering array of neuropeptides, often encoded by the same precursor molecule. We are just beginning to elucidate the mechanisms by which such a system has evolved through the identification of families of receptors (e.g., opioid,[12] neuropeptide Y (NPY) receptor family[13]), of peptides (e.g., oxytocin/vasopressin,[14] opioid/orphanin family[15]), and of processing enzymes (subtilisin/kexin family[16]).

It was commonly thought that during vertebrate evolution two or three genome duplications occurred.[17] Receptor duplication may have afforded protection from a lethal loss of receptor function, but once a duplicated receptor was present in an organism, it was also less restrained in conserving function and could assume a new role. For example, some neuropeptides can still bind to a number of receptor subtypes that are often expressed in a cell-specific manner (e.g., neuropeptide Y (NPY)).[18] Similarly, new peptides could evolve by gene duplication, and acquisition of mutations may have made them more active toward a specific receptor subtype. In addition, once a basic peptide processing system was in place, a new way of generating novel bioactive peptides was available by the generation of new processing sites in peptide precursor proteins. The complexity observed today most likely arose through this ability to achieve diversity without compromising the function of existing peptide/receptor systems and the viability of the organism. It is less likely that there was a particular need to have the same stretch of amino acids encode a peptide-mediating pain response (beta-endorphin, β-END), as well as a peptide-regulating eating behavior (alpha-melanin stimulating hormone, α-MSH) as for example in proopiomelanocortin (POMC). If such a view is correct, then we would expect important regulatory events to occur post-translationally. The processing pathway and the enzymes involved then assume particular importance.

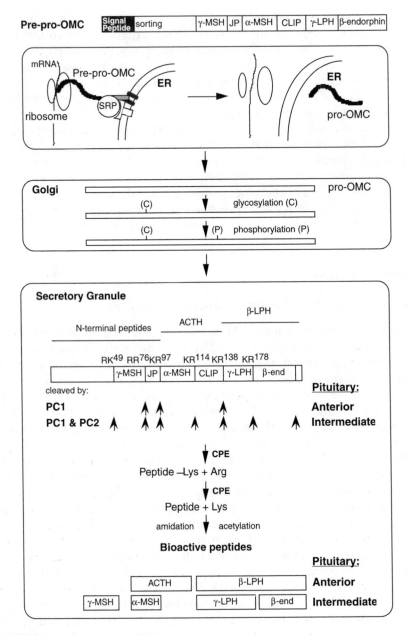

FIGURE 9.1

A schematic description of the major processing steps in the maturation of pituitary pre-proopiomelanocortin (POMC). POMC is synthesized by ribosomes, a preprohormone containing a hydrophobic signal peptide at the N-terminus. After targeting to the endoplasmic reticulum (ER) via binding to the signal recognition particle (SRP), this preprohormone associates with the ER membrane, the signal peptide traverses the membrane, and is cleaved off cotranslationally. POMC is then transported to the Golgi apparatus. The glycosylation of POMC begins in the rough ER and is completed in the Golgi apparatus with a number of modifications to the carbohydrate side chain.

9.2.1 The Prohormone Processing Pathway

Most secretory proteins are synthesized as precursors with an amino terminal signal peptide (amino acid residues)[15-25] that is necessary for the targeting of the protein to the membrane of the endoplasmic reticulum (ER). As soon as the first few N-terminal amino acids of the hydrophobic signal peptide have been synthesized, the ribosomes become associated with the ER membrane and continue translation. These targeting, attachment, and translocation events are thought to be mediated by the signal recognition particle, its receptor, and a protein-conducting channel.[19] While the protein chain is being inserted into the ER membrane the signal sequence is cleaved cotranslationally by a membrane-bound signal peptidase. After protein synthesis is finished the rest of the protein completes traversal through the membrane into the ER (Fig. 9.1).

From the ER, the proteins are transferred to the Golgi apparatus, and then are directed to their ultimate destination, the secretory vesicles or granules via the trans-Golgi network (TGN). It is also in the TGN that the proteins are sorted into a constitutive and a regulated secretory pathway. Precursor proteins in both pathways have to mature before they are released as bioactive peptides from the secretory vesicles, but maturation occurs in different compartments and is mediated by different enzymes.[20] In this review we are mainly concerned with the biosynthesis and action of neuro/endocrine peptides that are stored in the large dense-core vesicles (LDCV) of the regulated secretory pathway, from which they are exocytosed in response to a stimulus (secretagogue).[21] In many cases, the maturation process is initiated by cleavage at pairs of basic amino acids (Arg-Arg, Arg-Lys, Lys-Arg, or Lys-Lys) that in precursor proteins link sequences of the bioactive peptides. This cleavage occurs in an acidic milieu and is mediated by prohormone convertases (PCs) followed by removal of C-terminal basic residues by carboxypeptidase E (CPE, also known as enkephalin convertase and carboxypeptidase H).

Polyprotein precursors can be classified by their bioactive peptide compositions: (1) several copies of the same peptide (e.g., proenkephalin A and B);

FIGURE 9.1 (CONTINUED)
Within the Golgi apparatus, POMC is sorted and packaged into the secretory granule where it is proteolytically processed to biologically active peptides that are released from the cell upon stimulation. The major endoproteolytic cleavages of POMC, catalyzed by PC1 and PC2, occur at pairs of basic amino acid residues. PC1 preferentially cleaves at Glu-Gly-Lys-Arg97- and Glu-Phe-Lys-Arg138-generating ACTH and β-LPH which are normally observed in the anterior pituitary. In the intermediate lobe of the pituitary the PC1 cleavage products are further processed by PC2 to generate γ-MSH, α-MSH, γ-LPH, β-MSH, and β-endorphin. Completion of POMC processing in the pituitary requires removal of Lys and Arg residues from the carboxy termini of the PC1 and PC2 cleavage products by the exopeptidase CPE. In addition to proteolytic modification, chemical modifications including amidation and acetylation take place during POMC processing, altering the biological activity of the modified peptide. PC1, prohormone convertase 1; PC2, prohormone convertase 2; ACTH, adrenal corticotropin hormone; β-LPH; β-lipotropic hormone; MSH, melanocyte-stimulating hormone; β-end, β-endorphin; CLIP, corticotropin-like intermediate lobe peptide.

(2) two or more different, yet homologous, peptides (e.g., proglucagon and provasoactive intestinal peptide (VIP); (3) only one peptide (e.g., the pancreatic polypeptide-neuropeptide Y family, insulin, oxytocin-vasopressin precursors); (4) only one bioactive peptide released at varying lengths (e.g., cholecystokinin (CCK)-83, -58, -39, -33, -22, -8, and -5); and (5) entirely different types of bioactive peptides (e.g., proopiomelanocortin).[5]

9.2.2 Proopiomelanocortin, an Example of Prohormone Processing

An illustrative example of key features of prohormone processing is presented by proopiomelanocortin (POMC), a precursor molecule which encodes a number of different neuropeptides that are produced by differential post-translational processing (Fig. 9.1).

POMC is processed differently in various tissues. In the anterior pituitary, POMC is mainly converted to adrenal corticotropin hormone (ACTH), β-lipotropic hormone (lipotropin; β-LPH), and N-POMC. In the intermediate pituitary, ACTH is further processed to produce α-melanocyte-stimulating hormone (α-MSH) and a corticotropin-like intermediate lobe peptide (CLIP); β-LPH is further processed to β-endorphin and γ-LPH, and N-POMC yields γ-MSH and an N-terminal fragment. The major endoproteolytic cleavages of POMC occur at pairs of dibasic amino acid residues and are catalyzed by PC1 (also known as PC3) and PC2.[20,22,23] PC1 preferentially cleaves POMC at residues Glu-Gly-Lys-Arg$^{97}\downarrow$ and Glu-Phe-Lys-Arg$^{138}\downarrow$ generating ACTH and β-LPH (Fig. 9.1, the amino acid numbering follows Reference 24). However, PC1 also cleaves at Lys-Asp-Lys-Arg$^{178}\downarrow$ and Ala-Gln-Arg-Arg$^{76}\downarrow$ producing β-endorphin and joining peptide (JP), respectively .

On the other hand, PC2 is able to efficiently cleave POMC at Ala-Gln-Arg-Arg$^{76}\downarrow$, Glu-Gly-Lys-Arg$^{97}\downarrow$, Gly-Lys-Lys-Arg$^{114}\downarrow$, Glu-Phe-Lys-Arg$^{138}\downarrow$, and Lys-Asp-Lys-Arg$^{178}\downarrow$ generating α-MSH and β-endorphin (Fig. 9.1). Although PC2 has a broader substrate specificity than PC1, both PC1 and PC2 appear to be required for full cleavage of POMC. Lowering the endogenous expression of PC1 without a change in PC2 levels, by expressing PC1 antisense RNA in AtT20 cells, results in secretion of large amounts of unprocessed POMC and less of the smaller peptides.[25] It appears that the initial steps of POMC processing in the intermediate pituitary are carried out by PC1; PC2 then catalyzes the later steps.[26] However, the factors which regulate the preferential sites of cleavage by PC2 have yet to be determined. This tissue-specific differential proteolytic processing of POMC is possibly directed by a distinct distribution of PC1 and PC2 mRNAs. There is evidence that PC1 mRNA is expressed in both the anterior and intermediate pituitary, while PC2 mRNA is mainly expressed in the intermediate pituitary.[27–29]

The exopeptidase carboxypeptidase E (CPE) completes POMC maturation by removal of Lys and Arg residues from the carboxy-termini of the PC1 and PC2 cleavage products.[30]

9.2.3   The Major Processing Enzymes

9.2.3.1   *Endoproteases*

In mammals, seven endoproteases currently have been identified. These include furin/PACE (paired-basic-amino-acid-cleaving enzyme, *Pcsk3*), PC1/PC3 (*Pcsk1*), PC2 (*Pcsk2*), PACE4 (*Pcsk6*), PC4 (*Pcsk4*), PC5/PC6 (*Pcsk5*), and PC7/PC8/LPC (*Pcsk7*).[16,31,32] PC1/3, PC2, PC4, and PC5/6A are soluble forms of endoproteases, while the furin/PACE, PACE4, PC5/6B, and PC7/8 have transmembrane-spanning domains. Furin/PACE[33] and PACE4[34] are ubiquitously distributed, while PC1/3 and PC2 are found mainly in neural and endocrine cells.[35,36] PC4 is primarily expressed in testis.[37] PC5/6 isoforms A and B are generated from a single gene by alternative splicing. PC5/6A is widely distributed in endocrine and non-endocrine tissues, and is particularly abundant in intestinal and adrenal cells, while PC5/6B is restricted to tissues including the lungs, intestines, and adrenals.[16,38] PC7/8/LPC, which is expressed in the brain and many other tissues, appears to be a functional homologue of furin/PACE.[39-41] PC1/3, PC2, PC4, PC5/6A are sorted to and activated in the regulated secretory pathway, while furin/PACE, PACE4, PC5/6B, and PC7/8 are involved in the processing of proproteins in the constitutive pathway.[42]

Each endoprotease is synthesized as an inactive precursor (i.e., zymogen) and has both unique and conserved structural motifs. They commonly have an N-terminal signal peptide followed by an amino-terminal prodomain (about 80 to 90 aa); a catalytic domain with an active triad of aspartic acid, histidine, and serine residues; and a downstream domain (about 150 aa) called the P domain/homo B-domain with a conserved pentapeptide motif, RRDGL.[31] The N-terminal prodomain appears to act as an intramolecular chaperone that assists in the folding of the zymogen within the ER. The activation of these enzymes begins with an autocatalytic cleavage of the amino-terminal prodomain at a preferred Arg-X-Lys/Arg-Arg ↓ motif.[42,43] The P domain appears to be important for the correct folding of the endoprotease within the ER, as alteration of this domain prohibits the intramolecular cleavage of the prodomain.[44] The prodomain remains attached noncovalently even after cleavage, preventing cleavage of heterologous substrates. The cleaved convertase is then transferred to the Golgi and the trans-Golgi network (TGN), where the prodomain is completely dissociated from the catalytic domain, thereby, fully activating the enzyme.[43]

The major convertases that function in the secretory granules of the regulated secretory pathway in neuroendocrine cells and some other tissues are PC1/PC3 and PC2. Unlike the PC1/3 activation described above, PC2 has a more complex mechanism of transport and activation. PC2 requires a neuroendocrine secretory peptide, 7B2, for its maturation. 7B2 is itself derived from a precursor protein which, when proteolytically cleaved at a multibasic site by a furin-like protease, produces a ~21 kDa N-terminal domain and a small C-terminal fragment (CT-peptide). Pro-7B2 is usually coexpressed with PC2 in most neuroendocrine cells and has chaperonin-like properties.[45] However, 7B2 does not assist in proPC2 folding, but instead binds to completely folded PC2. The N-terminal domain of 7B2 facilitates the maturation of proPC2, and the C-terminal peptide inhibits PC2 activity. In the ER, pro7B2 binds to the catalytic domain of proPC2 through a proline-rich segment in the N-terminal fragment of the pro7B2 protein that is predicted to form a polyproline helix-like structure.[46] This facilitates the transport of the pro7B2/proPC2 complex to the Golgi apparatus. In the TGN, pro7B2 is rapidly cleaved by furin or PC3, generating its 21-kDa form. Once the 21-kDa 7B2 has been generated, the PC2 propeptide is processed intramolecularly. Upon autocatalytic processing of proPC2, the liberated inhibitory CT-peptide moves to the site previously occupied by the prodomain. The inhibitory effect of the CT-peptide is terminated by exoproteolytic removal of the two carboxyterminal lysine residues in the CT-peptide by carboxypeptidase E.[31,47]

9.2.3.2   Carboxypeptidases

There have been eleven members of the metallocarboxypeptidase gene family identified in mammals. Based on both function and homology, these carboxypeptidases (CPs) are generally divided into two groups. One group includes the digestive enzymes CPA (mast cell), CPA1, CPA2, CPU (plasma) and CPB (pancreas). The other group includes enzymes whose endoproteolytic activity is restricted to one or two C-terminal basic amino acids of substrate peptides and proteins. The latter group includes secretory granule CPE, plasma CPN, extracellular membrane-bound CPM, CPD, and CPZ.[48]

CPN acts in plasma to remove basic residues from a variety of peptides and proteins.[49] CPM is widely expressed on plasma membranes and proposed to process peptide hormones at the cell surface.[50] CPE has previously been thought to be the only secretory granule carboxypeptidase.[30] However, lack of functional CPE in Cpe^{fat}/Cpe^{fat} mice does not cause complete elimination of mature peptides,[8] indicating that other carboxypeptidases might compensate for the CPE defect. As a result, these additional activities were unmasked, and subsequently the CPE-like proteins, CPD[51,52] and CPZ[53] were cloned. CPD is present mainly in the Golgi and/or trans-Golgi network but not in the secretory granules where the majority of propeptide processing occurs, and CPZ does not function in an acidic milieu as it exists in the secretory granule. It is, therefore, an open question whether these newly identified enzymes are responsible for the residual carboxyterminal processing in Cpe^{fat}/Cpe^{fat} mice.

9.2.4   Regulation of Prohormone Processing

Why do organisms possess such an elaborate system for producing neuro/endocrine peptides or peptide hormones? An attractive hypothesis is that a large pool of inactive precursors may facilitate a rapid release of peptides through enzymatic cleavage rather than undergoing *de novo* synthesis.[54] Experiments testing this hypothesis have been sparse. However, it has been found that procholecystokinin (CCK) and progastrin accumulate in pituitary corticotrophs[55] and enkephalin precursor molecules accumulate in the adrenal medulla.[56] In the latter case, it was also shown that treatment of adrenal chromaffin cells with reserpine leads to the appearance of enkephalin pentapeptides concomitant with a decrease of the precursor molecules.[57] Overall, however, the importance of posttranslational attenuation in stimulated secretion has not yet been demonstrated. Nevertheless, cell-specific attenuation has been shown to occur and can be achieved by modulating the activity of the processing enzymes, either by their transcriptional regulation or through the action of protease inhibitors.[58]

Regulation of PC1, PC2, and furin expression in several cell lines treated with activators of the cyclic AMP (cAMP) and protein kinase C (PKC) second messenger pathways shows that prohormone convertases may be differentially regulated by cAMP and PKC mechanisms. This regulation may be tissue specific, as activation of the cAMP pathway increases mRNA levels of PC1, but not PC2 or furin, in SK-N-MCIXC cells, but increases all three mRNAs in WE 4/2 cells.[59,60] Such differential expression of the convertases should give rise to different sets of neuropeptides derived from given precursors.

Finally, the role of protease inhibitors in prohormone processing has just begun to be explored. Recently it was shown that the Kunitz protease inhibitor of the amyloid precursor protein (KPI/APP) can inhibit enkephalin processing enzyme (PTP) *in vitro* and that KPI/APP and PTP colocalize in the regulated secretory vesicles.[61] A role of the C-terminal fragment of the chaperone 7B2 in the inhibition of PC2 has been proposed,[46] and an *in vivo* role for this inhibition is suggested by the proinsulin processing pattern with the accumulation of diarginyl extended des-31,32 proinsulin observed in the Cpe^{fat} mutation.[8] However, expression of CT peptide alone has so far failed to lead to PC2 inhibition.[62]

9.2.5 Precursor Molecules and Peptides Important in Energy Homeostasis

The emerging picture indicates a complex pattern of neurotransmitter interaction in the control of food intake and energy homeostasis in the CNS. Many of the neurotransmitters have turned out to be neuropeptides, and novel peptides are likely to be found in the coming years. In Table 9.1, we present a short listing of precursor proteins and selected bioactive peptides derived from them that are thought to play a role in energy homeostasis.

9.3 Animal Models with Defects in the Processing Pathway

Despite the undoubted success of previous research carried out on prohormone processing, the recent identification of the molecular defects in genetic

TABLE 9.1

Peptides Involved in Regulation of Food Intake

Precursors	Peptides	Food Intake	Proposed CNS Sites of Action	Ref.
POMC	α-MSH	↓	Cortex, striatum, bed nucleus of the stria terminalis, PVN and ARC	105
			PVN, SON, CEA, AP, and PBN	106
	ACTH	↓	VMH	107, 108
	β-endorphin	↑	VMH and DMH	109, 110
ProNPY	NPY	↑	ARC and PVN	111–114
ProCRH	CRH	↓	PVN and ARC	112, 115
			PVN	116
ProTRH	TRH	↓	PVN	117, 118
ProGalanin	Galanin	↑	PVN	119, 120
			PVN and AG	121
			PVN and SON	122
ProCCK	CCK-8	↓	AP	123
			PVN	124
			NTS, AP, CeA, and PVN	125, 126
ProNT	NT	↓	VMH	127, 128
			PVN	129, 130
ProMCH	MCH	↑	LHA	131, 132
			VMH and DMH	133, 134

POMC, Proopiomelanocortin; NPY, Neuropeptide Y; CRH, Corticotropin releasing hormone; TRH, Thyrotoropin releasing hormone; CCK, cholecystokinin; NT, Neurotensin; MCH, Melanin-concentrating hormone; PVN, Paraventricular nucleus of the hypothalamus; LHA, Lateral hypothalamic area; SON, Supraoptic nuclus; ARC, Arcuate nucleus; DMH, Dorsomedial hypothalamic nuclei; VMH, Ventromedial hypothalamic nuclei; CEA, Central nucleus of the amygdala; AP, Area postrema; PBN, Lateral parabrachial nucleus; GAL-R1-R, galanin-R1 receptor; AG, amygdala; NTS, nucleus of the solitary tract; CeA, Central nucleus of the amygdala.

animal models has contributed new insights. Examination of peptide intermediates in null mutants for the various processing enzymes has told us which peptides are processed by what enzyme *in vivo*, as well as provided information about the temporal order of processing. Also, as in the example of the *Cpe^fat* mutation, a null allele has lead to the discovery of previously masked activities (e.g., carboxypeptidase D). Finally, animal models have shown for the first time that prohormone-processing defects can lead to misregulation of energy homeostasis.

9.3.1   *Cpe^fat*

The mutation *fat*, first described in 1990[63] as a late onset, moderate obesity without hyperglycemia, arose on the inbred HRS/J (HRS) strain. HRS-*fat/fat* mice were chronically hyperinsulinemic from weaning, but never developed overt diabetes. The mutation has been backcrossed onto C57BLKS/J (BKS), an inbred strain whose background genes can interact with mutations like Lep^{ob} (*ob*) or $Lepr^{db}$ (*db*) to result in hyperglycemia.[64] At early backcross generations, the *fat* mutation was not diabetogenic. However, development of maturity-onset hyperglycemia, primarily in males, has been observed in generations beyond F6.[65]

The hyperinsulinemia previously described as the earliest phenotypic characteristic caused by the *fat* mutation is primarily a hyperproinsulinemia.[8] Hyper(pro)insulinemia is demonstrable well before the development of overt obesity and is independent of the glycemic status of mutant *fat/fat* mice. Furthermore, one of the insulin-processing enzymes, CPE, is severely reduced in amount and activity in BKS-*fat/fat* mice compared to littermate controls. In BKS-*fat/fat* mice the reduction of CPE activity is associated with a reduced processing and accumulation of des-31,32 diarginyl extended proinsulin I and II. Since proinsulins and C-terminally extended insulins are less active than fully processed insulins, this reduction in biologically active insulins is thought to lead to an increased physiologic demand, producing β-cell hypersecretion.

The *fat* mutation had been previously mapped to mouse Chr 8. It was subsequently demonstrated that *fat* represents a missense mutation (Ser202Pro) in *Cpe*.[8] This mutation renders the protein unstable, leading to its degradation in the ER.[66]

The relationship between hyperproinsulinemia and the appearance of a later-developing obesity and diabetes on specific genetic backgrounds remains unclear. Hyperproinsulinemia is present in mice both with and without hyperglycemia (unpublished results) and hyperproinsulinemia in itself does not seem to be associated with gross obesity in humans.[67,68] The observation that the CPE defect is not limited to islet tissue, but also is present in the pituitary as well as the brain (unpublished observations) suggests that the obesity and diabetes in *fat/fat* mice may develop as a result of widespread defects in the exopeptidase processing step required for full maturation of a number of neuroendocrine/endocrine prohormones in addition to proinsulin. Indeed, a number of laboratories have meanwhile confirmed such defects in the processing of gastrin,[69,70] CCK,[71–73] POMC, enkephalin, dynorphin,[66] luteinizing hormone release hormone (LHRH) (Dr. W.C. Wetsel, pers. comm.), neurotensin, melanin concentrating hormone,[74] and substance P[75] in this model.

Like the *db* and *ob* mutants, *fat/fat* mice are infertile, indicative of defects in the neuroendocrine axis. Yet the fact that hypercorticism, a feature of BKS-*db/db* and *ob/ob* mutants, is not observed in BKS-*fat/fat* mice indicates that the CPE defect affects the neuroendocrine system at a level different from that of the defects encoded by *db* and *ob*. The low corticosterone levels found in *fat/fat* mice may be due to the defect in POMC processing and consequent lack of ACTH.

Due to the lack of CPE activity, *fat/fat* mice have secondary defects in the prohormone processing pathway as well. As described below, CPE appears to be necessary in the activation process of PC2, so that *fat/fat* mice also have reduced PC2 activity. Such a defect would explain the presence of des-31,32. diarginyl extended insulins in this model. Data have also been presented suggesting that CPE acts as a receptor that targets propeptides, such as POMC, to the regulated secretory pathway. In the absence of CPE, some propeptides may be mistargeted to the constitutive pathway, where they would not undergo correct processing.[76]

Considering the widespread abnormalities in prohormone processing in vital systems it seems puzzling that these mice only show an obesity syndrome but otherwise continue to be quite healthy compared to models such as *ob* and *db*. Also, since PC2 acts upstream of CPE, one might expect a similar obesity phenotype in PC2 knockout mice. However, as described below, PC2 null mice are not obese. It is possible that the obesity is the result of an interaction between the *Cpe^fat* mutation and the specific genetic background of BKS or HRS, respectively. Preliminary evidence indicates that this may be the case. As described further below, in genetic crosses, *fat/fat* animals can have normal body weights. And *Cpe^fat* made congenic on the Castaneus inbred background causes no overt obesity but the mice die prematurely between 12 and 16 weeks of age (Naggert et al., unpublished). Because obese BKS-*fat/fat* mice still produce at least a small amount of mature peptides, it has been suggested that perhaps other carboxypeptidases can substitute for the CPE defect. Indeed, the search for such activities has yielded several new candidates such as carboxypeptidase D,[51] CPZ,[53] CPX-1,[77] and CPX-2.[78] Although CPD is not found in secretory granules, it is a good candidate for a redundant activity in *fat/fat* mice based on cellular co-localization studies with CPE.[79] It is conceivable then that in certain genetic backgrounds such redundant enzymes are less active and can no longer compensate for the CPE defect, resulting in a more severe phenotype.

9.3.2 PC2 Null Mutant

A mouse model *Pesk2^tm/Dfs* lacking active (PC2^-/-) was generated by disrupting the third exon of the *Pcsk2* (PC2) gene which contains the C-terminal end of the prodomain and the beginning of the catalytic domain including the site for proteolytic autoactivation.[80] Homozygous null mice appeared normal at birth, but their growth rate was slightly reduced compared to wild-type mice. No dramatic disturbances in body proportions, adiposity, or major organs were observed. PC2^-/- mice exhibited chronic fasting hypoglycemia and a diminished rise in blood glucose levels during an intraperitoneal glucose tolerance test (GTT).

Morphologically, the α-, δ-, and γ-cells in the islets of Langerhans were hypertrophic and hyperplastic, while the β-cells were hypotrophic. Furthermore, electron microscopy studies revealed large numbers of imma-ture-appearing secretory granules in both α- and β-cells. The proportion of proinsulin to insulin was significantly increased in the pancreas of PC2^-/-

mice compared with wild type (30 to 35% vs. 6%), indicating defective pro-insulin processing.

PC2[-/-] mice also had high levels of circulating and pancreatic proglucagon with no detectable mature glucagon. This is in contrast to insulin levels that were too low to be detectable. Proglucagon processing in α-cells is normally carried out by PC2.[81,82] Because no sign of disturbed pancreatic islet morphology was observed in newborn PC2[-/-] mice, this suggests that the α-cell hyperplasia was probably due to chronic severe glucagon deficiency rather than the result of aberrant developmental processes.

The partial processing of proinsulin in PC2[-/-] mice may be ascribed to the normal coexpression of PC3 in β-cells. Although PC1/3 and PC2 have their preferential cleavage site in the proinsulin molecule, it has been demonstrated that PC3 can cleave at both sites, B-chain/C-peptide and C-peptide/A-chain junctions, in proinsulin to yield insulin.[83] PC2[-/-] mice accumulate des-31,32 proinsulin intermediates which are the product of PC1/3 cleavage.[84,85,47] There was also a complete absence of the major somatostatin peptide, somatostatin 14 (SS-14), in the pancreas of PC2[-/-] mice. Instead, SS-28 was present as a major end-product of prosomatostatin processing. In addition to alterations in pancreatic hormone processing, the PC2[-/-] mice also exhibited abnormalities in other neuro/endocrine tissues including marked reductions of enkephalins and dynorphins in the brain, and γ-MSH in the intermediate lobe of the pituitary.[31]

9.3.3   7B2 Null Mutant

7B2 null mutant mice (7B2[-/-]) were created by a transposon-facilitated knock-out technique. Exon 3 of the *Sgne1* (7B2) gene was interrupted by random integration of a transposon and subsequent introduction of a *neo* cassette.[86]

In 7B2[-/-] mice, maturation of proPC2 was severely impaired and catalytic activity of PC2 was completely absent. The PC2-dependent processing of polypeptide hormones including proglucagon, proinsulin, and proenkephalin was significantly diminished, as was observed in PC2[-/-] mice. Only 11% of 7B2[-/-] mice survived to weaning and, unlike PC2[-/-] mice, were runted, pale, and ecchymotic in appearance. 7B2[-/-] mice were hypoglycemic with elevated circulating insulin-like material by 4 to 5 weeks of age. Morphologically, pancreatic architecture was disorganized and both β and non-β cells were hyperplastic. Striking increases (10- to 20-fold) in the levels of intact ACTH and minimal conversion of this peptide to α-MSH were observed in the pituitaries of 7B2[-/-] mice. Circulating ACTH levels were also increased, accompanied by elevated corticosterone levels and adreno-cortical hyperplasia. These phenotypes, together with others such as skin thinning and dermal atrophy with hyperkeratosis, make these mice a model for a Cushing's-like syndrome.

Compared to PC2-deficient mice, the 7B2[-/-] mice appear to have more severe phenotypes, suggesting that 7B2 has additional *in vivo* functions apart from activating PC2. Perhaps it acts as a chaperonin-like molecule for other, as yet, unidentified proteins in the secretory pathway.

9.3.4 The Murine Anorexia Mutation

Mice homozygous for the recessive anorexia mutation (*anx*, Chr 2) exhibit reduced food intake, a marked reduction in body weight, and an emaciated appearance. The mice have reduced stomach contents from about 5 days of age continuing until death at about 22 days. These findings suggest that these mice may be a model for anorexia, as they fail to ingest sufficient food to sustain life. However, other abnormal behaviors are observed, including head weaving, body tremors, uncoordinated gait, and hyperactivity.[87]

Some observed characteristics (head weaving and body tremors) are typical of elevated serotonergic stimulation. Hyperinnervation of central serotonergic neurons in *anx* homozygotes has been demonstrated, while catecholaminergic innervation is normal, and normal laminar organization of the brain is retained.[88] Serotonergic mechanisms have also been implicated in modulating suckling behavior in newborns.[89]

Although the defect in *anx* mice has not been identified at the molecular level, recent findings suggest that prohormone processing and/or trafficking may be affected.[90] One central pathway important in inducing feeding behavior involves elevated production of NPY in neurons of the hypothalamic arcuate nucleus. These NPY neurons project to the paraventricular nucleus where they synapse with neurons carrying NPY receptors. This projection is thought to mediate the powerful stimulation of hyperphagia by NPY. In *anx/anx* mice, NPY immunoreactivity accumulates in the perikarya of arcuate NPY neurons; however, decreased staining is observed in NPY terminals in the paraventricular, arcuate, and other hypothalamic nuclei compared to control littermates. This reduction in terminal NPY appears to be specific to the hypothalamus as other NPY systems in the striatum, hippocampus, and cortex were unaffected. However, the reduction in terminal NPY is not likely the sole cause of the anorexia phenotype since NPY knockout mice do not exhibit reduced food intake.[91] It is probable then that *anx/anx* mice show a more generalized defect in axonal transport and/or prohormone processing of at least a subset of neuropeptides, including NPY. It is interesting to note in this context that Broberger et al. also reported a tendency toward reduced somatostatin in arcuate fibers, whereas CCK and 5-HT staining was unchanged.[90]

9.4 Human Disease Associated with Processing Defects

Ultimately, we study animal models to give us insights into human conditions. The mouse, with its close genetic and physiological similarities to humans, has contributed much to the understanding of human disease. After the first insights into the molecular causes of obesity had been gained in the mouse, mutations in the homologous genes in humans have been found to lead to similar obesity phenotypes.[92]

9.4.1 PC1 Mutations

The first human disorder thought to be due to impaired prohormone processing, multiple endocrinopathy, was reported in 1995 at about the same time as the *fat* mutation in mouse.[93] The two diseases, caused by PC1 and CPE mutations, respectively, are remarkably similar in appearance. The 43-year-old-female proband was obese (89.2 kg body weight and 34.4 kg/m² body mass index (BMI) from childhood (36 kg at 3 years of age)). The proband had come to clinical attention because of infertility and hypogonadotropic hypogonadism was diagnosed. In addition to obesity, other clinical abnormalities shown in this patient included impaired glucose tolerance, post-prandial hyperglycemia, and hypocortisolism. Notably, this patient had markedly increased circulating proinsulin levels while levels of mature insulin in the plasma were barely detectable, indicating a defect in proinsulin processing.

Molecular genetic analysis showed that the proband was a compound heterozygote, having two different mutations in her PCSK1 gene which lead to a severe deficiency in active PC1/3.[9] One mutation was a Gly483Arg missense mutation, which prevents processing of proPC1 and leads to retention of proPC1 in the ER. The other mutation was an A to C transversion at position +4 of the intron-5 donor splice site. This mutation causes skipping of exon 5, leading to a loss of 26 amino acid residues, a frameshift, and creation of a premature stop codon within the catalytic domain.

Although plasma insulin levels are low in PC2 null mice, they are, nevertheless, detectable.[84] PC1/3 deficiency, therefore, appears to cause more severe defects in proinsulin processing than PC2 deficiency. The elevated proinsulin in this human patient with PC1 mutations was accompanied by increased amounts of Des-64,65 proinsulin intermediates, as would be expected from a lack of PC1/3 which facilitates cleavage at the B-chain C-peptide junction generating Des-31,32 proinsulin. The patient was not diabetic, but had developed transient gestational diabetes during pregnancy of quadruplets (ovulation was induced with gonadotropins at the age of 30). While no elevation in proglucagon levels was observed in this patient, altered corticotropin precursor processing was reported to lead to a mild hypocortisolemia.

Unlike PC2 or 7B2 deficiency, but similar to the *Cpe^fat* mutation in mice, the lack of PC1/3 activity in humans leads to an obesity syndrome, consistent with a role of PC1/3 in the processing of hypothalamic neuropeptides controlling energy homeostasis and appetite. Nevertheless, the discrepancy in phenotype between the known mutations in the processing pathway requires further explanation. Specifically, the role of genetic background on expression of the runting and obesity phenotypes needs to be examined. A

PC1/3 null mutation on different mouse genetic backgrounds should help to further understand the mechanism of energy imbalance mediated by a PC1/3 defect.

9.4.2   POMC Mutations

Although not due to defects in the prohormone-processing machinery, two human cases of POMC deficiency caused by genetic defects are of interest[94] because mutations in the POMC gene also lead to early onset morbid obesity. The phenotypic attributes of one female patient were obesity (>30kg at 3 years of age), ACTH deficiency, and red hair pigmentation. Symptoms of increased appetite had been observed since 4 months of age. Direct sequencing of PCR products containing the entire coding region of the POMC gene revealed that this patient was a compound heterozygote for two different mutations in the third exon. One was a paternally transmitted transversion of G to T at nucleotide (nt) position 7013, which leads to a premature stop codon at amino acid 79.[95,96] This truncated POMC protein is predicted to have lost bioactive POMC-derived peptides, including ACTH, α-MSH and β-endorphin. The other mutation in this patient was a one base pair (bp) deletion at nt 7133 (C) leading to a frame-shift which is predicted to disturb the structure of the receptor-binding core motif of ACTH and α-MSH (His-Phe-Arg-Trp to His-Phe-Ala-Gly) and introduces a premature stop codon at amino acid 131. Therefore, this compound heterozygous patient had a complete loss of ACTH, α-MSH, and β-endorphin, while the levels of other anterior- and pituitary-derived hormones were normal.

A second, male patient who was homozygous for a transversion of C to A at nt 3804 in exon 2 within the 5′-untranslated region developed early onset severe obesity (>40 kg at 8 years of age). This point mutation creates an extra out-of-frame initiation codon (ATG) and is predicted to interfere with normal POMC translation, leading to a complete lack of POMC protein.

Other variants of the POMC gene have been identified during screening of obese and underweight patients, but it is less clear in these cases whether the mutation is the cause for the observed obesity.[97]

An in-frame insertion of 9-bp (AGC AGC GGC) or 18-bp (AGC AGC GGC AGC AGC GGC) between codons 73 and 74 of POMC, carboxy-terminal to γ-MSH, has been identified. One male patient, homozygous for the 9-bp insertion, was extremely obese at the age of 14 (BMI 32.2 kg/m², waist/hip ratio 0.97), and a female who was heterozygous for the 18-bp insertion had a BMI of 36.4 kg/m². In addition, a female obese adolescent was identified who carried two mutations in γ-LPH transmitted from her mother, an out-of-frame insertion of 6-bp (CCC GGG) within codon 176 introducing two amino acids, and a transversion of G → T at nt 7316 introducing a premature termination at codon 180. These mutations are predicted to cause loss of β-MSH and β-endorphin. The heterozygous mother was not obese (BMI 28.3 kg/m² at age 35.6). The patient also carried a missense mutation (A-7341-G, Glu-188-Gly) transmitted from the father. Because the father was obese (BMI 30.4 kg/m², age 35.7 years) but presumably heterozyous, it is likely that mutations in other genes contributed to the obesity in the female patient (BMI 35.9 kg/m², waist/hip ratio 0.83, age 16.5 years).

9.4.3 Processing Defects in the Human Population

The discovery of rare forms of obesity syndromes caused by defects in prohormone processing prompted a search for such defects as causes for more common forms of obesity and non-insulin-dependent diabetes mellitus (NIDDM). Limited population studies have been carried out in which polymorphisms in the PCSK1 (PC1/3)[98,99] and CPE genes[100] were examined in case-control studies. No significant associations with obesity or NIDDM were observed. For a microsatellite repeat polymorphism in intron 2 of the PCSK2 (PC2) gene, a higher frequency of one allele was found in Japanese NIDDM patients compared to controls.[101] However, no difference in fasting glucose, insulin, or proinsulin levels were found when carriers of the associated allele were compared to noncarriers. Furthermore, only one mutation affecting the PC2 coding sequence was found in an NIDDM patient from this study cohort. Although mutations within the promoter region affecting expression levels cannot be excluded at this time, association with an NIDDM gene close to the PC2 gene is also a possibility.

Currently it does not appear as if mutations in prohormone processing genes can explain significant portions of obesity or Type II diabetes (NIDDM) in the general population; however, broader population-based screens are necessary to exclude these genes. In addition, the upstream control regions of these genes must be examined as well.

9.5 A Genetic Approach for Identifying Distal Effects on Energy Homeostasis

Much of our knowledge about the function of neuro/endocrine peptides stems from studies on localization, expression, observing changes in disease or healthy states, and administration of the peptides by nonphysiological means (intravenous or intracerebroventricular injections). While such studies have provided invaluable information about the possible functions of these peptides, they provide limited knowledge about their direct and indirect *in vivo* action. For example, injection of a single peptide in a single site may not reflect its *in vivo* action. It is entirely possible that the particular peptide is not released in isolation, but normally co-released with others in the same or different tissues. Additionally, the phenotypic effects of a peptide may not be due to changes in its presence or expression, but may be controlled by its

effects on downstream molecules. The *in vivo* function of many neuropeptides is still controversial.[102]

A potentially powerful approach to revealing downstream factors that are
important in mediating the effects of a mutation on the phenotype of a whole
animal is quantitative trait locus (QTL) analysis. QTL analysis in mice makes
use of the genetic variation between two inbred strains of mice. If the two
genomes are mixed by carrying out backcrosses or F2 intercrosses, the new
genetic combinations can give rise to measurable phenotypes. These traits
can then be genetically mapped to QTLs. If only QTLs that interact epistati-
cally with a particular mutation are considered, i.e., in the absence of the
mutation no QTL can be detected, then these QTLs must represent genes in a
pathway that connects the mutant gene with the observed phenotype. For
example, the *fat* mutation is due to a loss of CPE activity, so that normal prohormone processing is impaired. However, because many neuropeptides are
misprocessed, the etiology of the obese phenotype in *fat*/*fat* mice is not clear;
e.g., is one peptide such as MSH critical or do multiple defects contribute to
the observed obesity syndrome.

In order to determine which critical genes determine the obese/diabetic phenotype, a QTL mapping cross was carried out. A hyperglycemic BKS-*fat*/*fat*
female was mated to a HRS-+/+ male and the resulting (BKS/HRS)F1-*fat*/+
offspring were intercrossed to obtain an F2 generation. The (BKS/HRS)F2-
fat/*fat* animals were the experimental group and (BKS/HRS)F2-*fat*/+ and
(BKS/HRS)F2-+/+ the controls. It was found that many of the obesity-related
phenotypes such as body weight and adiposity, plasma glucose, insulin and
serum lipid levels segregated in the (BKS/HRS)F2-*fat*/*fat* population.[103]
From our preliminary analyses, several conclusions can be drawn.[104] First,
there are one or more loci determining each of the subphenotypes that had
been measured in this cross. Second, as has been found in other QTL analyses, some loci influence several phenotypes, while others affect only one specific phenotype. Third, the percentage of genetic variance explained by QTLs
is generally high, so that a few major genes appear to control each trait. And
fourth, importantly, the presence of these QTLs is entirely dependent on the
presence of the *Cpe^{fat}* defect; they are not detected in its absence. For example,
in F2-*fat*/*fat* mice, a QTL for adiposity on Chr 11 was detected ($F = 11.7$, $p =
0.003$), whereas no QTL was detected at this marker in F2-+/+ mice from the
same cross ($F = 0.2$, $p = 0.905$). *Cpe^{fat}*, therefore, can be called a disease gene,
i.e., a gene that is necessary, but not sufficient for the phenotype to develop.
It has to interact with susceptibility genes, genes that are in themselves neither necessary nor sufficient to cause disease, but which in conjunction with
the disease gene determine the observed phenotype.

The genetic mapping of such QTLs, followed by the construction of congenic strains to isolate the individual QTLs in a common genetic background, will eventually allow the identification of the underlying genes.
Congenic strains are constructed by transferring a susceptibility allele onto
a resistant strain background by repeated backcrossing to the resistant
strain. It provides a convenient way of separating unlinked genes and is

particularly useful in assessing the nature and strength of the phenotypic contribution of individual genes in complex traits caused by multiple genes (Serreze et al. 1994).[135] These congenic strains can then be used in genetic fine mapping and positional (candidate) cloning of the gene determining the trait.

Extending such QTL analyses to the knockout mice for *Pcsk2* (PC2) and *Sgne1* (7B2) should shed light on the molecular reasons for the difference in phenotype compared to the *Cpe^fat* mice.

9.6 Conclusion

We have learned a great deal about prohormone processing during the past 50 years; however, major questions remain to be answered. Prominent among these is the question of the cell-specific and temporal regulation of neuropeptide synthesis, maturation, and secretion. New tools available, such as genetic analysis in animals and humans, and conditional inactivation of genes in intact organisms, will help to approach these questions.

Although the proximal actions of many neuropeptides and peptide hormones are known, understanding how these actions are translated into an observable phenotype in an intact organism is still in its infancy. With the identification of the melanocortin pathway over the past few years the first insights have been gained into the pathways controlling food intake and energy homeostasis. Others remain to be discovered.

References

1. Naggert, J., Harris, T., and North, M., The genetics of obesity, *Curr. Opin. Genet. Dev.*, 7, 398, 1997.
2. Woods, S. C. and Stricker, E. M., Food intake and metabolism, in *Fundamental Neuroscience*, M. J. Zigmond, F. E. Bloom, S. C. Landis, J. L. Roberts, and L. R. Squire, Eds., Academic Press, San Diego, 1999, 1091.
3. Levin, B. E. and Routh, V. H., Role of the brain in energy balance and obesity [editorial], *Am. J. Physiol.*, 271, R491, 1996.
4. Strand, F. L., Neuropeptides: Regulators of Physiological Processes, *Cellular and Molecular Neuroscience*, C. F. Stevens, Ed., MIT Press, Cambridge, MA, 1999.
5. Rehfeld, J. F., Bardram, L., Cantor, P., Cerman, J., Hilsted, L., Johnsen, A. H., Mogensen, N., and Odum, L., Peptide hormone expression and precursor processing, *Acta Oncol.*, 28, 315, 1989.
6. Neurath, H., Proteolytic processing and regulation, *Enzyme*, 45, 239, 1991.

7. Seidah, N. G., Day, R., Marcinkiewicz, M., and Chretien, M., Precursor convertases: an evolutionary ancient, cell-specific, combinatorial mechanism yielding
   diverse bioactive peptides and proteins, *Ann. NY Acad. Sci.*, 839, 9, 1998.

8. Naggert, J. K., Fricker, L. D., Varlamov, O., Nishina, P. M., Rouille, Y., Steiner,
   D. F., Carroll, R. J., Paigen, B. J., and Leiter, E. H., Hyperproinsulinaemia in
   obese *fat/fat* mice associated with a carboxypeptidase E mutation which reduces enzyme activity, *Nat. Genet.*, 10, 135, 1995.

9. Jackson, R. S., Creemers, J. W., Ohagi, S., Raffin-Sanson, M. L., Sanders, L.,
   Montague, C. T., Hutton, J. C., and O'Rahilly, S., Obesity and impaired prohormone processing associated with mutations in the human prohormone convertase 1 gene, *Nat. Genet.*, 16, 303, 1997.

10. Civelli, O., Nothacker, H. P., and Reinscheid, R., Reverse physiology: discovery
    of the novel neuropeptide, orphanin FQ/nociceptin, *Crit. Rev. Neurobiol.*, 12,
    163, 1998.

11. Hinuma, S., Onda, H., and Fujino, M., The quest for novel bioactive peptides
    utilizing orphan seven-transmembrane-domain receptors, *J. Mol. Med.*, 77, 495,
    1999.

12. Li, X., Keith, Jr., D. E., and Evans, C. J., Multiple opioid receptor-like genes are
    identified in diverse vertebrate phyla, *FEBS Lett.*, 397, 25, 1996.

13. Larhammar, D., Structural diversity of receptors for neuropeptide Y, peptide
    YY and pancreatic polypeptide, *Regul. Pept.*, 65, 165, 1996.

14. Hoyle, C. H., Neuropeptide families: evolutionary perspectives, *Regul. Pept.*,
    73, 1, 1998.

15. Danielson, P. B. and Dores, R. M., Molecular evolution of the opioid/orphanin
    gene family, *Gen. Comp. Endocrinol.*, 113, 169, 1999.

16. Seidah, N. G., Chretien, M., and Day, R., The family of subtilisin/kexin like
    pro-protein and pro-hormone convertases: divergent or shared functions, *Bio-
    chimie*, 76, 197, 1994.

17. Lundin, L. G., Evolution of the vertebrate genome as reflected in paralogous
    chromosomal regions in man and the house mouse, *Genomics*, 16, 1, 1993.

18. Hokfelt, T., Broberger, C., Zhang, X., Diez, M., Kopp, J., Xu, Z., Landry, M.,
    Bao, L., Schalling, M., Koistinaho, J., DeArmond, S. J., Prusiner, S., Gong, J.,
    and Walsh, J. H., Neuropeptide Y: some viewpoints on a multifaceted peptide
    in the normal and diseased nervous system, *Brain Res. Rev.*, 26, 154, 1998.

19. Rapoport, T. A., Jungnickel, B., and Kutay, U., Protein transport across the
    eucaryotic endoplasmic reticulum and bacterial inner membranes, in *Annual
    Review Biochemistry*, C. C. Richardson, J. N. Abelson, and C. R. H. Raetz, Eds.,
    Annual Reviews, Palo Alto, CA, 1996, 271.

20. Halban, P. A. and Irminger, J. C., Sorting and processing of secretory proteins,
    Biochem. J., 299, 1, 1994.

21. De Camilli, P. and Jahn, R., Pathways to regulated exocytosis in neurons, *Annu.
    Rev. Physiol.*, 52, 625, 1990.

22. Benjannet, S., Rondeau, N., Day, R., Chretien, M., and Seidah, N. G., PC1 and
    PC2 are proprotein convertases capable of cleaving proopiomelanocortin at
    distinct pairs of basic residues, *Proc. Natl. Acad. Sci. USA*, 88, 3564, 1991.

23. Thomas, L., Leduc, R., Thorne, B. A., Smeekens, S. P., Steiner, D. F., and Thomas,
    G., Kex2-like endoproteases PC2 and PC3 accurately cleave a model prohor-
    mone in mammalian cells: evidence for a common core of neuroendocrine
    processing enzymes, *Proc. Natl. Acad. Sci. USA*, 88, 5297, 1991.

24. Uhler, M. and Herbert, E., Complete amino acid sequence of mouse pro-opi-omelanocortin derived from the nucleotide sequence of pro-opiomelanocortin cDNA, *J. Biol. Chem.*, 258, 257, 1983.

25. Bloomquist, B. T., Eipper, B. A., and Mains, R. E., Prohormone-converting enzymes: regulation and evaluation of function using antisense RNA, *Mol. Endocrinol.*, 5, 2014, 1991.

26. Zhou, A., Bloomquist, B. T., and Mains, R. E., The prohormone convertases PC1 and PC2 mediate distinct endoproteolytic cleavages in a strict temporal order during proopiomelanocortin biosynthetic processing, *J. Biol. Chem.*, 268, 1763, 1993.

27. Smeekens, S. P., Avruch, A. S., LaMendola, J., Chan, S. J., and Steiner, D. F., Identification of a cDNA encoding a second putative prohormone convertase related to PC2 in AtT20 cells and islets of Langerhans, *Proc. Natl. Acad. Sci. USA*, 88, 340, 1991.

28. Seidah, N. G., Marcinkiewicz, M., Benjannet, S., Gaspar, L., Beaubien, G., Mattei, M. G., Lazure, C., Mbikay, M., and Chretien, M., Cloning and primary sequence of a mouse candidate prohormone convertase PC1 homologous to PC2, Furin, and Kex2: distinct chromosomal localization and messenger RNA distribution in brain and pituitary compared to PC2, *Mol. Endocrinol.*, 5, 111, 1991.

29. Smeekens, S. P. and Steiner, D. F., Identification of a human insulinoma cDNA encoding a novel mammalian protein structurally related to the yeast dibasic processing protease Kex2, *J. Biol. Chem.*, 265, 2997, 1990.

30. Fricker, L. D., Carboxypeptidase E, *Annu. Rev. Physiol.*, 50, 309, 1988.

31. Steiner, D. F., The proprotein convertases, *Curr. Opin. Chem. Biol.*, 2, 31, 1998.

32. Lindberg, I., The new eukaryotic precursor processing proteinases, *Mol. Endocrinol.*, 5, 1361, 1991.

33. Roebroek, A. J., Schalken, J. A., Leunissen, J. A., Onnekink, C., Bloemers, H. P., and Van de Ven, W. J., Evolutionary conserved close linkage of the c-fes/fps proto-oncogene and genetic sequences encoding a receptor-like protein, *EMBO J.*, 5, 2197, 1986.

34. Kiefer, M. C., Tucker, J. E., Joh, R., Landsberg, K. E., Saltman, D., and Barr, P. J., Identification of a second human subtilisin-like protease gene in the fes/fps region of chromosome 15, *DNA Cell. Biol.*, 10, 757, 1991.

35. Seidah, N. G., Gaspar, L., Mion, P., Marcinkiewicz, M., Mbikay, M., and Chretien, M., cDNA sequence of two distinct pituitary proteins homologous to Kex2 and furin gene products: tissue-specific mRNAs encoding candidates for prohormone processing proteinases [published erratum appears in *DNA Cell. Biol.* 1990 Dec., 9, 10, 789], *DNA Cell. Biol.*, 9, 415, 1990.

36. Day, R., Schafer, M. K., Watson, S. J., Chretien, M., and Seidah, N. G., Distribution and regulation of the prohormone convertases PC1 and PC2 in the rat pituitary, *Mol. Endocrinol.*, 6, 485, 1992.

37. Seidah, N. G., Day, R., Hamelin, J., Gaspar, A., Collard, M. W., and Chretien, M., Testicular expression of PC4 in the rat: molecular diversity of a novel germ cell-specific Kex2/subtilisin-like proprotein convertase, *Mol. Endocrinol.*, 6, 1559, 1992.

38. Lusson, J., Vieau, D., Hamelin, J., Day, R., Chretien, M., and Seidah, N. G., cDNA structure of the mouse and rat subtilisin/kexin-like PC5: a candidate proprotein convertase expressed in endocrine and nonendocrine cells, *Proc. Natl. Acad. Sci. USA*, 90, 6691, 1993.

39. Meerabux, J., Yaspo, M. L., Roebroek, A. J., Van de Ven, W. J., Lister, T. A., and Young, B. D., A new member of the proprotein convertase gene family (LPC) is located at a chromosome translocation breakpoint in lymphomas, *Cancer Res.*, 56, 448, 1996.

40. Seidah, N. G., Hamelin, J., Mamarbachi, M., Dong, W., Tardos, H., Mbikay, M., Chretien, M., and Day, R., cDNA structure, tissue distribution, and chromosomal localization of rat PC7, a novel mammalian proprotein convertase closest to yeast kexin-like proteinases, *Proc. Natl. Acad. Sci. USA*, 93, 3388, 1996.

41. Bruzzaniti, A., Goodge, K., Jay, P., Taviaux, S. A., Lam, M. H., Berta, P., Martin, T. J., Moseley, J. M., and Gillespie, M. T., PC8 [corrected], a new member of the convertase family [published erratum appears in *Biochem J.*, 316, 1007, 1996], *Biochem. J.*, 314, 727, 1996.

42. Beinfeld, M. C., Prohormone and proneuropeptide processing. Recent progress and future challenges, *Endocrine*, 8, 1, 1998.

43. Anderson, E. D., VanSlyke, J. K., Thulin, C. D., Jean, F., and Thomas, G., Activation of the furin endoprotease is a multiple-step process: requirements for acidification and internal propeptide cleavage, *EMBO J.*, 16, 1508, 1997.

44. Gluschankof, P. and Fuller, R. S., A C-terminal domain conserved in precursor processing proteases is required for intramolecular N-terminal maturation of pro-Kex2 protease, *EMBO J.*, 13, 2280, 1994.

45. Braks, J. A., and Martens, G. J., 7B2 is a neuroendocrine chaperone that transiently interacts with prohormone convertase PC2 in the secretory pathway, *Cell*, 78, 263, 1994.

46. Zhu, X., Lamango, N. S., and Lindberg, I., Involvement of a polyproline helix-like structure in the interaction of 7B2 with prohormone convertase 2, *J. Biol. Chem.*, 271, 23582, 1996.

47. Rouille, Y., Duguay, S. J., Lund, K., Furuta, M., Gong, Q., Lipkind, G., Oliva, Jr., A. A., Chan, S. J., and Steiner, D. F., Proteolytic processing mechanisms in the biosynthesis of neuroendocrine peptides: the subtilisin-like proprotein convertases, *Front. Neuroendocrinol.*, 16, 322, 1995.

48. Skidgel, R. A., Structure and function of mammalian zinc carboxypeptidases, in Zinc Metalloproteases in *Health and Disease*, N. M. Hooper, Ed., Taylor and Francis, London, 1996, 241.

49. Skidgel, R. A., Basic carboxypeptidases: regulators of peptide hormone activity, *Trends Pharmacol. Sci.*, 9, 299, 1988.

50. Tan, F., Chan, S. J., Steiner, D. F., Schilling, J. W., and Skidgel, R. A., Molecular cloning and sequencing of the cDNA for human membrane-bound carboxypeptidase M. Comparison with carboxypeptidases A, B, H, and N, *J. Biol. Chem.*, 264, 13165, 1989.

51. Song, L. and Fricker, L. D., Purification and characterization of carboxypeptidase D, a novel carboxypeptidase E-like enzyme, from bovine pituitary, *J. Biol. Chem.*, 270, 25007, 1995.

52. Song, L. and Fricker, L. D., Tissue distribution and characterization of soluble and membrane-bound forms of metallocarboxypeptidase D, *J. Biol. Chem.*, 271, 28884, 1996.

53. Song, L. and Fricker, L. D., Cloning and expression of human carboxypeptidase Z, a novel metallocarboxypeptidase, *J. Biol. Chem.*, 272, 10543, 1997.

54. Rehfeld, J. F., Posttranslational attenuation of peptide gene expression, *FEBS Lett.*, 268, 1, 1990.

55. Rehfeld, J. F., Accumulation of nonamidated preprogastrin and preprocholecystokinin products in porcine pituitary corticotrophs. Evidence of post-translational control of cell differentiation, *J. Biol. Chem.*, 261, 5841, 1986.

56. Liston, D., Patey, G., Rossier, J., Verbanck, P., and Vanderhaeghen, J. J., Processing of proenkephalin is tissue-specific, *Science*, 225, 734, 1984.

57. Wilson, S. P., Unsworth, C. D., and Viveros, O. H., Regulation of opioid peptide synthesis and processing in adrenal chromaffin cells by catecholamines and cyclic adenosine 3':5'- monophosphate, *J. Neurosci.*, 4, 2993, 1984.

58. Hook, V. Y., Azaryan, A. V., Hwang, S. R., and Tezapsidis, N., Proteases and the emerging role of protease inhibitors in prohormone processing, *Faseb J.*, 8, 1269, 1994.

59. Mania-Farnell, B. L., Botros, I., Day, R., and Davis, T. P., Differential modulation of prohormone convertase mRNA by second messenger activators in two cholecystokinin-producing cell lines, *Peptides*, 17, 47, 1996.

60. Jansen, E., Ayoubi, T. A., Meulemans, S. M., and Van de Ven, W. J., Neuroendocrine-specific expression of the human prohormone convertase 1 gene. Hormonal regulation of transcription through distinct cAMP response elements, *J. Biol. Chem.*, 270, 15391, 1995.

61. Hook, V. Y., Sei, C., Yasothornsrikul, S., Toneff, T., Kang, Y. H., Efthimiopoulos, S., Robakis, N. K., and Van Nostrand, W., The kunitz protease inhibitor form of the amyloid precursor protein (KPI/APP) inhibits the proneuropeptide processing enzyme prohormone thiol protease (PTP). Colocalization of KPI/APP and PTP in secretory vesicles, *J. Biol. Chem.*, 274, 3165, 1999.

62. Fortenberry, Y., Liu, J., and Lindberg, I., The role of the 7B2 CT peptide in the inhibition of prohormone convertase 2 in endocrine cell lines, *J. Neurochem.*, 73, 994, 1999.

63. Coleman, D. L. and Eicher, E. M., Fat (*fat*) and tubby (*tub*): two autosomal recessive mutations causing obesity syndromes in the mouse, *J. Hered.*, 81, 424, 1990.

64. Coleman, D. L., Obese and diabetes: two mutant genes causing diabetes-obesity syndromes in mice, *Diabetologia*, 14, 141, 1978.

65. Leiter, E. H., Kintner, J., Flurkey, K., Beamer, W. G., and Naggert, J. K., Physiologic and endocrinologic characterization of male sex-biased diabetes in C57BLKS/J mice congenic for the *fat* mutation at the carboxypeptidease E locus, *Endocrine*, 10, 57, 1999.

66. Fricker, L. D., Berman, Y. L., Leiter, E. H., and Devi, L. A., Carboxypeptidase E activity is deficient in mice with the *fat* mutation. Effect on peptide processing, *J. Biol. Chem.*, 271, 30619, 1996.

67. Kahn, S. E., Leonetti, D. L., Prigeon, R. L., Boyko, E. J., Bergstrom, R. W., and Fujimoto, W. Y., Relationship of proinsulin and insulin with noninsulin-dependent diabetes mellitus and coronary heart disease in Japanese-American men: impact of obesity — clinical research center study, *J. Clin. Endocrinol. Metab.*, 80, 1399, 1995.

68. Birkeland, K. I., Torjesen, P. A., Eriksson, J., Vaaler, S., and Groop, L., Hyperproinsulinemia of type II diabetes is not present before the development of hyperglycemia, *Diabetes Care*, 17, 1307, 1994.

69. Udupi, V., Gomez, P., Song, L., Varlamov, O., Reed, J. T., Leiter, E. H., Fricker, L. D., and Greeley, Jr., G. H., Effect of carboxypeptidase E deficiency on progastrin processing and gastrin messenger ribonucleic acid expression in mice with the *fat* mutation, *Endocrinology*, 138, 1959, 1997.

70. Lacourse, K. A., Friis-Hansen, L., Rehfeld, J. F., and Samuelson, L. C., Disturbed progastrin processing in carboxypeptidase E-deficient fat mice, *FEBS Lett.*, 416, 45, 1997.

71. Cain, B. M., Wang, W., and Beinfeld, M. C., Cholecystokinin (CCK) levels are greatly reduced in the brains but not the duodenums of Cpe(*fat*)/Cpe(*fat*) mice: a regional difference in the involvement of carboxypeptidase E (Cpe) in pro-CCK processing, *Endocrinology*, 138, 4034, 1997.

72. Wang, W., Cain, B. M., and Beinfeld, M. C., Adult carboxypeptidase E-deficient fat/fat mice have a near-total depletion of brain CCK 8 accompanied by a massive accumulation of glycine and arginine extended CCK: identification of CCK 8 Gly as the immediate precursor of CCK 8 in rodent brain, *Endocrine*, 9, 329, 1998.

73. Lacourse, K. A., Friis-Hansen, L., Samuelson, L. C., and Rehfeld, J. F., Altered processing of procholecystokinin in carboxypeptidase E-deficient fat mice: differential synthesis in neurons and endocrine cells, *FEBS Lett.*, 436, 61, 1998.

74. Rovere, C., Viale, A., Nahon, J., and Kitabgi, P., Impaired processing of brain proneurotensin and promelanin-concentrating hormone in obese *fat/fat* mice, *Endocrinology*, 137, 2954, 1996.

75. Perloff, M. D., Kream, R. M., and Beinfeld, M. C., Reduced levels of substance P in the brains of Cpe(fat)/Cpe(*fat*) mice, *Peptides*, 19, 1115, 1998.

76. Cool, D. R., Normant, E., Shen, F., Chen, H. C., Pannell, L., Zhang, Y., and Loh, Y. P., Carboxypeptidase E is a regulated secretory pathway sorting receptor: genetic obliteration leads to endocrine disorders in Cpe(*fat*) mice, *Cell*, 88, 73, 1997.

77. Lei, Y., Xin, X., Morgan, D., Pintar, J. E., and Fricker, L. D., Identification of mouse CPX-1, a novel member of the metallocarboxypeptidase gene family with highest similarity to CPX-2, *DNA Cell. Biol.*, 18, 175, 1999.

78. Xin, X., Day, R., Dong, W., Lei, Y., and Fricker, L. D., Identification of mouse CPX-2, a novel member of the metallocarboxypeptidase gene family: cDNA cloning, mRNA distribution, and protein expression and characterization, *DNA Cell. Biol.*, 17, 897, 1998.

79. Dong, W., Fricker, L. D., and Day, R., Carboxypeptidase D is a potential candidate to carry out redundant processing functions of carboxypeptidase E based on comparative distribution studies in the rat central nervous system, *Neuroscience*, 89, 1301, 1999.

80. Furuta, M., Yano, H., Zhou, A., Rouille, Y., Holst, J. J., Carroll, R., Ravazzola, M., Orci, L., Furuta, H., and Steiner, D. F., Defective prohormone processing and altered pancreatic islet morphology in mice lacking active SPC2, *Proc. Natl. Acad. Sci. USA*, 94, 6646, 1997.

81. Rouille, Y., Martin, S., and Steiner, D. F., Differential processing of proglucagon by the subtilisin-like prohormone convertases PC2 and PC3 to generate either glucagon or glucagon-like peptide, *J. Biol. Chem.*, 270, 26488, 1995.

82. Rouille, Y., Bianchi, M., Irminger, J. C., and Halban, P. A., Role of the prohormone convertase PC2 in the processing of proglucagon to glucagon, *FEBS Lett.*, 413, 119, 1997.

83. Irminger, J. C., Meyer, K., and Halban, P., Proinsulin processing in the rat insulinoma cell line INS after overexpression of the endoproteases PC2 or PC3 by recombinant adenovirus, *Biochem. J.*, 320, 11, 1996.

84. Furuta, M., Carroll, R., Martin, S., Swift, H. H., Ravazzola, M., Orci, L., and Steiner, D. F., Incomplete processing of proinsulin to insulin accompanied by elevation of des-31,32 proinsulin intermediates in islets of mice lacking active PC2, *J. Biol. Chem.*, 273, 3431, 1998.

85. Smeekens, S. P., Montag, A. G., Thomas, G., Albiges-Rizo, C., Carroll, R., Benig, M., Phillips, L. A., Martin, S., Ohagi, S., and Gardner, P., Proinsulin processing by the subtilisin-related proprotein convertases furin, PC2, and PC3, *Proc. Natl. Acad. Sci. USA*, 89, 8822, 1992.

86. Westphal, C. H., Muller, L., Zhou, A., Zhu, X., Bonner-Weir, S., Schambelan, M., Steiner, D. F., Lindberg, I., and Leder, P., The neuroendocrine protein 7B2 is required for peptide hormone processing *in vivo* and provides a novel mechanism for pituitary Cushing's disease, *Cell*, 96, 689, 1999.

87. Maltais, L. J., Lane, P. W., and Beamer, W. G., Anorexia, a recessive mutation causing starvation in preweanling mice, *J. Hered.*, 75, 468, 1984.

88. Son, J. H., Baker, H., Park, D. H., and Joh, T. H., Drastic and selective hyperinnervation of central serotonergic neurons in a lethal neurodevelopmental mouse mutant, anorexia (*anx*), *Brain Res. Mol. Brain Res.*, 25, 129, 1994.

89. Williams, C. L., Rosenblatt, J. S., and Hall, W. G., Inhibition of suckling in weaning-age rats: a possible serotonergic mechanism, *J. Comp. Physiol. Psychol.*, 93, 414, 1979.

90. Broberger, C., Johansen, J., Schalling, M., and Hokfelt, T., Hypothalamic neurohistochemistry of the murine anorexia (*anx/anx*) mutation: altered processing of neuropeptide Y in the arcuate nucleus, *J. Comp. Neurol.*, 387, 124, 1997.

91. Erickson, J. C., Clegg, K. E., and Palmiter, R. D., Sensitivity to leptin and susceptibility to seizures of mice lacking neuropeptide Y, *Nature*, 381, 415, 1996.

92. Perusse, L., Chagnon, Y. C., Weisnagel, J., and Bouchard, C., The human obesity gene map: the 1998 update, *Obes. Res.*, 7, 111, 1999.

93. O'Rahilly, S., Gray, H., Humphreys, P. J., Krook, A., Polonsky, K. S., White, A., Gibson, S., Taylor, K., and Carr, C., Brief report: impaired processing of prohormones associated with abnormalities of glucose homeostasis and adrenal function, *N. Engl. J. Med.*, 333, 1386, 1995.

94. Krude, H., Biebermann, H., Luck, W., Horn, R., Brabant, G., and Gruters, A., Severe early-onset obesity, adrenal insufficiency and red hair pigmentation caused by POMC mutations in humans, *Nat. Genet.*, 19, 155, 1998.

95. Takahashi, H., Hakamata, Y., Watanabe, Y., Kikuno, R., Miyata, T., and Numa, S., Complete nucleotide sequence of the human corticotropin-beta-lipotropin precursor gene, *Nucleic Acids Res.*, 11, 6847, 1983.

96. Takahashi, H., Teranishi, Y., Nakanishi, S., and Numa, S., Isolation and structural organization of the human corticotropin — beta-lipotropin precursor gene, *FEBS Lett.*, 135, 97, 1981.

97. Hinney, A., Becker, I., Heibult, O., Nottebom, K., Schmidt, A., Ziegler, A., Mayer, H., Siegfried, W., Blum, W. F., Remschmidt, H., and Hebebrand, J., Systematic mutation screening of the pro-opiomelanocortin gene: identification of several genetic variants including three different insertions, one nonsense and two missense point mutations in probands of different weight extremes, *J. Clin. Endocrinol. Metab.*, 83, 3737, 1998.

98. Ohagi, S., Sakaguchi, H., Sanke, T., Tatsuta, H., Hanabusa, T., and Nanjo, K., Human prohormone convertase 3 gene: exon-intron organization and molecular scanning for mutations in Japanese subjects with NIDDM, *Diabetes*, 45, 897, 1996.

99. Kalidas, K., Dow, E., Saker, P. J., Wareham, N., Halsall, D., Jackson, R. S., Chan, S. P., Gelding, S., Walker, M., Kousta, E., Johnston, D. G., O'Rahilly, S., and McCarthy, M. I., Prohormone convertase 1 in obesity, gestational diabetes mellitus, and NIDDM: no evidence for a major susceptibility role, *Diabetes*, 47, 287, 1998.

100. Utsunomiya, N., Ohagi, S., Sanke, T., Tatsuta, H., Hanabusa, T., and Nanjo, K., Organization of the human carboxypeptidase E gene and molecular scanning for mutations in Japanese subjects with NIDDM or obesity, *Diabetologia*, 41, 701, 1998.

101. Yoshida, H., Ohagi, S., Sanke, T., Furuta, H., Furuta, M., and Nanjo, K., Association of the prohormone convertase 2 gene (PCSK2) on chromosome 20 with NIDDM in Japanese subjects, *Diabetes*, 44, 389, 1995.

102. van Dijk, G., Thiele, T. E., Seeley, R. J., Woods, S. C., and Bernstein, I. L., Glucagon-like peptide 1 and satiety, *Nature*, 385, 214, 1997.

103. Kim, J. H., Nishina, P. M., and Naggert, J. K., Genetic models for non insulin dependent diabetes mellitus in rodents, *J. Basic Clin. Physiol. Pharmacol.*, 9, 325, 1998.

104. Naggert, J. K., North, M. A., and Nishina, P. M., Central gene defects causing obesity-*fat* and *tub.*, in *Nutrition, Genetics and Obesity*, Bray, G.A. and Ryan, D.H., Eds., Louisiana State University Press, Baton Rouge, 1999, 320.

105. Brown, K. S., Gentry, R. M., and Rowland, N. E., Central injection in rats of alpha-melanocyte-stimulating hormone analog: effects on food intake and brain Fos, *Regul. Pept.*, 78, 89, 1998.

106. Thiele, T. E., van Dijk, G., Yagaloff, K. A., Fisher, S. L., Schwartz, M., Burn, P., and Seeley, R. J., Central infusion of melanocortin agonist MTII in rats: assessment of c-Fos expression and taste aversion, *Am. J. Physiol.*, 274, R248, 1998.

107. Ninan, I. and Kulkarni, S. K., Dopamine receptor sensitive effect of dizocilpine on feeding behaviour, *Brain Res.*, 812, 157, 1998.

108. Vergoni, A. V., Poggioli, R., and Bertolini, A., Corticotropin inhibits food intake in rats, *Neuropeptides*, 7, 153, 1986.

109. Grandison, L. and Guidotti, A., Stimulation of food intake by muscimol and beta endorphin, *Neuropharmacology*, 16, 533, 1977.

110. Khawaja, X. Z., Chattopadhyay, A. K., and Green, I. C., Increased beta-endorphin and dynorphin concentrations in discrete hypothalamic regions of genetically obese (*ob/ob*) mice, *Brain Res.*, 555, 164, 1991.

111. Morley, J. E., Hernandez, E. N., and Flood, J. F., Neuropeptide Y increases food intake in mice, *Am. J. Physiol.*, 253, R516, 1987.

112. McCarthy, H. D., McKibbin, P. E., Perkins, A. V., Linton, E. A., and Williams, G., Alterations in hypothalamic NPY and CRF in anorexic tumor-bearing rats, *Am. J. Physiol.*, 264, E638, 1993.

113. Kalra, S. P., Dube, M. G., Sahu, A., Phelps, C. P., and Kalra, P. S., Neuropeptide Y secretion increases in the paraventricular nucleus in association with increased appetite for food, *Proc. Natl. Acad. Sci. USA*, 88, 10931, 1991.

114. Beck, B., Jhanwar-Uniyal, M., Burlet, A., Chapleur-Chateau, M., Leibowitz, S. F., and Burlet, C., Rapid and localized alterations of neuropeptide Y in discrete hypothalamic nuclei with feeding status, *Brain Res.*, 528, 245, 1990.

115. Krahn, D. D., Gosnell, B. A., Levine, A. S., and Morley, J. E., Behavioral effects of corticotropin-releasing factor: localization and characterization of central effects, *Brain Res.*, 443, 63, 1988.

116. Menzaghi, F., Heinrichs, S. C., Pich, E. M., Tilders, F. J., and Koob, G. F., Functional impairment of hypothalamic corticotropin-releasing factor neurons with immunotargeted toxins enhances food intake induced by neuropeptide Y, *Brain Res.*, 618, 76, 1993.

117. Blake, N. G., Eckland, D. J., Foster, O. J., and Lightman, S. L., Inhibition of hypothalamic thyrotropin-releasing hormone messenger ribonucleic acid during food deprivation, *Endocrinology*, 129, 2714, 1991.

118. Karydis, I. and Tolis, G., Orexins, anorexia, and thyrotropin-releasing hormone, *Thyroid*, 8, 947, 1998.

119. Crawley, J. N., Austin, M. C., Fiske, S. M., Martin, B., Consolo, S., Berthold, M., Langel, U., Fisone, G., and Bartfai, T., Activity of centrally administered galanin fragments on stimulation of feeding behavior and on galanin receptor binding in the rat hypothalamus, *J. Neurosci.*, 10, 3695, 1990.

120. Kyrkouli, S. E., Stanley, B. G., Seirafi, R. D., and Leibowitz, S. F., Stimulation of feeding by galanin: anatomical localization and behavioral specificity of this peptide's effects in the brain, *Peptides*, 11, 995, 1990.

121. Corwin, R. L., Robinson, J. K., and Crawley, J. N., Galanin antagonists block galanin-induced feeding in the hypothalamus and amygdala of the rat, *Eur. J. Neurosci.*, 5, 1528, 1993.

122. Gorbatyuk, O. and Hokfelt, T., Effect of inhibition of glucose and fat metabolism on galanin-R1 receptor mRNA levels in the rat hypothalamic paraventricular and supraoptic nuclei, *Neuroreport*, 9, 3565, 1998.

123. van der Kooy, D., Area postrema: site where cholecystokinin acts to decrease food intake, *Brain Res.*, 295, 345, 1984.

124. Rinaman, L., Hoffman, G. E., Dohanics, J., Le, W. W., Stricker, E. M., and Verbalis, J. G., Cholecystokinin activates catecholaminergic neurons in the caudal medulla that innervate the paraventricular nucleus of the hypothalamus in rats, *J. Comp. Neurol.*, 360, 246, 1995.

125. Dorre, D. and Smith, G. P., Cholecystokinin-B receptor antagonist increases food intake in rats, *Physiol. Behav.*, 65, 11, 1998.

126. Wang, L., Martinez, V., Barrachina, M. D., and Tache, Y., Fos expression in the brain induced by peripheral injection of CCK or leptin plus CCK in fasted lean mice, *Brain Res.*, 791, 157, 1998.

127. Luttinger, D., King, R. A., Sheppard, D., Strupp, J., Nemeroff, C. B., and Prange, Jr., A. J., The effect of neurotensin on food consumption in the rat, *Eur. J. Pharmacol.*, 81, 499, 1982.

128. Hawkins, M. F., Central nervous system neurotensin and feeding, *Physiol. Behav.*, 36, 1, 1986.

129. Beck, B., Stricker-Krongrad, A., Richy, S., and Burlet, C., Evidence that hypothalamic neurotensin signals leptin effects on feeding behavior in normal and fat-preferring rats, *Biochem. Biophys. Res. Commun.*, 252, 634, 1998.

130. Stanley, B. G., Hoebel, B. G., and Leibowitz, S. F., Neurotensin: effects of hypothalamic and intravenous injections on eating and drinking in rats, *Peptides*, 4, 493, 1983.

131. Rossi, M., Choi, S. J., O'Shea, D., Miyoshi, T., Ghatei, M. A., and Bloom, S. R., Melanin-concentrating hormone acutely stimulates feeding, but chronic administration has no effect on body weight, *Endocrinology*, 138, 351, 1997.

132. Bittencourt, J. C., Presse, F., Arias, C., Peto, C., Vaughan, J., Nahon, J. L., Vale, W., and Sawchenko, P. E., The melanin-concentrating hormone system of the rat brain: an immuno- and hybridization histochemical characterization, *J. Comp. Neurol.,* 319, 218, 1992.
133. Ludwig, D. S., Mountjoy, K. G., Tatro, J. B., Gillette, J. A., Frederich, R. C., Flier, J. S., and Maratos-Flier, E., Melanin-concentrating hormone: a functional melanocortin antagonist in the hypothalamus, *Am. J. Physiol.,* 274, E627, 1998.
134. Chambers, J., Ames, R. S., Bergsma, D., Muir, A., Fitzgerald, L. R., Hervieu, G., Dytko, G. M., Foley, J. J., Martin, J., Liu, W. S., Park, J., Ellis, C., Ganguly, S., Konchar, S., Cluderay, J., Leslie, R., Wilson, S., and Sarau, H. M., Melanin-concentrating hormone is the cognate ligand for the orphan G-protein-coupled receptor SLC-1, *Nature,* 400, 261, 1999.
135. Serreze, D. V., Prochazka, M., Reifsnyder, P. C., Bridgett, M. M., and Leiter, E. H., Use of recombinant congenic and congenic strains of NOD mice to identify a new insulin-dependent diabetes resistance gene, *J. Exp. Med.,* 180, 1553, 1994.

10

The Agouti Gene in Obesity: Central and Peripheral Mechanisms, and Therapeutic Implications

Michael B. Zemel, Bingzhong Xue, and Hang Shi

CONTENTS

10.1 Introduction 205
10.2 Agouti Mutations 207
10.3 Yellow Mouse Characteristics..208
10.4 Molecular Characterization of Agouti..209
10.5 Agouti Signaling: Role of Melanocortin Receptors 212
10.6 Role of POMC-Derived Peptides 214
10.7 Agouti Interactions with Mahogany and Mahganoid......................215
10.8 Agouti–Leptin Interactions..216
10.9 Peripheral Actions of Agouti 217
10.10 Role of Calcium 217
10.11 Modulation of Intracellular Calcium by Dietary Calcium:
       Implications for Obesity..220
References 222

10.1 Introduction

The cloning and characterization of several mouse obesity genes as well as their human homologues over the last 8 years have not only resulted in a quantum leap in our insight into the pathophysiology of obesity, but also present opportunities to identify new cellular targets for the development of novel therapeutic strategies. Although the *ob* and *db* genes have been the most widely studied of these, *agouti* was the first obesity gene cloned,[1] and in the ensuing 8 years, both central and peripheral mechanisms of agouti action have been studied extensively. This chapter focuses on these mechanisms of agouti action and their application to the development of intervention strategies.

Variations in mouse coat color have long provided phenotypic markers for genotypic variation and mutations associated with disease. Mutations in the mouse coat color gene agouti were recognized to cause an adult-onset obesity by 1905,[2] and the agouti gene was finally cloned and characterized nearly a century later.[1,3] The gene, mapped to mouse chromosome 2, encodes a 131-amino acid molecule with a consensus signal peptide.

Agouti is transiently expressed in neonatal skin, where it controls the relative amount and distribution of melanin produced by the hair follicle melanocytes. These melanocytes produce a black pigment, eumelanin, in response to α-melanocyte-stimulating hormone (α-MSH) stimulation, while in the absence of α-MSH they produce a default yellow pigment, phaeomelanin[4] [Fig. 10.1]. Follicular melanocytes produce eumelanin under the influence of α-MSH at the beginning of the hair growth cycle. During the mid-portion of this cycle, there is transient expression of agouti, which competitively antagonizes α-MSH receptor binding, resulting in a temporary synthesis of phaeomelanin. As agouti expression ceases, eumelanin synthesis is restored under the influence of α-MSH, which is again able to bind to its receptor.[5] This produces the characteristic pigmentation pattern of wild-type mice, a predominantly black hair shaft with a subapical yellow segment.[4] There are two different wild-type alleles at the agouti locus: agouti (*A*) and

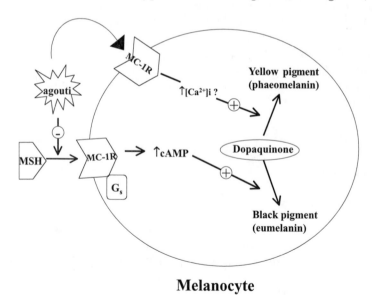

Melanocyte

FIGURE 10.1

Agouti regulation of pigmentation. Agouti competitively antagonizes α-MSH binding to its receptor (MC1-R), thereby preventing MC1-R-G_s coupled synthesis of cAMP. Consequently, phaeomelanin is synthesized. Agouti may also serve as an inverse agonist of MC1-R independently of α-MSH antagonism.

light-bellied agouti (A^w). In agouti (A) mice, yellow pigment is synthesized only during the mid-portion of the hair growth cycle, as described above, resulting in characteristic agouti hair (i.e., black hair with a subapical band of yellow). In contrast, the A^w mice have yellow hair on the ventral surface due to the expression of a ventral-specific agouti transcript, while their dorsal hairs have the characteristic agouti coloration due to the dorsal expression of the hair-cycle-specific agouti transcript noted above.[6,7]

10.2 Agouti Mutations

At least 34 different dominant and recessive agouti alleles have been reported, resulting in a phenotypic dominance hierarchy in which phaeomelanin synthesis is generally dominant over eumelanin synthesis.[8] A number of dominant mutations at the agouti locus result in ectopic agouti expression in virtually all tissues throughout the life of the mouse. The most dominant mutations are lethal yellow (A^y) and viable yellow (A^{vy}). These, along with sienna yellow (A^{sy}), intermediate yellow (A^{iy}), hypervariable yellow (A^{hvy}), and intracisternal A-particle yellow (A^{iapy}), are regulatory mutations in the promoter region, all of which result in ectopic expression of normal agouti transcripts. These mutations result in a uniformly yellow fur in A^y and variable coat colors in the other mutations, ranging from completely yellow to various degrees of yellow and black mottling to a black coat color, referred to as pseudoagouti, which closely resembles wild-type agouti.[9–13] In addition, mice carrying these dominant mutations develop a pleiotropic syndrome which includes obesity, insulin resistance, hyperinsulinemia, hyperphagia, increased linear growth, and decreased thermogenesis.[5,9,14] In general, the degree of agouti overexpression is correlated to the degree of mutant phenotype observed in terms of both coat color and metabolic derangements.[15] This produces a spectrum from the yellow mice with the most pronounced obesity, to mottled mice that frequently exhibit a more attenuated syndrome, to pseudoagouti mice that exhibit minimal agouti expression (detectable via reverse transcriptase polymerase chain reaction (RT-PCR), but not via northern blot), a wild-type coat color and no apparent metabolic derangements.[11,12,15]

Although the mechanism of somatic reversion to the lean phenotype in pseudoagouti animals is not fully defined, the detection of agouti transcripts indicates that epigenetic inactivation of regulatory sequences is responsible for the somatic reversion.[13] Differences in the methylation status of the long terminal repeat (LTR) within the intracisternal A particle (IAP) responsible for ectopic agouti expression (see molecular characterization below) are associated with differential phenotypic expression, as the IAP LTR is methylated in pseudoagouti, but not yellow, mice.[9,15] In addition, expression is influenced by maternal genotype and epigenetic phenotype at the agouti locus[15–17], and pseudoagouti dams produce pseudoagouti offspring more frequently than do dams with yellow phenotypes.[17]

Each of the dominant agouti mutations results in ubiquitous expression of normal agouti protein.[1,15,18] The concept that this ectopic expression is sufficient to induce the pleiotropic disease syndrome was confirmed in transgenic mice overexpressing agouti under the control of the promoters of one of two ubiquitously expressed genes, β-actin or phosphglycerate kinase.[19] Analysis of several lines of transgenic mice expressing agouti under the control of either promoter demonstrates agouti expression in every tissue examined, yellow fur, maturity-onset obesity, hyperinsulinemia, and marked increases in plasma leptin.[19–21] Thus, ectopic expression of agouti is directly responsible for the metabolic derangements observed, as the transgenic animals recapitulate the phenotype of dominant agouti mutants.

10.3　Yellow Mouse Characteristics

Dominant agouti mutants exhibit maturity-onset obesity. Increases in body weight are first observed around 4 weeks of age, and peak between 8 and 17 months.[5,22] Body fat approaches 25 to 26% of body fat in adult yellow mice, or approximately 4-fold higher than wild-type mice.[23] This increase in adiposity is characterized by adipocyte hypertrophy without hyperplasia, and adipose tissue transplantation studies demonstrate that this is largely due to host characteristics.[24,25] In addition to their adiposity, yellow mice exhibit an overall increase in anabolic characteristics, with increased linear growth, muscle mass, and fat-free dry weight.[26–29]

Although yellow obese mice do exhibit hyperphagia, this is not the primary cause of their obesity, as they exhibit a 4-fold increase in body fat but only a 30% increase in food intake. Accordingly, obesity in these mice is primarily due to increased metabolic efficiency, with a preferential partitioning of food energy into fat storage.[30] Yellow mice also exhibit increases in the expression and activity of lipogenic enzymes in both liver and adipose tissue.[31,32] Further, lipolysis is reduced in adipose tissue of yellow mice compared to wild-type mice, and the lipolytic response to epinephrine, theophylline, and the β-agonists LY79771 and LY104119 is suppressed,[33–35] while the response to dibutyryl cyclic AMP is normal. However, cAMP responses to stimulation with LY79771 or LY104119 are impaired, suggesting a defect in generation or maintenance of cAMP.[34,35] Although one early report demonstrated a defect in adaptive thermogenesis in yellow obese mice,[36] there is no difference in brown adipose tissue thermogenic enzyme activity or thermogenic response to a β-adrenergic agonist in yellow vs. wild-type mice.[35,37] Moreover, weight changes in A^{vy} mice subjected to energy restriction are not accompanied by changes in thermogenesis.[35] Accordingly, decreased thermogenesis does not account for the increased metabolic efficiency characteristic of these animals. Instead, the observed coordinated augmentation of lipogenesis and inhibition of lipolysis may contribute to this increase in metabolic efficiency.

Early experiments demonstrated that parabiosis between yellow mice and normal littermates failed to affect body weight or composition in either group, demonstrating that the primary defect in yellow mouse obesity is not in a circulating factor that could be shared in the circulation of parabiotic partners.[38] Further, although both hypophysectomy and adrenalectomy attenuate obesity in yellow mice, differences in body composition persist.[39–41] Thus, neither pituitary- nor adrenal-mediated endocrine pathways have a primary role in yellow mouse obesity. In contrast, given the role of insulin in promoting nutrient partitioning into adipose tissue, hyperinsulinemia may contribute to the enhanced metabolic efficiency of yellow mice. Elevations in insulin are first apparent at approximately 6 weeks of age and peaks at approximately 6 months of age,[42,43] and there is a positive correlation between weight gain and insulinemia and between insulin levels and lipogenic enzyme activity in obese yellow mice.[32] Moreover, pancreatic β-cell hyperplasia precedes the development of obesity in yellow mice. Finally, studies in transgenic mice demonstrate that excess weight gain is, in part, dependent upon insulin.[44] Nonetheless, the relationship among insulin resistance, hyperinsulinemia, and obesity is complex and yellow mouse obesity is clearly not solely due to hyperinsulinemia. Indeed, hyperinsulinemia induced in lean littermates failed to produce a comparable degree of weight gain to that found in agouti transgenic mice.[44] Thus, while hyperinsulinemia may promote the increased metabolic efficiency characteristic of obese yellow mice, it is not sufficient to produce the obesity observed. Instead, agouti and insulin appear to exhibit a synergistic interaction, discussed subsequently in this chapter, which results in the development of obesity.

10.4 Molecular Characterization of Agouti

Agouti was the first obesity gene to be cloned and characterized.[1,3] The gene has three coding exons (exons 2, 3 and 4). The utilization of different promoters and alternative splicing of the first (non-coding) exon results in ventral-specific and hair-cycle-specific transcripts, discussed earlier in this chapter, that vary in size from 0.7 to 0.8 kb despite their identical coding sequences.[6,7] The murine agouti gene is located on chromosome 2 and encodes a 131-amino acid protein.[1,3] Agouti protein contains a 22-amino acid signal sequence, a highly basic central region in which 16 of the 29 amino acids are lysine or arginine residues, a poly-proline-rich region that follows the basic region, and a cysteine-rich carboxyl-terminal region (Fig. 10.2). Asn 39 is a putative N-linked glycosylation site, consistent with the purified protein having a larger apparent mass than predicted (18.5 vs. 11.8 kDa)[3,45](Fig. 10.2).

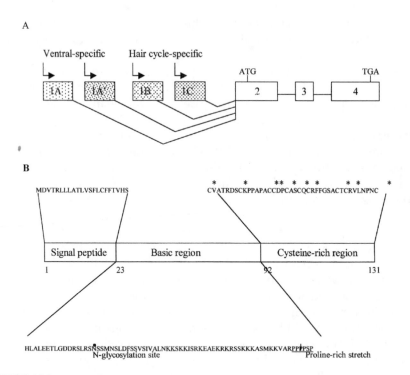

FIGURE 10.2
Genomic and protein structure of agouti. (A) Genomic structure of the mouse agouti gene. Alternative splicing of the first non-coding exon gives rise to ventral-specific (1A and 1A′) and hair cycle-specific (1B and 1C) transcripts. The start and stop codons have been indicated in exons 2 and 4. (B) Agouti protein structure. • Putative N-glycosylation site. *Cysteine residues. Underline: Proline-rich stretch.

All 10 cysteine residues in the carboxyl terminal region are involved in forming disulfide bonds.[45] There is a strong spatial homology between this pattern of cysteine residues in agouti and those found in the venom of primitive hunting spiders and cone snails (plectoxins and conotoxins), toxins which primarily target calcium channels.[45,46] It is noteworthy that the carboxyl-terminal region of agouti retains biological activity *in vitro*, while other constructs do not.[45,47]

Lethal yellow (*A^y*) homozygotes die around the time of implantation, while heterozygotes express a larger than expected 1.1-kb agouti transcript in adult tissues. This increase in size is due to the replacement of novel sequences at the 5′ untranslated region of the *A^y* agouti transcript, while exons 2 to 4 contain the 131-amino acid open reading frame identical to wild-type agouti transcripts.[1,3] These novel 5′ untranslated sequences correspond to the upstream untranslated region of a gene called *Raly* (*Ribonucleoprotein Associated with Lethal Yellow*), a ubiquitously expressed heterogeneous nuclear ribonucleoprotein which normally maps 280 kb proximal to agouti on mouse chromosome 2.[18,48] This chimeric Raly/agouti transcript results from a 170-kb

A

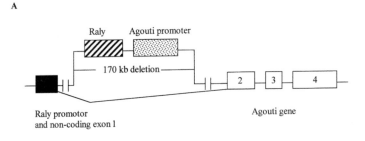

B

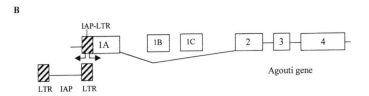

FIGURE 10.3

Proposed models for agouti dominant mutations. (A) The A^y mutation results from the 170 kb deletion which removes agouti promoter and most of the Raly gene except the first non-coding exon. (B) The A^{vy} mutation results from the insertion of an IAP element in exon 1A. IAP: intracisternal A particle. LTR: long terminal repeats.

deletion that removes all but the first non-coding exon of Raly, thereby resulting in splicing of the Raly upstream non-coding region to the agouti coding exons and ubiquitous expression of agouti driven by the Raly promoter[48] (Fig. 10.3). The deletion of Raly is responsible for the embryonic lethality of the homozygote.

In contrast, homozygotes of the other dominant agouti mutations are viable. Ubiquitous expression of agouti in A^{vy} mice results from insertion of an intracisternal A particle (IAP) into exon 1 of agouti, producing a chimeric agouti in which the normal splicing pattern, and hence the normal size, is preserved (Fig. 10.3). The promoter/enhancer within the long terminal repeat (LTR) of the IAP, which has bi-directional promoter activity, is responsible for the ectopic expression of normal agouti protein.[49] Similarly, molecular analysis of A^{iy}, A^{hvy}, and A^{iapy} demonstrates that they also result from insertion of an IAP upstream of the coding region, resulting in ectopic expression of normal agouti protein.[49,50]

The human homologue of agouti, also referred to as agouti signaling protein (ASIP), maps to chromosome 20 and encodes a 132-amino acid protein which is 80% identical to murine agouti protein.[51,52] Although the 3′ and 5′ untranslated regions of human and murine agouti are not similar, the nucleotide sequence of the open reading frames are 85% identical between the two species.[51,52] The amino terminus signal sequence, central basic domain, and cysteine-rich carboxyl terminal regions are also highly conserved between the mouse and human proteins.[51,52] ASIP is expressed primarily in adipose tissue and pancreas;[51,53] it is also found in heart, ovary, and testis and, to a lesser extent in foreskin, kidney, and liver.[51,52] Although its function in humans has not yet been established, human agouti protein retains full functionality when expressed in transgenic mice under the control of the β-actin promoter.[52]

10.5 Agouti Signaling: Role of Melanocortin Receptors

Although the genetic defect in the agouti yellow mouse syndrome clearly involves ectopic expression of the agouti gene, the actual mechanism of the yellow obese syndrome is not clear. Both central and peripheral effects of agouti have been explored extensively, and available evidence suggests central effects on appetite regulation, mediated by melanocortin receptors, as well as peripheral effects on adipocytes and pancreatic islets, which will be discussed in a later section of this chapter. The initial observation that agouti modulation of pigmentation is mediated by antagonism of α-MSH binding to its melanocortin receptor (melanocortin 1 receptor (MC1-R))[45,54,55] has led to the proposal, now widely accepted, that melanocortin receptor antagonism may be responsible for many of the metabolic effects of agouti (Fig. 10.1). However, caution is warranted in extrapolating this observation, as a growing body of evidence demonstrates that agouti also exerts effects on melanocytes independent of α-MSH.[55-60] Indeed, agouti has been proposed to act as an inverse agonist for MC1-R, as it appears to antagonize the constitutive activity of the receptor in the absence of α-MSH.[60] In addition, agouti stimulates Ca^{2+} signaling in several cell types via a mechanism that is dependent upon melanocortin receptors but is not mediated by their antagonism[61] (Fig. 10.4).

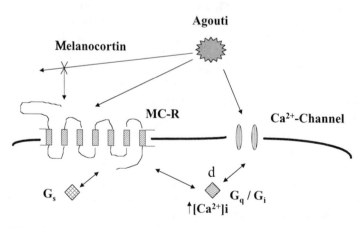

FIGURE 10.4
Agouti stimulation of Ca^{2+} influx is dependent upon the presence of melanocortin receptors, but is not mediated by melanocortin receptor antagonism.

MC1-R belongs to the melanocortin receptor family of 7-transmembrane G-coupled receptors which includes five known members.[62] MC1-R, whose ligand is α-MSH, is primarily expressed in melanocytes and melanoma cells and is involved in the regulation of pigmentation.[63,64] MC2-R, the adrenocorticotropin (ACTH) receptor, is expressed in the adrenal cortex, adipose tissue, and skin.[65-69] MC3-R is expressed in the hypothalamus and limbic system,[70] and a high degree of expression has been noted in the dorsomedial part of the ventromedial nucleus of the hypothalamus and the arcuate nucleus; expression is also found in the septum, hippocampus, thalamus, and midbrain.[71] MC3-R expression is also detectable via RT-PCR in human stomach, duodenum, and rat pancreas.[70] MC4-R expression is widely distributed throughout the brain, with a high degree of expression in hypothalamic centers involved in appetite and body weight regulation.[72-74] MC5-R is a widely distributed receptor found in skeletal muscle and several endocrine and exocrine organs. Although its function is not fully understood, it appears to be involved in thermoregulation and immunomodulation.[2,75,76]

The five melanocortin receptors exhibit 39 to 61% amino acid homology with one another, with MC3-R, MC4-R and MC5-R more closely related to one another (55 to 61%) than to MC1-R and MC2-R (43 to 46%). MC1-R and MC2-R exhibit the least homology (39%) in this receptor family. Each of the melanocortin receptors couples to activation of adenylyl cyclase, although MC3-R is also coupled to G_q, with a consequent stimulation of inositol 1, 3, 4-phosphage production.[77]

The HEK-293 human embryonic kidney cell line does not express melanocortin receptors and, accordingly, transfection of these cells with each melanocortin receptor has served as a useful tool to study the agouti–melanocortin receptor interaction.[61,78] Lu et al.[78] used this approach to demonstrate that agouti is a high affinity antagonist of MC1-R, MC2-R, and MC4-R but exerts little or no effect on MC5-R. Of the receptors antagonized by agouti, loss or gain of function mutations at MC1-R predictably affects pigmentation without causing significant metabolic derangements, while loss of MC2-R function results in familial glucocorticoid deficiency.[2,14,62] Thus, only MC4-R remains as a target for contributing to the agouti-induced obesity syndrome.

Indeed, several studies now suggest that MC4-R may play a role in human obesity. In the Quebec Family Study, Chagnon et al.[79] demonstrated a significant association between restriction fragment length polymorphisms (RFLP) of MC4-R and obesity-related phenotypes. Moreover, two recent reports describe a severely obese child and an adult who were heterozygous for a deletion or insertion-induced frameshift mutation, respectively, in the MC4-R gene.[80,81] In addition, three allelic variants have been identified in obese humans by polymorphism analysis.[82] One variant from an extremely obese individual was cloned and found to be severely impaired in ligand binding and signaling, raising the possibility that it may contribute to the development of obesity.[82] Moreover, several mutations, including base deletion-induced frameshift, base substitution (both resulting in truncated MC4-R), missense and haploid sufficiency, have been identified in extremely obese patients.[83,84]

MC4-R is abundantly expressed in the paraventricular nucleus, dorsmedial nucleus, and ventromedial nucleus, major hypothalamic regions involved in the regulation of feeding, energy homeostasis, and body weight.[85–88] Huszar et al.[89] reported that MC4-R knockout mice exhibit adult-onset obesity associated with hyperphagia, hyperinsulinemia, and insulin resistance, recapitulating many of the metabolic features of dominant agouti mutants. Further intracerebroventricular administration of MTII, a potent MC4-R antagonist, caused a dose-dependent suppression of food intake in four murine models of obesity and hyperphagia.[90] This effect of MC4-R in controlling feeding behavior was confirmed with the demonstration that MC4-R-deficient mice failed to respond to the anorectic actions of MTII.[91] Moreover, food restriction results in selective upregulation of MC4-R density in rat hypothalamus, while diet-induced obesity leads to a downregulation of MC4-R, further suggesting an important role for MC4-R in the control of feeding behavior.[92]

Although agouti is not normally expressed in the brain, an agouti homologue called Agouti Related Protein (AGRP) is expressed in the brain and serves as an endogenous antagonist of α-MSH at MC4-R.[93] AGRP is abundantly expressed in the arcuate nucleus, where its expression is markedly elevated in obese (*ob/ob*) mice.[93] Ubiquitous expression of AGRP in transgenic mice recapitulates the phenotype of obesity found in MC4-R knockout mice.[94,95] These transgenic mice do not exhibit a yellow coat color, suggesting that AGRP does not antagonize MC1-R.[94] AGRP exhibits 25% homology to agouti, with the highest degree of identity found in the cysteine-rich carboxyl terminus.[93] Since the carboxyl terminus of agouti is responsible for its antagonistic role at MC4-R, this homology with AGRP predicts a similar function for this domain, and this function has been verified.[96–98] Further, intracerebroventricular administration of a c-terminal fragment of AGRP increased food intake in rats, an effect that was mimicked by treatment with SHU9119, a potent MC4-R antagonist.[98]

10.6   Role of POMC-Derived Peptides

The endogenous ligand for MC4-R is α-MSH, a peptide cleaved from proopiomelanocortin (POMC); sequential cleavage of this precursor also generates the melanocortin peptides β-MSH, γ-MSH, ACTH and β-endorphin.[85] Expression of the *pomc* gene in the hypothalamus and brainstem produces melanocortigenic neurotransmitters, and expression in the pituitary gland produces melanocortin hormones.[2] α-MSH binds to MC4-R with a high affinity and appears to act as a strong agonist in food intake and body weight regulation. Yaswen et al.[99] recently generated *pomc* knockout mice lacking all POMC-derived peptides. These mice develop hyperphagia and obesity with a time course and severity comparable to the aforementioned MC4-R knockout mice.[89] Interestingly, however, loss of α-MSH produced a much more subtle effect on pigmentation than was expected based on the yellow coat color seen both in agouti mutants and loss of function mutations at the MC1-R locus. The authors suggest that the failure of ligand deprivation to produce the same phenotype as loss of receptor function or receptor antagonism results from either other ligands acting at MC1-R or, more likely, some degree of basal activity of the MC1-receptor even in the absence of ligand.

To confirm the role of α-MSH in the control of body weight regulation, a stable agonist, [Ac-Cys[4], D-Phe[7], Cys[10]] α-MSH, was administered daily via intraperitoneal injection. MSH administration resulted in marked weight loss: 38% of the knockout-induced weight gain within 1 week and 46% within 2 weeks in the mutant mice but was without significant effect in wild-type littermates. These data clearly implicate POMC peptides in body weight regulation. However, several cautionary notes are warranted in extending this conclusion. First, the observation that loss of α-MSH produces a different effect on pigmentation than loss or antagonism of receptor function suggests the salutary effects of MSH on weight loss found in POMC-deficient animals may be attenuated in POMC-replete animals, even in the presence of agouti, AGRP, or other potential melanocortin receptor antagonists. Indeed, twice-daily administration of comparable doses of a stable MSH analogue (norleucine[4], D-phenylalanine[7], α-MSH) failed to alter any aspect of the obese phenotype (body weight, fat weight, core temperature, adipocyte lipid metabolism, circulating glucose, and insulin) of either dominant agouti mutant mice (*A^y*) or transgenic mice ubiquitously expressing agouti.[100] Thus, the effects of MSH administration in *pomc* knockouts may not necessarily extrapolate to other models. Nonetheless, abundant evidence now clearly implicates POMC peptides and MC4-R in agouti and AGRP-induced obesity.

10.7 Agouti Interactions with Mahogany and Mahoganoid

The mouse mutations *mahogany* (*mg*) and *mahoganoid* (*md*) are negative modifiers of agouti,[101] as mutations at *mg* or *md* suppress the effects of *A^y* on both coat color and obesity.[101,102] These effects are specific for agouti, as mutations of mahogany did not suppress weight gain in other models of obesity.[102,103] Mahogany acts along the agouti–melanocortin pathway, and mutations at *mg* do not reverse obesity in MC4-R knockout mice, although *mg* does reverse diet-induced obesity.[103] Further, *mg* mice are resistant to diet-induced obesity and eat significantly more than normal mice without gaining weight, presumably due to increases in metabolic rate and spontaneous motor activity.[102]

The gene encoding *mg* encodes a 1428 amino acid, single-transmembrane-domain protein that is expressed in several tissues, including the hypothalamus.[103,104] The cytoplasmic tail of mahogany is short and contains no previously defined signaling domain,[103,104] while the extracellular domain is an orthologue of human attractin.[104,105] It has been suggested that mahogany may serve as a low affinity receptor for agouti, thereby reducing its local concentration,[103,104] and mahogany has been demonstrated to bind recombinant agouti protein, but not AGRP,[106] possibly by interactions between agouti and the C-type lectin domain and/or glycosaminoglycan side chains of mahogany.[104]

10.8   Agouti–Leptin Interactions

Recent data indicate that there is significant cross-talk between the leptin and agouti-ASIP-melanocortin signaling pathways. The leptin receptor is expressed in AGRP- and POMC-producing neurons in the hypothalamic arcuate nucleus,[107–109] and leptin has been demonstrated to regulate AGRP expression.[93,94,107,110] Further, *pomc* expression is significantly reduced in leptin-deficient *ob/ob* mice and leptin resistant *db/db* mice and is upregulated by leptin treatment.[111–113] Moreover, central administration of the MC4-R antagonist SHU9119 completely inhibits the anorexic response to leptin in mice, suggesting that MC4-R may, in part, also mediate leptin action.[114] However, obese MC4-R deficient mice do not respond the anorexic effects of leptin, while non-obese MC4-R-deficient mice do.[115] These data demonstrate that, although MC4-R plays a role in leptin signaling, it is clearly not an exclusive target of leptin action.

Plasma leptin levels are elevated in obese yellow mice, and agouti protein directly stimulates leptin expression and secretion in both 3T3-L1 adipocytes and human adipose tissue.[21] The marked elevations of circulating leptin accompanied by persistent obesity in dominant agouti mutants has led to the suggestion that these animals are leptin resistant. However, Boston et al.[116] studied the independent and interactive effects of agouti and leptin in mice by comparing a dominant agouti mutant (lethal yellow, A^y/a), leptin deficient (lep^{ob}/lep^{ob}) and double mutant (yellow/leptin-deficient; $A^y/a\ lep^{ob}/lep^{ob}$) mice with controls (C57BL/6J). The presence of the A^y allele produced similar degrees of weight gain in both the wild-type and leptin-deficient lep^{ob}/lep^{ob} mice, demonstrating that the effects of defective POMC signaling and leptin deficiency are independent and additive. To further evaluate the relationship between MC4-R signaling and leptin action, the effects of leptin administration on weight loss, food intake, and serum insulin were compared in the four mouse genotypes.[116] A^y mice exhibited significant resistance to leptin action relative to the $lep^{ob}lep^{ob}$ mice, as indicated by an inability of leptin to induce weight loss, suppress food intake, or lower serum insulin. However, this leptin resistance is likely to result from receptor desensitization secondary to increased circulating leptin, as removal of leptin from the A^y/a mice in the double mutant lethal yellow/leptin-deficient model ($A^y/a\ lep^{ob}/lep^{ob}$) completely restored the responsiveness of these animals to exogenous leptin. These data indicate that agouti-induced obesity is independent of leptin action, although elevated leptin in dominant agouti mutants is likely to serve as a counterregulatory mechanism to limit the degree of agouti-induced obesity.

10.9 Peripheral Actions of Agouti

An accumulating body of evidence indicates that, in addition to the aforementioned central effects of agouti, peripheral actions of agouti are likely to contribute to agouti-induced obesity and strongly suggest a role of agouti signaling in adipocytes and pancreatic β-cells. Although hyperphagia in obese yellow mice appears to be mediated by agouti antagonism of MC4-R, as discussed above, these mice also exhibit marked increases in the efficiency of energy utilization, with preferential energy partitioning into adipose tissue stores. Moreover, although there has been considerable focus on central MC4-R antagonism, MC4-R mRNA has also been detected in human adipose tissue and skeletal muscle.[79] Moreover, transgenic mice that selectively express agouti in adipose tissue under the control of the aP2 promoter develop mild obesity, especially if concomitant hyperinsulinemia is induced, while their non-transgenic littermates do not.[44-46] Thus, agouti expression in adipose tissue results in an increase in energy partitioning into adipose tissue, leading to accelerated accretion of adipose tissue mass. This demonstrates that agouti-induced obesity includes a significant peripheral component. Recent data indicate that these effects are mediated by modulation of intracellular Ca^{2+}.

10.10 Role of Calcium

The C-terminal region of the agouti protein retains full functional activity relative to the intact protein in an *in vitro* assay system,[45] as discussed previously. Further, the agouti C-terminus bears a striking spatial homology in both number and spacing of cysteine residues to spider and snail venoms (ω-conotoxins, plectoxins) which target Ca^{2+} channels.[46] Accordingly, the C-terminus may form a three-dimensional structure that is functionally similar to these venoms and may thereby serve to modulate Ca^{2+} transport. Indeed, we have reported that A^{vy} mice exhibit increases in both steady-state intracellular Ca^{2+} and Ca^{2+} influx in several tissues.[61,117] This increase in intracellular $(Ca^{2+})_i$ was closely correlated with both the degree of ectopic agouti expression and body weight,[117] suggesting the possibility of a causal mechanism between intracellular Ca^{2+} and obesity in these animals. Since A^{vy} mice exhibit elevated rates of adipocyte lipogenesis and increased adipocyte size relative to lean controls,[38,118] the links among agouti, intracellular Ca^{2+}, and regulatory enzymes in lipid metabolism have been explored further.

Recombinant agouti protein directly increased Ca^{2+} influx and steady-state intracellular Ca^{2+} in a variety of cell types, including both murine and human adipocytes.[61,117] This regulation occurs in response to physiologically meaningful concentrations of agouti (EC_{50} of 18 to 62 nM, depending upon cell type) and, although studies in HEK-293 cells demonstrate the dependence of this effect upon the presence of intact melanocortin receptors (MCRs), it is not dependent upon MCR antagonism.[61] The role of these increases in Ca^{2+} in lipogenesis has been explored using fatty acid synthase (FAS), as this multifunctional enzyme is highly regulated by nutrients and hormones and is a key enzyme in *de novo* lipogenesis. FAS expression and activity are markedly increased in A^{vy} relative to control mice,[31] and nanomolar concentrations of agouti protein stimulate ~two-fold increases in FAS gene expression and activity and triglyceride accumulation in 3T3-L1 adipocytes[31] as well as in human adipocytes, similar to the maximal increases stimulated by insulin. These increases are mediated by a distinct agouti/Ca^{2+} response sequence in the FAS promoter.[119] This sequence maps to the –435 to –415 region of the FAS promoter and is upstream of the insulin response element, which maps to –67 to –52, consistent with the observed additive effects of agouti and insulin on FAS gene transcription.[119] Further, recent evidence indicates that agouti exerts a regulatory effect on human FAS expression *in vivo*, and there is a strong correlation between agouti expression and FAS expression in adipose tissue obtained from normal volunteers.[120] This agouti modulation of FAS transcription appears to be mediated via intracellular Ca^{2+}, as it can be inhibited by Ca^{2+} antagonism[14,31] and can be mimicked in the absence of agouti by either receptor- or voltage-mediated Ca^{2+} channel activation.[121]

In addition to activating lipogenesis, recent data also indicate that increasing intracellular Ca^{2+} may also contribute to increased triglyceride stores by inhibiting lipolysis. Increasing Ca^{2+} influx with either arginine vasopressin or epidermal growth factor was reported to inhibit lipolysis in rat adipocytes in a Ca^{2+} dose-responsive fashion.[122] Further, we have shown that the agouti gene product similarly inhibits lipolysis in human adipocytes via a Ca^{2+}-dependent mechanism.[123] This inhibition can also be mimicked in the absence of agouti by either receptor- or voltage-mediated Ca^{2+} channel activation.[123] The anti-lipolytic effect of intracellular Ca^{2+} is due to a direct activation of phosphodiesterase 3B, resulting in a decrease in cAMP and, consequently, reduced ability of agonists to stimulate phosphorylation and activation of hormone-sensitive lipase[124]. Thus, agouti regulation of adipocyte intracellular Ca^{2+} appears to promote triglyceride storage in human adipocytes by exerting a coordinated control of lipogenesis and lipolysis, serving to simultaneously stimulate the former and inhibit the latter.

However, it is important to note that agouti interaction with insulin is required for the full expression of agouti-induced obesity. Agouti and insulin exert independent, additive effects on FAS transcription and lipogenesis.[119] Since increased intracellular Ca^{2+} is the proximate signal for insulin release, and agouti regulates Ca^{2+} in several cell types[61] (Fig. 10.4), it is reasonable to speculate that agouti may stimulate insulin release as well. Indeed, we have recently found that agouti is expressed in human pancreas and stimulates Ca^{2+} signaling in rat, hamster, and human pancreatic β cells.[53] Further, hyperplasia of β cells precedes the development of obesity in agouti mutant mice, suggesting that hyperinsulinemia may be a direct effect of agouti acting on the pancreas and that the combination of this hyperinsulinemia and agouti-stimulated adipocyte Ca^{2+} influx may lead to obesity. In support of this concept, transgenic mice expressing agouti at high levels in adipose tissue under the control of the aP2 promoter become obese if they are also hyperinsulinemic as a result of either exogenous insulin or a high sucrose diet, while hyperinsulinemia was without effect in non-transgenic littermate controls.[44,125,126] Since humans exhibit a similar pattern of adipocyte agouti expression,[51] similar agouti/insulin/Ca^{2+} interactions may result in excessive adipocyte triglyceride storage.

Taken together, these data indicate that regulation of adipocyte intracellular Ca^{2+}, possibly coupled with pancreatic Ca^{2+} and insulin release, may be an important target for the development of therapeutic strategies for the prevention and treatment of obesity[14] (Fig. 10.5). To evaluate this hypothesis, agouti-expressing transgenic mice were treated with high doses of a Ca^{2+} channel antagonist, nifedipine. This treatment resulted in an 18% reduction in fat pad mass and completely normalized the agouti-induced hyperinsulinemia over

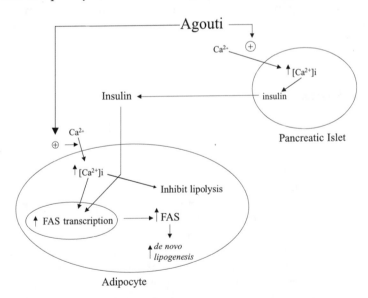

FIGURE 10.5
Agouti modulation of adiposity. Agouti stimulates Ca^{2+} influx in pancreatic β-cells, resulting in increased insulin release. Agouti stimulates Ca^{2+} influx in adipocytes, resulting in increased fatty acid synthase (FAS) transcription and activity and inhibition of lipolysis. The agouti-induced insulinemia augments the effects of agouti on adipocytes by independently increasing FAS transcription and inhibiting lipolysis.

a 4-week treatment period in the transgenic mice, but was without effect in the non-transgenic littermate controls.[20] Thus, adipocyte and/or pancreatic β-cell $(Ca^{2+})_i$ appear to be reasonable therapeutic targets for the treatment and/or prevention of obesity.

We recently extended this concept by demonstrating that human adipocytes express a sulfonylurea receptor (SUR) which exerts a regulatory effect on the Ca^{2+} channel and, consequently, modulates adipocyte lipid accumulation.[121,127] Compounds acting on the pancreatic SUR to increase (e.g., glinbenclamide) or decrease (e.g., diazoxide) intracellular Ca^{2+} (indirectly, via a K^+-ATP channel) cause corresponding increases and decreases in weight gain, although these effects have previously been attributed to the effects of these compounds on circulating insulin. However, the identification of SUR expression in human adipocytes[121] suggests that it may modulate adipocyte Ca^{2+} flux and thereby regulate lipid metabolism. Indeed, the SUR agonist glinbenclamide increases human adipocyte intracellular Ca^{2+} and thereby causes marked increases in lipogenic enzyme activity and inhibition of lipolysis. Moreover, inhibition of the adipocyte SUR-regulated Ca^{2+} channel with diazoxide completely prevented each of these effects. Accordingly, the adipocyte SUR may represent a new target for the development of therapeutic interventions in obesity.[121] In support of this concept, diazoxide has been demonstrated to exert significant anti-obesity effects in both obese Zucker rats and hyperinsulinemic obese adults.[128-130] Although this effect was attributed to actions on pancreatic β-cell insulin release, we subsequently found diazoxide treatment to significantly suppress adipose tissue fatty acid synthase and lipoprotein lipase in obese Zucker rats.[127]

10.11 Modulation of Intracellular Calcium by Dietary Calcium: Implications for Obesity

We recently reported that 1,25-dihydroxy-vitamin D [1,25-(OH_2)-D] stimulates Ca^{2+} influx, resulting in significant, sustained dose-responsive increases in steady-state intracellular Ca^{2+} in primary cultures of human adipocytes.[131] Moreover, 1,25-(OH_2)-D treatment of human adipocytes resulted in a coordinated activation of FAS and inhibition of lipolysis, similar to the action of agouti on these cells.[131] Consequently, suppression of 1,25-(OH_2)-D with high calcium diets would be anticipated to reduce adipocyte intracellular Ca^{2+}, inhibit FAS, and activate lipolysis, thereby exerting an anti-obesity effect.

This concept was confirmed in transgenic mice expressing agouti in adipose tissue under the control of the aP2 promoter. Mice placed on low calcium (0.4%)/high fat/high sucrose diets for 6 weeks exhibited marked increases in adipocyte lipogenesis, inhibited lipolysis, and accelerated increases in body weight and adipose tissue mass. However, high calcium (1.2%) diets reduced lipogenesis by 51% and stimulated lipolysis 3 to 5-fold, resulting in 26 to 39%

reductions in body weight and adipose tissue mass, respectively.[131] The magnitude of these effects depended upon the source of dietary calcium, with dairy sources of calcium exerting significantly greater effects than calcium carbonate.

Consistent with this finding, 12 months of yogurt supplementation, sufficient to raise daily calcium intake from approximately 400 to 1000 mg/day, resulted in a 4.9 kg reduction in body fat in obese African Americans without an accompanying reduction in caloric intake.[131] The relevance of this finding at the population level was assessed via analysis of the National Health and Nutrition Examination Survey (NHANES III); odds ratios for percent body fat as a function of calcium intake were estimated by logistic regression, with age, race/ethnicity, activity level, and caloric intake as covariates. The odds of being in the highest quartile of body fat were reduced from 1.0 for the first quartile of calcium intake to 0.75, 0.40, and 0.16 for the second, third, and fourth quartiles of calcium intake, respectively, for women.[131] The regression model for males similarly demonstrated a significant inverse relationship between dietary calcium and body fat, although the same simple dose-response relationship found in women was not evident.[131]

These data have significant implications for the prevention or attenuation of diet-induced obesity but do not directly address the issue of whether high calcium diets will exert any effect on established obesity. Accordingly, a follow-up study was conducted to determine whether increasing dietary calcium will reduce metabolic efficiency and accelerate fat loss secondary to caloric restriction following dietary induction of obesity.[132] Administration of the same low-calcium/high-fat/high-sucrose diet to aP2-agouti transgenic mice resulted in a ~100% increase in adipocyte intracellular Ca^{2+} and a corresponding weight gain of 29% and a 2-fold increase in total fat pad mass, demonstrating that dysregulation of adipocyte intracellular Ca^{2+} is associated with increased adiposity in aP2-agouti transgenic mice. The animals were then placed on energy restriction (70% of an *ad libitum* fed control group) for an additional 6 weeks. Energy restriction on the low-calcium diet failed to reduce intracellular Ca^{2+} and only reduced body weight and fat pad mass by 11 and 8%, respectively. In contrast, energy restriction in conjunction with high-calcium (1.2%) diets normalized intracellular calcium and resulted in 19 to 29% reductions in body weight and 42 to 69% decreases in fat pad mass, depending upon the calcium source (calcium carbonate vs. dairy). In addition, the high-calcium diets caused marked reductions in FAS expression and activity (35 to 81%), 2 to 3-fold increases in lipolysis and increases in core temperature (0.48 to 0.67° C) and uncoupling protein-2 expression.[132] These data demonstrate that high-calcium diets suppress adipocyte intracellular Ca^{2+} by suppressing 1,25-(OH_2)-D and thereby shifts the partitioning of dietary energy from energy storage to energy expenditure (Fig. 10.6).

Collectively, these data from agouti modulation of adipocyte Ca^{2+} flux, Ca^{2+}-channel antagonism experiments, adipocyte sulfonylurea receptor studies, and dietary calcium modulation of adipocyte lipid metabolism all demonstrate that adipocyte Ca^{2+} signaling is an attractive target for the development of obesity interventions.

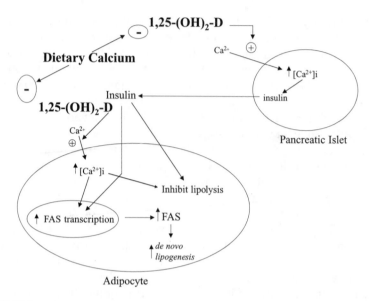

FIGURE 10.6

Dietary calcium modulation of adiposity. 1,25-dihyroxy-vitamin D [1,25-$(OH)_2$-D] stimulates Ca^{2+} influx in both pancreatic β-cells and adipocytes, resulting in increased insulin release, increased FAS transcription and activity, and reduced lipolysis. Increasing dietary calcium suppresses 1,25-$(OH)_2$-D release, thereby removing a stimulus for Ca^{2+} influx. Consequently, insulin release is reduced, FAS transcription and activity are reduced, and lipolysis is activated.

References

1. Bultman, S. J., Michaud, E. J., and Woychik, R. P., Molecular characterization of the mouse agouti locus, *Cell*, 71, 1195, 1992.
2. Barsh, G., From agouti to *pomc*-100 years of fat blonde mice, *Nature Med.*, 5, 984, 1999.
3. Miller, M. W., Duhl, D. M. J., Vrieling, H., Cordes, S. P., Ollmann, M. M., Winkes, B. M., and Barsh, G. S., Cloning of the mouse agouti gene predicts a secreted protein ubiquitously expressed in mice carrying the lethal yellow mutation, *Genes Dev.*, 7, 454, 1993.
4. Galbraith, D. B., The agouti pigment pattern of the mouse: a quantitative and experimental study, *J. Exp. Zool.*, 155, 71, 1964.
5. Wolff, G. L., Roberts, D. W., and Mountjoy, K. G., Physiological consequences of ectopic agouti gene expression: the yellow mouse syndrome, *Physiol. Genomics*, 1, 151, 1999.
6. Bultman, S., Kiebig, M. L., Michaud, E. J., Sweet, H. O., Davisson, M. T., and Woychik, R. P., Molecular analysis of reverse mutations from nonagouti (*a*) to black-and-tan (*aᵗ*) and white-bellied agouti (*Aʷ*) reveals alternative forms of agouti transcripts, *Genes Dev.*, 8, 481, 1994.

7. Vrieling, H., Duhl, D. M. J., Millar, S., Miller, K. A., and Barsh, G. S., Differences in dorsal and ventral pigmentation result from regional expression of the mouse *agouti* gene, *Proc. Natl. Acad. Sci. USA*, 91, 5667, 1994.

8. Siracusa, L. D., The agouti gene: turned on to yellow, *Trend. Genet.*, 10, 423, 1994.

9. Yen, T. T., Gill, A. M., Frigeri, L. G., Barsh, G. S., and Wolff, G. L., Obesity, diabetes, and neoplasia in yellow A^{vy}/- mice: ectopic expression of the agouti gene, *FASEB J.*, 8, 479, 1994.

10. Dickie, M. M., Mutations at the agouti locus in the mouse, *J. Hered.*, 60: 20, 1969.

11. Siracusa, L. D., Washburn, L. L., Swing, D. A., Argeson, A. C., Jenkins, N. A., and Copeland, N. G., Hypervariable yellow (A^{hvy}), a new murine agouti mutation: A^{hvy} displays the largest variation in coat color phenotypes of all known agouti alleles, *J. Hered.*, 86: 121, 1995.

12. Argeson, A. C., Nelson, K. K., and Siracusa, L. D., Molecular basis of the pleiotropic phenotype of mice carrying the hypervariable yellow (A^{hvy}) mutation at the agouti locus, *Genetics*, 142, 557, 1996.

13. Duhl, D. M. J., Vrieling, H., Miller, K. A., Wolff, G. L., and Barsh, G. S., Neomorphic agouti mutations in obese yellow mice, *Nat. Genet.*, 8, 59, 1994.

14. Zemel, M. B. and Xue, B., Agouti/melanocortin interactions with leptin pathways in obesity, *Nutr. Rev.*, 56, 271, 1998.

15. Michaud, E. J., van Vugt, M. J., Bultman, S. J., Sweet, H. O., Davisson, M. T., and Woychik, R. P., Differential expression of a new dominant agouti allele (A^{ispy}) is correlated with methylation state and is influenced by parental lineage, *Genes Dev.*, 8, 1463, 1994.

16. Wolff, G. L., Influence of maternal phenotype on metabolic differentiation of agouti locus mutants in the mouse, *Genetics*, 88, 529, 1978.

17. Wolff, G. L., Kodell, R. L., Moore, S. R., and Cooney, C. A., Maternal epigenetics and methyl supplements affect agouti gene expression in A^{vy}/a mice, *FASEB J.*, 12, 949, 1998.

18. Michaud, E. J., Bultman, S. J., Stubbs, L. J., and Woychik, R. P., The embryonic lethality of homozygous lethal yellow mice (A^y/A^y) is associated with the disruption of a novel RNA-binding protein, *Genes Dev.*, 7, 1203, 1993.

19. Klebig, M. L., Wilkinson, J. E., Geisler, J. G., and Woychik, R. P., Ectopic expression of the agouti gene in transgenic mice causes obesity, features of type II diabetes, and yellow fur, *Proc. Natl. Acad. Sci. USA*, 92, 4728, 1995.

20. Kim, J. H., Mynatt, R. L., Moore, J. W., Woychik, R. P., Moustaïd, N., and Zemel, M. B., The effects of calcium channel blockade on agouti-induced obesity, *FASEB J.*, 10, 1646, 1996.

21. Claycombe, K. J., Xue, B. Z., Mynatt, R. L., Zemel, M. B., and Moustaïd-Moussa, N., Regulation of leptin by agouti, *Physiol. Genomics*, 2, 101, 2000.

22. Dickie, M. M. and Woolley, G. W., The age factor in weight of yellow mice, *J. Hered.*, 37, 365, 1946.

23. Yen, T. T., Allan, J. A., Yu, P. L., Acton, M. A., and Pearson, D. V., Triacyglycerol contents and *in vivo* lipogenesis of ob/ob, db/db and A^{vy}/a mice, *Biochem. Biophys. Acta*, 441, 213, 1976.

24. Johnson, P. R. and Hirsch, J., Cellularity of adipose depots in six strains of genetically obese mice, *J. Lipid Res.*, 13, 2, 1972.

25. Meade, C. J., Ashwell, M., and Sowter, C., Is genetically transmitted obesity due to an adipose tissue defect?, *Proc. R. Soc. Lond. B.*, 205, 395, 1979.

26. Carpenter, K. J., and Mayer, J., Physiologic observations on yellow obesity in the mouse, *Am. J. Physiol.*, 193, 499, 1958.

27. Heston, W. E. and Vlahakis, G., Elimination of the effect of the A^y gene on pulmonary tumors in mice by alteration of its effect on normal growth, *J. Natl. Cancer Inst.*, 27, 1189, 1961.
28. Jackson, E., Stolz, D., and Martin, R., Effect of adrenalectomy on weight gain and body composition of yellow obese mice (A^y/a), *Horm. Metab. Res.*, 8, 452, 1976.
29. Wolff, G. L., Roberts, D. E., and Balbraith, D. B., Prenatal determination of obesity, tumor susceptibility, and coat color pattern in viable yellow (A^y/a) mice, *J. Hered.*, 77, 151, 1986.
30. Frigeri, L. G., Wolff, G. L., and Teguh, C., Differential responses of yellow mouse A^{vy}/a and agouti A/a (BALB/c X VY) F1 hybrid to the same diets: glucose tolerance, weight gain, and adipocyte cellularity, *Int. J. Obes.*, 12, 305, 1988.
31. Jones, B. H., Kim, J. H., Zemel, M. B., Woychik, R. P., Michaud, E. J., Wilkison, W. O., and Moustaïd, N., Upregulation of adipocyte metabolism by agouti protein: possible paracrine actions in yellow mouse obesity, *Am. J. Physiol.*, 270. E192, 1996.
32. Yen, T. T., Greenberg, M. M., Yu, P. L., and Pearson, D. V., An analysis of the relationships among obesity, plasma insulin, and hepatic lipogenic enzymes in "viable yellow obese" mice (A^{vy}/a), *Horm. Metab. Res.*, 8, 159, 1976.
33. Yen, T. T., Steinmetz, J., and Wolff, G. L., Lipolysis in genetically obese and diabetes-prone mice, *Horm. Metab. Res.*, 2, 200, 1970.
34. Yen, T. T., McKee, M. M., Stamm, N. B., and Bemis, K. G., Stimulation of cyclic AMP and lipolysis in adipose tissue of normal and obese A^{vy}/a mice by LY 79771, a phenethanolamine, and stereoisomers, *Life Sci.*, 32, 1515, 1983.
35. Yen, T. T., Mckee, M. M., and Stamm, N. B., Thermogenesis and weight control, *Int. J. Obes.*, 8, 65, 1984.
36. Turner, M. L., Hereditary obesity and temperature regulation, *Am. J. Physiol.*, 152, 197, 1948.
37. Matsushita, H. and Kobayashi, K., Studies on some thermogenetic enzymes in brown adipose tissue of genetically obese mice, *Experientia Suppl.*, 32, 277, 1978.
38. Wolff, G. L., Growth of inbred yellow (A^ya) and non-yellow (aa) mice in parabiosis, *Genetics*, 48, 1041, 1963.
39. Plocher, T. A. and Powley, T. L., Effect of hypophysectomy on weight gain and body composition in the genetically obese yellow (A^y/a) mouse, *Metabolism*, 25, 593, 1976.
40. Salem, M. A. M., Lewis, U. J., Haro, L. S., Kishi, K., McAllister, D. L., Seavey, B. K., Bee, G., and Wolff, G. L., Effects of hypophysectomy and the insulin-like and anti-insulin pituitary peptides on carbohydrate metabolism in yellow A^{vy}/A (BALB/c x VY) F_1 hybrid mice, *Proc. Soc. Exp. Biol. Med.*, 191, 408, 1989.
41. Shimizu, H., Shargill, N. S., and Bray, G. A., Adrenalectomy and response to corticosterone and MSH in the genetically obese yellow mouse, *Am. J. Physiol.*, 256, R494, 1989.
42. Frigeri, L. G., Wolff, G. L., and Robel, G., Impairment of glucose tolerance in yellow (A^{vy}/A) (BALB/c x VY) F-1 hybrid mice by hyperglycemic peptide(s) from human pituitary glands, *Endocrinology*, 113, 2097, 1983.
43. Gill, A. M. and Yen, T. T., Effects of ciglitazone on endogenous plasma islet amyloid polypeptide and insulin sensitivity in obese-diabetic viable yellow mice, *Life Sci.*, 48, 703, 1991.
44. Mynatt, R. L., Miltenberger, R. J., Klebig, M. L., Zemel, M. B., Wilkinson, J. E., Wilkison, W. O., and Woychik, R. P., Combined effects of insulin treatment and adipose tissue-specific agouti expression on the development of obesity, *Proc. Natl. Acad. Sci. USA*, 94, 919, 1997.

45. Willard, D. H., Bodnar, W., Harris, C., Kiefer, L., Nichols, J. S., Blanchard, S., Hoffman, C., Moyer, M., Burkhart, W., Weiel, J., Luther, M. A., Wilkison, W. O., and Rocque, W. J., Agouti structure and function: characterization of a potent α-melanocyte stimulating hormone receptor antagonist, *Biochemistry*, 34, 12341, 1995.

46. Manne, J., Argeson, A. C., and Siracusa, L. D., Mechanisms for the pleiotropic effects of the agouti gene, *Proc. Natl. Acad. Sci. USA*, 92, 4721, 1995.

47. Kieffer, L. L., Ittoop, O. R., Bunce, K., Truesdale, A. T., Willard, D. H., Nichols, J. S., Blanchard, S. G., Mountjoy, K., Chen, W. J., and Wilkison, W. O., Mutations in the carboxyl terminus of the agouti protein decrease inhibition of ligand binding to the melanocortin receptors, *Biochemistry*, 36, 2084, 1997.

48. Michaud, E. J., Bultman, S. B., and Klebig, M. L., A molecular model for the genetic and phenotypic characteristics of the mouse lethal yellow (A^y) mutation, *Proc. Natl. Acad. Sci. USA*, 91, 2562, 1994.

49. Klebig, M. L., Wilkinson, J. E., and Woychik, R. P., Molecular analysis of the mouse agouti gene and the role of dominant agouti locus mutations in obesity and insulin resistance, in *Molecular and Genetic Aspects of Obesity*, Bray, G., Ed., Louisiana State Univ. Press, Baton Rouge, 1994, 120.

50. Argeson, A. C., Nelson, K. K., and Siracusa, L. D., (1996) Molecular basis of the pleiotropic phenotype of mice carrying the hypervariable yellow (A^{hvy}) mutation at the agouti locus, *Genetics*, 142, 557, 1996.

51. Kwon, H. Y., Bultman, S. J., Loffler, C., Chen, W. J., Furdon, P. J., Powell, J. G., Usala, A. L., Wilkison, W., Hansmann, I., and Woychik, R. P., Molecular structure and chromosomal mapping of the human homolog of the agouti gene, *Proc. Natl. Acad. Sci. USA*, 91, 9760, 1994.

52. Wilson, B. D., Ollmann, M. M., Kang, L., Stoffel, M., Bell, G. I., and Barsh, G. S., Structure and function of ASP, the human homolog of the mouse agouti gene, *Hum. Mol. Genet.*, 4, 223, 1995.

53. Xue, B. Z., Wilkison, W. O., Mynatt, R. L., Moustaïd, N., Goldman, M., and Zemel, M. B., The agouti gene product stimulates pancreatic β-cell Ca^{2+} signaling and insulin release, *Physiol. Genomics*, 1, 11, 1999.

54. Lu, D., Willard, D., Patel, I. R., Kadwell, S., Overton, L., Kost, T., Luther, M., Chan, W., Woychik, R. P., Wilkison, W. O., and Cone, R. D., Agouti protein is an antagonist of the melanocyte-stimulating-hormone receptor, *Nature*, 371, 799, 1994.

55. Blanchard, S. G., Harris, C. O., Ittoop, O., Nichols, J. S., Parks, D. J., Truesdale, A. T., and Wilkison, W. O., Characterization of the agouti antagonism of melanocortin binding and action in the $B_{16}F_{10}$ murine melanoma cell line, *Biochemistry*, 34, 10406, 1995.

56. Sakai, C., Ollmann, M., Kobayashi, T., Abdel-Malek, Z., Muller, J., Vieira, W. D., Imokawa, G., Barsh, G. S., and Hearing, V. J., Modulation of murine melanocyte function *in vitro* by agouti signal protein, *EMBO J.*, 16, 3544, 1997.

57. Suzuki, I., Tada, A., Ollmann, M. M., Barsh, G. S., Im, S., Lamoreux, M. L., Hearing, V. J., Nordlund, J. J., and Abdel-Malek, Z. A., Agouti signaling protein inhibits melanogenesis and the response of human melanocytes to α-melanotropin, *J. Invest. Dermatol.*, 108, 838, 1997.

58. Hunt, G. and Thody, A. J., Agouti protein can act independently of melanocyte-stimulating hormone to inhibit melanogenesis, *J. Endocrinol.*, 147, R1, 1995.

59. Graham, A., Wakamatsu, K., Hunt, G., Ito, S., and Thody, A. J., Agouti protein inhibits the production of eumelanin and phaeomelanin in the presence and absence of α-melanocyte stimulating hormone, *Pigment Cell Res.*, 10, 298, 1997.

60. Siegrist, W., Drozdz, R., Cotti, R., Willard, D. H., Wilkison, W. O., and Eberle, A. N., Interactions of α-melanotropin and agouti on B16 melanoma cells: evidence for inverse agonism of agouti, *J. Receptor Signal Transduction Res.*, 17, 75, 1997.

61. Kim, J. H., Kieffer, L. L., Woychik, R. P., Wilkison, W. O., Truesdale, A., Ittoop, O., Willard, D., Nichols, J., and Zemel, M. B., Agouti regulation of intracellular calcium. Role of melanocortin receptor, *Am. J. Physiol.*, 272, E379, 1997.

62. Cone, R. D., Lu, D., Koppula, S., Vage, D. I., Klungland, H., Boston, B., Chen, W., Orth, D. N., Pouton, C., and Kesterson, R. A., The melanocortin receptors: agonists, antagonists, and the hormonal control of pigmentation, *Recent Prog. Horm. Res.*, 51, 287, 1996.

63. Wikberg, J. E. S., Melanocortin receptors: perspectives for novel drugs, *Eur. J. Pharmacol.*, 375, 295, 1999.

64. Wikberg, J. E. S., Melacortin receptors: perspectives for novel drugs, *Eur. J. Pharmacol.*, 375, 295, 1999.

65. Mountjoy, K. G., Robbins, L. S., Mortrud, M. T., and Cone, R. D., The cloning of a family of genes that encode the melanocortin receptors, *Science*, 257, 1248, 1992.

66. Chjajlani, V., Distribution of cDNA for melanocortin receptor subtypes in human tissues, *Biochem. Mol. Biol. Int.*, 38, 73, 1996.

67. Xia, Y. and Wikberg, J. E. S., In situ hybridization histochemical localization of ACTH receptor mRNA in mouse adrenal gland, *Cell Tissue Res.*, 286, 63, 1996.

68. Slominski, A., Ermak, G., and Mihm, M., ACTH receptor, CYP11A1, CYP17 and CYP21A2 genes are expressed in skin, *J. Clin. Endocrinol. Metab.*, 81, 2746, 1996.

69. Ermak, G. and Slominski, A., Production of POMC, CRH-R1, MC1, and MC2 receptor mRNA and expression of tyrosinase gene in relation to hair cycle and dexamethasone treatment in the C57BL/6 mouse skin, *J. Invest. Dermatol.*, 108, 160, 1997.

70. Gantz, I., Konda, Y., Tashiro, T., Shimoto, Y., Miwa, H., Munzert, G., Watson, S. J., DelValle, J., and Yamada, T.Y., Molecular cloning of a novel melanocortin receptor, *J. Biol. Chem.*, 268, 8246, 1993.

71. Roselli-Rehfuss, L., Mountjoy, K. G., Robbins, L. S., Mortrud, M. T., Low, M. J., Tatro, J. B., Entwistle, M. L., Simerly, R. B., and Cone, R. D., Identification of a receptor for γ melanocotropin and other proopiomelanocortin peptides in the hypothalamus and limbic system, *Proc. Natl. Acad. Sci. USA*, 90, 8856, 1993.

72. Gantz, I., Miwa, H., Konda, Y., Shimoto, Y., Tashiro, T., Watson, S. J., DelValle, J., and Yamada, Y., Molecular cloning, expression, and gene localization of a fourth melanocortin receptor, *J. Biol. Chem.*, 268, 15174, 1993.

73. Mountjoy, K. G., Mortrud, M. T., Low, M. J., Simerly, R. B., and Cone, R. D., Localization of the melanocortin-4 receptor (MC4-R) in neuroendocrine and autonomic control circuits in the brain, *Mol. Endocrinol.*, 8, 1298, 1994.

74. Magenis, R. E., Smith, L., Nadeau, J. H., Hohnson, K. R., Mountjoy, K. G., and Cone, R., Mapping of the ACTH, MSH and neural MC3 and MC4 melanocortin receptors in the mouse and human, *Mammal. Genome*, 5, 503, 1994.

75. Van der Kraan, M., Adan, R. A., Entwistle, M. L., Gispen, W. H., Berbach, J. P. H., and Tatro, J. B., Expression of melanocortin-5 receptor in secretory epithelia supports a functional role in exocrine and endocrine glands, *Endocrinology*, 139, 2348, 1998.

76. Labbe, O., Desarnau, F., Eggerickx, D., Vassart, G., and Parmentier, M., Molecular cloning of a mouse melanocortin 5 receptor gene widely expressed in peripheral tissue, *Biochemistry*, 33, 4543, 1994.

77. Konda, Y., Gantz, I., DelValle, J., Shimoto, Y., Miwa, H., and Yamada, T., Interaction of dual intracellular signaling pathways activated by the melanocortin-3 receptor, *J. Biol. Chem.*, 269, 13162, 1994.

78. Lu, D., Willard, D., Patel, I. R., Kadwell, S., Overton, L., Kost, T., Luther, M., Chen, W., Woychik, R. P., Wilkison, W. O., and Cone, R. D., Agouti protein is an antagonist of the melanocyte-stimulating hormone receptor, *Nature*, 371, 799, 1994.

79. Chagnon, Y. C., Chen, W. J., Perusse, L., Chagnon, M., Nadeau, A., Wilkison, W. O., and Bouchard, C., Linkage and association studies between the melanocortin receptor 4 and 5 genes and obesity-related phenotypes in the Quebec family study, *Mol. Med.*, 3, 663, 1997.

80. Yeo, G. S. H., Farooqi, I. S., Aminian, S., Halsall, D. J., Stanhope, R. J., and O'Rahilly, S., A frameshift mutation in MC4R associated with dominantly inherited human obesity, *Nature Genet.*, 20, 111, 1998.

81. Vaisse, C., Clement, K., Guy-Grand, B., and Froguel, P., A frameshift mutation in human MC4R is associated with a dominant form of obesity, *Nature Genet.*, 20, 113, 1998.

82. Gu, W., Tu, Z., Kleyn, P. W., Kissebah, A., Duprat, L., Lee, J., Chin, W., Maruti, S., Deng, N., Fisher, S. L., Franco, L. S., Burn, P., Yagaloff, K. A., Nathan, J., Heymsfield, S., Albu, J., Pi-Sunyer, F. X., and Allison, D. B., Identification and functional analysis of novel human melanocortin-4 receptor variants, *Diabetes*, 48, 635, 1999.

83. Hinney, A., Schmidt, A., Nottebom, K., Heibult, O., Becker, I., Ziegler, A., Gerber, G., Sina, M., Gorg, T., Mayer, H., Siegfried, W., Fichter, M., Remschmidt, H., and Hebebrand, J., Several mutations in melanocortin-4 receptor gene including a nonsense and a frameshift mutation associated with dominantly inherited obesity in humans, *J. Clin. Endocr. Metab.*, 84, 1483, 1999.

84. Sina, M., Hinney, A., Ziegler, A., Neupert, T., Mayer, H., Siegfried, W., Blum, W. F., Remschmidt, H., and Hebebrand, J., Phenotypes in three pedigrees with autosomal dominant obesity caused by haploin sufficiency mutations in the melanocortin-4 receptor gene, *Am. J. Hum. Genet.*, 65, 1501, 1999.

85. Mountjoy, K. G. and Wong, J., Obesity, diabetes and functions for proopiomelanocortin-derived peptides, *Mol. Cell. Endocrinol.*, 128, 171, 1997.

86. Woods, S. C., Seeley, R. J., Porte, D., and Schwartz, M. W., Signals that regulate food intake and energy homeostasis, *Science*, 280, 1378, 1998.

87. Elmquist, J. K., Maratos-Flie, E., Saper, C., and Flier, J. S., Unraveling the central nervous system pathways underlying responses to leptin, *Nature Neurosci.*, 6, 445, 1998.

88. Friedman, J. M. and Halaas, J., Leptin and the regulation of body weight in mammals, *Nature*, 395, 763, 1998.

89. Huszar, D., Lynch, C. A., Fairchild-Huntress, V., Dumore, J. H., Fang, Q., Berke-meier, L. R., Gu, W., Kesterson, R. D., Boston, B. A., Cone, R. D., Smith, F. J., Campfield, L. A., Burn, P., and Lee, F., Targeted disruption of the melanocortin-4 receptor results in obesity in mice, *Cell*, 88, 131, 1997.

90. Fan, W., Boston, B. A., Kesterson, R. A., Hruby, V. J., and Cone, R. D., Role of melanocortinergic neurons in feeding and the agouti obesity syndrome, *Nature*, 385, 165, 1997.

91. Marsh, D. J., Hollopeter, G., Huszar, D., Laufer, R., Yagaloff, K. A., Fisher, S. L., Burn, P., and Palmiter, R. D., Response of melanocortin-4-receptor-deficient mice to anorectic and orexigenic peptides, *Nature Genet.*, 21, 119, 1992.

92. Harrold, J. A., Widdowson, P. S., and Williams, G., Altered energy balance causes selective changes in melanocortin-4 (MC4-R), but not melanocortin-3 (MC3-R) receptors in specific hypothalamic regions, *Diabetes*, 48, 268, 1999.

93. Shutter, J. R., Graham, M., Kinsey, A. C., Scully, S., Luthy, R., and Stark, K., Hypothalamic expression of ART, a novel gene related to agouti, is up-regu-lated in obese and diabetic mutant mice, *Genes Dev.*, 11, 593, 1997.

94. Ollmann, M. M., Wilson, B. D., Yang, Y. K., Kerns, J. A., Chen, Y., Gantz, I., and Barsh, G. S., Antagonism of central melanocortin receptors *in vitro* and *in vivo* by agouti-related protein, *Science*, 278, 135, 1997.

95. Graham, M., Shutter, J. R., Sarmiento, U., Sarosi, I., and Stark, K. L., Overex-pression of Agrt leads to obesity in transgenic mice, *Nature Genet.*, 17, 273, 1997.

96. Quillan, J. M., Sadee, W., Wei, E. T., Jimenez, C., Ji, L., and Chang, J. K., A synthetic human agouti-related protein-(83-132)-NH$_2$ fragment is a potent in-hibitor of melanocortin receptor function, *FEBS Letters*, 428, 59, 1998.

97. Yang, Y. K., Thompson, D. A., Dickinson, C. J., Wilken, J., Barsh, G. S., Kent, S. B., and Gantz, I., Characterization of agouti-related protein binding to melano-cortin receptors, *Mol. Endocrinol.*, 13, 148, 1999.

98. Rossi, M., Kim, M. S., Morgan, D. G., Small, C. J., Edwards, C. M., Sunter, D., Abusnana, S., Goldstone, A. P., Russell, S. H., Stanley, S. A., Smith, D. M., Yagaloff, K., Ghatei, M. A., and Bloom, S. R., A C-terminal fragment of agouti-related protein increases feeding and antagonizes the effect of alpha-melano-cyte stimulating hormone *in vivo*, *Endocrinology*, 139, 4428, 1998.

99. Yaswen, L., Diehl, N., Brennan, M. B., and Hochgeschwender, U., Obesity in the mouse model of pro-opiomelanocortin deficiency responds to peripheral melanocortin, *Nature Med.*, 5, 1066, 1999.

100. Zemel, M. B., Moore, J. W., Moustaïd, N., Kim, J. H., Nichols, J. S., Blanchard, S. G., Parks, D. J., Harris, C., Lee, F. W., Grizzle, M., James, M., and Wilkison, W.O., Effects of a potent melanocortin agonist on the diabetic/obese phenotype in yellow mice, *Int. J. Obesity*, 98, 678, 1998.

101. Miller, K. A., Gunn, T. M., Carrasquillo, M. M., Lamoreux, M. L., Galbraith, D. B., and Barsh, G. S., Genetic studies of the mouse mutations mahogany and mahoganoid, *Genetics*, 146, 1407, 1997.

102. Dimulescu, D. M., Fan, W., Boston, B. A., McCall, K., Lamoreux, M. L., Moore, K. J., Montagno, J., and Cone, R. D., Mahogany (*mg*) stimulates feeding and increases basal metabolic fate independent of its suppression of agouti, *Proc. Natl. Acad. Sci. USA*, 95, 2707, 1998.

103. Nagle, D. L., McGrail, S. H., Vitale, J., Woolf, E. A., Dussault Jr, B. J., DiRocco, L., Holmgren, L., Montagno, J., Bork, P., Huszar, D., Fairchild-Huntress, V. G. P., Keilty, J., Ebeling, C., Baldini, L., Gilchrist, J., Burn, P., Carlson, G. A., and Moore, K. J., The mahogany protein is a receptor involved in suppression of obesity, *Nature*, 398, 148, 1999.

104. Gunn, T. M., Miller, K. A., He, L., Hyman, R. W., Davis, R. W., Azarani, A., Schlossman, S. F., Duke-Cohan, H. S., and Barsh, G. S., The mouse mahogany locus encodes a transmembrane form of human attractin, *Nature*, 398, 152, 1999.

105. Duke-Cohan, J. S., Gu, J., Mclaughlin, D. F., Xu, Y., Freeman, G. J., and Schlossman, S. F., Attractin (DPPT-L), a member of the CUB family of cell adhesion and guidance proteins, is secreted by activated human T lymphocytes and modulates immune cell interactions, *Proc. Natl. Acad. Sci. USA*, 95, 11336, 1998.

106. Jackson, I. J., The mahogany mouse mutation, further links between pigmentation, obesity and the immune system, *Trends Genet.*, 15, 429, 1999.

107. Wilson, B. D., Bagnol, D., Kaelin, C. B., Ollmann, M. M., Gantz, I., Watson, S. J., and Barsh, G. S., Physiological and anatomical circuitry between agouti related protein and leptin signaling, *Endocrinology*, 140, 2387, 1999.

108. Baskin, D. G., Breininger, J. F., and Schwartz, M. W., Leptin receptor mRNA identifies a subpopulation of neuropeptide Y neurons activated by fasting in rat hypothalamus, *Diabetes*, 48, 828, 1999.

109. Cheung, C. C., Clifton, D. K., and Steiner, R. A., Proopiomelanocortin neurons are direct targets for leptin in the hypothalamus, *Endocrinology*, 138, 4489, 1997.

110. Mizuno, T. M. and Mobbs, C. V., Hypothalamic agouti-related protein messenger ribonucleic acid is inhibited by leptin and stimulated by fasting, *Endocrinology*, 140, 814, 1999.

111. Schwartz, M. W., Seeley, R. J., Woods, S. C., Weigle, D. S., Campfield, L. A., Burn, P., and Baskin, D. G., Leptin increases hypothalamic pro-opiomelanocortin mRNA expression in the rostral arcuate nucleus, *Diabetes*, 46, 2119, 1997.

112. Thornton, J. E., Cheung, C. C., Clifton, D. K., and Steiner, R. A., Regulation of hypothalamic proopiomelanocortin mRNA by leptin in *ob/ob* mice, *Endocrinology*, 138, 5063, 1997.

113. Mizuno, T. M., Kleopoulos, S. P., Bergen, H. T., Roberts, J. L., Priest, C. A., and Mobbs, C. V., Hypothalamic pro-opiomelanocortin mRNA is reduced by fasting in *ob/ob* and *db/db* mice, but is stimulated by leptin, *Diabetes*, 47, 294, 1997.

114. Seeley, R. J., Yagaloff, K. A., Fisher, S. L., Burn, P., Thiele, T. E., Dijk, G., Baskin, D. G., and Schwartz, M. W., Melanocortin receptors in leptin effects, *Nature*, 290, 349, 1997.

115. Marsh, D. J., Hollopeter, G., Huszar, D., Laufer, R., Yagaloff, K. A., Fisher, S. L., Burn, P., and Palmiter, R. D., Response of melanocortin-4 receptor-deficient mice to anorectic and orexigenic peptides, *Nature Genet.*, 21, 119, 1999.

116. Boston, B. A., Blaydon, K. M., Varnerin, J., and Cone, R. D., Independent and additive effects of central POMC and leptin pathways on murine obesity, *Science*, 278, 1641, 1997.

117. Zemel, M. B., Kim, J. H., Woychik, R. P., Michaud, E. J., Kadwell, S. H., Patel, I. R., and Wilkison, W. O., Agouti regulation of intracellular calcium: Role in the insulin resistance of viable yellow mice, *Proc. Natl. Acad. Sci. USA*, 92, 4733, 1995.

118. Johnson, P. R. and Hirsch, J., Cellularity of adipose depot in six strains of genetically obese mice, *J. Lipid.*, 13, 2, 1972.

119. Claycombe, K. J., Wang, Y., Jones, B. H., Kim, S., Wilkison, W. O., Zemel, M. B., Chun, J., and Moustaïd-Moussa, N., Transcriptional regulation of the adipocyte fatty acid synthase gene by the agouti gene product: Interaction with insulin, *FASEB J.*, 11, A352 (Abstr.), 1997.

120. Xue, B. and Zemel, M. B., (2000) Relationship between human adipose tissue agouti and fatty acid synthase (FAS), *J. Nutr.*, 130, 2478, 2000.

121. Shi, H., Moustaïd-Moussa, N., Wilkison, W. O., and Zemel, M. B., Role of the sulfonylurea receptor in regulating human adipocyte metabolism, *FASEB J.*, 13, 1833, 1999.

122. Tebar, F., Soley, M., and Ramirez, I., The antilipoytic effects of insulin and epidermal growth factor in rat adipocytes are mediated by different mechanisms, *Endocrinology*, 137, 4181, 1996.

123. Xue, B., Moustaïd-Moussa, N., Wilkison, W. O., and Zemel, M. B., The agouti gene product inhibits lipolysis in human adipocytes via a Ca^{2+} dependent mechanism, *FASEB J.*, 12, 1391, 1998.

124. Xue, B. and Zemel, M. B., Mechanism of intracellular calcium inhibition of lipolysis in human adipocytes, *FASEB J.*, 14, (Abstr.), A733, 2000.

125. Mynatt, R. L. and Truett, G. E., Influence of agouti protein on gene expression in mouse adipose tissue, *FASEB J.*, (Abstr.), 14, A733, 2000.

126. Zemel, M. B., Mynatt, R. L., and Dibling, D., Synergism between diet-induced hyperinsulinemia and adipocyte-specific agouti expression, *FASEB J.*, (Abstr.), 13, A873, 1999.

127. Standridge, M., Alemzadeh, R., Zemel, M., Koontz, J., and Moustaïd-Moussa, N., Diazoxide down-regulates leptin and lipid metabolizing enzymes in adipose tissue of Zucker rats, *FASEB J.*, 14, 455, 2000.

128. Alemzadeh, R., Slonim, A. E., Zdanowicz, M. M., and Maturo, J., Modification of insulin resistance by diazoxide in obese Zucker rats, *Endocrinology*, 133, 705, 1993.

129. Alemzadeh, R., Jacobs, A. W., and Pitukcheewnont, P. Antiobesity effect of diazoxide in obese Zucker rats, *Metabolism*, 45, 334, 1996.

130. Alemzadeh, R., Langley, G., Upchurch, L., Smith, P., and Slonim, A. E., Beneficial effect of diazoxide in obese hyperinsulinemic adults, *J. Clin. Endocr. Metab.*, 83, 1911, 1998.

131. Zemel, M. B., Shi, H., Greer, B., DiRienzo, D. and Zemel, P. C., Regulation of adiposity by dietary calcium, *FASEB J.*, 14, 1132, 2000.

132. Shi, H. and Zemel, M. B., Effects of dietary calcium on adipocyte lipid metabolism and body weight regulation in energy-restricted mice, *FASEB J.*, 14, (Abstr.), A790 2000.

11

Dietary Fats and APC-Driven Intestinal Tumorigenesis

Jay Whelan and Michael F. McEntee

CONTENTS

11.1 Introduction 231
11.2 Polyunsaturated Fatty Acid Metabolism...232
11.3 Cyclooxygenases 233
11.4 Intestinal Tumorigenesis and APC 234
11.5 Dietary Polyunsaturated Fatty Acids and Tumorigenesis 239
    11.5.1 N-3 Fatty Acids 240
    11.5.2 Conjugated Linoleic Acid (CLA) 243
    11.5.3 Gamma-Linolenic Acid (GLA)..243
11.6 Mechanisms of Action 245
    11.6.1 Arachidonic Acid vs. N-3 Fatty Acids 245
    11.6.2 Δ-6 Desaturase..245
    11.6.3 Prostaglandins..247
11.7 Summary and Conclusions...249
References 250

11.1 Introduction

Epidemiological evidence clearly links dietary fat intake with colorectal cancer risk.[1,2] As fat intake increases, the risk for colorectal cancer increases; however, the risk associated with individual fatty acids is less defined. This chapter is particularly interested in addressing what is known about the impact of dietary fatty acid composition on intestinal tumorigenesis.

11.2 Polyunsaturated Fatty Acid Metabolism

There are two major families of dietary polyunsaturated fatty acids (PUFAs): the n-3 and n-6 families. N-6 PUFAs are derived from the parent compound linoleic acid (LA, 18:2 n-6) (Fig. 11.1). LA is the major PUFA in the diet and accounts for ~6 to 7% of caloric intake. Following consumption of LA, it is converted to γ-linolenic (GLA, 18:3 n-6) acid via the Δ-6 desaturase, and subsequently converted to arachidonic acid (AA, 20:4 n-6) through the intermediate dihomo-γ-linolenic acid (DGLA, 20:3 n-6) via successive steps involving an elongase and the Δ-5 desaturase. AA is arguably the most important PUFA associated with membrane phospholipids.[3] In parallel (Fig. 11.1), PUFAs of the n-3 family are derived from the parent fatty acid α-linolenic acid (ALA, 18:3 n-3), the metabolic precursor of the more highly unsaturated n-3 PUFAs found in fish oils, e.g., stearidonic acid (SDA, 18:4 n-3), eicosapentaenoic acid (EPA, 20:5 n-3), and docosahexaenoic acid (DHA, 22:6 n-3). Utilizing the same enzymatic machinery as LA, ALA is metabolized to EPA. Unlike AA

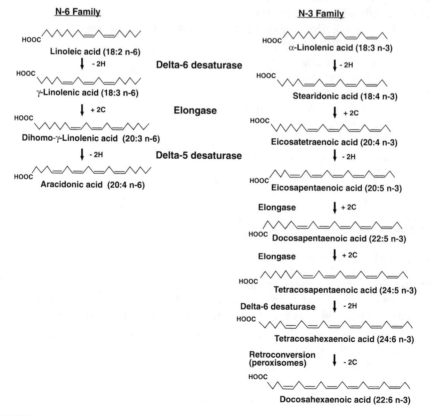

FIGURE 11.1
Metabolic pathways of n-6 and n-3 fatty acids.

which is poorly metabolized to longer more unsaturated fatty acids,[4-6] EPA is converted to DHA via a set of unique reactions previously attributed to a putative Δ-4 desaturase.[7,8] EPA undergoes two elongation steps to 24:5 n-3 at the endoplasmic reticulum and is subsequently desaturated to 24:6 n-3 via Δ-6 desaturase. Following the removal of two carbons via peroxisomal oxidation, 24:6 n-3 is retroconverted to DHA. PUFAs from the n-3 and n-6 families are not metabolically interconvertible, and as such, consumption of one family of fatty acids can attenuate the metabolism of the other.

It is the competition between these two fatty acid families that defines the role of dietary PUFAs and the risk of intestinal tumorigenesis. Indeed, establishing an appropriate mix of dietary n-3 and n-6 PUFAs in an effort to reduce chronic diseases has been a concern for a number of years. Dietary n-6 PUFAs appear to be pro-tumorigenic and it has been suggested that these effects are mediated via the AA cascade, in particular, via prostaglandins. N-3 PUFAs are potent antagonists to AA and its metabolism, suggesting a possible mechanism for their antitumorigenic effects. A direct comparison of each PUFA in the metabolic sequence could explicitly establish if their impact on tumorigenesis is mediated through the metabolism of AA. Certainly, determining the efficacy of these fatty acids is complicated by the fact that typical dietary intakes of LA and ALA (~15g/d and ~2g/d, respectively)[9] are far higher than those of AA (~200mg/d)[10,11] and EPA/DHA (~200mg/d),[9] but the highly unsaturated fatty acids are more biologically potent than their precursors because they bypass the initial Δ-6 desaturase step, the rate-limiting step in the metabolic pathways of n-3 and n-6 PUFAs.

11.3 Cyclooxygenases

Following release of AA from membrane phospholipids by a variety of phospholipase A_2s,[12-14] AA is enzymatically oxidized to prostaglandins (PGs) by a two-step process involving cyclooxygenases (also referred to as prostaglandin H synthases) (Fig. 11.2). Two known isozymes of cyclooxygenase (COX), COX-1 and COX-2, catalyze the committed step in PG biosynthesis (Table 11.1); however, a third form has been proposed.[15] These bifunctional enzymes exist as homodimers. They contain an epidermal growth factor domain, a membrane-binding domain, and two enzymatic activities with distinct active sites.[16] The initial activity, cyclooxygenase, oxidizes arachidonic acid through a free radical-generated mechanism to the endoperoxide intermediate PGG_2, which is subsequently reduced to PGH_2 by the protein-associated peroxidase which is located at the interface of the dimer.[17] PGH_2 is the common precursor for all the prostaglandins, prostacyclin, and thromboxanes. The COX enzymes are localized within the outer leaflet of the endoplasmic reticulum and the outer and inner membranes of the nuclear membrane.[18]

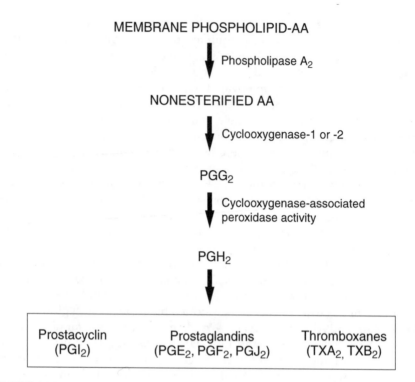

FIGURE 11.2
Metabolic pathway of cyclooxygenase-derived eicosanoids.

COX-1 is constitutively expressed in most tissues and appears to be important in housekeeping processes that modulate basic cellular functions, but has also been shown to be induced.[19,20] COX-2 is not normally expressed in most tissues and is considered to be the inducible form of the enzyme. Its expression is upregulated in monocytes/macrophages, fibroblasts, and endothelial cells in response to cytokines, growth factors, mitogens, and tumor promoters; however, basal expression has been observed in the macula densa of the kidney, the brain, testes, and tracheal epithelium (as reviewed in References 21 and 22) Importantly, COX-2 expression has been shown to be elevated in a number of cancers, including small intestinal, pancreatic, gastric, colorectal, and lung,[23–31] and that induction of COX-2 expression appears to play an important role in maintaining tumor integrity[32,33] and may contribute to the metastatic process.[34,35]

11.4 Intestinal Tumorigenesis and APC

Colorectal cancer, the third most common form of malignancy in both men and women, was attributed with over 57,000 deaths in 1995.[36] The disease

TABLE 11.1

Comparison of Cyclooxygenase-1 and -2. (See Refs. 18, 21, 142, 146–149)

	COX-1	COX-2
Temporal pattern of expression	Primarily constitutive, induction in some cell types	Primarily inducible in presence of cytokines, growth factors, tumor promoters (constitutively expressed in tumors, testes, trachea, kidney, brain)
Prominent tissue/cell type	Ubiquitous	Inflammatory cells, tumors, kidney, brain
Gene size	22 kb	8.3 kb
mRNA size	2.8 kb	4.5 kb
Protein size	~70 kDa	~70 kDa
Amino acid homology to COX-1	—	75%
Amino acid sequence identity with COX-1	—	63%
Structural forms	Homodimer	Homodimer
Heme-containing	Yes	Yes
Peroxidase activity	Yes	Yes
Catalytic mechanism involves free radicals	Yes	Yes
Peroxide activated	Yes	Yes
Inhibited by NSAIDs	Yes	Yes
Substrate specificity	AA>DGLA>>>LA,GLA,EPA > ALA	AA>DGLA>LA>ALA>GLA > EPA
K_m for AA as substrate	~5 μM	~5 μM
Product profile (substrate: arachidonic acid)	PGG_2, PGH_2, 11-HETE, 15-HETE	PGG_2, PGH_2, 11-HETE, 15-HETE, 15(R)-HETE (in presence of aspirin)
Subcellular localization	ER and nuclear envelope	Nuclear envelope, along with ER
Primary mode of action	Extracellular: paracrine, autocrine	Paracrine, autocrine, intracrine (nuclear)

progresses through defined pathologic stages that range from the earliest proliferation of neoplastic epithelium, referred to as an aberrant crypt focus (ACF),[37] to benign adenomas (or polyps), to metastatic cancer.[38] This morphologic progression of events has been associated with specific genetic and epigenetic abnormalities which can be used to model intestinal tumorigenesis and test the effects of dietary or pharmacologic intervention.[39,40] In most individuals, colorectal cancer occurs spontaneously (i.e., sporadic form) but a relatively small percentage of cases occur in individuals predisposed to the disease by inherited defects in either the adenomatous polyposis coli (*APC*) gene, where the syndrome is referred to as familial adenomatous polyposis (FAP), or in a DNA mismatch repair gene which results in hereditary non-polyposis colorectal cancer (HNPCC).[41] Mutations of the *APC* gene initiate formation of essentially all tumors in FAP patients, are present in most early cases of sporadic colorectal cancer, and may also contribute to tumorigenesis in HNPCC. *APC* is considered a tumor suppressor gene because oncogenic mutations result in loss of the full-length APC protein through truncation of the transcripts and/or genetic deletion.

Animal models used to study colorectal cancer fall into two categories: those that spontaneously develop intestinal tumors as a result of predisposing inheritable mutations, and those in which neoplasia is induced by chemical carcinogens (Table 11.2). The most commonly used genetic models carry a germline mutation in the murine *Apc* gene and develop intestinal tumors with spontaneous loss of the wild-type allele, whereas chemically induced tumors in mice and rats more often result from mutations in other genes, although dysregulation of β-catenin (a downstream protein regulated by Apc) still may have a seminal role.[42] A major advantage of the genetic models is the reproducible loss of *Apc* gene function, as occurs early in the development of most human colorectal cancers. A potential disadvantage is the propensity of these mice to develop more small intestinal than colorectal tumors. The chemically induced tumors are restricted to the colon of treated rodents and occur with formation of ACF, as is the case in humans. Whether a model is stronger for its molecular or anatomic characteristics is debatable, but we have chosen to use a genetic mouse model for our studies.

The Apc^Min/+ model was derived from a C57BL/6J male mouse which had been exposed to the mutagen ethyl nitrosourea.[43] Intestinal tumorigenesis in this strain has been well characterized and widely used to study the molecular and genetic pathogenesis of this disease as well as methods of chemotherapeutic and preventative intervention. Apc^Min/+ mice (available through Jackson Laboratories, Bar Harbor, Maine) carry a germline mutation in *Apc* that truncates the protein at 850 amino acids. The mutation is homozygous lethal *in utero* but heterozygotes develop adenomas throughout the intestinal tract. By approximately 60 to 80 days of age each mouse will harbor an average of 40 small intestinal tumors and up to 3 or 4 colonic polyps.[44] These tumors rarely, if ever, progress to invasive cancer presumably because of the restricted life span of the Apc^Min/+ mouse (~130 days). Aging Apc^Min/+ mice become anemic due to low-grade hemorrhage through the ulcerated surface of intestinal tumors.

To date, five other strains of Apc^+/- mice have been developed by targeted mutation of the gene at different locations, resulting in variable truncation of

TABLE 11.2

Rodent Models of Intestinal Tumorigenesis in Humans

	Genetic (Apc) Models	Carcinogen-Induced Models
Earliest genetic defect	Apc	β-catenin & Ras >> Apc
Tumor location	Small intestine > Colon	Colon
Tumor multiplicity	30+/mouse (< 4 colonic)	< 1 to 3/animal
Adherent crypt foci	No	Yes
Neoplastic progression	No	Yes — to invasive cancer

the encoded protein.[45] The incidence of intestinal tumors varies in these strains of mice with the germline mutation, and may progress to invasive carcinomas, but the phenotypes essentially duplicate the original Apc$^{Min/+}$ mutant. The only significant exception is the Apc^{1638T} mouse which survives as a homozygous mutant and does not develop intestinal tumors.[46] The Apc$^{Min/+}$ mouse phenotype is affected by at least one modifier gene.[43] Modifier of Min, (Mom)-1, is mutated in C57BL/6J mice and is believed to encode a secretory phospholipase (sPLA$_2$). When Apc$^{Min/+}$ mice on this background are crossed with AKR mice, which have wild-type Mom-1 alleles, the F1 progeny have a significantly reduced incidence of intestinal tumorigenesis and longer life span, attributed in large part (but not exclusively) to the effects of wild-type Mom-1. The biologic basis for this effect on intestinal tumorigenesis is unclear and the human sPLA$_2$ analog has not been found to be mutated in colorectal cancer.

Normally, Apc expression is upregulated as cells emerge from the small intestinal crypt or migrate up the colonic crypt to the mucosal surface. The wild-type protein downregulates the Wnt signaling pathway, contributes to microtubule function, and may affect other cell processes through interactions with less well-characterized proteins (reviewed by Nathke[47] and Polakis[48]). While the Apc protein may have multiple functions in a normal cell, loss of control in the Wnt signaling pathway appears to be most significant with respect to intestinal tumorigenesis.[46] As depicted in Fig. 11.3, a

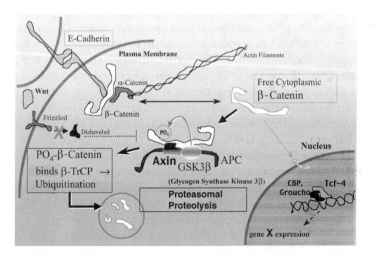

FIGURE 11.3
APC and the Wnt-signaling pathway. The tumor suppressor protein APC is a critical partner in controlling β-catenin nuclear localization and expression of downstream genes. APC acts in concert with axin to facilitate glycogen synthase kinase-3β-mediated phosphorylation of β-catenin, ear-marking it for ubiquitination. Inactivation of APC or stimulation of the Wnt-signaling pathway results in post-translational stabilization of β-catenin and subsequent nuclear localization. Interaction of β-catenin with the nuclear transcription factor TCF transforms epithelial cells from a normal to a neoplastic phenotype.[48]

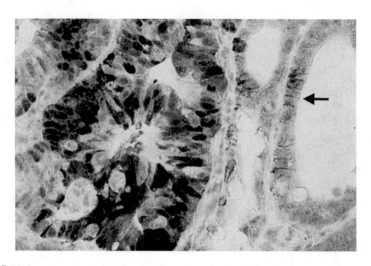

FIGURE 11.4
Photomicrograph of an Apc^Min/+ mouse small intestinal tumor immunohistochemically stained for β-catenin (intensely dark stained regions). β-catenin accumulates in the cytosol and nucleus of neoplastic epithelial cells (left portion of figure), but is restricted to cell membranes in non-neoplastic epithelial cells (arrow) as an integral component of adherens junctions.

Wnt signal inhibits the otherwise normal (default) destruction of free cytoplasmic β-catenin by inactivating axin.[49] As a result, β-catenin migrates into the nucleus (Fig. 11.4) where it initiates transcription of target genes with members of the T-cell factor/lymphoid enhancer factor (Tcf/Lef) nuclear transcription family. It is now clear that tumorigenesis is associated with the dysregulation of intracellular levels of β-catenin. In the absence of a Wnt signal, Apc, GSK-3β, axin, and β-catenin form a cytoplasmic complex which promotes phosphorylation of β-catenin, thereby targeting it for ubiquitination and subsequent proteasomal proteolysis.[48] Truncation or loss of Apc cripples formation of this cytoplasmic complex and the Wnt signal becomes constitutive with accumulation of β-catenin in the cytoplasm and nucleus of neoplastic cells. Therefore, with loss of full-length Apc the normal maturation processes associated with upregulation of the wild-type protein and migration of cells out of the crypt are lacking. The pivotal role of β-catenin in intestinal tumorigenesis is reflected by frequent mutations in this protein in tumors that contain wild-type Apc.[50,51] Such mutations result in loss of phosphorylation sites critical to β-catenin proteolysis and have the same effect as loss of full-length Apc on expression of Wnt-signaling targets which include upregulation of c-Myc, cyclin D1, matrix metalloproteinase-7 (MPP-7, matrilysin), PPARγ, CD44, and perhaps COX-2.[49] Although loss of carboxyl-terminus binding sites for EB1, DLG, and microtubules alone is not sufficient for intestinal tumorigenesis,[46] tumorigenic APC (or β-catenin) mutations that result in upregulation of Wnt/β-catenin signaling contribute to the abnormal cell migration, differentiation, apoptosis, and proliferation that characterize neoplastic cell behavior.

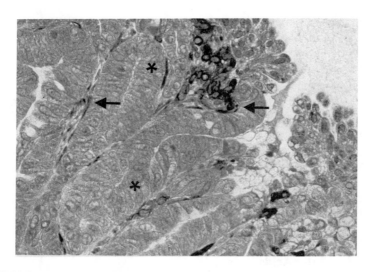

FIGURE 11.5

Histologic section of a small intestinal tumor from an Apc[Min/+] mouse immunohistochemically stained for COX-2. Only non-neoplastic stomal mesenchymal cells express the enzyme (arrows), whereas the neoplastic epithelial cells are negative (asterisk). (Original magnification, 400×)

Apc[Min/+] mice spontaneously develop tumors throughout the intestinal tract, but the induction of COX-2 expression is localized in the stroma of the tumors, not the epithelial cells and not the adjacent normal mucosa[52–54] (Fig. 11.5). Similarly, COX-2 expression in human colorectal tumors is also observed in both adenomas and carcinomas, with apparent preferential localization in the interstitial cells of early lesions.[55–58] Regression of intestinal tumors following treatment with sulindac, a non-selective inhibitor of COX-1 and COX-2, occurs in both FAP patients and Apc[Min/+] mice, and removal of treatment results in tumor regrowth.[44,52,59,60] Therefore, as a model for intestinal tumorigenesis, the Apc[Min/+] mouse possesses a number of characteristics that are similarly observed in human tumors.[43]

11.5 Dietary Polyunsaturated Fatty Acids and Tumorigenesis

Western style diets characterized by high intakes of energy, fat, meat, refined grains, and sugar combined with low intakes of fiber, calcium, and fruits and vegetables have been strongly linked to an increased risk of colorectal cancer.[2,61,62] Similar correlations have been observed in animal models with Apc gene defects. Increasing beef and fat content positively affects intestinal tumor load and some dietary fibers appear to be protective.[63–66] The feeding of a Western style diet has been shown to increase intestinal tumorigenesis in the Apc[1638] mouse model[67] and enhance hyperproliferation of epithelial cells (in various tissues) in null mice (wild type for Apc).[68,69]

Among the components of the diet, the amount and type of dietary fat consumed is of particular importance.[1,70–72] Certainly, a number of PUFAs have proved to be very promising as antitumorigenic lipids in both chemically induced tumor models and models containing germline mutations.[73–77] In an effort to systematically evaluate the efficacy of a variety of dietary PUFAs on intestinal tumorigenesis *in vivo*, we fed Apc[Min/+] mice selectively tailored diets containing individual fatty acid ethyl esters (1.5 to 3%, w/w). The strength of this dietary design allowed us to directly compare different fatty acids from different families.[78] The fatty acids evaluated included GLA and AA from the n-6 family, ALA, SDA, EPA and DHA from the n-3 family, and conjugated linoleic acid (CLA). CLA refers collectively to a number of positional and geometric isomers of LA whose double bonds are in conjugation (typically in the 9 and 11 or 10 and 12 positions).[20]

11.5.1   N-3 Fatty Acids

Recent studies have reported that not only is the amount of fat in the diet particularly important to intestinal tumorigenesis, but the type of dietary fat may even be of greater importance. Epidemiological studies indicate that consumption of fish oil-derived n-3 PUFAs (in particular, EPA and DHA) correlate with a reduced risk of colorectal cancer.[70–72] However, it has been unclear how EPA and DHA compare to other n-3 PUFAs, i.e., ALA and SDA.

The four major n-3 PUFAs, ALA, SDA, EPA and DHA, were evaluated side by side, with diets controlled for macro- and micronutrient composition (including fatty acid composition), with identical levels of n-6 and n-3 PUFAs. Figure 11.6 summaries the results of supplementing fatty acid ethyl esters (3% wt/wt) to the diets of Apc[Min/+] mice on intestinal tumor load. When mice were fed diets containing EPA, tumor multiplicity was reduced by 50% as compared to oleic acid controls.[78] Similarly, Paulsen et al. reported that diets containing n-3 PUFA-enriched fish oil concentrate (0, 0.4, 1.25, and 2.5%, w/w) reduced tumor multiplicity in female Apc[Min/+] mice in an dose-dependent manner, while the results in male mice were less consistent.[74] However, the authors point out an important flaw in the design of the study when they replaced corn oil (rich in pro-tumorigenic n-6 PUFAs) with the fish oil concentrate. In our study, not all n-3 fatty acids had the same effect. DHA was not as effective as EPA, reducing tumor number by only 30% ($P = 0.15$), and thus, it appears that EPA (vs. DHA) has the greater of the two effects on reducing tumor load. In the only other study examining the efficacy of dietary DHA in a similar animal model, DHA resulted in fewer tumors in female Apc[Δ716] knockout mice, but not in their male counterparts.[77] DHA could be acting via retroconversion to EPA,[7,78,79] thus accounting for its less-pronounced efficacy compared to EPA; however, independent effects of DHA cannot be ruled out.

When ALA was used as the n-3 fatty acid, it failed to reduce tumor number (Fig. 11.6). This is important because ALA is the major source of n-3

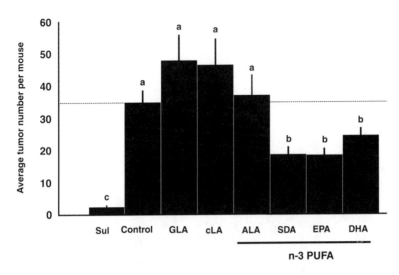

FIGURE 11.6

Effect of dietary fatty acids on tumor number. Apc[Min/+] mice were fed a variety of fatty acid ethyl esters (3%, w/w) for approximately 7 weeks and tumor number was determined following macroscopic evaluation.[78] Bars represent means ±SEM. Superscripts indicate a significant difference among groups by Fisher's least significant difference multiple comparison method at P < 0.05. Sulindac (Sul) at a dose of 400 ppm was used as a positive control. ALA, α-linolenic acid; cLA, conjugated linoleic acid; DHA, docosahexaenoic acid; EPA, eicosapentaenoic acid; GLA, γ-linolenic acid; SDA, stearidonic acid.

fatty acids in the U.S. diet. While we observed no effect with ALA, others have demonstrated protective effects with perilla oil (a source of ALA) on chemically induced colorectal tumors in rats;[80,81] however, these studies replaced safflower oil which is rich in the tumor-promoting PUFA LA.[82] One possible explanation for our lack of efficacy is an insufficient conversion of ALA to EPA because of the Δ-6 desaturase step, the rate-limiting step in the metabolic pathway (Fig. 11.1). However, the levels of EPA in intestinal phospholipids were 10 times higher with ALA than in control animals (3.2 mol vs. 0.3 mol%) (Table 11.3) and equivalent to those observed with the DHA-fed animals (2.8 mol%), suggesting that modification of phospholipid levels of EPA alone is not sufficient to reduce tumor multiplicity in this model.[78] Nevertheless, it appears that the Δ-6 desaturase is a limiting step for efficacy of n-3 fatty acids. This explanation is bolstered by the fact that SDA, the immediate product of Δ-6 desaturase activity, was as effective as EPA in reducing overall tumor number in this animal model.[78] Therefore, bypassing this rate-limiting step appears to be critical. These data suggest that ALA's ability to reduce tumor load is limited compared to its metabolic derivatives.

The ability of SDA to reduce tumor load could be related to its conversion to EPA rather than DHA given the fact that (1) the antitumorigenic effects of SDA were identical to EPA; (2) dietary SDA had no effect on tissue DHA levels compared to controls (5.3 vs. 5.0 mol%, respectively);[78] and (3) dietary

TABLE 11.3

Fatty Acid Composition of Apc[Min/+] Mouse Small Intestinal Phospholipids after Consumption of Diets Supplemented with Various Fatty Acid Ethyl Esters for 7 Weeks

Fatty Acid	Dietary Groups						
	Control	CLA	GLA	ALA	SDA	EPA	DHA
	(mol/100 mol total fatty acids)						
18:2 (n-6)	21.2 ± 0.4^e	22.6 ± 0.7^d	16.0 ± 0.4^f	28.2 ± 0.4^b	29.7 ± 0.4^a	21.0 ± 0.4^e	27.3 ± 0.4^b
20:3 (n-6)	1.4 ± 0.1^b	1.4 ± 0.1^b	2.7 ± 0.1^a	1.4 ± 0.0^b	1.2 ± 0.0^b	0.7 ± 0.0^c	0.7 ± 0.0^c
20:4 (n-6)	19.8 ± 0.5^b	18.4 ± 0.3^b	25.3 ± 0.7^a	9.2 ± 0.2^d	5.9 ± 0.1^f	7.6 ± 0.1^e	7.0 ± 0.2^{ef}
20:5 (n-3)	0.3 ± 0.0^e	0.4 ± 0.1^{de}	$<0.1^e$	3.2 ± 0.1^c	4.7 ± 0.2^b	12.9 ± 0.6^a	2.8 ± 0.1^c
22:6 (n-3)	5.0 ± 0.2^{cd}	5.0 ± 0.1^{bcd}	3.7 ± 0.2^f	5.6 ± 0.2^b	5.3 ± 0.2^{bc}	4.3 ± 0.2^{ef}	10.8 ± 0.1^a

Note: Values are means ±SEM. Superscripts within each row indicate a significant difference among groups by Fisher's least significant difference multiple comparison method at P < 0.05. Abbreviations: ALA, alpha-linolenic acid; CLA, conjugated linoleic acid; DHA, docosahexaenoic acid; EPA, eicosapentaenoic acid; GLA, g-linolenic acid; ND, none detected; SDA, stearidonic acid.[78]

DHA had only a modest impact on tumor number. In addition to SDA's ability to be efficiently converted to EPA, it has the added benefit of driving down tissue AA content by inhibiting the Δ-6 desaturase (as indicated by a 40% increase in tissue LA levels) and through EPA's competition with AA for incorporation into membrane phospholipids.

In summary, these studies clearly indicate that dietary n-3 PUFAs are antitumorigenic if they contain 4 or more double bonds, and SDA's equivalent impact on tumorigenesis as that of EPA suggests it possesses "pro-EPA" activity. What is not known is the mechanism of their action. Highly unsaturated n-3 PUFAs are 2.5 to 5 times more effective than ALA in modifying tissue AA levels and eicosanoid biosynthesis.[83] Are they acting as antagonists of AA, as inhibitors of prostaglandin biosynthesis, or as independent mediators? Some of these questions will be addressed later.

11.5.2 Conjugated Linoleic Acid (CLA)

CLA, predominantly as 9(Z),11(E)-18:2 (n-7), occurs naturally in small amounts in cooked meats and dairy products[84] and is potently antitumorigenic in chemically induced rat mammary tumors and in murine skin tumors at relatively low dietary levels (≥ 0.5%, w/w).[85,86] Compared to studies investigating the efficacy of CLA on mammary tumorigenesis, evidence for protection against colorectal cancer is less definitive. To date, gavage treatment with CLA has been shown to result in fewer chemically induced colonic ACF and gastric neoplasms in mice,[87,88] and CLA treatment reduced proliferation of human colon tumor cells *in vitro*.[89,90] In contrast to these encouraging results, supplementation of CLA to diets of Apc[Min/+] mice failed to reduce tumor multiplicity or alter average tumor size, even at dietary levels as high as 3% (w/w) (Fig. 11.6).[78] It has been suggested that CLA may exert its antitumorigenic effect by inhibiting the conversion of LA to AA and ultimately to eicosanoids.[91-94] Banni et al. showed that CLA at a level of 1% (w/w) in the diet maximally lowered GLA, DGLA, and AA levels as a percentage of total lipid in normal mammary tissue.[91] Others have detected conjugated AA derivatives of CLA in hepatic lipids of rats following intragastric CLA administration.[95] However, we did not observe any alterations in the small intestinal phospholipid content of LA or its derivatives nor did we detect conjugated AA and, concomitantly, did not observe any differences in prostaglandin formation (Fig. 11.7).[78]

11.5.3 Gamma-Linolenic Acid (GLA)

GLA, the Δ6-desaturase product of LA, is found predominantly in only a few dietary sources (evening primrose oil, borage oil, blackcurrant seed oil, and spirulina).[96] By bypassing the Δ6-desaturase reaction, dietary GLA is rapidly metabolized to dihomo-γ-linolenic acid (DGLA, 20:3 n-6) and

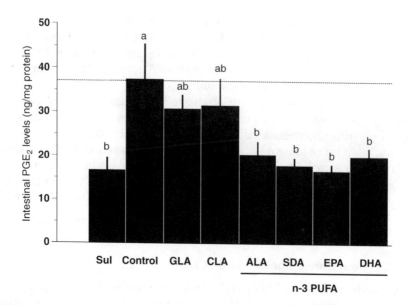

FIGURE 11.7

Effect of dietary fatty acids on intestinal PGE_2 levels. $Apc^{Min/+}$ mice were fed a variety of fatty acid ethyl esters (3%, w/w) for approximately 7 weeks and PGE_2 levels were determined in normal appearing mucosa.[78] Bars represent means ±SEM. Superscripts indicate a significant difference among groups by Fisher's least significant difference multiple comparison method at $P < 0.05$. Sulindac (Sul) at a dose of 400 ppm was used as a positive control. ALA, α-linolenic acid; cLA, conjugated linoleic acid; DHA, docosahexaenoic acid; EPA, eicosapentaenoic acid; GLA, γ-linolenic acid; SDA, stearidonic acid.

results in significant increases in tissue AA content as compared to control animals (25.3 vs. 19.8 mol%, respectively) (Table 11.3). To date, the efficacy of dietary GLA on intestinal tumorigenesis has not been determined and the actual antitumorigenicity of GLA has been only narrowly investigated thus far. Arterial GLA injections have been shown to inhibit growth of implanted hepatoma cells in rats,[97] and intra-tumoral injections of lithium-GLA resulted in smaller tumor volumes in mice implanted with pancreatic tumor cells.[98] Dietary GLA has demonstrated potential efficacy as an anti-tumorigenic agent only in 7,12-dimethylbenz(α)anthracene (DMBA)-induced mammary tumors in rats, where a diet containing evening prim-rose oil (20 g/100 g) resulted in a lower tumor incidence than did one containing corn oil.[99] Similar results were observed in nude mice bearing breast carcinoma xenografts.[100] A preventive role for dietary GLA in gastrointestinal tumorigenesis has yet to be established, although GLA treatment has been shown to limit the metastatic potential of human colon cancer cell lines and to block cell cycle progression *in vitro*.[101,102] However, the use of GLA at a dietary level of 3% (w/w) did not alter intestinal tumor load in $Apc^{Min/+}$ mice. In fact, GLA-treated mice had the highest tumor load of all dietary treatments (Fig. 11.6).

11.6 Mechanisms of Action

11.6.1 Arachidonic Acid vs. N-3 Fatty Acids

Studies in humans and in animal models overwhelmingly indicate a protective effect of n-3 fatty acids and the mechanism is largely thought to be related to a reduction in eicosanoid biosynthesis. In particular, PGE_2 has been widely implicated as a key mediator of tumorigenesis.[103–110] Prostaglandin biosynthesis is controlled by the availability of free AA and the activities of the two cyclooxygenase isozymes. Levels of free AA are influenced by the content of AA in cellular phospholipids and the activity of the various phospholipases responsible for its release. Cyclooxygenase activity is primarily controlled at the transcriptional level.

While it is clear that highly unsaturated n-3 fatty acids can potently reduce tumor multiplicity in $Apc^{Min/+}$ mice, it is less clear whether this effect is related to AA and/or its metabolism. Dietary AA (1 to 1.5%, w/w) has no effect on tumor load in $Apc^{Min/+}$ mice despite the fact that tissue AA content is increased by ~70% and PGE_2 formation doubles[44,73] (Table 11.4), implicating a lack of AA involvement. However, if the levels of PGE_2 formed and the amounts of AA in tissues were to exceed a threshold where maximal pro-neoplastic effects occur, augmentation of these levels would have little additional impact. Therefore, if n-3 fatty acids act by antagonizing AA and thus reducing AA signaling below the putative threshold, adding AA to the n-3 PUFA-containing diets should reverse the regression/loss of tumors. This hypothesis is based on our previous work that demonstrates dietary AA has the ability to completely abrogate the biochemical effects of EPA *in vivo*.[5,10,111] When $Apc^{Min/+}$ mice are fed diets containing EPA, tumor multiplicity is reduced by 50% and concomitant supplementation of AA rescued the tumors, annulling much of the effects of EPA (Table 11.4). These results suggest that the antitumorigenic effect of EPA and other n-3 fatty acids are, at least in part, via the antagonism of AA.[10,73]

11.6.2 Δ-6 Desaturase

It has been demonstrated that desaturation of ALA to SDA is critical to the antineoplastic efficacy of n-3 PUFAs. An extension of this reasoning would suggest that the pro-tumorigenic effect of n-6 PUFAs would also be dependent upon this same metabolic step. Indeed, selectively inhibiting Δ-6 desaturase[112] should significantly reduce tumor load in $Apc^{Min/+}$ mice. When $Apc^{Min/+}$ mice were treated with SC-26196, a selective inhibitor of Δ-6 desaturase, tumor number was significantly reduced by ~40% (Fig. 11.8). This reduction in tumors by SC-26196 is reversed when AA is added to the diet to bypass this inhibition (Fig. 11.8). Collectively, these results affirm the importance of AA and the Δ-6 desaturase step as key mediators influencing tumorigenesis and that the Δ-6 desaturase is an important regulatory step in the antitumorigenic properties of n-3 fatty acids.

TABLE 11.4

Tumor Load, Phospholipid Fatty Acid Composition, and PGE_2 Formation from Intestines of $Apc^{Min/+}$ Mice Whose Diets Were Supplemented with Arachidonic Acid and/or Eicosapentaenoic Acid

	Dietary Groups			
	Control	AA	EPA	AA+EPA
Tumors				
Tumor #/mouse	68 ± 9[a]	48 ± 9[a]	22 ± 1[b]	48 ± 6[a]
Selected fatty acids (mole%)				
18:2 n-6	23.7 ± 0.7[b]	15.3 ± 0.4[c]	26.7 ± 1.1[a]	17.3 ± 0.3[c]
20:4 n-6	16.7 ± 0.2[c]	28.2 ± 0.7[a]	6.2 ± 0.3[d]	25.1 ± 0.7[b]
20:5 n-3	0.3 ± 0.0[c]	0.2 ± 0.1[c]	7.1 ± 0.4[a]	1.0 ± 0.0[b]
Prostaglandins (ng/mg total protein)				
PGE_2	22.5 ± 7.6[bc]	53.6 ± 7.4[a]	6.1 ± 1.3[c]	28.0 ± 5.0[b]

Note: $Apc^{Min/+}$ mice were fed diet supplemented with the ethyl esters of arachidonic aid (AA), eicosapentaenoic acid (EPA) or oleic acid (Control) at a level of 1.5% (w/w) for approximately 8 weeks Data are presented as means ±SEM. Superscripts within each row indicate a significant difference among groups by Fisher's least significant difference multiple comparison method at P < 0.05.

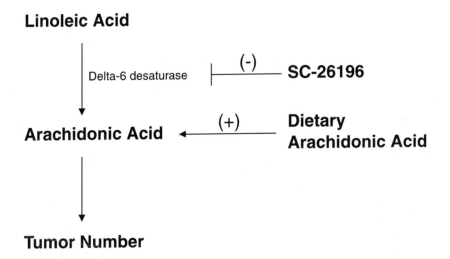

FIGURE 11.8

Effect of SC-26196 and/or dietary arachidonic acid (AA) on intestinal tumor number. Apc[Min/+] mice were fed diets supplemented with the Δ-6 desaturase inhibitor SC-26196 (100 mpk) and/or the ethyl ester of arachidonate (3%, w/w) for approximately 7 weeks and tumor number was determined following macroscopic evaluation. Tumor number was reduced by ~40% with SC-26196, and concomitant administration of arachidonic acid prevented tumor reduction.

GLA also bypasses the Δ-6 desaturase step, and it has been suggested that any antitumorigenic effects of GLA occur because of its conversion and modest accumulation of its metabolic derivative DGLA.[113] DGLA competes with AA for cyclooxygenase and 15-lipoxygenase (LOX) activity to produce PGE_1 and 15-hydroxyeicosatrienoic acid (15-HETrE), respectively.[114–116] These compounds reportedly have anti-proliferative properties. (See Reference 115 for review.) However, the inability of GLA to have an effect on tumorigenesis may be confounded by the fact that feeding GLA results in higher AA concentrations in intestinal phospholipids and does not significantly reduce AA-derived prostaglandins.[78] In addition, like PGE_2, the actions of PGE_1 are mediated via the G-protein-coupled EP receptors,[117,118] and recent evidence indicates that the EP1 receptor significantly contributes to tumorigenesis in this mouse model.[119,120]

11.6.3 Prostaglandins

The ability of dietary fatty acids to inhibit intestinal tumorigenesis has been explained by their effects on prostaglandin biosynthesis. This hypothesis was developed largely on the strength of epidemiological evidence demonstrating an inverse relationship between colorectal cancer mortality and the use of nonsteroidal antiinflammatory drugs (NSAIDs), both selective and nonselective inhibitors of the cyclooxygenase isozymes. NSAIDs reduce chemically induced and genetically predetermined colorectal tumors in experimental animal models, as well as the risk of human colorectal cancer.[44,52,121–126] Aspirin is the most widely used NSAID and many epidemiological studies report a 40 to 50% reduction in the incidence of colorectal cancer with regular sustained aspirin use.[125,126] Another NSAID, sulindac, is very effective in reducing colonic tumor number and size in FAP patients.[59,60]

A variety of NSAIDs, eg., sulindac, indomethacin, and piroxicam, reduce intestinal tumor load by 90 to 95% and the number of pre-existing tumors by 80 to 90% in Apc[Min/+] mice.[44,52,122,127,128] While NSAIDs like sulindac, indomethacin, and piroxicam are very effective in reducing tumor number in Apc[Min/+] mice, aspirin may not be as effective as other NSAIDs in this model,[127,129,130] and this effect may be due to its reduced ability to inhibit COX-2 derived prostaglandins.[131] There is compelling evidence for involvement of COX-2 in tumorigenesis. Cross-breeding Apc[Δ716] knockout mice with COX-2 knockout mice reduced tumor load by 86%.[132] Administration of the selective COX-2 inhibitors nimesulide and MF-tricyclic reduced intestinal tumor number by 50% in Apc[Min/+] mice[133] and 60% in Apc[Δ716] knockout mice.[132] However, differences in the ability to inhibit COX-2 may only provide a partial explanation because the efficacy of selective COX-2 inhibitors provides no advantage vs. less selective NSAIDs in Apc[Min/+] mice. Crossing COX-1 knockout mice with Apc[Min/+] mice results in 80 to 90% fewer tumors,[134] and may account for the efficacy observed with the nonselective inhibitors. Two recent articles discuss the importance of cyclooxygenase expression, in particular COX-2, by nontumor cells in the maintenance of tumor integrity and growth.[33,135] A number of studies also suggest prostaglandin-independent mechanisms may exist.[136–141]

The most recent data strongly implicate prostaglandin involvement in the reduction of intestinal tumorigenesis by dietary n-3 fatty acids. Intestinal prostaglandin levels are significantly lowered when n-3 fatty acids are supplemented to the diets of Apc[Min/+] mice regardless of unsaturation. However, lowering prostaglandin levels does not always equate with a lower tumor number. For example, ALA significantly attenuates PGE_2 levels, but does not alter tumor multiplicity, suggesting that prostaglandins play a partial role in tumorigenesis and the anti-neoplastic effects of n-3 PUFAs. Furthermore, regression analysis reveals a significant relationship between PGE_2 levels and tumor number.[78] It is possible that the degree of unsaturation associated with the n-3 fatty acids could differentially impact the expression, or more importantly, the activity of cyclooxygenase.[76,142,143] Intestinal tumors in Apc[Min/+] mice express both isozymes of COX where COX-2 is primarily expressed in the stroma and not the epithelial cells (Fig. 11.5).[54] Dietary fish oils (rich in EPA and DHA) reduce COX-2 expression in an azoxymethane (AOM)-induced rat colonic tumor model[76] and immunoreactive COX-1 and -2 protein levels in DMBA-induced mammary tumors,[143] whereas oils rich in n-6 fatty acids increase COX-2 expression.[76]

More importantly, prostaglandin involvement in intestinal tumorigenesis was recently demonstrated in a study using prostaglandin E receptor (EP) knockout mice and an EP receptor antagonist.[119] Watanabe et al. treated C57BL/6J mice with the colon carcinogen azoxymethane (AOM) and observed significantly fewer early neoplastic lesions (ACF) in EP1 receptor knockout mice compared to wild-type controls. Similarly, AOM-treated wild-type mice dose-dependently developed fewer ACF following administration of ONO-8711, an EP1-receptor antagonist. They also showed that ONO-8711 treatment resulted in 44% fewer tumors in Apc$^{Min/+}$ mice,[119] confirming the importance of EP1 and PGE$_2$ to Apc-mediated tumorigenesis. These results were replicated using another selective EP1 antagonist (ONO-8713) in an AOM-treated mouse model.[120] The EP1 receptor acts through a phospholipase C-mediated signaling pathway resulting in the potential activation of protein kinase C following the release of diacylglycerol. Overexpression of protein kinase Cβ_{II} results in downregulation of glycogen synthase kinase 3β (GSK-3β), an elevation in cellular β-catenin levels, and proliferation of colonic epithelium.[144] The Apc gene product acts in concert with GSK-3β to regulate the Wnt/β-catenin signaling pathway.[48] Loss of full-length Apc protein, as occurs in the Apc$^{Min/+}$ mouse model, disables the cell's ability to downregulate β-catenin and, as a result, free (not bound to E-cadherin) β-catenin increases in the cytoplasm and moves into the nucleus where it acts in conjunction with the nuclear transcription factors Tcf/Lef to induce expression of target genes.[48] Treatment with NSAIDs, inhibitors of prostaglandin biosynthesis, may reduce tumor loads in this model, at least in part, by attenuating β-catenin levels,[130,145] and n-3 PUFAs may also modulate this signaling pathway via reductions in AA and PKC activation.[102]

11.7   Summary and Conclusions

While numerous studies provide compelling evidence that dietary n-3 PUFAs abrogate intestinal tumorigenesis, the data presented here clearly establish that these effects are the result of their ability, at least in part, to antagonize arachidonic acid metabolism. That is not to say that augmenting arachidonic acid and its metabolism promotes tumorigenesis, as this is clearly not the case.[44,78,127] There appears to be a threshold for tissue AA levels where curtailing these levels results in an attenuation of tumorigenesis (Fig. 11.9), but we also present exceptions to this premise (i.e., ALA diet). Those dietary fatty acids that possess the greatest ability to minimize AA, its metabolism, and tumorigenesis have two things in common: (1) They are n-3 PUFAs, and (2) they possess at least 4 double bonds. Furthermore, the most recent data establish PGE$_2$ as a likely candidate involved in mediating much of the effects of dietary PUFAs.

It has recently been proposed that COX-2-derived PGE$_2$ is important for activating downstream growth factors, such as vascular endothelial growth factor (VEGF), and that the initial upregulation of COX-2 by tumor stromal

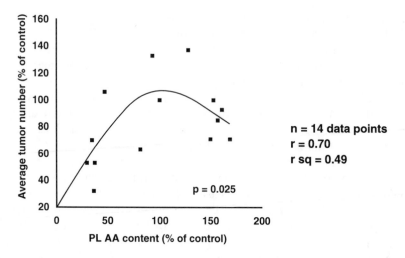

FIGURE 11.9

Intestinal tumor number as plotted against arachidonic acid (AA) content of intestinal phospholipids. Apc$^{Min/+}$ mice were fed a variety of diets containing different fatty acid compositions and tumor load was correlated with intestinal AA content.[44,71,78,127]

cells inaugurates this signaling pathway.[33,135] Thus, attenuating PGE$_2$ formation, by reducing tissue AA content, downregulating COX-2 expression, or inhibiting COX-2 activity (n-3 PUFAs are reported to do all three) could reduce angiogenesis and result in tumor regression.

References

1. Willett, W. C., Stampfer, M. J., Colditz, G. A., Rosner, B. A., and Speizer, F. E., Relation of meat, fat, and fiber intake to the risk of colon cancer in a prospective study among women, *N. Engl. J. Med.*, 323, 1664, 1990.
2. Giovannucci, E., Rimm, E. B., Stampfer, M. J., Colditz, G. A., Ascherio, A., and Willett, W. C., Intake of fat, meat, and fiber in relation to risk of colon cancer in men, *Cancer Res.*, 54, 2390, 1994.
3. German, J. B., Dillard, C. J., and Whelan, J., Biological effects of dietary arachidonic acid. Introduction, *J. Nutr.*, 126, 1076S, 1996.
4. Danon, A., Heimberg, M., and Oates, J. A., Enrichment of rat tissue lipids with fatty acids that are prostaglandin precursors, *Biochim. Biophys. Acta*, 388, 318, 1975.
5. Whelan, J., Surette, M. E., Hardardottir, I., Lu, G., Golemboski, K. A., Larsen, E., and Kinsella, J. E., Dietary arachidonate enhances tissue arachidonate levels and eicosanoid production in Syrian hamsters, *J. Nutr.*, 123, 2174, 1993.
6. Mohrhauer, H. and Holman, R. T., The effect of dose level of essential fatty acids upon the fatty acid composition of the rat liver, *J. Lipid Res.*, 4, 151, 1963.

7. Sprecher, H., An update on the pathways of polyunsaturated fatty acid metabolism, *Curr. Opin. Clin. Nutr. Metab. Care*, 2, 135, 1999.

8. Voss, A., Reinhart, M., Sankarappa, S., and Sprecher, H., The metabolism of 7,10,13,16,19-docosapentaenoic acid to 4,7,10,13,16,19-docosahexaenoic acid in rat liver is independent of a 4-desaturase, *J. Biol. Chem.*, 266, 19995, 1991.

9. Kris-Etherton, P. M., Taylor, D. S., Yu-Poth, S., Huth, P., Moriarty, K., Fishell, V., Hargrove, R. L., Zhao, G., and Etherton, T. D., Polyunsaturated fatty acids in the food chain in the United States, *Am. J. Clin. Nutr.*, 71, 179S, 2000.

10. Li, B., Birdwell, C., and Whelan, J., Antithetic relationship of dietary arachidonic acid and eicosapentaenoic acid on eicosanoid production *in vivo*, *J. Lipid Res.*, 35, 1869, 1994.

11. Taber, L., Chiu, C. H., and Whelan, J., Assessment of the arachidonic acid content in foods commonly consumed in the American diet, *Lipids*, 33, 1151, 1998.

12. Murakami, M., Shimbara, S., Kambe, T., Kuwata, H., Winstead, M. V., Tischfield, J. A., and Kudo, I., The functions of five distinct mammalian phospholipase A2s in regulating arachidonic acid release. Type IIa and type V secretory phospholipase A2s are functionally redundant and act in concert with cytosolic phospholipase A2, *J. Biol. Chem.*, 273, 14411, 1998.

13. Murakami, M., Kambe, T., Shimbara, S., and Kudo, I., Functional coupling between various phospholipase A2s and cyclooxygenases in immediate and delayed prostanoid biosynthetic pathways, *J. Biol. Chem.*, 274, 3103, 1999.

14. Dennis, E. A., Phospholipase A2 in eicosanoid generation, *Am. J. Respir. Crit. Care Med.*, 161, S32-S35, 2000.

15. Willoughby, D. A., Moore, A. R., and Colville-Nash, P. R., COX-1, COX-2, and COX-3 and the future treatment of chronic inflammatory disease, *Lancet*, 355, 646, 2000.

16. Marnett, L. J., Rowlinson, S. W., Goodwin, D. C., Kalgutkar, A. S., and Lanzo, C. A., Arachidonic acid oxygenation by COX-1 and COX-2. Mechanisms of catalysis and inhibition, *J. Biol. Chem.*, 274, 22903, 1999.

17. Kiefer, J. R., Pawlitz, J. L., Moreland, K. T., Stegeman, R. A., Hood, W. F., Gierse, J. K., Stevens, A. M., Goodwin, D. C., Rowlinson, S. W., Marnett, L. J., Stallings, W. C., and Kurumbail, R. G., Structural insights into the stereochemistry of the cyclooxygenase reaction, *Nature*, 405, 97, 2000.

18. Smith, W. L., Garavito, R. M., and DeWitt, D. L., Prostaglandin endoperoxide H synthases (cyclooxygenases)-1 and -2, *J. Biol. Chem.*, 271, 33157, 1996.

19. Brannon, T. S., North, A. J., Wells, L. B., and Shaul, P. W., Prostacyclin synthesis in ovine pulmonary artery is developmentally regulated by changes in cyclooxygenase-1 gene expression, *J. Clin. Invest.*, 93, 2230, 1994.

20. Samet, J. M., Fasano, M. B., Fonteh, A. N., and Chilton, F. H., Selective induction of prostaglandin G/H synthase I by stem cell factor and dexamethasone in mast cells, *J. Biol. Chem.*, 270, 8044, 1995.

21. Herschman, H. R., Prostaglandin synthase 2, *Biochim. Biophys. Acta*, 1299, 125, 1996.

22. Garavito, R. M. and DeWitt, D. L., The cyclooxygenase isoforms: structural insights into the conversion of arachidonic acid to prostaglandins, *Biochim. Biophys. Acta*, 1441, 278, 1999.

23. Zimmermann, K. C., Sarbia, M., Weber, A. A., Borchard, F., Gabbert, H. E., and Schror, K., Cyclooxygenase-2 expression in human esophageal carcinoma, *Cancer Res.*, 59, 198, 1999.

24. Ristimaki, A., Honkanen, N., Jankala, H., Sipponen, P., and Harkonen, M., Expression of cyclooxygenase-2 in human gastric carcinoma, *Cancer Res.*, 57, 1276, 1997.
25. Eberhart, C. E., Coffey, R. J., Radhika, A., Giardiello, F. M., Ferrenbach, S., and DuBois, R. N., Up-regulation of cyclooxygenase 2 gene expression in human colorectal adenomas and adenocarcinomas, *Gastroenterology*, 107, 1183, 1994.
26. Wolff, H., Saukkonen, K., Anttila, S., Karjalainen, A., Vainio, H., and Ristimaki, A., Expression of cyclooxygenase-2 in human lung carcinoma, *Cancer Res.*, 58, 4997, 1998.
27. Hida, T., Yatabe, Y., Achiwa, H., Muramatsu, H., Kozaki, K., Nakamura, S., Ogawa, M., Mitsudomi, T., Sugiura, T., and Takahashi, T., Increased expression of cyclooxygenase 2 occurs frequently in human lung cancers, specifically in adenocarcinomas, *Cancer Res.*, 58, 3761, 1998.
28. Bauer, A. K., Dwyer-Nield, L. D., and Malkinson, A. M., High cyclooxygenase 1 (COX-1) and cyclooxygenase 2 (COX-2) contents in mouse lung tumors, *Carcinogen*, 21, 543, 2000.
29. Tucker, O. N., Dannenberg, A. J., Yang, E. K., Zhang, F., Teng, L., Daly, J. M., Soslow, R. A., Masferrer, J. L., Woerner, B. M., Koki, A. T., and Fahey, T. J., Cyclooxygenase-2 expression is up-regulated in human pancreatic cancer, *Cancer Res.*, 59, 987, 1999.
30. Yip-Schneider, M. T., Barnard, D. S., Billings, S. D., Cheng, L., Heilman, D. K., Lin, A., Marshall, S. J., Crowell, P. L., Marshall, M. S., and Sweeney, C. J., Cyclooxygenase-2 expression in human pancreatic adenocarcinomas, *Carcinogen*, 21, 139, 2000.
31. DuBois, R. N., Review article: cyclooxygenase--a target for colon cancer prevention, *Aliment. Pharmacol. Ther.*, 14, 64, 2000.
32. Prescott, S. M. and Fitzpatrick, F. A., Cyclooxygenase-2 and carcinogenesis, *Biochim. Biophys. Acta*, 1470, M69-M78, 2000.
33. Prescott, S. M., Is cyclooxygenase-2 the alpha and the omega in cancer?, *J. Clin. Invest.*, 105, 1511, 2000.
34. Tsujii, M., Kawano, S., and DuBois, R. N., Cyclooxygenase-2 expression in human colon cancer cells increases metastatic potential, *Proc. Natl. Acad. Sci. USA*, 94, 3336, 1997.
35. Tsujii, M., Kawano, S., Tsuji, S., Sawaoka, H., Hori, M., and DuBois, R. N., Cyclooxygenase regulates angiogenesis induced by colon cancer cells, *Cell*, 93, 705, 1998.
36. Landis, S. H., Murray, T., Bolden, S., and Wingo, P. A., Cancer statistics, 1999, *CA Cancer J. Clin.*, 49, 8, 1999.
37. Siu, I. M., Robinson, D. R., Schwartz, S., Kung, H. J., Pretlow, T. G., Petersen, R. B., and Pretlow, T. P., The identification of monoclonality in human aberrant crypt foci, *Cancer Res.*, 59, 63, 1999.
38. Hamilton, S. R., The adenoma-adenocarcinoma sequence in the large bowel: variations on a theme, *J. Cell. Biochem. Suppl.*, 16G, 41, 1992.
39. Fearon, E. R. and Vogelstein, B., A genetic model for colorectal tumorigenesis, *Cell*, 61, 759, 1990.
40. Kinzler, K. W. and Vogelstein, B., Lessons from hereditary colorectal cancer, *Cell*, 87, 159, 1996.
41. Kinzler, K. W. and Vogelstein, B., Landscaping the cancer terrain, *Science*, 280, 1036, 1998.

42. Takahashi, M., Mutoh, M., Kawamori, T., Sugimura, T., and Wakabayashi, K., Altered expression of β-catenin, inducible nitric oxide synthase and cyclooxygenase-2 in azoxymethane-induced rat colon carcinogenesis, *Carcinogen*, 21, 1319, 2000.
43. Shoemaker, A. R., Gould, K. A., Luongo, C., Moser, A. R., and Dove, W. F., Studies of neoplasia in the Min mouse, *Biochim. Biophys. Acta*, 1332, F25-F48, 1997.
44. Chiu, C. H., McEntee, M. F., and Whelan, J., Sulindac causes rapid regression of preexisting tumors in Min/+ mice independent of prostaglandin biosynthesis, *Cancer Res.*, 57, 4267, 1997.
45. Heyer, J., Yang, K., Lipkin, M., Edelmann, W., and Kucherlapati, R., Mouse models for colorectal cancer, *Oncogene*, 18, 5325, 1999.
46. Smits, R., Kielman, M. F., Breukel, C., Zurcher, C., Neufeld, K., Jagmohan-Changur, S., Hofland, N., van Dijk, J., White, R., Edelmann, W., Kucherlapati, R., Khan, P. M., and Fodde, R., Apc1638T: a mouse model delineating critical domains of the adenomatous polyposis coli protein involved in tumorigenesis and development, *Genes Dev.*, 13, 1309, 1999.
47. Nathke, I. S., The adenomatous polyposis coli protein, *J. Clin. Pathol.: Mol. Pathol.*, 52, 169, 1999.
48. Polakis, P., The oncogenic activation of β-catenin, *Curr. Opin. Genet. Dev.*, 9, 15, 1999.
49. Peifer, M. and Polakis, P., Wnt signaling in oncogenesis and embryogenesis — a look outside the nucleus, *Science*, 287, 1606, 2000.
50. Miyaki, M., Iijima, T., Kimura, J., Yasuno, M., Mori, T., Hayashi, Y., Koike, M., Shitara, N., Iwama, T., and Kuroki, T., Frequent mutation of β-catenin and APC genes in primary colorectal tumors from patients with hereditary nonpolyposis colorectal cancer, *Cancer Res.*, 59, 4506, 1999.
51. Iwao, K., Nakamori, S., Kameyama, M., Imaoka, S., Kinoshita, M., Fukui, T., Ishiguro, S., Nakamura, Y., and Miyoshi, Y., Activation of the β-catenin gene by interstitial deletions involving exon 3 in primary colorectal carcinomas without adenomatous polyposis coli mutations, *Cancer Res.*, 58, 1021, 1998.
52. Boolbol, S. K., Dannenberg, A. J., Chadburn, A., Martucci, C., Guo, X. J., Ramonetti, J. T., Abreu-Goris, M., Newmark, H. L., Lipkin, M. L., DeCosse, J. J., and Bertagnolli, M. M., Cyclooxygenase-2 overexpression and tumor formation are blocked by sulindac in a murine model of familial adenomatous polyposis, *Cancer Res.*, 56, 2556, 1996.
53. Williams, C. S., Luongo, C., Radhika, A., Zhang, T., Lamps, L. W., Nanney, L. B., Beauchamp, R. D., and DuBois, R. N., Elevated cyclooxygenase-2 levels in Min mouse adenomas, *Gastroenterology*, 111, 1134, 1996.
54. Hull, M. A., Booth, J. K., Tisbury, A., Scott, N., Bonifer, C., Markham, A. F., and Coletta, P. L., Cyclooxygenase 2 is up-regulated and localized to macrophages in the intestine of Min mice, *Br. J. Cancer*, 79, 1399, 1999.
55. Chapple, K. S., Cartwright, E. J., Hawcroft, G., Tisbury, A., Bonifer, C., Scott, N., Windsor, A. C., Guillou, P. J., Markham, A. F., Coletta, P. L., and Hull, M. A., Localization of cyclooxygenase-2 in human sporadic colorectal adenomas, *Am. J. Pathol.*, 156, 545, 2000.
56. Bamba, H., Ota, S., Kato, A., Adachi, A., Itoyama, S., and Matsuzaki, F., High expression of cyclooxygenase-2 in macrophages of human colonic adenoma, *Int. J. Cancer*, 83, 470, 1999.

57. Shattuck-Brandt, R. L., Lamps, L. W., Heppner, G. K., DuBois, R. N., and Matrisian, L. M., Differential expression of matrilysin and cyclooxygenase-2 in intestinal and colorectal neoplasms, *Mol. Carcinog.,* 24, 177, 1999.

58. Hao, X., Bishop, A. E., Wallace, M., Wang, H., Willcocks, T. C., Maclouf, J., Polak, J. M., Knight, S., and Talbot, I. C., Early expression of cyclo-oxygenase-2 during sporadic colorectal carcinogenesis, *J. Pathol.,* 187, 295, 1999.

59. Giardiello, F. M., Offerhaus, J. A., Tersmette, A. C., Hylind, L. M., Krush, A. J., Brensinger, J. D., Booker, S. V., and Hamilton, S. R., Sulindac induced regression of colorectal adenomas in familial adenomatous polyposis: evaluation of predictive factors, *Gut,* 38, 578, 1996.

60. Waddell, W. R. and Loughry, R. W., Sulindac for polyposis of the colon, *J. Surg. Oncol.,* 24, 83, 1983.

61. Lipkin, M., Reddy, B., Newmark, H., and Lamprecht, S. A., Dietary factors in human colorectal cancer, *Annu. Rev. Nutr.,* 19, 545, 1999.

62. Slattery, M. L., Edwards, S. L., Boucher, K. M., Anderson, K., and Caan, B. J., Lifestyle and colon cancer: an assessment of factors associated with risk, *Am. J. Epidemiol.,* 150, 869, 1999.

63. Wasan, H. S., Novelli, M., Bee, J., and Bodmer, W. F., Dietary fat influences on polyp phenotype in multiple intestinal neoplasia mice, *Proc. Natl. Acad. Sci. USA,* 94, 3308, 1997.

64. Mutanen, M., Pajari, A. M., and Oikarinen, S. I., Beef induces and rye bran prevents the formation of intestinal polyps in Apc(Min) mice: relation to beta-catenin and PKC isozymes, *Carcinogen,* 21, 1167, 2000.

65. Pierre, F., Perrin, P., Champ, M., Bornet, F., Meflah, K., and Menanteau, J., Short-chain fructo-oligosaccharides reduce the occurrence of colon tumors and develop gut-associated lymphoid tissue in Min mice, *Cancer Res.,* 57, 225, 1997.

66. Hioki, K., Shivapurkar, N., Oshima, H., Alabaster, O., Oshima, M., and Taketo, M. M., Suppression of intestinal polyp development by low-fat and high-fiber diet in Apc(delta716) knockout mice, *Carcinogen,* 18, 1863, 1997.

67. Yang, K., Edelmann, W., Fan, K., Lau, K., Leung, D., Newmark, H., Kucherlapati, R., and Lipkin, M., Dietary modulation of carcinoma development in a mouse model for human familial adenomatous polyposis, *Cancer Res.,* 58, 5713, 1998.

68. Richter, F., Newmark, H. L., Richter, A., Leung, D., and Lipkin, M., Inhibition of Western-diet induced hyperproliferation and hyperplasia in mouse colon by two sources of calcium, *Carcinogen,* 16, 2685, 1995.

69. Xue, L., Lipkin, M., Newmark, H., and Wang, J., Influence of dietary calcium and vitamin D on diet-induced epithelial cell hyperproliferation in mice, *J. Natl. Cancer Inst.,* 91, 176, 1999.

70. Caygill, C. P., Charlett, A., and Hill, M. J., Fat, fish, fish oil and cancer, *Br. J. Cancer,* 74, 159, 1996.

71. Kato, I., Akhmedkhanov, A., Koenig, K., Toniolo, P. G., Shore, R. E., and Riboli, E., Prospective study of diet and female colorectal cancer: the New York University Women's Health Study, *Nutr. Cancer,* 28, 276, 1997.

72. Fernandez, E., Chatenoud, L., La Vecchia, C., Negri, E., and Franceschi, S., Fish consumption and cancer risk, *Am. J. Clin. Nutr.,* 70, 85, 1999.

73. Petrik, M. B., McEntee, M. F., Chiu, C. H., and Whelan, J., Antagonism of arachidonic acid is linked to the antitumorigenic effect of dietary eicosapentaenoic acid in Apc(Min/+) mice, *J. Nutr,* 130, 1153, 2000.

74. Paulsen, J. E., Elvsaas, I. K., Steffensen, I. L., and Alexander, J., A fish oil derived concentrate enriched in eicosapentaenoic and docosahexaenoic acid as ethyl ester suppresses the formation and growth of intestinal polyps in the Min mouse, *Carcinogen*, 18, 1905, 1997.
75. Paulsen, J. E., Stamm, T., and Alexander, J., A fish oil-derived concentrate enriched in eicosapentaenoic and docosahexaenoic acid as ethyl esters inhibits the formation and growth of aberrant crypt foci in rat colon, *Pharmacol. Toxicol.*, 82, 28, 1998.
76. Singh, J., Hamid, R., and Reddy, B. S., Dietary fat and colon cancer: modulation of cyclooxygenase-2 by types and amount of dietary fat during the postinitiation stage of colon carcinogenesis, *Cancer Res.*, 57, 3465, 1997.
77. Oshima, M., Takahashi, M., Oshima, H., Tsutsumi, M., Yazawa, K., Sugimura, T., Nishimura, S., Wakabayashi, K., and Taketo, M. M., Effects of docosahexaenoic acid (DHA) on intestinal polyp development in Apc delta 716 knockout mice, *Carcinogen*, 16, 2605, 1995.
78. Petrik, M. B., McEntee, M. F., Johnson, B. T., Obukowicz, M. G., and Whelan, J., Highly-unsaturated (n-3) fatty acids, but not α-linolenic, conjugated linoleic and gamma-linolenic acids, reduce tumorigenesis in Apc$^{Min/+}$ mice, *J. Nutr*, 130, 2434, 2000.
79. Cha, Y. S., Li, B., Sachan, D. S., and Whelan, J., Dietary docosahexaenoic acid decreases plasma triglycerides with mixed effects on indices of β-oxidation, *Korean J. Nutr.*, 30, 1067, 1997.
80. Hirose, M., Masuda, A., Ito, N., Kamano, K., and Okuyama, H., Effects of dietary perilla oil, soybean oil and safflower oil on 7,12-dimethylbenz[a]anthracene (DMBA) and 1,2-dimethyl-hydrazine (DMH)-induced mammary gland and colon carcinogenesis in female SD rats, *Carcinogen*, 11, 731, 1990.
81. Narisawa, T., Fukaura, Y., Yazawa, K., Ishikawa, C., Isoda, Y., and Nishizawa, Y., Colon cancer prevention with a small amount of dietary perilla oil high in alpha-linolenic acid in an animal model, *Cancer*, 73, 2069, 1994.
82. Reddy, B. S., Dietary fat and colon cancer: animal model studies, *Lipids*, 27, 807, 1992.
83. Whelan, J., Broughton, K. S., and Kinsella, J. E., The comparative effects of dietary alpha-linolenic acid and fish oil on 4- and 5-series leukotriene formation *in vivo*, *Lipids*, 26, 119, 1991.
84. Chin, S. F., Liu, W., Storkson, J. M., Ha, Y. L., and Pariza, M. W., Dietary sources of conjugated dienoic isomers of linoleic acid, a newly recognized class of anticarcinogens, *J. Food Compos. Anal.*, 5, 185, 1992.
85. Ip, C., Chin, S. F., Scimeca, J. A., and Pariza, M. W., Mammary cancer prevention by conjugated dienoic derivative of linoleic acid, *Cancer Res.*, 51, 6118, 1991.
86. Belury, M. A., Nickel, K. P., Bird, C. E., and Wu, Y., Dietary conjugated linoleic acid modulation of phorbol ester skin tumor promotion, *Nutr. Cancer*, 26, 149, 1996.
87. Ha, Y. L., Storkson, J., and Pariza, M. W., Inhibition of benzo(a)pyrene-induced mouse forestomach neoplasia by conjugated dienoic derivatives of linoleic acid, *Cancer Res.*, 50, 1097, 1990.
88. Liew, C., Schut, H. A., Chin, S. F., Pariza, M. W., and Dashwood, R. H., Protection of conjugated linoleic acids against 2-amino-3-methylimidazo[4,5-f]quinoline-induced colon carcinogenesis in the F344 rat: a study of inhibitory mechanisms, *Carcinogen*, 16, 3037, 1995.

89. O'Shea, M., Stanton, C., and Devery, R., Antioxidant enzyme defence responses of human MCF-7 and SW480 cancer cells to conjugated linoleic acid, *Anticancer Res.*, 19, 1953, 1999.
90. Shultz, T. D., Chew, B. P., Seaman, W. R., and Luedecke, L. O., Inhibitory effect of conjugated dienoic derivatives of linoleic acid and beta-carotene on the *in vitro* growth of human cancer cells, *Cancer Lett.*, 63, 125, 1992.
91. Banni, S., Angioni, E., Casu, V., Melis, M. P., Carta, G., Corongiu, F. P., Thompson, H., and Ip, C., Decrease in linoleic acid metabolites as a potential mechanism in cancer risk reduction by conjugated linoleic acid, *Carcinogen*, 20, 1019, 1999.
92. Kavanaugh, C. J., Liu, K. L., and Belury, M. A., Effect of dietary conjugated linoleic acid on phorbol ester-induced PGE2 production and hyperplasia in mouse epidermis, *Nutr. Cancer*, 33, 132, 1999.
93. Liu, K. L. and Belury, M. A., Conjugated linoleic acid reduces arachidonic acid content and PGE2 synthesis in murine keratinocytes, *Cancer Lett.*, 127, 15, 1998.
94. Belury, M. A. and Kempa-Steczko, A., Conjugated linoleic acid modulates hepatic lipid composition in mice, *Lipids*, 32, 199, 1997.
95. Sebedio, J. L., Juaneda, P., Gregoire, S., Chardigny, J. M., Martin, J. C., and Ginies, C., Geometry of conjugated double bonds of CLA isomers in a commercial mixture and in their hepatic 20:4 metabolites, *Lipids*, 34, 1319, 1999.
96. Phillips, J. C. and Huang, Y. S., Natural sources and biosynthesis of γ-linolenic acid: an overview, in *γ-Linolenic Acid: Metabolism and Its Roles in Nutrition and Medicine*, Huang, Y. -S. and Mills, D. E., Eds., AOCS Press, Champaign, IL, 1996, 1.
97. Kokura, S., Yoshikawa, T., Kaneko, T., Iinuma, S., Nishimura, S., Matsuyama, K., Naito, Y., Yoshida, N., and Kondo, M., Efficacy of hyperthermia and polyunsaturated fatty acids on experimental carcinoma, *Cancer Res.*, 57, 2200, 1997.
98. Ravichandran, D., Cooper, A., and Johnson, C. D., Effect of lithium gamma-linolenate on the growth of experimental human pancreatic carcinoma, *Br. J. Surg.*, 85, 1201, 1998.
99. el-Ela, S. H., Prasse, K. W., Carroll, R., and Bunce, O. R., Effects of dietary primrose oil on mammary tumorigenesis induced by 7,12-dimethylbenz(a)anthracene, *Lipids*, 22, 1041, 1987.
100. Pritchard, G. A., Jones, D. L., and Mansel, R. E., Lipids in breast carcinogenesis, *Br. J. Surg.*, 76, 1069, 1989.
101. Jiang, W. G., Hiscox, S., Hallett, M. B., Scott, C., Horrobin, D. F., and Puntis, M. C., Inhibition of hepatocyte growth factor-induced motility and *in vitro* invasion of human colon cancer cells by gamma-linolenic acid, *Br. J. Cancer*, 71, 744, 1995.
102. Jiang, Y. H., Lupton, J. R., and Chapkin, R. S., Dietary fish oil blocks carcinogen-induced down-regulation of colonic protein kinase C isozymes, *Carcinogen*, 18, 351, 1997.
103. Reddy, B. S. and Maruyama, H., Effect of dietary fish oil on azoxymethane-induced colon carcinogenesis in male F344 rats, *Cancer Res.*, 46, 3367, 1986.
104. Anti, M., Marra, G., Armelao, F., Bartoli, G. M., Ficarelli, R., Percesepe, A., De Vitis, I., Maria, G., Sofo, L., and Rapaccini, G. L., Effect of omega-3 fatty acids on rectal mucosal cell proliferation in subjects at risk for colon cancer, *Gastroenterology*, 103, 883, 1992.

105. Bartram, H. P., Gostner, A., Scheppach, W., Reddy, B. S., Rao, C. V., Dusel, G., Richter, F., Richter, A., and Kasper, H., Effects of fish oil on rectal cell proliferation, mucosal fatty acids, and prostaglandin E2 release in healthy subjects, *Gastroenterology*, 105, 1317, 1993.

106. Chang, W. L., Chapkin, R. S., and Lupton, J. R., Fish oil blocks azoxymethane-induced rat colon tumorigenesis by increasing cell differentiation and apoptosis rather than decreasing cell proliferation, *J. Nutr*, 128, 491, 1998.

107. Kim, D. Y., Chung, K. H., and Lee, J. H., Stimulatory effects of high-fat diets on colon cell proliferation depend on the type of dietary fat and site of the colon, *Nutr. Cancer*, 30, 118, 1998.

108. Minoura, T., Takata, T., Sakaguchi, M., Takada, H., Yamamura, M., Hioki, K., and Yamamoto, M., Effect of dietary eicosapentaenoic acid on azoxymethane-induced colon carcinogenesis in rats, *Cancer Res.*, 48, 4790, 1988.

109. Lindner, M. A., A fish oil diet inhibits colon cancer in mice, *Nutr. Cancer*, 15, 1, 1991.

110. Reddy, B. S., Burill, C., and Rigotty, J., Effect of diets high in omega-3 and omega-6 fatty acids on initiation and postinitiation stages of colon carcinogenesis, *Cancer Res.*, 51, 487, 1991.

111. Whelan, J., Broughton, K. S., Surette, M. E., and Kinsella, J. E., Dietary arachidonic and linoleic acids: comparative effects on tissue lipids, *Lipids*, 27, 85, 1992.

112. Obukowicz, M. G., Welsch, D. J., Salsgiver, W. J., Martin-Berger, C. L., Chinn, K. S., Duffin, K. L., Raz, A., and Needleman, P., Novel, selective delta6 or delta5 fatty acid desaturase inhibitors as antiinflammatory agents in mice, *J. Pharmacol. Exp. Ther.*, 287, 157, 1998.

113. Fan, Y. Y. and Chapkin, R. S., Importance of dietary gamma-linolenic acid in human health and nutrition, *J. Nutr*, 128, 1411, 1998.

114. Borgeat, P., Hamberg, M., and Samuelsson, B., Transformation of arachidonic acid and homo-gamma-linolenic acid by rabbit polymorphonuclear leukocytes. Monohydroxy acids from novel lipoxygenases, *J. Biol. Chem.*, 251, 7816, 1976.

115. Fan, Y. Y., Ramos, K. S., and Chapkin, R. S., Dietary gamma-linolenic acid enhances mouse macrophage-derived prostaglandin E1 which inhibits vascular smooth muscle cell proliferation, *J. Nutr*, 127, 1765, 1997.

116. Johnson, M. M., Swan, D. D., Surette, M. E., Stegner, J., Chilton, T., Fonteh, A. N., and Chilton, F. H., Dietary supplementation with gamma-linolenic acid alters fatty acid content and eicosanoid production in healthy humans, *J. Nutr*, 127, 1435, 1997.

117. Boie, Y., Stocco, R., Sawyer, N., Slipetz, D. M., Ungrin, M. D., Neuschafer-Rube, F., Puschel, G. P., Metters, K. M., and Abramovitz, M., Molecular cloning and characterization of the four rat prostaglandin E2 prostanoid receptor subtypes, *Eur. J. Pharmacol.*, 340, 227, 1997.

118. Funk, C. D., Furci, L., FitzGerald, G. A., Grygorczyk, R., Rochette, C., Bayne, M. A., Abramovitz, M., Adam, M., and Metters, K. M., Cloning and expression of a cDNA for the human prostaglandin E receptor EP1 subtype, *J. Biol. Chem.*, 268, 26767, 1993.

119. Watanabe, K., Kawamori, T., Nakatsugi, S., Ohta, T., Ohuchida, S., Yamamoto, H., Maruyama, T., Kondo, K., Ushikubi, F., Narumiya, S., Sugimura, T., and Wakabayashi, K., Role of the prostaglandin E receptor subtype EP1 in colon carcinogenesis, *Cancer Res.*, 59, 5093, 1999.

120. Watanabe, K., Kawamori, T., Nakatsugi, S., Ohta, T., Ohuchida, S., Yamamoto, H., Maruyama, T., Kondo, K., Narumiya, S., Sugimura, T., and Wakabayashi, K., Inhibitory effect of a prostaglandin E receptor subtype EP(1) selective antagonist, ONO-8713, on development of azoxymethane-induced aberrant crypt foci in mice, *Cancer Lett.*, 156, 57, 2000.

121. Alberts, D. S., Hixson, L., Ahnen, D., Bogert, C., Einspahr, J., Paranka, N., Brendel, K., Gross, P. H., Pamukcu, R., and Burt, R. W., Do NSAIDs exert their colon cancer chemoprevention activities through the inhibition of mucosal prostaglandin synthetase?, *J. Cell. Biochem. Suppl.*, 22, 18, 1995.

122. Jacoby, R. F., Marshall, D. J., Newton, M. A., Novakovic, K., Tutsch, K., Cole, C. E., Lubet, R. A., Kelloff, G. J., Verma, A., Moser, A. R., and Dove, W. F., Chemoprevention of spontaneous intestinal adenomas in the Apc Min mouse model by the nonsteroidal anti-inflammatory drug piroxicam, *Cancer Res.*, 56, 710, 1996.

123. Rao, C. V., Tokumo, K., Rigotty, J., Zang, E., Kelloff, G., and Reddy, B. S., Chemoprevention of colon carcinogenesis by dietary administration of piroxicam, alpha-difluoromethylornithine, 16 alpha-fluoro-5-androsten-17-one, and ellagic acid individually and in combination, *Cancer Res.*, 51, 4528, 1991.

124. Reddy, B. S., Rao, C. V., Rivenson, A., and Kelloff, G., Inhibitory effect of aspirin on azoxymethane-induced colon carcinogenesis in F344 rats, *Carcinogen*, 14, 1493, 1993.

125. Rosenberg, L., Palmer, J. R., Zauber, A. G., Warshauer, M. E., Stolley, P. D., and Shapiro, S., A hypothesis: nonsteroidal anti-inflammatory drugs reduce the incidence of large-bowel cancer, *J. Natl. Cancer Inst.*, 83, 355, 1991.

126. Thun, M. J., Namboodiri, M. M., and Heath, C. W. J., Aspirin use and reduced risk of fatal colon cancer, *N. Engl. J Med.*, 325, 1593, 1991.

127. Chiu, C. H., McEntee, M. F., and Whelan, J., Discordant effect of aspirin and indomethacin on intestinal tumor burden in Apc(Min/+)mice, *Prostaglandins Leukotr. Essen. Fatty Acids*, 62, 269, 2000.

128. Ritland, S. R. and Gendler, S. J., Chemoprevention of intestinal adenomas in the ApcMin mouse by piroxicam: kinetics, strain effects and resistance to chemosuppression, *Carcinogen*, 20, 51, 1999.

129. Barnes, C. J. and Lee, M., Chemoprevention of spontaneous intestinal adenomas in the adenomatous polyposis coli Min mouse model with aspirin, *Gastroenterology*, 114, 873, 1998.

130. Mahmoud, N. N., Dannenberg, A. J., Mestre, J., Bilinski, R. T., Churchill, M. R., Martucci, C., Newmark, H., and Bertagnolli, M. M., Aspirin prevents tumors in a murine model of familial adenomatous polyposis, *Surgery*, 124, 225, 1998.

131. Warner, T. D., Giuliano, F., Vojnovic, I., Bukasa, A., Mitchell, J. A., and Vane, J. R., Nonsteroid drug selectivities for cyclo-oxygenase-1 rather than cyclo-oxygenase-2 are associated with human gastrointestinal toxicity: a full *in vitro* analysis, *Proc. Natl. Acad. Sci. USA*, 96, 7563, 1999.

132. Oshima, M., Dinchuk, J. E., Kargman, S. L., Oshima, H., Hancock, B., Kwong, E., Trzaskos, J. M., Evans, J. F., and Taketo, M. M., Suppression of intestinal polyposis in Apc delta716 knockout mice by inhibition of cyclooxygenase 2 (COX-2), *Cell*, 87, 803, 1996.

133. Nakatsugi, S., Fukutake, M., Takahashi, M., Fukuda, K., Isoi, T., Taniguchi, Y., Sugimura, T., and Wakabayashi, K., Suppression of intestinal polyp development by nimesulide, a selective cyclooxygenase-2 inhibitor, in Min mice, *Jpn. J. Cancer Res.*, 88, 1117, 1997.

134. Langenbach, R., Loftin, C., Lee, C., and Tiano, H., Cyclooxygenase knockout mice: models for elucidating isoform-specific functions, *Biochem. Pharmacol.*, 58, 1237, 1999.
135. Williams, C. S., Tsujii, M., Reese, J., Dey, S. K., and DuBois, R. N., Host cyclooxygenase-2 modulates carcinoma growth, *J. Clin. Invest.*, 105, 1589, 2000.
136. Rigas, B., and Shiff, S. J., Is inhibition of cyclooxygenase required for the chemopreventive effect of NSAIDs in colon cancer? A model reconciling the current contradiction, *Med. Hypotheses*, 54, 210, 2000.
137. Piazza, G. A., Rahm, A. K., Finn, T. S., Fryer, B. H., Li, H., Stoumen, A. L., Pamukcu, R., and Ahnen, D. J., Apoptosis primarily accounts for the growth-inhibitory properties of sulindac metabolites and involves a mechanism that is independent of cyclooxygenase inhibition, cell cycle arrest, and p53 induction, *Cancer Res.*, 57, 2452, 1997.
138. Piazza, G. A., Alberts, D. S., Hixson, L. J., Paranka, N. S., Li, H., Finn, T., Bogert, C., Guillen, J. M., Brendel, K., Gross, P. H., Sperl, G., Ritchie, J., Burt, R. W., Ellsworth, L., Ahnen, D. J., and Pamukcu, R., Sulindac sulfone inhibits azoxymethane-induced colon carcinogenesis in rats without reducing prostaglandin levels, *Cancer Res.*, 57, 2909, 1997.
139. Stoner, G. D., Budd, G. T., Ganapathi, R., DeYoung, B., Kresty, L. A., Nitert, M., Fryer, B., Church, J. M., Provencher, K., Pamukcu, R., Piazza, G., Hawk, E., Kelloff, G., Elson, P., and van Stolk, R. U., Sulindac sulfone induced regression of rectal polyps in patients with familial adenomatous polyposis, *Adv. Exp. Med. Biol.*, 470, 45, 1999.
140. Chan, T. A., Morin, P. J., Vogelstein, B., and Kinzler, K. W., Mechanisms underlying nonsteroidal antiinflammatory drug-mediated apoptosis, *Proc. Natl. Acad. Sci. USA*, 95, 681, 1998.
141. Charalambous, D., Skinner, S. A., and O'Brien, P. E., Sulindac inhibits colorectal tumour growth, but not prostaglandin synthesis in the rat, *J. Gastroenterol. Hepatol.*, 13, 1195, 1998.
142. Laneuville, O., Breuer, D. K., Xu, N., Huang, Z. H., Gage, D. A., Watson, J. T., Lagarde, M., DeWitt, D. L., and Smith, W. L., Fatty acid substrate specificities of human prostaglandin-endoperoxide H synthase-1 and -2. Formation of 12-hydroxy-(9Z, 13E/Z, 15Z)-octadecatrienoic acids from alpha-linolenic acid, *J. Biol. Chem.*, 270, 19330, 1995.
143. Hamid, R., Singh, J., Reddy, B. S., and Cohen, L. A., Inhibition by dietary menhaden oil of cyclooxygenase-1 and -2 in N-nitrosomethylurea-induced rat mammary tumors, *Int. J. Oncol.*, 14, 523, 1999.
144. Murray, N. R., Davidson, L. A., Chapkin, R. S., Clay, G. W., Schattenberg, D. G., and Fields, A. P., Overexpression of protein kinase C betaII induces colonic hyperproliferation and increased sensitivity to colon carcinogenesis, *J. Cell. Biol.*, 145, 699, 1999.
145. McEntee, M. F., Chiu, C. H., and Whelan, J., Relationship of beta-catenin and Bcl-2 expression to sulindac-induced regression of intestinal tumors in Min mice, *Carcinogen*, 20, 635, 1999.
146. Otto, J. C. and Smith, W. L., Prostaglandin endoperoxide synthases-1 and -2, *J. Lipid Mediat. Cell Signal.*, 12, 139, 1995.
147. Vane, J. R., Bakhle, Y. S., and Botting, R. M., Cyclooxygenases 1 and 2, *Annu. Rev. Pharmacol. Toxicol.*, 38, 97, 1998.

148. Thuresson, E. D., Lakkides, K. M., and Smith, W. L., Different catalytically competent arrangements of arachidonic acid within the cyclooxygenase active site of prostaglandin endoperoxide H synthase-1 lead to the formation of different oxygenated products, *J. Biol. Chem.*, 275, 8501, 2000.
149. Laneuville, O., Breuer, D. K., DeWitt, D. L., Hla, T., Funk, C. D., and Smith, W. L., Differential inhibition of human prostaglandin endoperoxide H synthases-1 and -2 by nonsteroidal anti-inflammatory drugs, *J. Pharmacol. Exp. Ther.*, 271, 927, 1994.

12

Body Weight Regulation, Uncoupling Proteins, and Energy Metabolism

Sheila Collins, Wenhong Cao, Tonya M. Dixon, Kiefer W. Daniel,
Hiroki Onuma, and Alexander V. Medvedev

CONTENTS

12.1 Brief History of Discovery of Uncoupling Proteins 262
    12.1.1 UCP1 as a Brown Fat-Specific Modulator
        of Heat Production 262
    12.1.2 Overview of Defects in Thermogenesis in Rodents
        Models of Obesity 262
    12.1.3 Identity of UCP Homologs and Genetic Linkage
        with Body Weight Disorders 263
12.2 Overview of the β_3AR and Effects of Selective Agonists 264
    12.2.1 Unusual Thermogenic Properties of Atypical
        βAR Ligands 264
    12.2.2 The Third βAR is a Fat-Specific Gene 264
    12.2.3 Impaired Adipose Tissue Adrenergic Signaling
        in Obesity 265
    12.2.4 Selective β_3AR Agonists as Potential Thermogenic
        and Antiobesity Agents 268
    12.2.5 Novel Signaling Properties of the β_3AR 269
12.3 UCP2 and UCP3: Links to Resting Metabolic Rate, Fuel
    Metabolism, or Signal Transduction 270
    12.3.1 Regulation of UCP2 and UCP3 Expression
        by Dietary Manipulations 270
    12.3.2 Modulators of UCP2/3 Activity 271
    12.3.3 Tissue Distribution of UCP2 Implicates a Role
        in Immune Function 272
    12.3.4 Future Directions for UCP Research 273
References 274

12.1 A Brief History of Discovery of Uncoupling Proteins

12.1.1 UCP1 as a Brown Fat-Specific Modulator of Heat Production

The rich and varied history of brown adipose tissue as an anatomically discreet tissue type includes early speculations in the 17th century that it was part of the thymus. A century later it was thought to be an endocrine organ involved in blood formation or a form of fat acting as a reservoir for certain nutrients.[1] It was only in 1961 that brown adipose tissue was proposed to be thermogenic.[2,3] Since that time, an immense body of work has shown that brown adipose tissue is uniquely capable of responding to various environmental stimuli to generate heat from stored metabolic energy. In response to sympathetic nervous system activation, brown adipose tissue undergoes an orchestrated hyperplastic and hypertropic expansion, increased blood flow, and recruitment of lipid and carbohydrate fuels for oxidative metabolism.[4,5] A unique and critical element of this thermogenic machine was recognition of the presence of the brown-fat specific mitochondrial uncoupling protein (UCP), originally called thermogenin.[6] This mitochondrial protein allows controlled proton leakage for the purpose of heat generation at the expense of coupled ATP production (Fig. 12.1). The cloning of the brown fat UCP from rodents provided the opportunity to investigate the molecular mechanism of thermogenic uncoupling in mitochondria and regulation of the UCP gene by hormonal stimulation.[7–9]

12.1.2 Overview of Defects in Thermogenesis in Rodent Models of Obesity

From the earliest studies of the obese mouse (now called leptin-deficient C57BL/6J Lep^{ob}), there was evidence that these mice were not only obese, hyperglycemic, and hyperinsulinemic, but that they exhibited extreme sensitivity to the cold.[10] Histologically, brown adipose tissue in these obese animals appears inactive in that it is infiltrated by white adipocytes and does not possess the rich density of mitochondria expressing UCP1 as normally seen in lean animals. The blunted capacity for adrenergic stimulation of lipolysis in adipose tissue of these animals (described below) probably also hinders the activation of UCP1 function by free fatty acids. Other monogenic obesity models and hypothalamic lesioning studies in rodents indicated a complex set of neural and endocrine abnormalities, culminating in the loss of homeostatic mechanisms controlling both food intake and metabolic efficiency.[11]

The suggestive role for brown fat and thermogenesis in body weight regulation was strengthened further by the generation of mice lacking brown fat as a consequence of targeted expression of diptheria toxin in brown adipocytes.[12] These animals became obese and somewhat hyperphagic. Since the adipocyte-derived hormone leptin (the product of the *ob* locus[13]) regulates food intake, metabolic rate, and thermogenesis in brown fat,[14–17] the obesity

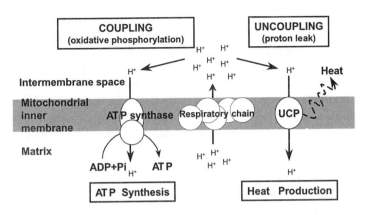

FIGURE 12.1

Schematic model of mitochondrial uncoupling. This simple cartoon compares the relationship between mitochondrial respiration that is coupled to the production of ATP via the ATP synthase vs. the UCP-dependent transfer of protons across the inner membrane down the electrochemical gradient, whose action yields heat as a result of a need for increased fuel consumption to maintain ATP levels.

in BAT-deficient mice may be a result of the inability of leptin to modulate brown fat thermogenesis. However, the metabolic capacity of brown fat may not be restricted to its expression of UCP1, since specific targeted disruption of the UCP1 gene clearly showed that this UCP is responsible for thermal regulation by brown fat, but the animals are not obese.[18]

12.1.3 Identity of UCP Homologs and Genetic Linkage with Body Weight Disorders

Sporadic observations that the brown fat UCP could be detected (primarily when using antisera to measure protein levels) in other tissues such as muscle,[19] led Ricquier and colleagues to search for homologues of the UCP. In 1997, Fleury et al.[20] reported the cloning of UCP2. In addition to significant homology (59%) with the brown fat UCP (now named UCP1) and the ability to uncouple respiration as efficiently as UCP1 in model systems, we found that UCP2 was broadly expressed in many tissues. This led to the hypothesis that UCP2 was the long-sought explanation for the relative inefficiency of oxidative respiration seen in most cell types. We also noted that the UCP2 gene resides in a chromosomal location on distal mouse chromosome 7 that is coincident with a quantitative trait locus (QTL) linkage to hyperinsulinemia and high plasma leptin levels (reflective of body fat stores). In addition, we showed that the expression of UCP2 was specifically elevated in white adipose tissue in strains of mice that are relatively resistant to the development of diet-induced obesity and diabetes, but not in obesity-prone mice.[20,21]

Other groups subsequently reported the discovery of UCP3, expressed predominantly in skeletal muscle and brown fat, and to a lesser extent in heart.[22,23] The structural homology between these UCPs and basic features about their regulation and expression in various rodent models and human populations have been recently reviewed.[24-26] The UCP3 gene is also located 8 to 10 kb 5' to the UCP2 gene in both the mouse and human genomes.[21,27] While this close linkage relationship means that either or both of these UCPs could be related to this QTL, we could not find evidence for changes in expression of UCP3 in the mouse models that originally defined this QTL.[21] It should be noted that increased expression of UCP2 in brown fat of UCP1$^{-/-}$ animals was observed,[18] but it is not yet clear whether this increase is related to the maintenance of normal body weight in these animals.

12.2 Overview of the β₃AR and Effects of Selective Agonists

12.2.1   Unusual Thermogenic Properties of Atypical βAR Ligands

The study of lipolysis and thermogenesis in white and brown adipose tissue by the β-adrenergic receptor (βAR) has witnessed episodic confusion and controversy as the number of adrenergic receptor subtypes has grown by molecular cloning, and new pharmacologic tools have become available. For many years it was generally accepted that a single βAR subtype controlled adipocyte metabolism.[28,29] This view began to erode as ever more selective sympathomimetic agents were developed that could discriminate between β₁AR and β₂AR. However, the adipocyte βAR could not be defined clearly as being one or the other of these two subtypes or a combination thereof (especially true in rodents), and it was postulated that an atypical βAR existed in this cell type, which was either a new receptor or a modified state of β₁AR or β₂AR. The most significant evidence for a new receptor subtype appeared when Arch and colleagues reported[30] that a series of new β-adrenergic ligands, which were clearly not classical β₁AR or β₂AR ligands, had the remarkable ability to reverse the severe obesity and diabetes of the C57BL/6J *Lep^{ob}* (*ob/ob*) mouse. These novel compounds increased oxygen consumption, eliminated the classic cold-intolerance of these animals and, importantly, reduced their excess adipose tissue stores.

12.2.2   The Third βAR is a Fat-Specific Gene

Additional pharmacological studies and molecular cloning eventually led to the identification of the β₃AR in 1989/1990 as a G protein-coupled receptor (GPCR) expressed predominantly in adipose tissue[31] and the target of the agents developed by Arch, Cawthorne and colleagues.[30] We now know that all three βAR subtypes: β₁AR, β₂AR, and β₃AR, are expressed in white and brown adipocytes,[32-35] and together they mediate the effects of noradrenaline-stimulated lipolysis and thermogenesis. The β₃AR is expressed in adipocytes as a

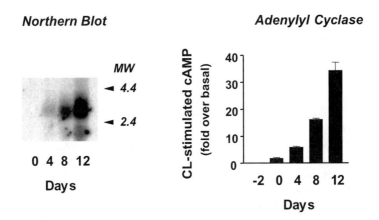

Northern Blot

Adenylyl Cyclase

FIGURE 12.2
Differentiation-dependent expression and activity of the β_3AR in 3T3-F442A adipocytes. As adipogenic cell lines such as 3T3-F442A differentiate, the expression and functional activity of the β_3AR appear. Left: Northern blot analysis of β_3AR mRNA levels. Right: Cyclic AMP production in cells differentiated for the indicated periods.

function of differentiation[36] (Fig. 12.2). Similar to certain other adipocyte-specific genes, the β_3AR requires the expression of C/EBPα for induction and maintenance of expression (Dixon et al.[37]), similar to certain other adipocyte-specific genes.[38a,38b]

Many studies have now documented the potent anti-obesity and anti-hyperglycemic properties of selective β_3AR agonists in a variety of animal models.[30,39–42] These observations have fueled intense investigation of these drugs as potential obesity and/or diabetes therapies for humans. The presence of β_3AR in human adipose tissue has been much debated. Part of the difficulty stems from the fact that agonists like BRL37344 and CL316,243 were used to assess functional β_3AR in fat samples from humans as well as non-human primates. The problem here is that these compounds are, *at best*, weak partial agonists for the human β_3AR,[31] so that many studies with negative results need to be carefully viewed in this light. There is now clear evidence of β_3AR in human adipose tissue, but the levels found in human fat cells are much lower than are observed in rodents,[43,44] and are most evident in brown adipocytes found clustered among white fat cells particularly within intra-abdominal depots. As a result of this visceral location, it has been difficult at best to quantify the relative abundance of these brown adipocytes among individuals and in response to drug treatments. The ability of newer compounds that are full agonists and antagonists for the human β_3AR[45] to directly modulate lipolysis in monkey or human fat cells should help to clarify these issues.

12.2.3 Impaired Adipose Tissue Adrenergic Signaling in Obesity

It was known for many years that obese C57BL/6J *Lep^{ob}* and C57KsJ *LepR^{db}* mice exhibited a marked inability to effectively mobilize triglycerides from white adipose tissue.[46–49] These animals are also unable to recruit brown adipose tissue for thermogenesis in response to cold temperature-induced adrenergic stimulation,[49,50] indicating that adrenergic mechanisms regulating metabolism in both white and brown fat are affected in obesity. While defects in sympathetic outflow have been shown to be associated with obesity,[51–53] other experiments also clearly indicated that there was impaired β-adrenergic receptor (βAR) function at the level of the adipocyte itself, independent of the availability of catecholamines.[48]

Because activation of adenylyl cyclase by catecholamines and the expected elevation in intracellular cAMP are depressed in C57BL/6J *Lep^{ob}* animals, in the late 1970s and early 1980s several investigators tried to determine the nature of the molecular defect in adipocytes from obese animals. The components of the adrenergic signal transduction pathway (at least those which were known at the time, which did *not* include β_3AR) were examined, and were not different between lean and obese animals despite a severe blunting of the β-adrenergic response, adenylyl cyclase itself, and other downstream effectors of the lipolytic process.[48,54,55] Collectively, these results led to the conclusion that the signal transduction mechanism of the β-adrenergic receptor(s) must be defective. It is now apparent that earlier βAR radioligand-binding results in adipose tissue were misleading because the classical βAR radioligands such as cyanopindolol exhibit a 20- to 50-fold weaker affinity for the β_3AR than for β_1AR and β_2AR.[31,56] Therefore, β_3AR levels were essentially undetected, and estimates of β_1AR and β_2AR were distorted. In 1989/1990 the first β_3AR clone was isolated from a human genomic DNA library.[57]

Figure 12.3 shows the impaired ability of white adipose tissue from genetically obese (C57BL/6J *Lep^{ob}*) mice to stimulate adenylyl cyclase activity in response to β-agonist stimulation, and the dramatic decrease in expression of the newly discovered β_3AR, as well as of the β_1AR. Although these adenylyl cyclase data are similar to many previous reports (e.g., Reference 46), a unique aspect of our method of analysis was the use of epinephrine and the very large number of data points. This allowed us to perform complex nonlinear curve-fitting routines[58] to dissect the contributions of the individual βAR subtypes to the adenylyl cyclase response. In normal lean animals, the high- and low-affinity populations correspond to {$\beta_1AR + \beta_2AR$} and β_3AR, respectively. By contrast, there is only one population of sites in the C57BL/6J *Lep^{ob}* mouse, and this corresponds to the high-affinity population. Through a series of pharmacologic analyses we showed that these reductions in βAR expression (Fig. 12.3) correspond functionally to the impaired stimulation of cAMP production, and appear to be largely responsible for the defects in catecholamine-stimulated lipolysis observed in the C57BL/6J *Lep^{ob}* mouse.[33] Similar findings of depressed β_3AR mRNA levels in the Zucker fatty (*fa/fa*) rat were reported by Muzzin et al.,[59] but the relationship to changes in the function of the receptor was not examined in that study. We have now extended our original findings to several other mouse models of obesity. We find significant deficits in the expression and function

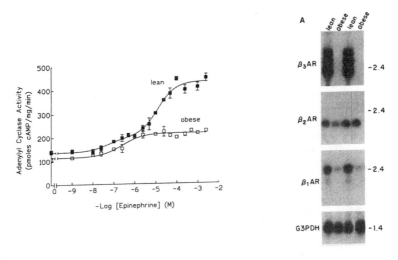

FIGURE 12.3
β-agonist-stimulated adenylyl cyclase and expression of βAR subtypes in white adipose tissue (WAT) of C57BL/6J (lean) and *Lep^ob* (obese) mice. Left: Dose-response curves of stimulation of cAMP production by epinephrine in WAT plasma membranes. Right: Northern blot of β_1-, β_2-, and β_3AR mRNA levels in WAT.[33] (Adapted from Collins et al., *Mol. Endocrinol.*, 8, 518, 1994. With permission.)

of adipocyte βARs in essentially every model of obesity that we have examined, including obesity induced by high-fat feeding in non-mutant mice.[60]

In considering the molecular basis for this dramatic impairment of βAR expression, an important connection may exist between the abnormal endocrine profiles that are observed in these models of obesity and the expression and function of individual βAR subtypes. For example, both the C57BL/6J *Lep^ob* and C57BL/6J *LepR^db* mice exhibit many endocrine abnormalities, including hyperinsulinemia, hypercorticoidism, infertility, and some evidence for perinatal hypothyroidism.[10,61-65] While glucocorticoids appear essential for the development of obesity in C57BL/6J *Lep^ob* and C57BL/6J *LepR^db* mice,[66-68] adrenalectomy does not completely restore body composition and circulating insulin levels to those of lean controls. Most of these endocrine patterns, including the corticosteroid axis, are normalized when *ob/ob* mice are administered recombinant leptin (reviewed in Reference 69). However, our results with two other mouse mutants, tubby (*tub/tub*) and fat (*fat/fat*), which have an intact leptin signaling system, as well as the diet-induced obese B/6J mouse, clearly show that there is reduced expression and function of adipocyte β_3AR and β_1AR in these animals,[60] despite their completely normal corticosteroid levels.[70-72] As in human obesity, all of these animal models of obesity are associated with hyperinsulinemia and insulin resistance. Therefore, considering these data together, it is evident that hyperinsulinemia is the single most common feature associated with both congenital and dietary obesity. Because of this strong association, we presently hypothesize that hyperinsulinemia contributes, either directly or indirectly, to the inhibition of adipocyte βAR expression and function in obesity, impairing catecholamine-stimulated lipolysis and exaggerating the excessive lipid storage in the adipocyte.

12.2.4 Selective β₃AR Agonists as Potential Thermogenic and Antiobesity Agents

Since the first reports by Arch and colleagues that atypical β-adrenergic ligands had thermogenic and weight-reducing properties in C57BL/6J *Lep^{ob}* mice,[30] there has been great interest in trying to understand their biochemical and physiological effects and to develop such compounds as therapeutic agents. In most species studied, including some studies in non-human primates, β₃AR-agonist treatment is associated with increased density of brown adipocytes expressing UCP1 within typical white adipose depots.[40–42,73,74] From our studies in various inbred strains of mice, the relative success of β₃-agonists as an anti-obesity therapy appears to parallel the extent of this expansion of brown adipocytes.[41] Others reported similar effects of cold-exposure as well as acute β₃-agonist stimulation in a series of recombinant inbred strains.[75] Importantly, in our studies we have observed that the beneficial effects of β₃AR agonists to decrease adipose tissue mass and improve glycemic control in mouse models of obesity and diabetes can persist, even after many weeks of chronic treatment.[41] This apparent lack of desensitization is rather unusual, particularly since tachyphylaxis is a hallmark of most receptor systems. Perhaps β₃AR activation and stimulation of downstream effectors can continue because the β₃AR is neither a target for phosphorylation[76] nor does it bind β-arrestin (Cao et al.[77]), an accessory protein involved in G protein-coupled receptor desensitization.[78]

One criticism frequently leveled against studies of the β₃AR and the effects of β₃AR agonists is that this phenomenon is peculiar to rodents. This view rests essentially on two arguments: first, that clearly detectable brown adipose tissue in adult humans is absent, and second, that initial studies employing β₃AR agonists such as BRL37344 in humans or non-human primates showed no effect for stimulating cAMP production or lipolysis. In fact, the situation is not so simple. To begin with, the problem with these initial pharmacologic studies is that these compounds are, *at best*, weak partial agonists at the human β₃AR.[31] Thus, negative results are not at all surprising. Regarding the presence of brown fat in humans, several studies of adult dogs and non-human primates provide an important comparison for consideration. Dogs and monkeys are essentially like humans in that, as newborns, there are discrete depots of brown fat that disappear with growth into adulthood. However, upon treatment with selective β₃AR agonists, each has been shown to exhibit increased metabolic rate, decreased fat mass, and the appearance of brown adipocytes scattered within the so-called typical white adipose depots.[42,73,74,79] Thus, in each case, whether rodent, canine, or primate, there is a link between efficacy and thermogenesis. Nevertheless, the mechanisms responsible for these effects of selective β_3AR agonists *in vivo* are still incomplete. This is an area of very active research, with the obvious question remaining as to whether there will be similar anti-diabetic/anti-obesity effects in humans. Preliminary studies suggest that these effects are at least possible in humans.[80] Whether there will be genetic predispositions to efficacy or complicating endocrine factors such as hyperinsulinemia that could impact therapeutic response to a β_3AR agonist will need to be examined.

12.2.5 Novel Signaling Properties of the β_3AR

Long before the discovery of the β_3AR and its recognition as a unique, adipocyte-specific receptor controlling lipolysis and thermogenesis, Rodbell made the observation that there was an unusual, biphasic stimulation of cAMP production in adipocytes in response to the βAR agonist isoproterenol.[81] Depending upon the concentration of GTP in the assay, isoproterenol could either stimulate or inhibit adenylyl cyclase activity in adipocyte plasma membranes. Murayama and Ui[82] showed that this inhibitory phase could be relieved by pretreatment of adipocytes with pertussis toxin (PTX). With the cloning of the β_3AR gene and the development of highly selective β_3AR agonists,[30,83] it was postulated that this novel adipocyte-specific βAR may be responsible for the biphasic adenylyl cyclase response in adipocytes.[84] In fact, we previously noted that despite the relatively high level of expression of the β_3AR in adipocytes, the efficiency of coupling of the β_3AR to stimulation of adenylyl cyclase is low.[33] However, until recently there has been no clear biochemical demonstration of physical coupling of the β_3AR to G_i, other than comparative functional experiments in the presence or absence of PTX.[85] Nor had there been any indication of what additional second messenger pathway may be activated as a consequence of this putative coupling of β_3AR to G_i. We recently reported that the β_3AR is simultaneously coupled to both Gs and G_i, with the consequent activation of the cAMP-dependent kinase (PKA) and mitogen-activated protein kinase (MAP) (ERK1/2) pathways, respectively.[85] Physical coupling of the β_3AR to Gs and G_i was demonstrated in cultured adipocytes using a photolabeling technique that relies upon the ability of agonist-activated receptor to trigger $G\alpha$ subunit dissociation and binding of GTP.[87] We showed that the restraining effect of G_i on cAMP production, and the dependence of MAP kinase signaling on G_i are indicated by the sensitivity to PTX.

More recent work in our lab now shows that novel sequence elements within the β_3AR itself are responsible for the direct recruitment to the receptor of SH3 domain-containing signaling molecules such as c-Src, and this interaction is required to trigger the ERK cascade.[77,88] This realization that the β_3AR in adipocytes is coupled to multiple signaling pathways has important implications for understanding the unique pharmacological properties of agonists at this receptor. Indeed, it is known that the adipogenic transcription factor PPARγ can be phosphorylated by ERK on Ser 112 and this modification

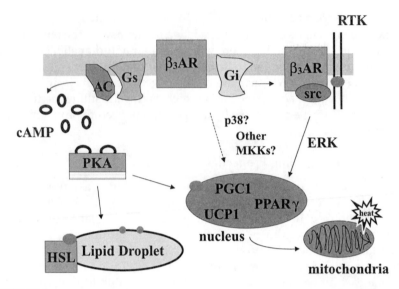

FIGURE 12.4

Hypothesis for the metabolic consequences of multiple signal transduction pathways elicited by the β_3AR in adipocytes. The β_3AR is simultaneously coupled to Gs and G_i, leading to stimulation of the protein kinase A (PKA) and the extracellular signal regulated kinase (ERK), respectively.[76] ERK activation by the β_3AR is, like other G_i-coupled receptors, dependent upon the recruitment of a receptor tyrosine kinase (RTK) and activated Src. Potential phosphorylation targets of the PKA and ERK pathways include hormone-sensitive lipase (HSL), perilipin (integral membrane protein of the lipid droplet), and nuclear proteins such as UCP1, PPARγ, PPARγ-coactivator 1 (PGC1). It is also possible that other MAP kinases (e.g., p38 MKKs) could be regulated by βARs.

serves to dampen the transcriptional capacity of peroxisome proliferator-activated receptors-γ (PPARγ).[89,90] Furthermore, the possibility that the combined activation of both the PKA and MAP kinase pathways could underlie the β_3AR agonist-dependent appearance of thermogenically active brown adipocytes in white fat depots needs to be explored, although this is admittedly only a speculation at this point (Fig. 12.4).

12.3 UCP2 and UCP3: Links to Resting Metabolic Rate, Fuel Metabolism, or Signal Transduction

12.3.1 Regulation of UCP2 and UCP3 Expression by Dietary Manipulations

The discovery of UCP2 and UCP3, exhibiting significant sequence and domain structural homology to UCP1 and capacity to uncouple mitochondrial respiration (at least in the yeast expression system),[20] immediately led to the notion that they might play a role in metabolic rate and fuel utilization. As described above, our initial observations that mRNA levels of UCP2 were differentially regulated in response to high-fat feeding in obesity-resistant and obesity-prone strains of mice supported this idea since this dietary upregulation occurred in at least two obesity-resistant strains. If UCP2 is an uncoupler of oxidative respiration, this would be consistent with increased expenditure of metabolic energy.[20,21]

The mechanism responsible for this upregulation of UCP2 gene expression was postulated to be due to increased fatty acids. In support of this idea we and others reported that ligands for the PPARγ and PPARα could increase UCP2 expression in adipocyte cell cultures.[91,92] (A follow-up study in human fat cells made similar conclusions.[93]) Not long after these original studies, several groups reported that fasting and/or starvation paradigms in rodents led to substantial increases in expression of both UCP2 and UCP3 in skeletal muscle and adipose tissue.[94,95] These observations initially led to a debate over the need to preserve body temperature vs. fuel stores. However, these studies of Dulloo and colleagues were pivotal in ultimately persuading the majority of investigators to conclude that, at least in peripheral tissues, these novel UCPs must be participating in the metabolic adaptations required during the fasted state, which requires a switch from predominantly glucose to predominantly fatty acids as a fuel source. They showed that blockading the fasting-induced rise in free fatty acids completely prevented the increase in UCP2 and UCP3 mRNA.[96–98] The molecular mechanisms regulating the UCP2 and UCP3 genes are currently under investigation, and yet the larger question that remains to be answered is the true physiologic role of these UCPs.

12.3.2 Modulators of UCP2/3 Activity

The uncoupling activity of UCP1 in brown adipocytes is inhibited by guanine nucleotides and stimulated by fatty acids, although there is still debate over the exact molecular mechanism whereby fatty acids stimulate UCP1 proton passage across the inner membrane (discussed in Reference 99). From studies in isolated brown fat mitochondria, Bouillaud and colleagues recently reported that the uncoupling activity of UCP1 is enhanced by retinoic acid[99,100] in a manner that is roughly equipotent to that of fatty acids. In addition, their comparative studies in yeast mitochondria expressing individual UCPs confirmed the effect of retinoids on UCP1, and they also showed that certain retinoids and analogs enhance the uncoupling activity of UCP2. However, unlike UCP1, there was no inhibition of UCP2 or UCP3 by GDP. Using a different approach, Garlid and colleagues compared the activity of recombinant UCP1, UCP2, UCP3 reconstituted in liposomes of defined composition.[101] They reported that proton flux via UCP2 and UCP3 could be inhibited by nucleotides, but at much higher concentrations (50 to 100 times) than for UCP1. Because of the magnitude of these differences, even after accounting for likely rightward shifts in the dose-response common in isolated systems, the physiologic significance of these nucleotide effects on UCP2 and UCP3 is unclear. Although unresolved at this time, the possibility remains that UCP2 and/or UCP3 are involved in the transport of lipids or other substrates across the mitochondrial inner membrane. When we consider the fact that it is many years after the discovery of UCP1 and the mechanism of uncoupling by UCP1 is still debated, perhaps we should not be surprised that efforts to determine the functions of UCP2 and UCP3 at the physiologic and molecular level are as yet unresolved.

12.3.3   Tissue Distribution of UCP2 Implicates a Role in Immune Function

At least at the mRNA level, the UCP2 gene is expressed in an enormous assortment of tissues and cell types. Some of these tissues, such as skeletal muscle, adipose tissue, and even certain brain regions such as hypothalamus, would be consistent with hypotheses that UCP2 has a role in energy expenditure and fuel metabolism. By contrast, the relative abundance of transcripts for UCP2 in tissues such as lung, spleen and intestine[20,99] immediately raised the question as to why there would be uncoupling in such tissues. It was then shown that in liver the expression of UCP2 was largely confined to resident Kupffer cells and not hepatocytes[102] (however, it appears that under certain circumstances hepatocytes can express UCP2).[103,104] The expression of UCP2 in Kupffer cells, which are phagocytes that serve to clear antigen entering the body from the gut, further raised the possibility that UCP2 might serve some function in macrophages, and macrophages are quite abundant in spleen, intestine, and lung. Since the major activity of macrophages involves the elimination of microorganisms/antigens by generation of reactive oxygen species (ROS), one could speculate on a role for UCP2 in this process.

An intriguing connection between mitochondrial uncoupling and ROS was proposed by Casteilla and colleagues,[104] based on their observation that inhibition of uncoupling activity of UCP1 in brown fat mitochondria by GDP was associated with a rise in H_2O_2 production; a similar effect was observed in spleen and thymus mitochondria (rich sources of UCP2) but not in hepatocytes (lacking UCP2). From these results the authors made the hypothesis that UCPs and mitochondrial uncoupling may indeed modulate the production of ROS. This idea has obvious implications for inflammation, apoptosis, and aging. Diehl and colleagues provided additional evidence linking ROS production and UCP2 expression from studies in which they showed coordinate changes in ROS levels and UCP2 expression in hepatocytes of regenerating rat liver.[104] The accumulation of ROS in hepatocytes was immediately followed by a significant increase in UCP2 expression, with the peak of UCP2 expression coinciding with the maximal decline in ROS production, leading to speculation of a cause and effect relationship. In addition, they showed that pretreatment of cultured hepatocytes with neutralizing anti-TNFα antibody inhibited ROS production and diminished UCP2 mRNA levels. Hence, these data implicated TNFα in the regulation of both ROS and UCP2 expression, and also hinted at a role for UCP2 in decreasing ROS production in support of the original hypothesis of Negre-Salvayre.

The relationship between TNFα or other cytokines and UCPs is still relatively unclear. For example, several studies have shown that treatment of mice and rats with LPS acutely increases UCP2 mRNA expression in liver, adipose tissue, and skeletal muscle, and that the mechanism is TNFα dependent.[103,106] A single treatment of rats with TNFα directly also was associated with a significant increase in UCP2 and UCP3 mRNA levels in skeletal muscle.[107] In contrast, treatment of cultured human adipose tissue with TNFα was reported to provoke a 2-fold decrease in UCP2 mRNA levels.[93]

Thus, while the relationship between cytokines, ROS, and UCPs is intriguing, there is a considerable amount of additional work required to clarify the link, if any, that exists. In the hope of understanding the physiologic role of the UCP2 gene, we recently generated mice with a targeted disruption of UCP2. Of the phenotypes exhibited by these mice, one interesting outcome is that they are completely resistant to certain infectious agents, and we find that UCP2 modulates the production of cytokines and ROS in macrophages.[108] This important observation will need to be explored in greater detail to understand the role of UCP2 in mechanisms of ROS sensing and signal transduction, and the possibility that pharmacologic modulation of UCP2 might play a role in septic and parasitic challenges, immunosuppression, as well as atherosclerosis.

12.3.4   Future Directions for UCP Research

The discovery of the novel UCPs (UCP2/UCP3) in 1997 led to an explosive reinvestigation of thermogenesis, the role of controlled wasting of metabolic energy, and the possibility that these new gene products might be genetically linked to certain metabolic disorders, or that the UCPs might be targets for therapeutic interventions for obesity, Type II diabetes, etc. However, after 2 to 3 years of research the situation is less clear. For a while there was much excitement surrounding the discovery of UCP3, since it is predominantly found in skeletal muscle, a major locus of metabolic fuel consumption and heat generation. Recently, the first reports describing the phenotypes of mice with targeted disruption of the UCP3 gene were, at the very least, disappointing from the perspective of metabolic control of body weight and glucose homeostasis.[109,110] Nevertheless, the studies of Dulloo and colleagues[96–98] indicate distinct changes in expression of UCP2 and UCP3 in response to shifts in metabolic fuel usage (carbohydrate vs. lipids), and should clearly point the way for us to try to decipher their meaning.

Other interesting developments in the study of UCPs, particularly UCP2 (because of its broad tissue distribution) may involve apoptosis. Participation of mitochondria in apoptosis is now widely accepted and supported by a number of studies describing mitochondrial alterations during apoptosis, such as the production of ROS, collapse of the inner mitochondrial membrane potential, opening of the mitochondrial permeability transition pore (MPTP), and the depletion of ATP (reviewed in Reference 111). The first direct hints that UCP2 may be specifically involved in apoptosis were obtained by microarray screening of changes in gene expression in apoptosis-resistant and apoptosis-sensitive clonal sublines of a B-cell mouse lymphoma.[112] Expression of UCP2 was significantly upregulated early in apoptosis-sensitive but not in apoptosis-resistant cells. Future studies in this area should be very exciting and illuminating, learning whether UCPs are involved in the process of apoptosis either directly or indirectly.

The role of UCPs in the brain, particularly UCP2, which displays extensive expression in the brain[113] including the hypothalamus, amygdala, and cerebellum, is at this point completely unknown. We can only speculate on the possibility that UCP2, if serving an uncoupling function in neurons, could shift relative production of ATP and hence impact ATP-sensitive ion channels and neurotransmission. In addition, if there is indeed any involvement of UCPs in apoptosis, ROS, etc., then alterations in UCP2 levels in the brain could possibly be involved in certain forms of neurodegeneration and dementia. The study of the novel UCPs over the past few years has certainly been an example of "the more we know, the less we understand." After this period of challenges and confusion, we can only expect future studies to shed more light, if not necessarily more heat!

Acknowledgments: This work was supported in part by NIH awards DK53092 and DK54024 to SC. We thank Claire Pecqueur for the basic design of Fig. 12.1.

References

1. Lindberg, O., Ed., *Brown Adipose Tissue*, Elsevier, New York, 1970.
2. Smith, R., Thermogenic activity of the hibernating gland in the cold-acclimated rat, *Physiologist*, 4, 113, 1961.
3. Ball, E. and Jungas, R., On the action of hormones which accelerate the rate of oxygen consumption and fatty acid release in rat adipose tissue *in vitro*, *Proc. Natl. Acad. Sci. USA*, 47, 932, 1961.
4. Bukowiecki, L., Collet, A., Follea, N., Guay, G., and Jahjah, L., Brown adipose tissue hyperplasia: a fundamental mechanism of adaptation to cold and hyperphagia, *Am. J. Physiol.*, 242, E353, 1982.
5. Géloën, A., Collet, A. J., and Bukowiecki, L. J., Role of sympathetic innervation in brown adipocyte proliferation, *Am. J. Physiol.*, 263, R1176, 1992.
6. Cannon, B., Hedin, A., and Nedergaard, J., Exclusive occurrence of thermogenin antigen in brown adipose tissue, *FEBS Lett.*, 150, 129, 1982.

7. Bouillaud, F., Ricquier, D., Mory, G., and Thibault, J., Increased level of mRNA for the uncoupling protein in brown adipose tissue of rats during thermogenesis induced by cold exposure or norepinephrine infusion, *J. Biol. Chem.*, 259, 11583, 1984.

8. Kozak, U. C., Kopecky, J., Teisinger, J., Enerback, S., Boyer, B., and Kozak, L. P., An upstream enhancer regulating brown-fat-specific expression of the mitochondrial uncoupling protein gene, *Mol. Cell. Biol.*, 14, 59, 1994.

9. Larose, M., Cassard-Doulcier, A.-M., Fleury, C., Serra, F., Champigny, O., and Bouillaud, F., Essential cis-acting elements in rat uncoupling protein gene are in an enhancer containing a complex retinoic acid response domain, *J. Biol. Chem.*, 271, 31533, 1996.

10. Bray, G. A., and York, D. A., Hypothalamic and genetic obesity in experimental animals: an autonomic and endocrine hypothesis, *Physiol. Rev.*, 59, 719, 1979.

11. Bray, G. A., Fisler, J., and York, D. A., Neuroendocrine control of the development of obesity: understanding gained from studies of experimental animal models, *Front. Neuroendocrinol.*, 11, 128, 1990.

12. Lowell, B. B., Susulic, V., Hamann, A., Lawitts, J. A., Himms-Hagen, J., and Boyer, B. B., Development of obesity in transgenic mice after genetic ablation of brown adipose tissue, *Nature*, 366, 740, 1993.

13. Zhang, Y., Proenca, R., Maffei, M., Barone, M., Leopold, L., and Friedman, J. M., Positional cloning of the mouse obese gene and its human homologue, *Nature*, 372, 425, 1994.

14. Halaas, J. L., Gajiwala, K. S., Maffei, M., Cohen, S. L., Chait, B. T., and Rabinowitz, D., Weight-reducing effects of the plasma protein encoded by the obese gene, *Science*, 269, 543, 1995.

15. Pelleymounter, M. A., Cullen, M. J., Baker, M. B., Hecht, R., Winters, D., and Boone, T., Effects of the obese gene product on body weight regulation in ob/ob mice, *Science*, 269, 540, 1995.

16. Campfield, L. A., Smith, F. J., Guisez, Y., Devos, R., and Burn, P., Recombinant mouse OB protein: evidence for a peripheral signal linking adiposity and central neural networks, *Science*, 269, 546, 1995.

17. Collins, S., Kuhn, C. M., Petro, A. E., Swick, A. G., Chrunyk, B. A., and Surwit, R. S., Role of leptin in fat regulation, *Nature*, 380, 677, 1996.

18. Enerback, S., Jacobsson, A., Simpson, E. M., Guerra, C., Yamashita, H., and Harper, M., Mice lacking mitochondrial uncoupling protein are cold-sensitive but not obese, *Nature*, 387, 90, 1997.

19. Yoshida, T., Sakane, N., Wakabayashi, Y., Umekawa, T., and Kondo, M., Anti-obesity and anti-diabetic effects of CL316,243, a highly specific β_3-adrenoceptor agonist, in yellow KK mice, *Life Sci.*, 54, 491, 1994.

20. Fleury, C., Neverova, M., Collins, S., Raimbault, S., Champigny, O., and Levi-Meyrueis, C., Uncoupling protein-2: a novel gene linked to obesity and hyperinsulinemia, *Nature Genet.*, 15, 269, 1997.

21. Surwit, R. S., Wang, S., Petro, A. E., Sanchis, D., Raimbault, S., and Ricquier, D., Diet-induced changes in uncoupling proteins in obesity-prone and obesity-resistant strains of mice, *Proc. Natl. Acad. Sci. USA*, 95, 4061, 1998.

22. Boss, O., Samec, S., Paoloni-Giacobino, A., Rossier, C., Dulloo, A., and Seydoux, J., Uncoupling protein-3: a new member of the mitochondrial carrier family with tissue-specific expression, *FEBS Lett.*, 408, 39, 1997.

23. Vidal-Puig, A., Solanes, G., Grujic, D., Flier, J. S., and Lowell, B. B., UCP3: an uncoupling protein homologue expressed preferentially and abundantly in skeletal muscle and brown adipose tissue, *Biochem. Biophys. Res. Comm.*, 235, 1, 79, 1997.

24. Fleury, C. and Sanchis, D., The mitochondrial uncoupling protein-2: current status, *Int. J. Biochem. Cell Biol.*, 31, 1261, 1999.

25. Boss, O., Muzzin, P., and Giacobino, J. P., The uncoupling proteins, a review, *Eur. J. Endocrinol.*, 139, 1, 1998.

26. Ricquier, D., Fleury, C., Larose, M., Sanchis, D., Pecqueur, C., and Raimbault, S., Contributions of studies on uncoupling proteins to research on metabolic diseases, *J. Intern. Med.*, 245, 637, 1999.

27. Solanes, G., Vidal-Puig, A., Grujic, D., Flier, J. S., and Lowell, B. B., The human uncoupling protein-3 gene-genomic structure, chromosomal localization, and genetic basis for short and long form transcripts, *J. Biol. Chem.*, 272, 25433, 1997.

28. Fain, J. and Garcia-Sainz, J., Adrenergic regulation of adipocyte metabolism, *J. Lipid Res.*, 24, 945, 1983.

29. Bahouth, S. W. and Malbon, C. C., Subclassification of β-adrenergic receptors of rat fat cells: a re-evaluation, *Mol. Pharmacol.*, 34, 318, 1988.

30. Arch, J. R. S., Ainsworth, A. T., Cawthorne, M. A., Piercy, V., Sennitt, M. V., and Thody, V. E., Atypical β-adrenoceptor on brown adipocytes as target for anti-obesity drugs, *Nature*, 309, 163, 1984.

31. Strosberg, A., Structure and function of the β₃-adrenergic receptor, *Ann. Rev. Pharmacol. Toxicol.*, 37, 421, 1997.

32. van Liefde, I., van Witzenberg, A., and Vauquelin, G., Multiple beta adrenergic receptor subclasses mediate the l-isoproteronol-induced lipolytic response in rat adipocytes, *J. Pharmacol. Exp. Ther.*, 262, 552, 1992.

33. Collins, S., Daniel, K. W., Rohlfs, E. M., Ramkumar, V., Taylor, I. L., and Gettys, T.W., Impaired expression and functional activity of the β₃- and β₁-adrenergic receptors in adipose tissue of congenitally obese (C57BL/6J ob/ob) mice, *Mol. Endocrinol.*, 8, 518, 1994.

34. Galitzky, J., Carpéné, C., Bousquet-Mélou, A., Berlan, M., and Lafontan, M., Differential activation of β₁-, β₂-, and β₃- adrenoceptors by catecholamines in white and brown adipocytes, *Fundam. Clin. Pharmacol.*, 9, 324, 1995.

35. Rohlfs, E. M., Daniel, K. W., Premont, R. T., Kozak, L. P., and Collins, S., Regulation of the uncoupling protein gene (Ucp) by β₁, β₂, β₃-adrenergic receptor subtypes in immortalized brown adipose cell lines, *J. Biol. Chem.*, 270, 10723, 1995.

36. Fève, B., Emorine, L. J., Lasnier, F., Blin, N., Baude, B., and Nahmias, C., Atypical β-adrenergic receptor in 3T3-F442A adipocytes. Pharmacological and molecular relationship with the human β₃-adrenergic receptor, *J. Biol. Chem.*, 266, 20329, 1991.

37. Dixon, T. M., Daniel, K. W., Farmer, S. R., and Collins, S., C/EBPα is required for transcription of the β₃AR gene during adipogenesis, *J. Biol. Chem.*, 276, 722, 2001.

38a. Wu, Z., Rosen, E. D., Brun, R., Hauser, S., Adelmant, G., and Troy, A. E., Cross-regulation of C/EBPα and PPARγ controls the transcriptional pathway of adipogenesis and insulin sensitivity, *Mol. Cell*, 3, 151, 1999.

38b. El-Jack, A. K., Hamm, J. K., Pilch, P. F., and Farmer, S.R., Reconstitution of insulin-sensitive glucose transport in fibroblasts requires expression of both PPARγ and C/EBPα, *J. Biol. Chem.*, 274, 7946, 1999.

39. Largis, E. E., Burns, M. G., Muenkel, H. A., Dolan, J. A., and Claus, T. H., Antidiabetic and antiobesity effects of a highly selective β3-adrenoceptor agonist (CL 316,243), *Drug Dev. Res.*, 32, 69, 1994.
40. Himms-Hagen, J., Cui, J., Danforth, Jr., E., Taatjes, D. J., Lang, S. S., and Waters, B.L., Effect of CL-316,243, a thermogenic β₃-agonist, on energy balance and brown and white adipose tissues in rats, *Am. J. Physiol.*, 266, R1371, 1994.
41. Collins, S., Daniel, K. W., Petro, A. E., and Surwit, R. S., Strain-specific response to β₃-adrenergic receptor agonist treatment of diet-induced obesity in mice, *Endocrinology*, 138, 405, 1997.
42. Sasaki, N., Uchida, E., Niiyama, M., Yoshida, T., and Saito, M., Anti-obesity effects of selective agonists to the β3-adrenergic receptor in dogs. II. Recruitment of thermogenic brown adipocytes and reduction of adiposity after chronic treatment with a β3-adrenergic agonist, *J. Vet. Med. Sci.*, 60, 465, 1998.
43. Krief, S., Lonnqvist, F., Raimbault, S., Baude, B., Van Spronsen, A., and Arner, P., Tissue distribution of β₃-adrenergic receptor mRNA in man, *J. Clin. Invest.*, 91, 344, 1993.
44. Weyer, C., Tataranni, P. A., Snitker, S., Danforth, Jr., E., and Ravussin, E., Increase in insulin action and fat oxidation after treatment with CL 316,243, a highly selective beta3-adrenoceptor agonist in humans, *Diabetes*, 47, 1555, 1998.
45. Candelore, M. R., Deng, L., Tota, L., Guan, X. M., Amend, A., and Liu, Y., Potent and selective human beta₃-adrenergic receptor antagonists, *J. Pharmacol. Exp. Ther.*, 290, 649, 1999.
46. Laudat, M. H. and Pairault, J., An impaired response of adenylate cyclase to stimulation by epinephrine in adipocyte plasma membranes from genetically obese mice (*ob/ob*), *Eur. J. Biochem.*, 56, 583, 1975.
47. Dehaye, J. P., Winand, J., and Christophe, J., Lipolysis and cyclic AMP levels in epididymal adipose tissue of obese hyperglycemic mice, *Diabetologia*, 13, 553, 1977.
48. Shepherd, R. E., Malbon, C. C., Smith, C. J., and Fain, J. N., Lipolysis and adenosine 3':5'-monophosphate metabolism in isolated white fat cells from genetically obese-hyperglycemic mice (*ob/ob*), *J. Biol. Chem.*, 252, 7243, 1977.
49. Trayhurn, P. and James, W. P. T., Thermoregulation and non-shivering thermogenesis in the genetically obese (*ob/ob*) mouse, *Pflugers Arch. Eur. J. Physiol.*, 373, 189, 1978.
50. Cox, J. E. and Powley, T. L., Development of obesity in diabetic mice pair-fed with lean siblings, *J. Comp. Physiol. Psychol.*, 91, 347, 1977.
51. Levin, B.E., Triscari, J., and Sullivan, A.C., Altered sympathetic activity during development of diet-induced obesity in rats, *Am. J. Physiol.*, 244, R347, 1983.
52. Levin, B. E., Triscari, J., and Sullivan, A. C., Relationship between sympathetic activity and diet-induced obesity in two rat strains, *Am. J. Physiol.*, 245, R364, 1983.
53. Takeuchi, H., Matsuo, T., Tokuyama, K., Shimomura, Y., and Suzuki, M., Diet-induced thermogenesis is lower in rats fed a lard diet than in those fed a high oleic acid safflower oil diet, a safflower oil diet or a linseed oil diet, *J. Nutr.*, 125, 920, 1994.
54. Bégin-Heick, N. and Heick, H. M. C., Increased response of adipose tissue of the *ob/ob* mouse to the action of adrenaline after treatment with thyroxin, *Can. J. Physiol. Pharmacol.*, 55, 1320, 1977.
55. Begin-Heick, N., Adenylate cyclase in lean and obese (*ob/ob*) mouse epididymal white adipocytes, *Can. J. Biochem. Cell Biol.*, 58, 1033, 1980.

56. Tate, K. M., Briend-Sutren, M.-M., Emorine, L. M., Delavier-Klutchko, C., Marullo, S., and Strosberg, A. D., Expression of three human β-adrenergic receptor subtypes in transfected Chinese hamster ovary cells, *Eur. J. Biochem.*, 196, 357, 1991.
57. Emorine, L. J., Marullo, S., Briend-Sutren, M. M., Patey, G., Tate, K., and Delavier-Klutchko, C., Molecular characterization of the human β$_3$-adrenergic receptor, *Science*, 245, 1118, 1989.
58. DeLean, A., Munson, P. J., and Rodbard, D., Simultaneous analysis of families of sigmoidal dose-response curves: application to bioassay, radioligand binding, and physiological dose-response curves, *Am. J. Physiol.*, 235, E97, 1978.
59. Muzzin, P., Revelli, J. P., Kuhne, F., Gocayne, J. D., McCombie, W. R., and Venter, J. C., An adipose tissue-specific β-adrenergic receptor. Molecular cloning and down-regulation in obesity, *J. Biol. Chem.*, 266, 24053, 1991.
60. Collins, S., Daniel, K. W., and Rohlfs, E. M., Depressed expression of adipocyte β-adrenergic receptors is a common feature of congenital and dietary obesity in rodents, *Int. J. Obesity*, 23, 669, 1999.
61. Saito, M. and Bray, G.A., Diurnal rhythm for corticosterone in obese (ob/ob) diabetes (*db/db*) and gold-thioglucose-induced obesity in mice, *Endocrinology*, 113, 2181, 1983.
62. Mobley, P. W., and Dubuc, P. U., Thyroid hormone levels in the developing obese-hyperglycemic syndrome, *Horm. Metab. Res.*, 11, 37, 1979.
63. van der Kroon, P. H. W., Wittgen-Struik, G., and Vermeulen, L., The role of hyperphagia and hypothyroidism in the development of the obese-hyperglycemic syndrome in mice (*ob/ob*), *Int. J. Obesity*, 5, 353, 1981.
64. van der Kroon, P. H. W., Boldewijn, H., and Langeveld-Soeter, N., Congenital hypothyroidism in latent obese (*ob/ob*) mice, *Int. J. Obesity*, 6, 83, 1982.
65. van der Kroon, P. H. W., Van Vroonhoven, T. M., and Douglas, L. T., Lowered oxygen consumption and heart rate as early symptoms of the obese-hyperglycemic syndrome in mice (*ob/ob*), *Int. J. Obesity*, 1, 325, 1977.
66. Solomon, J. and Mayer, J., The effect of adrenalectomy on the development of the obese-hyperglycemic syndrome in *ob/ob* mice, *Endocrinology*, 93, 510, 1973.
67. Yukimura, Y. and Bray, G. A., Effects of adrenalectomy on body weight and the size and number of fat cells in the Zucker rat, *Endocr. Res. Commun.*, 5, 189, 1978.
68. Freedman, M. R., Horwitz, B. A., and Stern, J. S., Effect of adrenalectomy and glucocorticoid replacement on development of obesity, *Am. J. Physiol.*, 250, R595, 1986.
69. Friedman, J. M. and Halaas, J. L., Leptin and the regulation of body weight in mammals, *Nature*, 395, 763, 1998.
70. Naggert, J. K., Fricker, L. D., Varlamov, O., Nishina, P. M., Rouille, Y., and Steiner, D. F., Hyperproinsulinaemia in obese fat/fat mice associated with a carboxypeptidase E mutation which reduces enzyme activity, *Nature Genet.*, 10, 135, 1995.
71. Noben-Trauth, K., Naggert, J. K., North, M. A., and Nishina, P. M., A candidate gene for the mouse mutation tubby, *Nature*, 380, 534, 1996.
72. Surwit, R. S., Kuhn, C. M., Cochrane, C., McCubbin, J. A., and Feinglos, M.N., Diet-induced type II diabetes in C57BL/6J mice, *Diabetes*, 37, 1163, 1988.
73. Champigny, O., Ricquier, D., Blondel, O., Mayers, R. M., Briscoe, M. G., and Holloway, B. R., β$_3$-Adrenergic receptor stimulation restores message and expression of brown-fat mitochondrial uncoupling protein in adult dogs, *Proc. Natl. Acad. Sci. USA*, 88, 10774, 1991.

74. Fisher, M. H., Amend, A. M., Bach, T. J., Barker, J. M., Brady, E. J., and Candelore, M. R., A selective human beta3 adrenergic receptor agonist increases metabolic rate in rhesus monkeys, *J. Clin. Invest.*, 101, 2387, 1998.

75. Guerra, C., Koza, R. A., Yamashita, H., Walsh, K., and Kozak, L. P., Emergence of brown adipocytes in white fat in mice is under genetic control: effects on body weight and adiposity, *J. Clin. Invest.*, 102, 412, 1998.

76. Liggett, S., Freedman, N. J., Schwinn, D. A., and Lefkowitz, R. J., Structural basis for receptor subtype-specific regulation revealed by a chimeric β_3-/β_2-adrenergic receptor, *Proc. Natl. Acad. Sci. USA*, 90, 3665, 1993.

77. Cao, W., Luttrell, L. M., Medvedev, A. V., Pierce, K. L., Lefkowitz, R. J., and Collins, S., Direct binding of activated c-Src to the β_3-adrenergic receptor is required for MAP kinase activation, *J. Biol. Chem.*, 275, 38131, 2000.

78. Lefkowitz, R. J., G protein-coupled receptors. III. New roles for receptor kinases and β-arrestins in receptor signaling and desensitization, *J. Biol. Chem.*, 273, 18677, 1998.

79. Shih, T. L., Candelore, M. R., Cascieri, M. A., Chiu, S. H., Colwell, Jr., L. F., and Deng, L., L-770,644: a potent and selective human beta3 adrenergic receptor agonist with improved oral bioavailability, *Bioorg. Med. Chem. Lett.*, 9, 1251, 1999.

80. Weyer, C., Gautier, J. F., and Danforth, Jr., E., Development of beta 3-adrenoceptor agonists for the treatment of obesity and diabetes — an update, *Diabetes Metab.*, 25, 11, 1999.

81. Cooper, D., Schlegel, W., Lin, M., and Rodbell, M., The fat cell adenylate cyclase system, *J. Biol. Chem.*, 254, 8927, 1979.

82. Murayama, T. and Ui, M., Loss of the inhibitory function of the guanine nucleotide regulatory component of adenylate cyclase due to its ADP ribosylation by islet-activating protein, pertussins toxin, in adipocyte membranes, *J. Biol. Chem.*, 258, 3319, 1983.

83. Bloom, J. D., Dutia, M. D., Johnson, B. D., Wissner, A., Burns, M. G., and Largis, E. E., Disodium (R, R)-5-[2[[2-(3-chlorophenyl)-2-hydroxyethyl]-amino]propyl]-1,3-benzodioxole-2,2-dicarboxylate(CL 316, 243). A potent β-adrenergic agonist virtually specific for β_3 receptors. A promising antidiabetic and anti-obesity agent, *J. Med. Chem.*, 35, 3081, 1992.

84. Begin-Heick, N., β_3-adrenergic activation of adenylyl cyclase in mouse white adipocytes: modulation by GTP and effect of obesity, *J. Cell. Biochem.*, 58, 464, 1995.

85. Chaudhry, A., MacKenzie, R. G., Georgic, L. M., and Granneman, J. G., Differential interaction of β_1- and β_3-adrenergic receptors with G_i in rat adipocytes, *Cell. Signaling*, 6, 457, 1994.

86. Soeder, K. S., Snedden, S. K., Cao, W., Della Rocca, G. J., Daniel, K. W., and Luttrell, L. M., The β_3-adrenergic receptor activates mitogen-activated protein kinase in adipocytes through a Gi-dependent mechanism, *J. Biol. Chem.*, 274, 12017, 1999.

87. Fields, T. A., Linder, M. E., and Casey, P. J., Subtype-specific binding of azidoanilido-GTP by purified G protein α subunits, *Biochemistry*, 33, 6877, 1994.

88. Collins, S., Cao, W., Soeder, K. J., and Snedden, S. K., β-Adrenergic receptor signaling in adipocytes, in *Adipocyte Biology and Hormone Signaling*, Ntambi, J. M., Ed., IOS Press, Washington, D.C., 2000, 51.

89. Hu, E., Kim, J. B., Sarraf, P., and Spiegelman, B. M., Inhibition of adipogenesis through MAP kinase-mediated phosphorylation of PPARγ, *Science,* 274, 2100, 1996.

90. Adams, M., Reginato, M., Shao, D., Lazar, M., and Chatterjee, V., Transcriptional activation by peroxisome proliferator-activated receptor γ is inhibited by phosphorylation at a consensus mitogen-activated protein kinase site, *J. Biol. Chem.,* 272, 5128, 1997.

91. Aubert, J., Champigny, O., Saint-Marc, P., Negrel, R., Collins, S., and Ricquier, D., Up-regulation of UCP-2 gene expression by PPAR agonists in preadipose and adipose cells, *Biochem. Biophys. Res. Commun.,* 238, 606, 1997.

92. Camirand, A., Marie, V., Rabelo, R., and Silva, J. E., Thiazolidinediones stimulate uncoupling protein-2 expression in cell lines representing white and brown adipose tissues and skeletal muscle, *Endocrinology,* 139, 428, 1998.

93. Viguerie-Bascands, N., Saulnier-Blache, J. S., Dandine, M., Dauzats, M., Daviaud, D., and Langin, D., Increase in uncoupling protein-2 mRNA expression by BRL49653 and bromopalmitate in human adipocytes, *Biochem. Biophys. Res. Commun.,* 256, 138, 1999.

94. Boss, O., Samec, S., Dulloo, A., Seydoux, J., Muzzin, P., and Giacobino, J., Tissue-dependent upregulation of rat uncoupling protein-2 expression in response to fasting or cold, *FEBS Lett.,* 142, 111, 1997.

95. Weigle, D., Selfridge, L., Schwartz, M., Seeley, R., Cummings, D., and Havel, P., Elevated free fatty acids induce uncoupling protein 3 expression in muscle, *Diabetes,* 47, 208, 1998.

96. Samec, S., Seydoux, J., and Dulloo, A. G., Role of UCP homologues in skeletal muscles and brown adipose tissue: mediators of thermogenesis or regulators of lipids as fuel substrate, *FASEB J.,* 12, 715, 1998.

97. Samec, S., Seydoux, J., and Dulloo, A. G., Skeletal muscle UCP3 and UCP2 gene expression in response to inhibition of free fatty acid flux through mitochondrial beta-oxidation, *Pflugers Arch.,* 438, 452, 1999.

98. Cadenas, S., Buckingham, J. A., Samec, S., Seydoux, J., Din, N., and Dulloo, A. G., UCP2 and UCP3 rise in starved rat skeletal muscle but mitochondrial proton conductance is unchanged, *FEBS Lett.,* 462, 257, 1999.

99. Ricquier, D. and Bouillaud, F., The uncoupling protein homologues: UCP1, UCP2, UCP3, StUCP and AtUCP, *Biochem. J.,* 345, 161, 2000.

100. Rial, E., Gonzalez-Barroso, M., Fleury, C., Iturrizaga, S., Sanchis, D., and Jimenez-Jimenez, J., Retinoids activate proton transport by the uncoupling proteins UCP1 and UCP2, *EMBO J.,* 18, 5827, 1999.

101. 100.Jaburek, M., Varecha, M., Gimeno, R. E., Dembski, M., Jezek, P., and Zhang, M., Transport function and regulation of mitochondrial uncoupling proteins 2 and 3, *J. Biol. Chem.,* 274, 26003, 1999.

102. Larrouy, D., Laharrague, P., Carrera, G., Viguerie-Bascands, N., Levi-Meyrueis, C., and Fleury, C., Kupffer cells are a dominant site of uncoupling protein 2 expression in rat liver, *Biochem. Biophys. Res. Commun.,* 235, 760, 1997.

103. Cortez-Pinto, H., Yang, S. Q., Lin, H. Z., Costa, S., Hwang, C. S., and Lane, M. D., Bacterial lipopolysaccharide induces uncoupling protein-2 expression in hepatocytes by a tumor necrosis factor-alpha-dependent mechanism, *Biochem. Biophys. Res. Commun.,* 251, 313, 1998.

104. Lee, F. Y., Li, Y., Zhu, H., Yang, S., Lin, H. Z., and Trush, M., Tumor necrosis factor increases mitochondrial oxidant production and induces expression of uncoupling protein-2 in the regenerating mice liver, *Hepatology,* 29, 677, 1999.

105. Negre-Salvayre, A., Hirtz, C., Carrera, G., Cazenave, R., Troly, M., and Salvayre, R., A role for uncoupling protein-2 as a regulator of mitochondrial hydrogen peroxide generation, *FASEB J.*, 11, 809, 1997.
106. Faggioni, R., Shigenaga, J., Moser, A., Feingold, K., and Grunfeld, C., Induction of UCP2 gene expression by LPS: a potential mechanism for increased thermogenesis during infection, *Biochem. Biophys. Res. Commun.*, 244, 75, 1998.
107. Busquets, S., Sanchis, D., Alvarez, B., Ricquier, D., Lopez-Soriano, F. J., and Argiles, J. M., In the rat, tumor necrosis factor alpha administration results in an increase in both UCP2 and UCP3 mRNAs in skeletal muscle: a possible mechanism for cytokine-induced thermogenesis, *FEBS Lett.*, 440, 348, 1998.
108. Arsenijevic, D., Onuma, H., Pecqueur, C., Raimbault, S., Manning, B. S., Miroux, B., Couplan, E., Alves-Guerra, M.-C., Surwit, R. S., Bouillaud, F., Richard, D., Collins, S., and Ricquier, D., Disruption of uncoupling protein-2 (UCP2) reveals a role in immunity and production of reactive oxygen species, *Nat. Genet.*, 26, 435, 2000.
109. Gong, D. W., Monemdjou, S., Gavrilova, O., Leon, L. R., Marcus-Samuels, B., Chou, C. J., Everett, C., Kozak, L. P., Li, C., Deng, C., Harper, M. E., and Reitman, M. L., Lack of obesity and normal response to fasting and thyroid hormone in mice lacking uncoupling protein-3, *J. Biol. Chem.*, 275, 16251, 2000.
110. Vidal-Puig, A. J., Grujic, D., Zhang, C. Y., Hagen, T., Boss, O., Ido, Y., Szczepanik, A., Wade, J., Mootha, V., Cortright, R., Muoio, D. M., and Lowell, B. B., Energy metabolism in uncoupling protein 3 gene knockout mice, *J. Biol. Chem.*, 275, 16258, 2000.
111. Green, D.R., and Reed, J. C., Mitochondria and apoptosis, *Science*, 281, 1309, 1998.
112. Voehringer, D. W., Hirschberg, D. L., Xiao, J., Lu, Q., Roederer, M., and Lock, C. B., Gene microarray identification of redox and mitochondrial elements that control resistance or sensitivity to apoptosis, *Proc. Natl. Acad. Sci. USA*, 97, 2680, 2000.
113. Richard, D., Rivest, R., Huang, Q., Bouillaud, F., Sanchis, D., and Champigny, O., Distribution of the uncoupling protein 2 mRNA in the mouse brain, *J. Comp. Neurol.*, 397, 549, 1998.

13

Vitamin A and Gene Expression

Peter McCaffery, Fausto Andreola, Valeria Giandomenico,
and Luigi M. De Luca

CONTENTS

13.1   Introduction 284
13.2   Aspects of Vitamin A Homeostasis...284
13.3   RBP 287
13.4   Gene Transcription Regulated by the Retinoic Acid Receptors
       and Their Interactions with the Orphan Nuclear Receptors..............288
       13.4.1   Retinoic Acid Receptors and Their Response Elements.........288
                13.4.1.1   Characteristics of the Retinoic Acid
                          Response Elements 288
                13.4.1.2   Receptor Binding to Response Elements..................289
                13.4.1.3   The Role of Nuclear Receptor Cofactors 292
       13.4.2   Orphan Receptors and Their Interactions
                with RA Signaling..293
                13.4.2.1   COUP-TFs 294
                13.4.2.2   ROR/RZR 296
                13.4.2.3   NUR77 and NURR1...297
                13.4.2.4   HNF-4 298
                13.4.2.5   PPAR 299
13.5   Discussion 300
References 302

Keywords: *retinoid receptors, orphan receptors, retinoid binding proteins,
retinoid metabolism, transcriptional regulation*

0-8493-2216-2/01/$0.00+$1.50
© 2001 by CRC Press LLC

13.1 Introduction

The fundamental observation (reviewed in Ref. 40) that vitamin A deficiency leads to a profound change in the differentiation of epithelial tissues has led investigators to suggest[204,231] and eventually prove[62,167] that the action of the vitamin is similar to that of steroid hormones, i.e., that retinoic acid activates gene expression through nuclear receptors in a variety of tissues. It should be noted that this concept has also included mesenchymal tissues and, in fact, the most well-known clinical application of retinoic acid is in differentiation therapy of acute promyelocytic leukemic cells to mature granulocytes.[33,41,224,225] Further, this differentiation concept has guided efforts to prevent epithelial carcinogenesis by dietary as well as topical application of retinoids[32,75,91,205] and continues to generate considerable enthusiasm as a viable approach to controlling malignant progression.[73,74,90,146]

These considerations explain the tremendous interest in this family of compounds from fields as diverse as dermatology, nutrition, epidemiology, carcinogenesis, toxicology and embryogenesis.[39]

In this review we will mainly concern ourselves with vitamin A homeostasis, plasma and cellular retinoid binding proteins, metabolism and, finally and mostly importantly, recent advances in gene activation processes which involve the RARs and the RXRs and their cognate receptors.

13.2 Aspects of Vitamin A Homeostasis

Vitamin A and its derivatives regulate fundamental physiological functions, including growth, reproduction, vision, and epithelial differentiation.[18,39,68,161,230]

Once absorbed from dietary sources, vitamin A, i.e., retinol, is carried in the blood stream bound to serum retinol-binding protein (holo-RBP complex), which eventually delivers it to the target cells.[64] In the cytoplasm of these cells, retinol is mainly bound to cellular retinol-binding proteins (CRBPs, types I and II) to form the retinol-CRBP (holo-CRBP) complex.[162] The subsequent fate of retinol is finely controlled by the vitamin A status of the animal; depending on reserves and peripheral demand, retinol can either be stored as retinyl esters or pushed into the oxidation pathway to eventually generate retinoic acid.[57,132,153,196] The esterification reaction is catalyzed by lecithin:retinol acyltransferase (LRAT)[132,185] and/or acyl-CoA:retinol acyltransferase (ARAT)[19] and yields highly hydrophobic retinyl esters, which are then stored as depot resources for eventual utilization, depending on homeostatic control. The first reaction in the utilization-oxidation pathway is catalyzed by the cytosolic alcohol dehydrogenases (ADHs) and/or the microsomal short-

(a) RAREhspLacZ   (b) COUP-TFII   (c) RAREhspLacZ
                                          + COUP-TFII

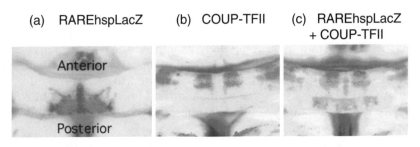

FIGURE 13.1
Comparison of RAREhsplacZ and COUP-TF-II distribution in postnatal day 0.3 mouse cerebellum.

chain dehydrogenase/reducatase (SDR)[17,50] and results in the formation of retinal, which in turn is further irreversibly oxidized to retinoic acid (RA) by members of the aldehyde dehydrogenase (AHD) family.[135] Retinoic acid, the physiologically active retinoid that interacts with two families of nuclear receptors (RARs and RXRs), can also be oxidized to more polar metabolites, 4-hydroxy and 4-oxo-RA by cytochrome P450s.[227]

A complex homeostatic mechanism controls the fate of intracellular retinol. Under vitamin A deficiency conditions, retinol is pushed to the oxidation pathway in order to overcome the reduction of RA levels associated with this condition. Conversely, any accumulation of RA prevents retinol from being oxidized and causes its sequestration into the esterification pathway. LRAT has been shown to play an important role in this autoregulative system described in human keratinocytes; in fact, in these cells, RA treatment induces LRAT activity and causes a 50% reduction in the conversion of retinol to RA.

Recently, particular attention has been focused on the role played by CRBP in vitamin A homeostasis. Even though this cellular protein had been shown to be involved in the esterification of retinol with long-chain fatty acids by LRAT, in the hydrolysis of retinyl esters to retinol, and finally in the oxidation of retinol to retinal, its actual physiological function *in vivo* remained unclear. Two independent groups have used different molecular approaches in an attempt to elucidate the function of CRBP, i.e., the generation of transgenic mice either expressing high levels of hCRBP-I or a disrupted form of the mouse CRBP-I gene.

Troen et al.[215] tested whether high expression of hCRBPI could induce a phenotype resembling vitamin A toxicity as a result of increased production of RA, or alternatively a phenotype of vitamin A deficiency at the target tissue level, as a result of an increased sequestration of vitamin A in storage cells because of large amounts of CRBP in them. Neither phenotype occurs in tissues overexpressing hCRBP-I, thus demonstrating that excess CRBP-I does not interfere with normal retinol metabolism and function.

In contrast, a biochemical phenotype is obtained when the mCRBP-I gene is knocked out.[61] The mutant mice are clearly borderline for vitamin A content. Even though healthy and fertile, they showed reduced liver retinyl palmitate levels, due to a decreased capacity to esterify incoming retinol and faster turnover of the retinoid pool. When kept on a vitamin A-deficient diet, the CRBP-I-null mice completely exhausted their liver retinyl esters store and developed abnormalities typical of a postnatal hypovitaminosis A syndrome within a very short time compared to wild type mice. So, clearly, CRBP-I is necessary for maintenance of normal homeostatic functions for this important vitamin and its absence precipitates the vitamin A-deficiency syndrome.

Other intracellular proteins fundamental in the retinoid signaling pathways are the cellular RA-binding proteins I and II (CRABP-I and CRABP-II).[56,152,163] These two isoforms show differential expression patterns in cells and tissues, thus suggesting that they may play distinct functions. CRABP-I is ubiquitously expressed in adult tissues, whereas CRABP-II localizes mainly in skin and female reproductive apparatus (uterus and ovaries).

CRABP-I, the better characterized isoform, has been proposed to modulate cellular response to retinoids; in fact, it may control the homeostasis of free intracellular RA available to the nuclear receptors by facilitating its catabolism and/or sequestering it.

On the other hand, little is known about the biological function(s) of CRABP-II. Even though different investigators have credited this protein with a nuclear function, no clear evidence for this role has been given until recently. Two interesting papers have been published, both indicating a nuclear function for CRABP-II. Delva et al.[42] have shown that CRABP-II is present both in the cytoplasm and the nucleus and that it interacts *in vivo* and *in vitro* with RARs (RARα and RXRα) and participates with the DR5-bound nuclear receptor complex to transactivate RA target genes. Further, its positive transcriptional control is RAR/RXR heterodimer-dependent as it cannot bind by itself to the RARE. CRABP-II is, therefore, a unique coactivator, in the sense that it binds the ligand although it has no structural homology with other currently known co-regulators.

In order to clarify a functional difference between CRABP-I and II in regulating the transcriptional activities of RA, Dong et al.[47]over-expressed both isoforms in COS-7 cells and showed that CRABP-II, but not CRABP-I, can markedly enhance RAR-mediated transcriptional activation of a reporter gene. As the two isoforms have almost the same affinity for the ligand (there is only a 2-fold difference in the Kd values for complex formation between RA and CRABP-I and II), a differential mechanism of delivery of RA to RAR could be the alternative explanation for the observed functional differences between the CRABPs. In this regard CRABP-I (donor) was shown to transfer RA (ligand) to RAR (acceptor) through a mechanism which requires prior dissociation of the ligand/donor (RA/CRABP-I) complex, followed by formation of the ligand/acceptor (RA/RAR) complex. In contrast, when CRABP-II was the donor, RA was shown to be transferred from the donor to the acceptor by a process which requires direct interactions of the two proteins. Therefore, the authors concluded that CRABP-II enhances the transcriptional activity of RAR by directly interacting with the receptor, thus facilitating the formation of active RAR-RA complexes. In contrast to the work of Delva et al.,[42] Dong and collaborators[48] could neither detect nor isolate a stable CRABP-II–RAR complex using several approaches. This failure to isolate the complex led them to hypothesize that the CRABP-II–RAR interactions are unstable and that the actual complex is a short-lived intermediate.

13.3 RBP

Thus far, the only function attributed to RBP is to transport retinol in the circulation from the vitamin A stores in the liver to peripheral tissues.[64,202] Retinol–RBP complexes are secreted by the liver into the blood stream where they circulate in a 1:1 molar complex with another protein, transthyretin (TTR). The formation of the RBP–TTR complex in the plasma is required for preventing glomerular filtration and renal catabolism of RBP.[64] Based on its very early expression during embryogenesis[206] and its highly regulated levels in the serum, RBP is also thought to be fundamental in maintaining the retinoid signaling pathways in the body.

For a better understanding of the physiological function of RBP, RBP$^{-/-}$ mice were generated.[174] Unexpectedly, these mice were found to be viable and fertile; nevertheless, they showed reduced retinol plasma levels and, during the first months of life, a markedly impaired retinal function not caused by any developmental retinal defect. When fed a vitamin A sufficient diet, RBP$^{-/-}$ mice acquired normal vision by 5 months, thus showing that RBP-independent pathway(s) for acquiring eye retinol must exist. The authors also postulate that the main responsible factor for the impaired retinal function is the absence of circulating retinol–RBP complexes in the plasma, rather than the low retinol levels; nevertheless, if this is the case, why do the RBP$^{-/-}$ mice show insufficient retinol levels in the eyes but appear normal in other tissue? A possible explanation could be the expression of a receptor for RBP in the retinal pigmental epithelium (RPE), which has been long suggested and might indeed play an important role in retinol delivery to the retina, but not to other tissues.[13] However, if this were the case it still remains unclear why dietary retinol re-establishes retinal function in the knockout animals.

The data from these studies, however, clearly demonstrate an RBP-independent mechanism for the accumulation of eye retinol. Finally, it is also noteworthy that by 5 months of age the liver retinol levels found in the RBP$^{-/-}$ mice are higher than those in the control counterparts; however, the hepatic retinoid stores in the knockout animals cannot be mobilized, as their liver retinol levels do not fall after a short exposure to a vitamin A-deficient diet. Taken together, these data clearly suggest that the major physiological role for RBP is to insure, under inadequate vitamin A intake, availability of retinol to maintain normal cellular functions.

13.4 Gene Transcription Regulated by the Retinoic Acid Receptors and Their Interactions with the Orphan Nuclear Receptors

Retinoic acid (RA) is the transcriptionally active derivative of vitamin A (retinol) and is required for both embryonic development and adult function.[49,121,143] Its transcriptional activity is mediated through specific receptors of the nuclear receptor superfamily. Like other ligands of this family, RA is lipophilic and can diffuse a significant distance from its site of synthesis. In the embryo, the creation of spatial gradients of transcriptional activation may be important for the function of RA in regulating pattern formation.[49,124] Unlike other ligands of the nuclear receptor family, however, RA is not a paracrine hormone acting at a distance from its site of synthesis but is synthesized in the local area of its action and hence is analogous to a growth factor.[136] As a result, local control of synthesis and catabolism of this receptor ligand provides an important level of regulation of RA-mediated transcription.[121]

A second tier of control occurs at the level of the receptor itself. Since the discovery of the RA receptors as nuclear receptor family members it has become increasingly evident that the RA receptors heterodimerize with many partners of the same superfamily. These interactions influence the level of transcriptional activation of the RA receptors, or convert the heterodimeric complex to a transcriptional repressor. Competition between nuclear receptors for shared response elements adds an additional level of interaction. The activity of RA can thus be regulated by the complement of nuclear receptors present when RA enters the nucleus and binds to its receptor. A subtle change in the ratios of the nuclear receptor may alter the transcriptional outcome.

This segment of the review will describe the nuclear receptors that interact with the RA signaling pathway, with an emphasis on the orphan receptors and their role in embryonic development.

13.4.1   Retinoic Acid Receptors and Their Response Elements

13.4.1.1   Characteristics of the Retinoic Acid Response Elements

The response elements present in the promoter or enhancers of RA-responsive genes have been extensively investigated. Two classes of RA receptors exist: the RARs (α, β, γ), activated by the all-*trans* or 9-*cis* isomers of RA, and the RXRs (α, β, γ) activated only by 9-*cis* RA.[126] These receptors bind to DNA as dimers which is reflected in the paired nature of the DNA response elements, termed RARE and RXRE, respectively, for RAR and RXR. The nucleotide sequence archetype upon which the RARE and RXREs are based has been described in accordance with a direct repeat (DR) 1 to 5 rule. This pattern was first suggested by Umesono et al.[218] The response elements were based on a direct repeat of the sequence AGGTCA, separated by between 3 and 5 nucleotides. The original 3-4-5 rule was extended to include a separation of 1 or 2 nucleotides according to the following framework: RAREs were DR2 and DR5, the RXREs DR1, and the response elements for vitamin D and thyroid hormone DR3 and DR4, respectively. This guideline worked well to describe several of the strongest RA-response elements, including the DR5 type that is the most prevalent of the simple direct repeats.

The DR1-5 rule is only a framework, however, and a series of additional factors also influences the effectiveness of each response element. The three critical factors are the nature of the spacing sequences, the type of 5′ flanking sequence, and the actual sequence of the repeated motif (based on PuG(G/T)TCA rather than simply AGGTCA). The repeated motif can also vary in its orientation and can be palindromic or a mixture of direct repeat and palindromic.[127] Hence the DR1-5 rule, although a useful foundation for the description of response elements, is not necessarily predictive for what will be a response element for the RA receptor dimers. Numerous modifications on this theme create a multitude of response elements that may react variably to a particular RA receptor dimer. A list of genes containing the DR1, 2, 5 or complex response elements is given in Table 13.1.

13.4.1.2 Receptor Binding to Response Elements

The differences between the two classes of RA receptors (RAR and RXR) go beyond their ligand specificities; the two receptor classes can perform quite separate functions. The RARs are ligand-regulated receptors that function similarly to the vitamin D and thyroid hormone receptors; once ligand bound they become transcriptional activators. The RXRs can also act in a ligand-activated manner; however, the RXRs perform a second essential function as accessory factors for many members of the nuclear receptor family. RXRs can heterodimerize to other nuclear receptors and, without requiring a 9-*cis* RA ligand, increase the affinity of these receptors for their respective response elements. Although the number of permutations of receptors appears limitless, there are some principles which, although not always rigidly adhered to, allow some grasp of what combinations are likely to regulate transcription.

1. The RAR/RXR heterodimers bind much more efficiently to any of the DR motifs than do the RAR/RAR homodimers.[97,112] Work with the combinational null mutants of RAR and RXR suggests that the RAR/RXR heterodimers are, indeed, an important functional unit activating RA-mediated transcription *in vivo*.[87,184]

2. The RXR/RXR homodimer is an effective unit for the activation of the DR-1 type response element.[97,128] In this case, although the RAR/RXR heterodimer binds with greater affinity to the DR1 element, it is incapable of activating transcription.[112] This RAR/RXR heterodimer will block RXR-dependent transcription at DR1 by virtue of the RAR half of the heterodimer sitting at the upstream

TABLE 13.1

RAREs

Gene	Ref.
DR1	
CRBP-II	128
CRABP-II[a]	55
Phosphoenolpyruvate carboxykinase	44, 195
PTH/PTH-related peptide receptor[b]	86
Apolipoprotein A-11	221
Lactoferrin	108
DR2	
CRABP-II[a]	55
CRBP-I	77
Hoxb1+	130
Alpha-fetoprotein	118
DR5	
RAR alpha 2	113
RAR beta 2	209
RAR gamma 2	111
Alcohol dehydrogenase 3	51
Hoxa-1 (3′)	105
Hepatocyte Nuclear Factor-3 alpha	79
Tissue-type plasminogen activator	22
MGP[b]	23
Hoxb4	66
Hoxd4	142
17 Beta-hydroxysteroid dehydrogenase type 1	168
ADP-ribosyl cyclase (CD38)	94
Sonic hedgehog	30
Beta 1-adrenergic receptor	7
Complex, Palindromic, or Unusual Direct Repeat	
Medium-chain acyl-coenzyme A dehydrogenase	176
Oxytocin	178
Laminin B1	220
Growth hormone	228
Uncoupling protein	175
H2Kb	80
Zif268	211
Oct3/4 (repression)	170
Stat1	101
Cholesteryl ester transfer	81
Transglutaminase type II	148
Glutathione S-transferase-pi	121
Dopamine D2 receptor	188
Gonadotropin-releasing hormone	36

TABLE 13.1 (CONTINUED)

RAREs

Gene	Ref.
Alpha 1 collagen	138
Apolipoprotein C-III	106
Complement factor H	147

ᵃ The CRABP-II promoter contains both DR1 and DR2 elements
ᵇ Parathyroid hormone/parathyroid hormone-related protein receptor
ᶜ Matrix Gla protein

end of the direct repeat and allosterically blocking the binding of the 9-*cis* RA ligand to RXR.[103]

3. The RXR receptors can heterodimerize with a variety of other nuclear receptor partners.[96, 97] This places the RXR in a key regulatory role since this class of receptor is the only type that will heterodimerize with the vitamin D receptor, thyroid hormone receptor, and RARs, creating heterodimers of high affinity for DR3, DR4, and DR5 (or DR2), respectively.

   a. On binding of the RXR-containing heterodimer to DR3, DR4, or DR5 elements, RXR is then situated at the upstream end of the repeated sequence and its partner at the downstream end.[104,243]

   b. In the case of RXR heterodimers of the vitamin D and thyroid hormone receptors and, for the most part, RAR, the RXR becomes a "silent" partner and does not require the 9-*cis* RA ligand. The very formation of the heterodimer prevents RXR from binding to 9-*cis* RA.[59,103]

   c. Exceptions exist to the above rule when RXR heterodimerizes with partners outside the vitamin D receptor, thyroid hormone receptor, and RAR groups. The PPAR[98] and farnesoid X receptors (FXR) heterodimers[58] with RXR are responsive to RXR ligands. RXR heterodimers with orphan receptors such as the liver X receptor (LXR)[229] or Nur77 (NGFI-B)[166] are also 9-*cis* RA responsive.

   d. Although 9-*cis* RA does not activate the unliganded RAR/RXR heterodimer, if RAR is bound to its all-*trans* RA ligand then 9-*cis* RA can bind to RXR and potentiate transcription. The likely explanation for this phenomenon is that allosteric inhibition that normally prevents 9-*cis* RA from binding to RXR is released when all-*trans* RA binds to RAR.[226] In some[114] but not all[212] circumstances this is also true for heterodimers of RXR and vitamin D receptors acting on the DR3 element. Likewise the heterodimerization of the thyroid hormone receptor and RXR has been reported to be augmented by 9-*cis* RA.[85] It is of note in regard to these receptor-activating roles of 9-*cis* RA that a splicing varient of RXR exists that can only perform the ligand-independent functions of RXR.[60]

It is evident from its heterodimerization properties that RXR is a pivotal element in the action of many nuclear receptors. Although, as described above, 9-*cis* RA is not always required for heterodimer activation, this RXR ligand may be necessary for all RXR signaling. 9-*cis* RA can initiate RXR-mediated signaling by inducing the release of RXR receptors from the tertrameric complexes which exist in solution.[92] Monomeric RXR is then available to heterodimerize, for instance, with the vitamin D receptor.[46] The importance of 9-*cis* RA in activating RXR heterodimers has clearly been demonstrated in the embryo. In *xenopus* the RXRs are known to be essential for the developmental functions of thyroid hormone receptors.[173] In the chick embryo, liganded RXR can mediate retinoid signal transduction.[122]

The differing roles of RAR and RXR mean that the availability and ratios of their ligands (9-*cis* and all-*trans* RA) as well as the receptors themselves will control which response element is active or repressed.[127] For instance, under circumstances of high 9-*cis* RA the RXR-RXR homodimer will be stabilized and will activate DR1 elements. High all-*trans* RA or high RAR will promote RAR-RXR heterodimerization and the activation of DR2 or DR5 elements. Low ligand concentrations can result in active repression because unliganded RAR can repress promoter activity.[10]

13.4.1.3   *The Role of Nuclear Receptor Cofactors*

The intermediaries between the RA receptor heterodimers and the basal transcriptional machinery are a set of co-activators and co-repressors.[31] Co-activators include the closely related CREB-binding protein (CBP) and P300[63] that possesses histone acetyltransferase activity resulting in acetylation of the histones, destabilizing the nucleosomes and allowing access of the transcriptional machinery to the DNA. The co-repressors include SMRT (silencing mediator for RARs and TRs) and N-CoR (nuclear receptor co-repressor) which act by promoting chromatin deacetylation and nucelosome reassembly. SMRT or N-CoR binds to the unliganded nuclear receptor heterodimer and hence, when the RARs are not bound to ligand, they repress transcription. When the ligand is bound to the receptors, the co-repressors are released, allowing transcription. An example of these co-repressors in action is evident in the RA receptor fusion proteins which result from the t(15;17) chromosomal translocation of acute promeylocytic leukemia.[67,116] These proteins consist of a fusion of RARα and promyelocytic leukemia (PML) protein or RARα and promyelocytic leukemia zinc-finger (PLZF) protein. Proliferation of leukemic cells with the PML-RAR alpha protein can be inhibited by RA, whereas cells with the PLZF-RAR alpha protein are resistant to RA. The crucial difference between these proteins is the ability of RA to release histone deacetylase activity from these fusion proteins while it is only the PML-RARα protein from which RA can induce histone deacetylase release.

13.4.2 Orphan Receptors and Their Interactions with RA Signaling

The orphan nuclear receptors are a default classification of nuclear receptors, characterized only by their lack of an identifiable high affinity ligand. Several of these receptors, with relatively restricted domains of expression, have a modulatory influence on the RA receptors. The RARα, RXRα, and RXRβ receptors have a very broad range of distribution in the embryo and this extensive range, together with a level complementary function, probably accounts for the relative minor phenotype apparent in the single receptor null mutant mice.[88] For instance, null mutations of the RXRs have shown that there is functional redundancy among the three RXRs (α, β, and γ) and that RXRα, during development, can perform most of the functions of the RXRs.[181] Because of this rather diffuse nature of the RA receptors, interactions with localized nuclear receptors are likely to be a critical factor in determining the specificity of RA transcriptional regulation. We describe below 5 groups of orphan receptors: COUP-TF-I/II; Nur77/Nurr1; ROR/RZR; PPAR α, β, and γ and HNF-4α, β, and γ, which may refine the action of nuclear receptors, including the RARs and RXRs, in the embryo and adult.

The COUP-TFs are the best characterized of the orphan receptors which modulate nuclear receptor signaling and can inhibit RA-mediated transcription. They can modulate the action of other nuclear receptors either by competing with their hormone response elements, by heterodimerizing and sequestering the receptors, or by directly inhibiting transcription. For the remaining orphan nuclear receptors, cross-talk via heterodimerization with RXR is known for the PPARs[89] and Nur77/Nurr1.[166] The PPAR/RXR heterodimer contrasts with the RAR/RXR heterodimer in that the former responds to the ligand of both partners, whereas RAR/RXR is non-reponsive to 9-*cis* RA. The difference in responsiveness of the heterodimers to RXR ligand has suggested that this may act as a 9-*cis* RA switch in cells that express PPAR. The ratio of RAR to PPAR, and hence the proportion of RAR/RXR to PPAR/RXR heterodimers, would determine whether the RXR signaling pathway is active.[45] The HNF-4 receptors, in contrast to the other orphan receptors described above, only form homodimers and do not bind to RXR.[82] However, HNF-4 can compete with other nuclear receptors for the DR1 element[156] and HNF-4 can also activate RAREs, as in the case of the complex RARE in the medium chain acyl-CoA dehydrogenase gene.[25] The RORs can function as monomers, binding to one half of the direct repeat and ROR-alpha signaling can be blocked by competitive binding of RAR/RXR heterodimers.[213]

All five classes of receptors can play an essential role in the developing embryo. The first three, COUP-TF-I/II, Nur77/Nurr1, ROR/RZR, are involved in CNS development while PPAR and HNF-4 are, respectively, vital for adipocyte and hepatocyte development. The primary response elements of COUP-TF, PPAR, and HNF-4 are based on the DR1 element, but a certain amount of specificity is resolved by the sequence of the direct repeat element itself, in addition to the identity of the spacer nucleotide.[151] Another element providing specificity to the PPARs is the 5′-extension of the direct repeat, which is patterned on a consensus of A(A/T)CT,[83] creating the PPREs. A 5′-extension also lends specificity to the DR1 modification that constitutes the RORE. It is the carboxy-terminal end of the ROR[133] and PPAR[76] that likely interacts with the 5′-extensions of their respective response elements.

13.4.2.1   COUP-TFs

The unique feature of the chick ovalbumin upstream promotor-transcription factors I and II (COUP-TF-I/Ear-3, COUP-TF-II/Arp-1) amongst the nuclear receptors is that these receptors are generally dominant repressors of both basal transcription and transactivation.[216] They will inhibit several nuclear receptors including the RAR, RXR, vitamin D, and thyroid hormone receptors. This inhibitory action is not absolute and the COUP-TFs can also activate gene transcription. COUP-TF-I and II may act as homodimers or heterodimerize with each other or other nuclear receptors such as ear-2 (COUP-TF-III),[4] a more distant member of the COUP family. The COUP-TFs bind with greatest affinity to the DR1 type response element[84] and can be grouped with the PPAR and HNF-4 nuclear receptors which bind to variations of this element. The COUP-TFs, however, can also bind to direct repeat or palindromes with spacers greater than 1 and this provides one mode of transcriptional repression for the COUP-TFs: direct competition with the DR3, 4, and 5 response elements of vitamin D, thyroid hormone, or RA receptors. COUP-TF-I has also been shown to bind to the estrogen response element.[100]

The inhibitory actions of the COUP-TFs have been extensively described. RXR-mediated activation has been shown to be completely repressed by COUP-TF-I[96] and this negative regulator can also block the induction of PCC7 differentiation by RA.[155] COUP-TF-II can also strongly inhibit transcriptional activation by PPAR/RXR[129] and HNF-4.[156] Four routes have been described by which the COUP-TFs interfere with nuclear receptor induced transcription.

1. Direct competition of the COUP-TF receptor and nuclear receptors for the HRE. This occurs, for instance, in the regulation of Oct 3 and 4 by COUP-TF-1 and II, where the COUP-TFs are able to displace RAR:RXR heterodimer binding to the Oct 3 and 4 RAREs.[16] COUP-TFs can also bind to the direct repeats DR3, DR4, and DR5, the HREs for the vitamin D receptor, thyroid hormone receptor and RAR, respectively, and hence the inhibitory action of the COUP-TFs is quite comprehensive for the nuclear receptors.

2. Sequestering of RXR by COUP-TFs. The COUP-TFs are able to effectively heterodimerize with RXR when bound to DNA (although not when free in solution),[37] preventing RXR from forming stimulatory heterodimers with other nuclear receptors.

3. Active repression. Active gene repression by COUP-TF-I is mediated by the transcriptional co-repressors N-CoR and SMRT.[197]

4. Transrepression. A second region of the COUP-TFs has transrepressor activity, acting independently of DNA binding. This route has been suggested as the main inhibitory mechanism employed by COUP-TF-II.[1]

Other genes transcriptionally repressed by the COUP-TFs include those for the Purkinje cell-protein-2 in the cerebellum,[2] CYP17,[9] alpha-fetoprotein,[119] and aromatase.[244] COUP-TF-I and II can repress transcriptional activation by the estrogen receptor,[99,154] while COUP-TF-I can repress the activation of angiotensinogen by HNF-4.[240]

Although transcriptional repression is a well-characterized role for the COUPs, their action is by no means restricted to this. Transactivation has been reported for the COUP-TFs, including activation of the genes for arrestin[123] and vHNF-1,[172] phosphoenolpyruvate carboxykinase,[210] NGFI-A,[171] and cholesterol 7alpha-hydroxylase.[208] COUP-TF-I has been described to generally promote RARE activation by RA in lung cancer cells, an effect that is counteracted by nur77.[233] Curiously, COUP-TF-I may also promote RA induced by RAR beta expression in cancer cells via a DR8 element.[115]

The action of the COUP-TFs as transcriptional modulators renders them essential for development. The overexpression of the COUP-TFs (in xenopus),[219] as well as the null mutations in mouse, results in drastic effects on embryonic development. The overexpression of COUP-TF-I in xenopus leads to general malformations in the brain and loss of the eyes.[193] COUP-TF-II is required for angiogenesis and heart development.[165] While both COUP-TF-I and II are present in the CNS, COUP-TF-I exhibits the highest levels of expression. In the developing brain, null mutations of COUP-TF-I lead to loss of neurons that normally form the subplate layer of the cortex. Loss of this layer may explain the failure of neurons in the thalamus to innervate their correct target in the cortex of this mutant. Loss of these projections, in turn, leads to cell death of the neurons of cortical layer IV in their target.[246] Abnormalities also occur in the development of the ganglia of the IXth cranial nerve (glossopharyngeal), as well as aberrations in the development of axonal connections between ganglion IX and the hindbrain. COUP-TF-I regulates a number of neurotransmitters including the glutamate receptor subunit KA2[35] as well as the N-methyl-d-aspartate (NMDA) receptor channel subunit NR2C.[169] In the developing embryo, a feedback pathway exists between RA and the COUP-TFs, and RA regulates the expression of both COUP-TF-I and II.[21] The embryonic signaling factor sonic hedgehog has been reported to activate COUP-TF-II gene transcription.[102] The COUP gene promoter contains a sonic hedgehog response element, independent of the Gl_i transcription factor generally associated with sonic hedgehog signaling.

An example of embryonic patterning generated by COUP-TF-II's interaction with RA may be evident in the cerebellum. The cerebellum is a region of the hindbrain in which several genes reveal a segmented pattern in the form of parasagittal stripes running along the anterior to posterior length (or partial length) of the cerebellum.[69,71,158] The developing cerebellum is believed to be a region of the CNS where RA signaling occurs[236,237,239] and we have shown (unpublished observation) that a RAREhsplacZ reporter transgene in a transgenic mouse line delineates a subset of these stripes. This mouse line was originally generated by Dr. J. Rossant[182] and the transgene construct consists of three copies of the DR5 RARE from RAR beta upstream of the promoter from the mouse heat-inducible hsp68 gene. The result of this transgene is that mice respond to endogenous retinoic acid by synthesizing the lacZ reporter gene and they can be used to identify regions of endogenous retinoic acid synthesis and retinoic acid signal transduction.

The stripes of transgene expression are predominantly in a midline structure of the cerebellum known as the vermis and are localized to the posterior half (Fig. 13.1). A number of genes are expressed in the developing cerebellum in a similar or complementary pattern in the cerebellar Purkinje cells and these are believed to set up the postnatal cerebellar parasagittal domains which form part of the intrinsic organization of the adult cerebellum.[5,141] The RAREhsplacZ reporter transgene is also localized to stripes in the Purkinje cells suggesting that RA signaling may play a role in the set up of these stripes. It was noted in this study of RAREhsplacZ distribution that the midline stripe at postnatal day 0.5 extended to a greater extent into the anterior cerebellum than did the lacZ positive regions on either side of the stripe, which appear to be skewed into horizontal curves with upturned edges (Fig. 13.1a). This pattern was very reminiscent, but reciprocal, of that of COUP-TF-II in the same region (Fig. 13.1b).[238] The most anterior regions of RAREhsplacZ expression lie immediately posterior to the two large COUP-TF-II patches that are situated on either side of the midline and the RAREhsplacZ response curves around the posterior edge of COUP-TF-II. This close juxtaposition is evident when the cerebellum was double labeled for both RAREhsplacZ and COUP-TF-II (Fig. 13.1c). In more posterior cerebellar regions there are also hints of alternating stripes of RAREhsplacZ and COUP-TF-II, although the more diffuse RAREhsplacZ stripes make this more difficult to discern. Since COUP-TF-II is a potent repressor of RA-mediated transcriptional activation, and is expressed in the same cell type as the RAREhsplacZ response, this suggests that COUP-TF-II may play a role in patterning RAREhsplacZ expression by inhibiting the lacZ response in those domains in which it is expressed.

13.4.2.2 ROR/RZR

The ROR/RZRs are a group of related orphan receptors that bind as monomers and hence do not require a direct or palindromic repeat as their response element but bind to a single hexameric motif. The two or four 5' nucleotides flanking the hexameric half-sites are crucial for specificity.[24] This type of response element is present in the promoter of a number of genes including cellular retinol binding protein, RAR beta, 5-lipoxygenase, bone sialoprotein, and Purkinje cell protein-2.[192] Four splicing varients of RORs alpha exist: alpha1, alpha2, alpha 3, and RZRalpha. Although ROR alpha is widely expressed, in the developing brain its strongest expression is in the cerebellar Purkinje cells from embryonic day 15 onward.[149] A mutation in ROR alpha creates the staggerer mutant mouse (sg/sg) in which Purkinje cells fail to develop correctly, resulting in tremor and body imbalance. The animals are also small in size and generally die within 3 to 4 weeks. Although ROR alpha is distributed evenly throughout the cerebellar Purkinje cells, the cells are disrupted in the staggerer mouse in a parasagittal fashion, as indicated by the distribution of calbindin.[150] Pcp-2, one of the genes downstream of ROR alpha,[131] is also distributed parasagittally and is approximately complementary to RAREhsplacZ in the Purkinje cells. ROR alpha functionally interacts with the RA receptors to regulate PCP-2[131] suggesting that RA may play some role in determining ROR alpha's parasagittal signaling.

Of the other two members of this orphan receptor group, RZR/ROR gamma is highly expressed in skeletal muscle[72] while RZR/ROR beta is specific to the brain. RZR/ROR beta is present in a number of regions generally known to be involved in receiving and processing sensory input, such as the dorsal horn of the spinal cord, layers IV and V of the sensory cortex, and the thalamus.[190] RZR/ROR beta is also expressed in several regions involved in the regulation of circadian rhythms, including the retina, suprachiasmatic nuclei, and the pineal gland. It had been suggested that melatonin was a ligand for RZR/ROR beta;[15] however, this now seems to be in doubt.[14] Nevertheless, the light/dark cyclic changes in RZR/ROR beta in the pineal gland and the retina suggest that this gene plays some role in circadian timing.[3] That RZR/ROR beta has an essential role in development is demonstrated by the phentoype of the null mutants which exhibit ataxia, retinal degeneration, and male infertility.[3]

13.4.2.3 NUR77 and NURR1

Nur77 and Nurr1 are two related orphan nuclear receptors. Both receptors bind as monomers to a non-repeating response element, but can also heterodimerize with RXR to activate gene transcription via a DR5 element. This heterodimerization creates an overlap with the RA signaling pathway and is promoted by the 9-*cis* RA RXR ligand.[166] Nur77 has also been reported to enhance ligand-independent transactivation of RAREs and reduce their responsiveness to RA.[233] Nur77 and Nurr1 themselves can heterodimerize and these dimers enhance transcription.[125] A third member of this group also exists and is termed neuron-derived orphan receptor (NOR-1).[160]

Nur77 (NGFI-B) was the first of this group to be identified, recognized as a gene induced by NGF following the neural differentiation of the PC12 pheochromocytoma cell line.[140] The induction of Nur77 by NGF is very rapid, placing it in the category of immediate early genes, i.e., rapidly inducible by growth factors or membrane depolarization.[242] Nurr-1 is also quickly induced by membrane depolarization in PC12 cells, but is unresponsive to NGF.[107] In the brain Nurr77 can be induced by events such as seizures,[234] ischemia,[117] and stress,[217] while in the immune system, Nur77 is likely important for apototic cell death and negative selection of T-cells.[120,232]

In the CNS, Nur77 is widely distributed whereas Nurr-1 is more localized in its expression pattern and is present in several sensory regions of the brain associated with the limbic system as well as the cerebellum in the internal granular cell and Purkinje cell layers.[189] A role for Nurr-1 in the differentiation of midbrain dopaminergic neurons was first suggested from its expression in that neuronal cell type. These dopaminergic cells are the neurons progressively lost in Parkinson's disease and in the null mutant of Nurr-1 these neurons fail to be born.[245] Nurr-1 is specific only for the dopaminergic neurons of the midbrain and is absent, for instance, in dopaminergic neurons of the hypothalamus[6] and these neurons are not lost in the Nurr-1 null mutant.[29] Nurr-1 transcriptionally activates the dopamine transporter gene[186] as well as the tyrosine hydroxylase gene required for dopamine synthesis[187] and Nurr-1 can induce a midbrain dopaminergic phenotype in neural stem cells.[222] Nurr-1 hence plays a determining role in the development of the midbrain dopaminergic neurons.

13.4.2.4   HNF-4

Hepatocyte nuclear factor-4 (HNF-4) is an orphan receptor first recognized for its role in liver development and adult hepatic function.[198] The actions of HNF-4 lie within a network of two other hepatic transcription factors, HNF-1 and HNF-3, which are not nuclear receptors. Together they regulate each other and coordinately regulate genes required for hepatic differentiation and metabolism.[54] The role of HNF-4 in development, however, is more fundamental; it is expressed as early as embryonic day 4.5 in primary endoderm[52] and its null mutation results in the failure of gastrulation.[34] At embryonic day 8.5 HNF-4 is expressed in the liver diverticulum and the hindgut and later is present in the kidney, pancreas, stomach, and intestine.[52] In the liver, HNF-4 promotes the determination of the hepatic phenotype from its progenitor cells[203] and induces the expression of many hepatic genes.[53] In the adult, HNF-4 regulates a series of genes involved in glucose, cholesterol, and fatty acid metabolism. These orphan receptors are not specific to the liver and involvement of HNF-4 alpha in glucose metabolism in the pancreas is demonstrated by the development of a form of non-insulin-dependent diabetes mellitus in HNF-4 alpha mutations.[235]

HNF-4 binds as a homodimer[82] to DR1 elements as well as the PPRE.[70] As described for the PPAR, the sequences surrounding the DR1 element, as well as the precise sequence of the DR1, can be important for HNF-4 binding and activation.[151,207] HNF-4-regulated genes in the liver include apolipoprotein A-II,[177] alpha1-microglobulin,[183] hepatocyte growth factor-like protein,[223] and steroid 15alpha-hydroxylase.[241] The supression of HNF-4-regulated transcriptional activation by the COUP-TFs has been reported in a number of circumstances. COUP-TI and II antagonize the effects of HNF-4 on apolipoprotein CIII[139] and the cytochrome P450 CYP3A1;[159] while COUP-TF-I represses HNF-4 activation of both ornithine transcarbamylase[93] and sex hormone-binding globulin.

13.4.2.5 PPAR

The peroxisome proliferator-activated receptors (PPARs alpha, beta, and gamma) can act as receptors for polyunsaturated fatty acids and several eicosanoids. These are natural ligands and hence the PPARs do not fit under the strict heading of orphan receptors; however, the relatively low affinity that these ligands have for the receptors suggests that the genuine ligands may remain to be identified. The PPARs are known to regulate glucose and lipid homeostasis and can also guide adipocyte differentiation.[43,191] It has been suggested that the function of PPAR alpha may be related to fatty acid metabolism while PPAR gamma may be more important for adipogenesis. That PPAR gamma is essential for glucose homeostasis was demonstrated by the finding that dominant negative mutations in this receptor are associated with insulin resistance and type 2 diabetes.[12] Because the PPAR/RXR heterodimer is reponsive to ligands for both receptor partners,[194] antidiabetic activity is found for both PPAR gamma[110] and RXR agonists.[145]

During embryonic development, the null mutant of this same receptor, PPAR gamma, is lethal at embryonic day 10 due to inadequate placental vascularization. Correction of the placental maldevelopment does not protect against embryonic death due to later hemorrhages and lipodystrophy.[11] Null mutants of PPAR alpha, in contrast, develop relatively normally[109] although the mice do exhibit abnormalities in lipid homeostasis.[38] In the embryo, PPAR alpha, as well as PPAR gamma, is expressed in the CNS at embryonic day 13.5 and is gone by 18.5.[20] Of all the receptors, PPAR gamma exhibits the most restricted distribution and at embryonic day 18.5 it is localized to and very strongly expressed in the brown adipose tissue. PPAR alpha is expressed at embryonic day 18.5 in the liver, digestive tract mucosa, epidermis, and brown adipose tissue while PPAR beta is relatively ubiquitous.[20]

The PPAR response element is similar to the DR1 repeat but is distinguished by a characteristic upstream flanking sequence.[27,164] The PPARs are similar to the nuclear receptors RAR, thyroid hormone and vitamin D receptors, in that they bind with high affinity to their response element as a heterodimer with RXR. They differ from these other two RXR partners in that the PPAR binds to the 5' half-site of the response element and RXR occupies the 3' half-site.[78] RXR/PPAR heterodimers have also been described as activating the estrogen response element.[157] The RXR/PPAR heterodimer regulates numerous genes involved in glucose and lipid homeostasis and RXR/PPAR-reponsive PPREs are present in the genes for hepatic phosphoenolpyruvate carboxykinase,[26] CYP4A6,[144] phosphoenolpyruvate carboxykinase,[214] malic enzyme[28] and acyl-CoA oxidase.[89] The PPRE of HMG-CoA synthase is a site acted upon by a number of nuclear receptors members, and is activated by PPAR and RXR, repressed by HNF-4,[180] and repressed or activated by COUP-TF.[179]

13.5 Discussion

Traditionally, hormones were identified on the basis of their physiological effects, i.e., they were purified, characterized chemically, and their physiological effects determined. The identification of their specific receptor(s) followed, through ligand–receptor interaction studies, utilizing radioactive ligands. Finally, the gene and its chromosomal location were characterized. A more recent approach, termed "reverse endocrinology,"[95] has permitted the identification of orphan receptors first, and subsequently, their specific ligands. In this manner, new synthetic ligands can be tested in reporter gene activation assays to eventually open up possibilities and suggest selective ligands as new drugs in endocrine and related diseases. The potential of this approach is realized if one considers that many of these pathways interact at the transcription level.

Cross-talk between the RA, thyroid hormone, and vitamin D receptors has been extensively investigated. Recently it has been shown that these interactions can even extend to the estrogen receptors.[201] This review has described several of the orphan nuclear receptors that interact with the RA receptors and hence modulate the RA signaling pathway. New orphan nuclear receptors are still being discovered and the list of receptors that modify RA signaling is likely to expand. In an organism as simple as the nematode worm more than 200 nuclear receptor genes are estimated, this family being the most prevalent of the transcription factors.[200] It seems likely that there will be an equivalent diversity in mammals. It has been noted that several orphan receptors are relatively specific in the control of restricted cell types, and these nuclear receptors impart identity to the cell lineage, e.g., HNF-4 for hepatocytes, PPAR gamma for adipocytes, RAR for neurons,[65,134] and Nurr-1 for dopaminergic neurons. If the variety of nuclear receptors is comparable to that found in the nematode then it may be expected that other such cell lineage regulatory receptors exist, and perhaps one role for the nuclear receptors during embryonic development is to initiate the identity of distinct cell lineages. Several metabolic enzymes are induced as part of this cell-specific differentiation program and they continue to be transcriptionally regulated by the same nuclear receptors in the adult. For this reason the orphan receptors, such as PPAR are HNF-4, are considered essential metabolic regulators.[199]

As with all ligand/receptor signaling events, at each progressive step of the RA signaling pathway there is an increase in the number of elements that contribute to the final signaling consequence (transcriptional modulation). In series, these steps include

1. The receptor ligand, RA, that can be synthesized and catabolized locally to create a concentration differential of ligand resulting in a gradation of transcriptional activation. Such is the case in the

developing retina where differential synthesis or catabolism of RA creates zones of differing RA transactivation.[137]

2. The individual RAR and RXR receptors that distinguish the transcriptional activity of all-*trans* and 9-*cis* RA as well as determine which DNA response element (DR1, DR2, or DR5) will be activated.

3. The nuclear receptor combinations, present at any given time, that will determine which heterodimers will form and which set of receptor species will be transcriptionally active. For instance, the high expression of COUP-TF-II would favor heterodimerization with RXR to create a transcriptional repressor. Alternatively, a high proportion of PPAR to RAR would favor the formation of PPAR/RXR, rather than RAR/RXR heterodimers, allowing PPAR ligand or 9-*cis* RA signaling to occur instead of the all-*trans* RA RAR ligand.[45] Because PPAR/RXR is responsive to the ligands of both heterodimeric partners, this provides a dual switch that is at its peak potency only when the cell is exposed to both ligands.

4. The RAREs, which bring together the nuclear receptors, co-activators and polymerases, resulting in transcription. The RAREs can range from the relatively simple direct repeats to HREs with complex series of overlapping direct repeats (e.g., glutathione S-transferase with seven repeat retinoic acid response element (RARE) consensus half-sites[121] or combinations of direct and palindromic repeats).

The modulators of RA-mediated transcription that act at these steps provide the necessary levels of refinement for RA transcriptional activation of each RA responsive gene. RA is known to be able to regulate transcription with broad brushstrokes, for instance, inducing neural gene expression in stem cells,[8] or precisely modulating, either up or down, the expression of single genes, as in the case of hoxb-1.[130] The combination of modulating factors which act on the receptors and response elements allows RA to act either as a broad regulator or fine manipulator of transcription.

Abbreviations

RA   retinoic acid

RAR   retinoic acid receptors

RXRs   9-*cis*-retinoic acid receptors

RBP   retinol binding protein

CRBP   cellular retinol binding protein

CRABP   cellular retinoic acid binding protein

RARE   retinoic acid response element
ThR   thyroid hormone receptor
COUP-TF chicken ovalbumin upstream promoter-transcription factor
CYP   cytochrome P450
RXRE   RXR response element
MGP   matrix Gla protein
PTH   parathyroid hormone
PPAR   peroxisome proliferator-activated receptor
PPRE   peroxisome proliferator-activated receptor response element
N-CoR nuclear receptor corepressor
SMRT   silencing mediator for RARs and TRs
CBP   CREB-binding protein
PML   promyelocytic leukemia
PLZF   promyelocytic leukemia zinc-finger
HNF   Hepatocyte nuclear factor-4
RORE   ROR response element
NMDA N-methyl-d-aspartate
Pcp-2   Purkinje cell protein-2.

References

1. Achatz, G., Holzl, B., Speckmayer, R., Hauser, C., Sandhofer, F., and Paulweber, B., Functional domains of the human orphan receptor ARP-1/COUP-TF-II involved in active repression and transrepression, *Mol. Cell Biol.*, 17, 4914, 1997.
2. Anderson, G. W., Larson, R. J., Oas, D. R., Sandhofer, C. R., Schwartz, H. L., Mariash, C. N., and Oppenheimer, J. H., Chicken ovalbumin upstream promoter-transcription factor (COUP-TF) modulates expression of the Purkinje cell protein-2 gene. A potential role for COUP-TF in repressing premature thyroid hormone action in the developing brain, *J. Biol. Chem.*, 273, 16391, 1998.
3. Andre, E., Conquet, F., Steinmayr, M., Stratton, S. C., Porciatti, V., and Becker-Andre, M., Disruption of retinoid-related orphan receptor beta changes circadian behavior, causes retinal degeneration and leads to vacillans phenotype in mice, *EMBO J.*, 17, 3867, 1998.
4. Avram, D., Ishmael, J. E., Nevrivy, D. J., Peterson, V. J., Lee, S. H., Dowell, P., and Leid, M., Heterodimeric interactions between chicken ovalbumin upstream promoter-transcription factor family members ARP1 and ear2, *J. Biol. Chem.*, 274, 14331, 1999.
5. Baader, S. L., Vogel, M. W., Sanlioglu, S., Zhang, X., and Oberdick, J., Selective disruption of "late onset" sagittal banding patterns by ectopic expression of engrailed-2 in cerebellar Purkinje cells, *J. Neurosci.*, 19, 5370, 1999.

6. Backman, C., Perlmann, T., Wallen, A., Hoffer, B. J., and Morales, M., A selective group of dopaminergic neurons express Nurr1 in the adult mouse brain, *Brain Res.*, 851, 125, 1999.

7. Bahouth, S. W., Beauchamp, M. J., and Park, E. A., Identification of a retinoic acid response domain involved in the activation of the beta 1-adrenergic receptor gene by retinoic acid in F9 teratocarcinoma cells, *Biochem. Pharmacol.*, 55, 215, 1998.

8. Bain, G., Kitchens, D., Yao, M., Huettner, J. E., and Gottlieb, D. I., Embryonic stem cells express neuronal properties *in vitro*, *Dev. Biol.*, 168, 342, 1995.

9. Bakke, M. and Lund, J., Transcriptional regulation of the bovine CYP17 gene: two nuclear orphan receptors determine activity of cAMP-responsive sequence 2, *Endocr. Res.*, 21, 509, 1995.

10. Baniahmad A., Kohne, A. C., and Renkawitz, R., A transferable silencing domain is present in the thyroid hormone receptor, in the v-erbA oncogene product and in the retinoic acid receptor, *Embo J.*, 11, 1015, 1992.

11. Barak, Y., Nelson, M. C., Ong, E. S., Jones, Y. Z., Ruiz-Lozano, P., Chien, K. R., Koder, A., and Evans, R. M., PPAR gamma is required for placental, cardiac, and adipose tissue development, Mol.Cell, 4, 585, 1999.

12. Barroso, I., Gurnell, M., Crowley, V. E., Agostini, M., Schwabe, J. W., Soos, M. A., Maslen, G. L., Williams, T. D., Lewis, H., Schafer, A. J., Chatterjee, V. K., and O'Rahilly, S., Dominant negative mutations in human PPAR gamma associated with severe insulin resistance, diabetes mellitus and hypertension [see comments], *Nature*, 402, 880, 1999.

13. Bavik, C. O., Busch, C., and Eriksson, U., Characterization of a plasma retinol-binding protein membrane receptor expressed in the retinal pigment epithelium, *J. Biol. Chem.*, 267, 23035, 1992.

14. Becker-Andre, M., Wiesenberg, I., Schaeren-Wiemers, N., Andre, E., Missbach, M., Saurat, J. H., and Sairat, J. H., Erratum to Pineal gland hormone melatonin binds and activates an orphan of the nuclear receptor superfamily, *J. Biol. Chem.*, 272, 16707, 1998.

15. Becker-Andre, M., Wiesenberg, I., Schaeren-Wiemers, N., Andre, E., Missbach, M., Saurat, J. H., and Carlberg, C., Pineal gland hormone melatonin binds and activates an orphan of the nuclear receptor superfamily [published erratum appears in *J. Biol. Chem.* 1997, June 27; 272(26): 16707], *J. Biol. Chem.*, 269, 28531, 1994.

16. Ben Shushan, E., Sharir, H., Pikarsky, E., and Bergman, Y., A dynamic balance between ARP-1/COUP-TF-II, EAR-3/COUP-TF-I, and retinoic acid receptor:retinoid X receptor heterodimers regulates Oct-3/4 expression in embryonal carcinoma cells, *Mol. Cell Biol.*, 15, 1034, 1995.

17. Blaner, W. S. and Olson, J. A., 5 / Retinol and retinoic acid metabolism, in *The Retinoids: Biology, Chemistry, and Medicine*, 2nd edition, Sporn, M. B., Roberts, A. B., and Goodman, D. S., Eds., Raven Press, New York, 1994.

18. Blomhoff, R., Green, M. H., Berg, T., and Norum, K. R., Transport and storage of vitamin A, *Science*, 250, 399, 1990.

19. Blomhoff, R., Green, M. H., Green, J. B., Berg, T., and Norum, K. R., Vitamin A metabolism: new perspectives on absorption, transport, and storage, *Physiol. Rev.*, 71, 951, 1991.

20. Braissant, O. and Wahli, W., Differential expression of peroxisome proliferator-activated receptor-alpha, -beta, and -gamma during rat embryonic development, *Endocrinology*, 139, 2748, 1998.

21. Brubaker, K., McMillan, M., Neuman, T., and Nornes, H. O., All-*trans* retinoic acid affects the expression of orphan receptors COUP- TF I and COUP-TF II in the developing neural tube, *Brain Res. Dev. Brain Res.*, 93, 198, 1996.

22. Bulens, F., Ibanez-Tallon, I., Van Acker, P., De Vriese, A., Nelles, L., Belayew, A., and Collen, D., Retinoic acid induction of human tissue-type plasminogen activator gene expression via a direct repeat element (DR5) located at -7 kilobases, *J. Biol. Chem.*, 270, 7167, 1995.

23. Cancela, M. L. and Price, P. A., Retinoic acid induces matrix Gla protein gene expression in human cells, *Endocrinology*, 130, 102, 1992.

24. Carlberg, C., Hoof van Huijsduijnen, R., Staple, J. K., Delamarter, J. F., and Becker-Andre, M., RZRs, a new family of retinoid-related orphan receptors that function as both monomers and homodimers, *Mol. Endocrinol.*, 8, 757, 1994.

25. Carter, M. E., Gulick, T., Raisher, B. D., Caira, T., Ladias, J. A., Moore, D. D., and Kelly, D. P., Hepatocyte nuclear factor-4 activates medium chain acyl-CoA dehydrogenase gene transcription by interacting with a complex regulatory element, *J. Biol. Chem.*, 268, 13805, 1993.

26. Cassuto, H., Aran, A., Cohen, H., Eisenberger, C. L., and Reshef, L., Repression and activation of transcription of phosphoenolpyruvate carboxykinase gene during liver development, *FEBS Lett.*, 457, 441, 1999.

27. Castelein, H., Declercq, P. E., and Baes, M., DNA binding preferences of PPAR alpha/RXR alpha heterodimers, *Biochem. Biophys. Res. Commun.*, 233, 91, 1997.

28. Castelein, H., Gulick, T., Declercq, P. E., Mannaerts, G. P., Moore, D. D., and Baes, M. I., The peroxisome proliferator activated receptor regulates malic enzyme gene expression, *J. Biol. Chem.*, 269, 26754, 1994.

29. Castillo, S. O., Baffi, J. S., Palkovits, M., Goldstein, D. S., Kopin, I. J., Witta, J., Magnuson, M. A., and Nikodem, V. M., Dopamine biosynthesis is selectively abolished in substantia nigra/ventral tegmental area but not in hypothalamic neurons in mice with targeted disruption of the Nurr1 gene, *Mol. Cell Neurosci.*, 11, 36, 1998.

30. Chang, B. E., Blader, P., Fischer, N., Ingham, P. W., and Strahle, U., Axial (HNF3beta) and retinoic acid receptors are regulators of the zebrafish sonic hedgehog promoter, *EMBO J.*, 16, 3955, 1997.

31. Chen, J. D. and Li, H., Coactivation and corepression in transcriptional regulation by steroid/nuclear hormone receptors, *Crit. Rev. Eukaryot. Gene Expr.*, 8, 169, 1998.

32. Chen, L. C. and De Luca, L. M., Retinoids and skin cancer, in *Skin Cancer: Mechanisms and Human Relevance*, Mukhtar, H., Ed., CRC Press, Boca Raton, 1995.

33. Chen, S. J., Wang, Z. Y., and Chen, Z., Acute promyelocytic leukemia: from clinic to molecular biology, *Stem Cells (Dayt).*, 13, 22, 1995.

34. Chen, W. S., Manova, K., Weinstein, D. C., Duncan, S. A., Plump, A. S., Prezioso, V. R., Bachvarova, R. F., and Darnell, J. E., Jr., Disruption of the HNF-4 gene, expressed in visceral endoderm, leads to cell death in embryonic ectoderm and impaired gastrulation of mouse embryos, *Genes Dev.*, 8, 2466, 1994.

35. Chew, L. J., Huang, F., Boutin, J. M., and Gallo, V., Identification of nuclear orphan receptors as regulators of expression of a neurotransmitter receptor gene, *J. Biol. Chem.*, 274, 29366, 1999.

36. Cho, S., Cho, H., Geum, D., and Kim, K., Retinoic acid regulates gonadotropin-releasing hormone (GnRH) release and gene expression in the rat hypothalamic fragments and GT1-1 neuronal cells *in vitro*, *Brain Res. Mol. Brain Res.*, 54, 74, 1998.

37. Cooney, A. J., Tsai, S. Y., O'Malley, B. W., and Tsai, M. J., Chicken ovalbumin upstream promoter transcription factor (COUP-TF) dimers bind to different GGTCA response elements, allowing COUP-TF to repress hormonal induction of the vitamin D3, thyroid hormone, and retinoic acid receptors, *Mol. Cell Biol.*, 12, 4153, 1992.

38. Costet, P., Legendre, C., More, J., Edgar, A., Galtier, P., and Pineau, T., Peroxisome proliferator-activated receptor alpha-isoform deficiency leads to progressive dyslipidemia with sexually dimorphic obesity and steatosis, *J. Biol. Chem.*, 273, 29577, 1998.

39. De Luca, L. M., Retinoids and their receptors in differentiation, embryogenesis, and neoplasia, *FASEB J.*, 5, 2924, 1991.

40. De Luca, L. M., Darwiche, N., Jones, C. S., and Scita, G., Retinoids in differentiation and neoplasia, *Scient. Am. Sci. Med.*, 2, 28, 1995.

41. de The, H., Chomienne, C., Lanotte, M., Degos, L., and Dejean, A., The t(15;17) translocation of acute promyelocytic leukaemia fuses the retinoic acid receptor alpha gene to a novel transcribed locus, *Nature*, 347, 558, 1990.

42. Delva, L., Bastie, J. N., Rochette-Egly, C., Kraiba, R., Balitrand, N., Despouy, G., Chambon, P., and Chomienne, C., Physical and functional interactions between cellular retinoic acid binding protein II and the retinoic acid-dependent nuclear complex, *Mol. Cell Biol.*, 19, 7158, 1999.

43. Devchand, P. R., Ijpenberg, A., Devesvergne, B., and Wahli, W., PPARs: nuclear receptors for fatty acids, eicosanoids, and xenobiotics, *Adv. Exp. Med. Biol.*, 469, 231, 1999.

44. Devine, J. H., Eubank, D. W., Clouthier, D. E., Tontonoz, P., Spiegelman, B. M., Hammer, R. E., and Beale, E. G., Adipose expression of the phosphoenolpyruvate carboxykinase promoter requires peroxisome proliferator-activated receptor gamma and 9-*cis*- retinoic acid receptor binding to an adipocyte-specific enhancer *in vivo*, *J. Biol. Chem.*, 274, 13604, 1999.

45. DiRenzo, J., Soderstrom, M., Kurokawa, R., Ogliastro, M. H., Ricote, M., Ingrey, S., Horlein, A., Rosenfeld, M. G., and Glass, C. K., Peroxisome proliferator-activated receptors and retinoic acid receptors differentially control the interactions of retinoid X receptor heterodimers with ligands, coactivators, and corepressors, *Mol. Cell Biol.*, 17, 2166, 1997.

46. Dong, D. and Noy, N., Heterodimer formation by retinoid X receptor: regulation by ligands and by the receptor's self-association properties, *Biochemistry*, 37, 10691, 1998.

47. Dong, D., Ruuska, S. E., Levinthal, D. J., and Noy, N., Distinct roles for cellular retinoic acid-binding proteins I and II in regulating signaling by retinoic acid, *J. Biol. Chem.*, 274, 23695, 1999.

48. Crabb, J. W., Nie, Z., Chen, Y., Hulmes, J. D., West, K. A., Kapron, J. T., Ruuska, S. E., Noy, N., and Saari, J. C., Cellular retinaldehyde-binding protein ligand interactions. Gln and Lys-221 are in the retinoid-binding pocket, *J. Biol. Chem.*, 273, 20712, 1998.

49. Dong, D., Ruuska, S. E., Levinthal, D. J., and Noy, N., Distinct roles for cellular retinoic acid-binding proteins I and II in regulating signaling by retinoic acid, *J. Biol. Chem.*, 274, 23695, 1999.

50. Drager, U. C. and McCaffery, P., Retinoic acid and development of the retina, *Prog. Retinal Eye Res.*, 16, 323, 1997.

51. Duester, G., Involvement of alcohol dehydrogenase, short-chain dehydrogenase/reductase, aldehyde dehydrogenase, and cytochrome P450 in the control of retinoid signaling by activation of retinoic acid synthesis, *Biochemistry*, 35, 12221, 1996.

52. Duester, G., Shean, M. L., McBride, M. S., and Stewart, M. J., Retinoic acid response element in the human alcohol dehydrogenase gene ADH3: implications for regulation of retinoic acid synthesis, *Mol. Cell Biol.*, 11, 1638, 1991.

53. Duncan, S. A., Manova, K., Chen, W. S., Hoodless, P., Weinstein, D. C., Bachvarova, R. F., and Darnell, J. E., Jr., Expression of transcription factor HNF-4 in the extraembryonic endoderm, gut, and nephrogenic tissue of the developing mouse embryo: HNF-4 is a marker for primary endoderm in the implanting blastocyst, *Proc. Natl. Acad. Sci. USA*, 91, 7598, 1994.

54. Duncan, S. A., Nagy, A., and Chan, W., Murine gastrulation requires HNF-4 regulated gene expression in the visceral endoderm: tetraploid rescue of Hnf-4(-/-) embryos, *Development*, 124, 279, 1997.

55. Duncan, S. A., Navas, M. A., Dufort, D., Rossant, J., and Stoffel, M., Regulation of a transcription factor network required for differentiation and metabolism, *Science*, 281, 692, 1998.

56. Durand, B., Saunders, M., Leroy, P., Leid, M., and Chambon, P., All-*trans* and 9-*cis* retinoic acid induction of mouse CRABPII gene transcription is mediated by RAR-RXR heterodimers, *Cell*, 71, 73, 1992.

57. Fiorella, P. D., Giguere, V., and Napoli, J. L., Expression of cellular retinoic acid-binding protein (type II) in Escherichia coli. Characterization and comparison to cellular retinoic acid-binding protein (type I), *J. Biol. Chem.*, 268, 21545, 1993.

58. Fiorella, P. D. and Napoli, J. L., Microsomal retinoic acid metabolism. Effects of cellular retinoic acid- binding protein (type I) and C18-hydroxylation as an initial step, *J. Biol. Chem.*, 269, 10538, 1994.

59. Forman, B. M., Goode, E., Chen, J., Oro, A. E., Bradley, D. J., Perlmann, T., Noonan, D. J., Burka, L. T., McMorris, T., and Lamph, W. W., Identification of a nuclear receptor that is activated by farnesol metabolites, *Cell*, 81, 687, 1995.

60. Forman, B. M., Umesono, K., Chen, J., and Evans, R. M., Unique response pathways are established by allosteric interactions among nuclear hormone receptors, *Cell*, 81, 541, 1995.

61. Fujita, A. and Mitsuhashi, T., Differential regulation of ligand-dependent and ligand-independent functions of the mouse retinoid X receptor beta by alternative splicing, *Biochem. Biophys. Res. Commun.*, 255, 625, 1999.

62. Ghyselinck, N. B., Bavik, C., Sapin, V., Mark, M., Bonnier, D., Hindelang, C., Dierich, A., Nilsson, C. B., Hakansson, H., Sauvant, P., Azais-Braesco, V., Frasson, M., Picaud, S., and Chambon, P., Cellular retinol-binding protein I is essential for vitamin A homeostasis, *EMBO J.*, 18, 4903, 1999.

63. Giguere, V., Ong, E. S., Segui, P., and Evans, R. M., Identification of a receptor for the morphogen retinoic acid, *Nature*, 330, 624, 1987.

64. Giordano, A. and Avantaggiati, M. L., p300 and CBP: partners for life and death, *J. Cell Physiol.*, 181, 218, 1999.

65. Goodman, D. S., Plasma retinol binding protein, in *The Retinoids, Vol. 2*, Sporn, M. B., Roberts, A. B., and Goodman, D. S., Eds., Academic Press, Orlando, FL, 1984.

66. Gottlieb, D. I. and Huettner, J. E., An *in vitro* pathway from embryonic stem cells to neurons and glia, *Cells, Tissues, Organs*, 165, 165, 1999.

67. Gould, A., Itasaki, N., and Krumlauf, R., Initiation of rhombomeric Hoxb4 expression requires induction by somites and a retinoid pathway, *Neuron*, 21, 39, 1998.

68. Grignani, F., De Matteis, S., Nervi, C., Tomassoni, L., Gelmetti, V., Cioce, M., Fanelli, M., Ruthardt, M., Ferrara, F. F., Zamir, I., Seiser, C., Lazar, M. A., Minucci, S., and Pelicci, P. G., Fusion proteins of the retinoic acid receptor-α recruit histone deacetylase in promyelocytic leukaemia, *Nature*, 391, 815, 1998.

69. Gudas, L. J., Sporn, M. B., and Roberts, A. B., Cellular Biology and Biochemistry of the Retinoids, in *Their Retinoids*, Sporn, M. B., Roberts, A. B., and Goodman, D. S., Eds., Raven Press, New York, 1994.

70. Hawkes, R. and Eisenman, L. M., Stripes and zones: the origins of regionalization of the adult cerebellum, *Perspect. Dev. Neurobiol.*, 5, 95, 1997.

71. Hegardt, F. G., Transcriptional regulation of mitochondrial HMG-CoA synthase in the control of ketogenesis, *Biochimie*, 80, 803, 1998.

72. Herrup, K. and Kuemerle, B., The compartmentalization of the cerebellum, *Annu. Rev. Neurosci.*, 20, 61, 1997.

73. Hirose, T., Smith, R. J., and Jetten, A. M., ROR gamma: the third member of ROR/RZR orphan receptor subfamily that is highly expressed in skeletal muscle, *Biochem. Biophys. Res. Commun.*, 205, 1976, 1994.

74. Hong, W. K., Endicott, J., Itri, L. M., Doos, W., Batsakis, J. G., Bell, R., Fofonoff, S., Byers, R., Atkinson, E. N., and Vaughan, C., 13-*cis*-retinoic acid in the treatment of oral leukoplakia, *N. Engl. J. Med.*, 315, 1501, 1986.

75. Hong, W. K., Lippman, S. M., Itri, L. M., Karp, D. D., Lee, J. S., Byers, R. M., Schantz, S. P., Kramer, A. M., Lotan, R., Peters, L. J., Dimery, I. W., Brown, B. W., and Goepfert, H., Prevention of second primary tumors with isotretinoin in squamous-cell carcinoma of the head and neck, *N. Engl. J. Med.*, 323, 795, 1990.

76. Hong, W. K. and Sporn, M. B., Recent advances in chemoprevention of cancer, *Science*, 278, 1073, 1997.

77. Hsu, M. H., Palmer, C. N., Song, W., Griffin, K. J., and Johnson, E. F., A carboxyl-terminal extension of the zinc finger domain contributes to the specificity and polarity of peroxisome proliferator-activated receptor DNA binding, *J. Biol. Chem.*, 273, 27988, 1998.

78. Husmann, M., Hoffmann, B., Stump, D. G., Chytil, F., and Pfahl, M., A retinoic acid response element from the rat CRBPI promoter is activated by an RAR/RXR heterodimer, *Biochem. Biophys. Res. Commun.*, 187, 1558, 1992.

79. Ijpenberg, A., Jeannin, E., Wahli, W., and Desvergne, B., Polarity and specific sequence requirements of peroxisome proliferator-activated receptor (PPAR)/retinoid X receptor heterodimer binding to DNA. A functional analysis of the malic enzyme gene PPAR response element, *J. Biol. Chem.*, 272, 20108, 1997.

80. Jacob, A., Budhiraja, S., and Reichel, R. R., The HNF-3alpha transcription factor is a primary target for retinoic acid action, *Exp. Cell Res.*, 250, 1, 1999.

81. Jansa, P. and Forejt, J., A novel type of retinoic acid response element in the second intron of the mouse H2Kb gene is activated by the RAR/RXR heterodimer, *Nucleic Acids Res.*, 24, 694, 1996.

82. Jeoung, N. H., Jang, W. G., Nam, J. I., Pak, Y. K., and Park, Y. B., Identification of retinoic acid receptor element in human cholesteryl ester transfer protein gene, *Biochem. Biophys. Res. Commun.*, 258, 411, 1999.

83. Jiang, G., Nepomuceno, L., Hopkins, K., and Sladek, F. M., Exclusive homodimerization of the orphan receptor hepatocyte nuclear factor 4 defines a new subclass of nuclear receptors, *Mol. Cell Biol.,* 15, 5131, 1995.

84. Johnson, E. F., Palmer, C. N., Griffin, K. J., and Hsu, M. H., Role of the peroxisome proliferator-activated receptor in cytochrome P450 4A gene regulation, *FASEB J.,* 10, 1241, 1996.

85. Kadowaki, Y., Toyoshima, K., and Yamamoto, T., Ear3/COUP-TF binds most tightly to a response element with tandem repeat separated by one nucleotide, *Biochem. Biophys. Res. Commun.,* 183, 492, 1992.

86. Kakizawa, T., Miyamoto, T., Kaneko, A., Yajima, H., Ichikawa, K., and Hashizume, K., Ligand-dependent heterodimerization of thyroid hormone receptor and retinoid X receptor, *J. Biol. Chem.,* 272, 23799, 1997.

87. Karperien, M., Farih-Sips, H., Hendriks, J. A., Lanske, B., Papapoulos, S. E., Abou-Samra, A. B., Lowik, C. W., and Defize, L. H., Identification of a retinoic acid-inducible element in the murine PTH/PTHrP (parathyroid hormone/parathyroid hormone-related peptide) receptor gene, *Mol. Endocrinol.,* 13, 1183, 1999.

88. Kastner, P., Grondona, J. M., Mark, M., Gansmuller, A., LeMeur, M., Decimo, D., Vonesch, J. L., Dolle, P., and Chambon, P., Genetic analysis of RXRα developmental function: convergence of RXR and RAR signaling pathways in heart and eye morphogenesis, *Cell,* 78, 987, 1994.

89. Kastner, P., Mark, M., and Chambon, P., Nonsteroid nuclear receptors: what are genetic studies telling us about their role in real life?, *Cell,* 83, 859, 1995.

90. Keller, H., Dreyer, C., Medin, J., Mahfoudi, A., Ozato, K., and Wahli, W., Fatty acids and retinoids control lipid metabolism through activation of peroxisome proliferator-activated receptor-retinoid X receptor heterodimers, *Proc. Natl. Acad. Sci. USA,* 90, 2160, 1993.

91. Kelloff, G. J., Crowell, J. A., Hawk, E. T., Steele, V. E., Lubet, R. A., Boone, C. W., Covey, J. M., Doody, L. A., Omenn, G. S., Greenwald, P., Hong, W. K., Parkinson, D. R., Bagheri, D., Baxter, G. T., Blunden, M., Doeltz, M. K., Eisenhauer, K. M., Johnson, K., Longfellow, D. G., Knapp, G. G., Malone, W. F., Nayfield, S. G., Seifreid, H. E., Swall, L. M., and Sigman, C. C., Clinical development plan: 13-*cis*-Retinoic acid, *J. Cell. Biochem.,* 26, Suppl., 168, 1996.

92. Kelloff, G. J., Crowell, J. A., Hawk, E. T., Steele, V. E., Lubet, R. A., Boone, C. W., Covey, J. M., Doody, L. A., Omenn, G. S., Greenwald, P., Hong, W. K., Parkinson, D. R., Bagheri, D., Baxter, G. T., Blunden, M., Doeltz, M. K., Eisenhauer, K. M., Johnson, K., Longfellow, D. G., Knapp, G. G., Malone, W. F., Nayfield, S. G., Seifreid, H. E., Swall, L. M., and Sigman, C. C., Clinical development plan: Vitamin A., *J. Cell. Biochem.,* 26, Suppl., 269, 1996.

93. Kersten, S., Pan, L., Chambon, P., Gronemeyer, H., and Noy, N., Role of ligand in retinoid signaling. 9-*cis*-retinoic acid modulates the oligomeric state of the retinoid X receptor, *Biochemistry,* 34, 13717, 1995.

94. Kimura, A., Nishiyori, A., Murakami, T., Tsukamoto, T., Hata, S., Osumi, T., Okamura, R., Mori, M., and Takiguchi, M., Chicken ovalbumin upstream promoter-transcription factor (COUP-TF) represses transcription from the promoter of the gene for ornithine transcarbamylase in a manner antagonistic to hepatocyte nuclear factor-4 (HNF-4), *J. Biol. Chem.,* 268, 11125, 1993.

95. Kishimoto, H., Hoshino, S., Ohori, M., Kontani, K., Nishina, H., Suzawa, M., Kato, S., and Katada, T., Molecular mechanism of human CD38 gene expression by retinoic acid. Identification of retinoic acid response element in the first intron, *J. Biol. Chem.*, 273, 15429, 1998.

96. Kliewer, S. A., Lehmann, J. M., and Willson, T. M., Orphan nuclear receptors: shifting endocrinology into reverse, *Science*, 284, 757, 1999.

97. Kliewer, S. A., Umesono, K., Heyman, R. A., Mangelsdorf, D. J., Dyck, J. A., and Evans, R. M., Retinoid X receptor-COUP-TF interactions modulate retinoic acid signaling, *Proc. Natl. Acad. Sci. USA*, 89, 1448, 1992.

98. Kliewer, S. A., Umesono, K., Mangelsdorf, D. J., and Evans, R. M., Retinoid X receptor interacts with nuclear receptors in retinoic acid, thyroid hormone and vitamin D_3 signalling, *Nature*, 355, 446, 1992.

99. Kliewer, S. A., Umesono, K., Noonan, D. J., Heyman, R. A., and Evans, R. M., Convergence of 9-*cis* retinoic acid and peroxisome proliferator signalling pathways through heterodimer formation of their receptors, *Nature*, 358, 771, 1992.

100. Klinge, C. M., Role of estrogen receptor ligand and estrogen response element sequence on interaction with chicken ovalbumin upstream promoter transcription factor (COUP-TF), *J. Steroid Biochem. Mol. Biol.*, 71, 1, 1999.

101. Klinge, C. M., Silver, B. F., Driscoll, M. D., Sathya, G., Bambara, R. A., and Hilf, R., Chicken ovalbumin upstream promoter-transcription factor interacts with estrogen receptor, binds to estrogen response elements and half-sites, and inhibits estrogen-induced gene expression, *J. Biol. Chem.*, 272, 31465, 1997.

102. Kolla, V., Weihua, X., and Kalvakolanu, D. V., Modulation of interferon action by retinoids. Induction of murine STAT1 gene expression by retinoic acid [published erratum appears in *J. Biol. Chem.* 1997 June 20; 272(25): 16068], *J. Biol. Chem.*, 272, 9742, 1997.

103. Krishnan, V., Pereira, F. A., Qiu, Y., Chen, C. H., Beachy, P. A., Tsai, S. Y., and Tsai, M. J., Mediation of Sonic hedgehog-induced expression of COUP-TF-II by a protein phosphatase, *Science*, 278, 1947, 1997.

104. Kurokawa, R., DiRenzo, J., Boehm, M., Sugarman, J., Gloss, B., Rosenfeld, M. G., Heyman, R. A., and Glass, C. K., Regulation of retinoid signalling by receptor polarity and allosteric control of ligand binding, *Nature*, 371, 528, 1994.

105. Kurokawa, R., Yu, V. C., Naar, A., Kyakumoto, S., Han, Z., Silverman, S., Rosenfeld, M. G., and Glass, C. K., Differential orientations of the DNA-binding domain and carboxy-terminal dimerization interface regulate binding site selection by nuclear receptor heterodimers, *Genes Dev.*, 7, 1423, 1993.

106. Langston, A. W. and Gudas, L. J., Identification of a retinoic acid responsive enhancer 3' of the murine homeobox gene Hox-1.6, *Mech. Dev.*, 38, 217, 1992.

107. Lavrentiadou, S. N., Hadzopoulou-Cladaras, M., Kardassis, D., and Zannis, V. I., Binding specificity and modulation of the human ApoCIII promoter activity by heterodimers of ligand-dependent nuclear receptors, *Biochemistry*, 38, 964, 1999.

108. Law, S. W., Conneely, O. M., DeMayo, F. J., and O'Malley, B. W., Identification of a new brain-specific transcription factor, NURR1, *Mol. Endocrinol.*, 6, 2129, 1992.

109. Lee, M. O., Liu, Y., and Zhang, X. K., A retinoic acid response element that overlaps an estrogen response element mediates multihormonal sensitivity in transcriptional activation of the lactoferrin gene, *Mol. Cell Biol.*, 15, 4194, 1995.

110. Lee, S. S., Pineau, T., Drago, J., Lee, E. J., Owens, J. W., Kroetz, D. L., Fernandez-Salguero, P. M., Westphal, H., and Gonzalez, F. J., Targeted disruption of the alpha isoform of the peroxisome proliferator-activated receptor gene in mice results in abolishment of the pleiotropic effects of peroxisome proliferators, *Mol. Cell Biol.*, 15, 3012, 1995.

111. Lehmann, J. M., Moore, L. B., Smith-Oliver, T. A., Wilkison, W. O., Willson, T. M., and Kliewer, S. A., An antidiabetic thiazolidinedione is a high affinity ligand for peroxisome proliferator-activated receptor gamma (PPAR gamma), *J. Biol. Chem.*, 270, 12953, 1995.

112. Lehmann, J. M., Zhang, X. K., and Pfahl, M., RAR gamma 2 expression is regulated through a retinoic acid response element embedded in Sp1 sites, *Mol. Cell Biol.*, 12, 2976, 1992.

113. Leid, M., Kastner, P., Lyons, R., Nakshatri, H., Saunders, M., Zacharewski, T., Chen, J., Staub, A., Garnier, J., Mader, S., and Chambon, P., Purification, cloning, and RXR identity of the HeLa cell factor with which RAR or TR heterodimerizes to bind target sequences efficiently, *Cell*, 68, 377, 1992.

114. Leroy, P., Nakshatri, H., and Chambon, P., Mouse retinoic acid receptor α2 isoform is transcribed from a promoter that contains a retinoic acid response element, *Proc. Natl. Acad. Sci. USA*, 88, 10138, 1991.

115. Li, X. Y., Xiao, J. H., Feng, X., Qin, L., and Voorhees, J. J., Retinoid X receptor-specific ligands synergistically upregulate 1, 25-dihydroxyvitamin D3-dependent transcription in epidermal keratinocytes *in vitro* and *in vivo*, *J. Invest Dermatol.*, 108, 506, 1997.

116. Lin, B., Chen, G. Q., Xiao, D., Kolluri, S. K., Cao, X., Su, H., and Zhang, X. K., Orphan receptor COUP-TF is required for induction of retinoic acid receptor beta, growth inhibition, and apoptosis by retinoic acid in cancer cells, *Mol. Cell Biol.*, 20, 957, 2000.

117. Lin, R. J., Nagy, L., Inoue, S., Shao, W., Miller, W. H., Jr., and Evans, R. M., Role of the histone deacetylase complex in acute promyelocytic leukaemia, *Nature*, 391, 811, 1998.

118. Lin, T. N., Chen, J. J., Wang, S. J., Cheng, J. T., Chi, S. I., Shyu, A. B., Sun, G. Y., and Hsu, C. Y., Expression of NGFI-B mRNA in a rat focal cerebral ischemia-reperfusion model, *Brain Res. Mol. Brain Res.*, 43, 149, 1996.

119. Liu, Y., Chen, H., and Chiu, J. F., Identification of a retinoic acid response element upstream of the rat alpha-fetoprotein gene, *Mol. Cell Endocrinol.*, 103, 149, 1994.

120. Liu, Y. and Chiu, J. F., Transactivation and repression of the alpha-fetoprotein gene promoter by retinoid X receptor and chicken ovalbumin upstream promoter transcription factor, *Nucleic Acids Res.*, 22, 1079, 1994.

121. Liu, Z. G., Smith, S. W., McLaughlin, K. A., Schwartz, L. M., and Osborne, B. A., Apoptotic signals delivered through the T-cell receptor of a T-cell hybrid require the immediate-early gene nur77, *Nature*, 367, 281, 1994.

122. Lo, H. and Ali-Osman, F., Structure of the human allelic glutathione S-transferase-pi gene variant, hGSTP1 C, cloned from a glioblastoma multiforme cell line, *Chem. Biol. Interact.*, 111-112, 91, 1998.

123. Lu, H. C., Eichele, G., and Thaller, C., Ligand-bound RXR can mediate retinoid signal transduction during embryogenesis, *Development*, 124, 195, 1997.

124. Lu, X. P., Salbert, G., and Pfahl, M., An evolutionary conserved COUP-TF binding element in a neural-specific gene and COUP-TF expression patterns support a major role for COUP-TF in neural development, *Mol. Endocrinol.*, 8, 1774, 1994.

125. Maden, M., The role of retinoids in developmental mechanisms in embryos, *Subcell. Biochem.*, 30, 81, 1998.

126. Maira, M., Martens, C., Philips, A., and Drouin, J., Heterodimerization between members of the Nur subfamily of orphan nuclear receptors as a novel mechanism for gene activation, *Mol. Cell Biol.*, 19, 7549, 1999.

127. Mangelsdorf, D. J. and Evans, R. M., Retinoid receptors as transcription factors, in *Transcriptional Regulation*, McKnight, S. L. and Yamamoto, K. R., Eds., Cold Spring Harbor Laboratory Press, Plainview, NY, 1993.

128. Mangelsdorf, D. J., Umesono, K., and Evans, R. M., The retinoid receptors, in *The Retinoids: Biology, Chemistry, and Medicine*, 2nd edition, Sporn, M. B., Roberts, A. B., and Goodman, D. S., Eds., Raven Press, New York, 1994.

129. Mangelsdorf, D. J., Umesono, K., Kliewer, S. A., Borgmeyer, U., Ong, E. S., and Evans, R. M., A direct repeat in the cellular retinol-binding protein type II gene confers differential regulation by RXR and RAR, *Cell*, 66, 555, 1991.

130. Marcus, S. L., Capone, J. P., and Rachubinski, R. A., Identification of COUP-TF-II as a peroxisome proliferator response element binding factor using genetic selection in yeast: COUP-TF-II activates transcription in yeast but antagonizes PPAR signaling in mammalian cells, *Mol. Cell Endocrinol.*, 120, 31, 1996.

131. Marshall, H., Studer, M., Popperl, H., Aparicio, S., Kuroiwa, A., Brenner, S., and Krumlauf, R., A conserved retinoic acid response element required for early expression of the homeobox gene hoxb-1, *Nature*, 370, 567, 1994.

132. Matsui, T., Transcriptional regulation of a Purkinje cell-specific gene through a functional interaction between ROR alpha and RAR, *Genes Cells*, 2, 263, 1997.

133. Matsuura, T. and Ross, A. C., Regulation of hepatic lecithin: retinol acyltransferase activity by retinoic acid, *Arch. Biochem. Biophys.*, 301, 221, 1993.

134. McBroom, L. D., Flock, G., and Giguere, V., The nonconserved hinge region and distinct amino-terminal domains of the ROR alpha orphan nuclear receptor isoforms are required for proper DNA bending and ROR alpha-DNA interactions, *Mol. Cell Biol.*, 15, 796, 1995.

135. McBurney, M. W., P19 embryonal carcinoma cells, *Int. J. Dev. Biol.*, 37, 135, 1993.

136. McCaffery, P. and Drager, U. C., Retinoic acid synthesizing enzymes in the embryonic and adult vertebrate, in *Enzymology and Molecular Biology of Carbonyl Metabolism*, Weiner, H., Crabb, D. W., and Flynn, T. G., Eds., Plenum Press, New York, 1995.

137. McCaffery, P. and Drager, U. C., Regulation of retinoic acid signaling in the embryonic nervous system: a master differentiation factor, *Cytokine Growth Factor Rev.*, 11, 233, 2000.

138. McCaffery, P., Wagner, E., O'Neil, J., Petkovich, M., and Drager, U. C., Dorsal and ventral retinal territories defined by retinoic acid synthesis, break-down and nuclear receptor expression, *Mech. Dev.*, 85, 203, 1999.

139. Meisler, N. T., Parrelli, J., Gendimenico, G. J., Mezick, J. A., and Cutroneo, K. R., All-*trans*-retinoic acid inhibition of Pro alpha1(I) collagen gene expression in fetal rat skin fibroblasts: identification of a retinoic acid response element in the Pro alpha1(I) collagen gene, *J. Invest Dermatol.*, 108, 476, 1997.

140. Mietus-Snyder, M., Sladek, F. M., Ginsburg, G. S., Kuo, C. F., Ladias, J. A., Darnell, J. E., Jr., and Karathanasis, S. K., Antagonism between apolipoprotein AI regulatory protein 1, Ear3/COUP- TF, and hepatocyte nuclear factor 4 modulates apolipoprotein CIII gene expression in liver and intestinal cells, *Mol. Cell Biol.*, 12, 1708, 1992.

141. Milbrandt, J., Nerve growth factor induces a gene homologous to the glucocorticoid receptor gene, *Neuron*, 1, 183, 1988.

142. Millen, K. J., Hui, C. C., and Joyner, A. L., A role for En-2 and other murine homologues of *Drosophila* segment polarity genes in regulating positional information in the developing cerebellum, *Development*, 121, 3935, 1995.

143. Moroni, M. C., Vigano, M. A., and Mavilio, F., Regulation of the human HOXD4 gene by retinoids, *Mech. Dev.*, 44, 139, 1993.

144. Morriss-Kay, G. and Ward, S. J., Retinoids and mammalian development, *Int. Rev. Cytol.*, 188, 73, 1999.

145. Muerhoff, A. S., Griffin, K. J., and Johnson, E. F., The peroxisome proliferator-activated receptor mediates the induction of CYP4A6, a cytochrome P450 fatty acid omega-hydroxylase, by clofibric acid, *J. Biol. Chem.*, 267, 19051, 1992.

146. Mukherjee, R., Davies, P. J., Crombie, D. L., Bischoff, E. D., Cesario, R. M., Jow, L., Hamann, L. G., Boehm, M. F., Mondon, C. E., Nadzan, A. M., Paterniti, J. R., Jr., and Heyman, R. A., Sensitization of diabetic and obese mice to insulin by retinoid X receptor agonists, *Nature*, 386, 407, 1997.

147. Mulshine, J. L., De Luca, L. M., and Dedrick, R. L., Regional delivery of retinoids: a new approach to early lung cancer intervention, in *Clinical and Biological Basis of Lung Cancer Prevention*, Martinet, Y., Hirsch, F. R., Martinet, N., and Vignaud, J. M., Eds., Birkhäuser, Basel, 1998.

148. Munos-Canores, Vik, D. P., and Tack, B. F., Mapping of a retinoic acid-responsive element in the promoter region of the complement factor H gene, *J. Biol. Chem.*, 265, 20065, 1990.

149. Nagy, L., Saydak, M., Shipley, N., Lu, S., Basilion, J. P., Yan, Z. H., Syka, P., Chandraratna, R. A., Stein, J. P., Heyman, R. A., and Davies, P. J., Identification and characterization of a versatile retinoid response element (retinoic acid receptor response element-retinoid X receptor response element) in the mouse tissue transglutaminase gene promoter, *J. Biol. Chem.*, 271, 4355, 1996.

150. Nakagawa, S., Watanabe, M., and Inoue, Y., Prominent expression of nuclear hormone receptor ROR alpha in Purkinje cells from early development, *Neurosci. Res.*, 28, 177, 1997.

151. Nakagawa, S., Watanabe, M., Isobe, T., Kondo, H., and Inoue, Y., Cytological compartmentalization in the staggerer cerebellum, as revealed by calbindin immunohistochemistry for Purkinje cells, *J. Comp. Neurol.*, 395, 112, 1998.

152. Nakshatri, H. and Bhat-Nakshatri, P., Multiple parameters determine the specificity of transcriptional response by nuclear receptors HNF-4, ARP-1, PPAR, RAR and RXR through common response elements, *Nucleic Acids Res.*, 26, 2491, 1998.

153. Napoli, J. L., Biochemical pathways of retinoid transport, metabolism, and signal transduction, *Clin. Immunol. Immunopathol.*, 80, S52, 1996.

154. Napoli, J. L., Boerman, M. H., Chai, X., Zhai, Y., and Fiorella, P. D., Enzymes and binding proteins affecting retinoic acid concentrations, *J. Steroid Biochem. Mol. Biol.*, 53, 497, 1995.

155. Narayanan, C. S., Cui, Y., Zhao, Y. Y., Zhou, J., and Kumar, A., Orphan receptor Arp-1 binds to the nucleotide sequence located between TATA box and transcriptional initiation site of the human angiotensinogen gene and reduces estrogen induced promoter activity, *Mol. Cell Endocrinol.*, 148, 79, 1999.
156. Neuman, K., Soosaar, A., Nornes, H. O., and Neuman, T., Orphan receptor COUP-TF-I antagonizes retinoic acid-induced neuronal differentiation, *J. Neurosci. Res.*, 41, 39, 1995.
157. Nishiyama, C., Hi, R., Osada, S., and Osumi, T., Functional interactions between nuclear receptors recognizing a common sequence element, the direct repeat motif spaced by one nucleotide (DR-1), *J. Biochem. (Tokyo)*, 123, 1174, 1998.
158. Nunez, S. B., Medin, J. A., Braissant, O., Kemp, L., Wahli, W., Ozato, K., and Segars, J. H., Retinoid X receptor and peroxisome proliferator-activated receptor activate an estrogen responsive gene independent of the estrogen receptor, *Mol. Cell Endocrinol.*, 127, 27, 1997.
159. Oberdick, J., Baader, S. L., and Schilling, K., From zebra stripes to postal zones: deciphering patterns of gene expression in the cerebellum, *Trends Neurosci.*, 21, 383, 1998.
160. Ogino, M., Nagata, K., Miyata, M., and Yamazoe, Y., Hepatocyte nuclear factor 4-mediated activation of rat CYP3A1 gene and its modes of modulation by apolipoprotein AI regulatory protein I and v-ErbA-related protein 3, *Arch. Biochem. Biophys.*, 362, 32, 1999.
161. Ohkura, N., Hijikuro, M., Yamamoto, A., and Miki, K., Molecular cloning of a novel thyroid/steroid receptor superfamily gene from cultured rat neuronal cells, *Biochem. Biophys. Res. Commun.*, 205, 1959, 1994.
162. Olson, J. A., Formation and Function of Vitamin A, in *Biostatins of Isoprenoid Compounds*, Vol. 2, Porter, J. W. and Spurgeon, S. L., Eds., Wiley-Interscience, New York, 1983.
163. Ong, D. E., Newcomer, M. E., and Chytil, F., Cellular retinoid-binding proteins, in *The Retinoids: Biology, Chemistry, and Medicine*, 2nd ed., Sporn, M. B., Roberts, A. B., and Goodman, D. S., Eds., Raven Press, New York, 1994.
164. Ong, D. E., Newcomer, M. E., and Chytil, F., Cellular retinoid-binding proteins, in *The Retinoids: Biology, Chemistry, and Medicine*, 2nd ed., Sporn, M. B., Roberts, A. B., and Goodman, D. S., Eds., Raven Press, New York, 1994.
165. Palmer, C. N., Hsu, M. H., Griffin, H. J., and Johnson, E. F., Novel sequence determinants in peroxisome proliferator signaling, *J. Biol. Chem.*, 270, 16114, 1995.
166. Pereira, F. A., Qiu, Y., Zhou, G., Tsai, M. J., and Tsai, S. Y., The orphan nuclear receptor COUP-TF-II is required for angiogenesis and heart development, *Genes Dev.*, 13, 1037, 1999.
167. Perlmann, T. and Jansson, L., A novel pathway for vitamin A signaling mediated by RXR heterodimerization with NGFI-B and NURR1, *Genes Dev.*, 9, 769, 1995.
168. Petkovich, M., Brand, N. J., Krust, A., and Chambon, P., A human retinoic acid receptor which belongs to the family of nuclear receptors, *Nature*, 330, 444, 1987.
169. Piao, Y. S., Peltoketo, H., Oikarinen, J., and Vihko, R., Coordination of transcription of the human 17 beta-hydroxysteroid dehydrogenase type 1 gene (EDH17B2) by a cell-specific enhancer and a silencer: identification of a retinoic acid response element, *Mol. Endocrinol.*, 9, 1633, 1995.

170. Pieri, I., Klein, M., Bayertz, C., Gerspach, J., van der Ploeg, P. A., Pfizenmaier, K., and Eisel, U., Regulation of the murine NMDA-receptor-subunit NR2C promoter by Sp1 and fushi tarazu factor1 (FTZ-F1) homologues, *Eur. J. Neurosci.*, 11, 2083, 1999.

171. Pikarsky, E., Sharir, H., Ben Shushan, E., and Bergman, Y., Retinoic acid represses Oct-3/4 gene expression through several retinoic acid-responsive elements located in the promoter-enhancer region, *Mol. Cell Biol.*, 14, 1026, 1994.

172. Pipaon, C., Tsai, S. Y., and Tsai, M. J., COUP-TF upregulates NGFI-A gene expression through an Sp1 binding site, *Mol. Cell Biol.*, 19, 2734, 1999.

173. Power, S. C. and Cereghini, S., Positive regulation of the vHNF1 promoter by the orphan receptors COUP- TF1/Ear3 and COUP-TF-II/Arp1, *Mol. Cell Biol.*, 16, 778, 1996.

174. Puzianowska-Kuznicka, M., Damjanovski, S., and Shi, Y. B., Both thyroid hormone and 9-*cis* retinoic acid receptors are required to efficiently mediate the effects of thyroid hormone on embryonic development and specific gene regulation in *Xenopus laevis*, *Mol. Cell Biol.*, 17, 4738, 1997.

175. Quadro, L., Blaner, W. S., Salchow, D. J., Vogel, S., Piantedosi, R., Gouras, P., Freeman, S., Cosma, M. P., Colantuoni, V., and Gottesman, M. E., Impaired retinal function and vitamin A availability in mice lacking retinol-binding protein, *EMBO J.*, 18, 4633, 1999.

176. Rabelo, R., Reyes, C., Schifman, A., and Silva, J. E., A complex retinoic acid response element in the uncoupling protein gene defines a novel role for retinoids in thermogenesis, *Endocrinology*, 137, 3488, 1996.

177. Raisher, B. D., Gulick, T., Zhang, Z., Strauss, A. W., Moore, D. D., and Kelly, D. P., Identification of a novel retinoid-responsive element in the promoter region of the medium chain acyl-coenzyme A dehydrogenase gene, *J. Biol. Chem.*, 267, 20264, 1992.

178. Ribeiro, A., Pastier, D., Kardassis, D., Chambaz, J., and Cardot, P., Cooperative binding of upstream stimulatory factor and hepatic nuclear factor 4 drives the transcription of the human apolipoprotein A-II gene, *J. Biol. Chem.*, 274, 1216, 1999.

179. Richard, S. and Zingg, H. H., Identification of a retinoic acid response element in the human oxytocin promoter, *J. Biol. Chem.*, 266, 21428, 1991.

180. Rodriguez, J. C., Ortiz, J. A., Hegardt, F. G., and Haro, D., Chicken ovalbumin upstream-promoter transcription factor (COUP-TF) could act as a transcriptional activator or repressor of the mitochondrial 3-hydroxy-3-methylglutaryl-CoA synthase gene, *Biochem. J.*, 326 (Pt 2), 587, 1997.

181. Rodriguez, J. C., Ortiz, J. A., Hegardt, F. G., and Haro, D., The hepatocyte nuclear factor 4 (HNF-4) represses the mitochondrial HMG-CoA synthase gene, *Biochem. Biophys. Res. Commun.*, 242, 692, 1998.

182. Ross, S. A., McCaffery, P. J., Drager, U. C., and DeLuca, L. M., Retinoid in embryonal development, *Physiol. Revs.*, 80, 1021, 2000.

183. Rossant, J., Zirngibl, R., Cado, D., Shago, M., and Giguere, V., Expression of a retinoic acid response element-hsplacZ transgene defines specific domains of transcriptional activity during mouse embryogenesis, *Genes Dev.*, 5, 1333, 1991.

184. Rouet, P., Raguenez, G., Ruminy, P., and Salier, J. P., An array of binding sites for hepatocyte nuclear factor 4 of high and low affinities modulates the liver-specific enhancer for the human alpha1-microglobulin/bikunin precursor, *Biochem. J.*, 334, 577, 1998.

185. Roy, B., Taneja, R., and Chambon, P., Synergistic activation of retinoic acid (RA)-responsive genes and induction of embryonal carcinoma cell differentiation by an RA receptor alpha (RAR alpha)-, RAR beta-, or RAR gamma-selective ligand in combination with a retinoid X receptor-specific ligand, *Mol. Cell Biol.*, 15, 6481, 1995.

186. Ruiz, A., Winston, A., Lim, Y. H., Gilbert, B. A., Rando, R. R., and Bok, D., Molecular and biochemical characterization of lecithin retinol acyltransferase, *J. Biol. Chem.*, 274, 3834, 1999.

187. Sacchetti, P., Brownschidle, L. A., Granneman, J. G., and Bannon, M. J., Characterization of the 5'-flanking region of the human dopamine transporter gene, *Brain Res. Mol. Brain Res.*, 74, 167, 1999.

188. Sakurada, K., Ohshima-Sakurada, M., Palmer, T. D., and Gage, F. H., Nurr1, an orphan nuclear receptor, is a transcriptional activator of endogenous tyrosine hydroxylase in neural progenitor cells derived from the adult brain, *Development*, 126, 4017, 1999.

189. Samad, T. A., Krezel, W., Chambon, P., and Borrelli, E., Regulation of dopaminergic pathways by retinoids: activation of the D2 receptor promoter by members of the retinoic acid receptor-retinoid X receptor family, *Proc. Natl. Acad. Sci. USA*, 94, 14349, 1997.

190. Saucedo-Cardenas, O. and Conneely, O. M., Comparative distribution of NURR1 and NUR77 nuclear receptors in the mouse central nervous system, *J. Mol. Neurosci.*, 7, 51, 1996.

191. Schaeren-Wiemers, N., Andre, E., Kapfhammer, J. P., and Becker-Andre, M., The expression pattern of the orphan nuclear receptor RORbeta in the developing and adult rat nervous system suggests a role in the processing of sensory information and in circadian rhythm, *Eur. J. Neurosci.*, 9, 2687, 1997.

192. Schoonjans, K., Staels, B., and Auwerx, J., The peroxisome proliferator activated receptors (PPARs) and their effects on lipid metabolism and adipocyte differentiation, *Biochim. Biophys. Acta*, 1302, 93, 1996.

193. Schraeder, M., Danielsson, C., Wiesenberg, I., and Carlberg, C., Identification of natural monomeric response elements of the nuclear receptor RZR/ROR: interference with COUP-TF, *J. Biol. Chem.*, 271, 19732, 1996.

194. Schuh, T. J. and Kimelman, D., COUP-TF-I is a potential regulator of retinoic acid-modulated development in *Xenopus* embryos, *Mech. Dev.*, 51, 39, 1995.

195. Schulman, I. G., Shao, G., and Heyman, R. A., Transactivation by retinoid X receptor-peroxisome proliferator- activated receptor gamma (PPARgamma) heterodimers: intermolecular synergy requires only the PPARgamma hormone-dependent activation function, *Mol. Cell Biol.*, 18, 3483, 1998.

196. Scott, D. K., Mitchell, J. A., and Granner, D. K., Identification and characterization of the second retinoic acid response element in the phosphoenolpyruvate carboxykinase gene promoter, *J. Biol. Chem.*, 271, 6260, 1996.

197. Shankar, S. and De Luca, L. M., Retinoic acid supplementation of a vitamin A deficient diet inhibits retinoid loss from hamster liver and serum pools, *J. Nutr.*, 118, 675, 1988.

198. Shibata, H., Nawaz, Z., Tsai, S. Y., O'Malley, B. W., and Tsai, M. J., Gene silencing by chicken ovalbumin upstream promoter-transcription factor I (COUP-TF-I) is mediated by transcriptional corepressors, nuclear receptor-corepressor (N-CoR) and silencing mediator for retinoic acid receptor and thyroid hormone receptor (SMRT), *Mol. Endocrinol.*, 11, 714, 1997.

199. Sladek, F. M., Orphan receptor HNF-4 and liver-specific gene expression [published erratum appears in *Receptor,* 1994 Spring; 4(1):following 63], *Receptor,* 3, 223, 1993.
200. Sladek, R. and Giguere, V., Orphan nuclear receptors: an emerging family of metabolic regulators, *Adv. Pharmacol.,* 47, 23, 2000.
201. Sluder, A. E., Mathews, S. W., Hough, D., Yin, V. P., and Maina, C. V., The nuclear receptor superfamily has undergone extensive proliferation and diversification in nematodes, *Genome Res.,* 9, 103, 1999.
202. Song, M. R., Lee, S. K., Seo, Y. W., Choi, H. S., Lee, J. W., and Lee, M. O., Differential modulation of transcriptional activity of oestrogen receptors by direct protein-protein interactions with retinoid receptors, *Biochem. J.,* 336, 711, 1998.
203. Soprano, D. R. and Blaner, W. S., Plasma retinol-binding protein, in *The Retinoids: Biology, Chemistry, and Medicine,* 2nd ed., Sporn, M. B., Roberts, A. B., and Goodman, D. S., Eds., Raven Press, New York, 1994.
204. Spath, G. F. and Weiss, M. C., Hepatocyte nuclear factor 4 provokes expression of epithelial marker genes, acting as a morphogen in dedifferentiated hepatoma cells, *J. Cell Biol.,* 140, 935, 1998.
205. Sporn, M. B. and Newton, D. L., Chemoprevention of cancer with retinoids, *Fed. Proc.,* 38, 2528, 1979.
206. Sporn, M. B., Roberts, A. B., and Goodman, D. S., *The Retinoids,* Academic Press, Orlando, 1984.
207. Sporn, M. B., Roberts, A. B., and Goodman, D. S., Biology, Chemistry, and Medicine, in *The Retinoids,* Raven Press, New York, 1994.
208. Stroup, D. and Chiang, J. Y., HNF4 and COUP-TF-II interact to modulate transcription of the cholesterol 7alpha-hydroxylase gene (CYP7A1), *J. Lipid Res.,* 41, 1, 2000.
209. Stroup, D., Crestani, M., and Chiang, J. Y., Orphan receptors chicken ovalbumin upstream promoter transcription factor II (COUP-TF-II) and retinoid X receptor (RXR) activate and bind the rat cholesterol 7alpha-hydroxylase gene (CYP7A), *J. Biol. Chem.,* 272, 9833, 1997.
210. Sucov, H. M., Murakami, K. K., and Evans, R. M., Characterization of an autoregulated response element in th mouse retinoic acid receptor type b gene, *Proc. Natl. Acad. Sci. USA,* 87, 5392, 1990.
211. Sugiyama, T., Wang, J. C., Scott, D. K., and Granner, D. K., Transcription activation by the orphan nuclear receptor, chicken ovalbumin upstream promoter-transcription factor I (COUP-TF-I). Definition of the domain involved in the glucocorticoid response of the phosphoenolpyruvate carboxykinase gene, *J. Biol. Chem.,* 275, 3446, 2000.
212. Suva, L. J., Towler, D. A., Harada, S., Gaub, M. P., and Rodan, G. A., Characterization of retinoic acid- and cell-dependent sequences which regulate zif268 gene expression in osteoblastic cells, *Mol. Endocrinol.,* 8, 1507, 1994.
213. Thompson, P. D., Jurutka, P. W., Haussler, C. A., Whitfield, G. K., and Haussler, M. R., Heterodimeric DNA binding by the vitamin D receptor and retinoid X receptors is enhanced by 1,25-dihydroxyvitamin D3 and inhibited by 9-*cis*-retinoic acid. Evidence for allosteric receptor interactions, *J. Biol. Chem.,* 273, 8483, 1998.

214. Tini, M., Fraser, R. A., and Giguere, V., Functional interactions between retinoic acid receptor-related orphan nuclear receptor (ROR alpha) and the retinoic acid receptors in the regulation of the gamma F-crystallin promoter, *J. Biol. Chem.*, 270, 20156, 1995.

215. Tontonoz, P., Hu, E., Devine, J., Beale, E. G., and Spiegelman, B. M., PPAR gamma 2 regulates adipose expression of the phosphoenolpyruvate carboxykinase gene, *Mol. Cell Biol.*, 15, 351, 1995.

216. Troen, G., Eskild, W., Fromm, S. H., De Luca, L. M., Ong, D. E., Wardlaw, S. A., Reppe, S., and Blomhoff, R., Vitamin A-sensitive tissues in transgenic mice expressing high levels of human cellular retinol-binding protein type i are not altered phenotypically, *J. Nutr.*, 129, 1621, 1999.

217. Tsai, S. Y. and Tsai, M. J., Chick ovalbumin upstream promoter-transcription factors (COUP-TFs): coming of age, *Endocr. Rev.*, 18, 229, 1997.

218. Umemoto, S., Kawai, Y., Ueyama, T., and Senba, E., Chronic glucocorticoid administration as well as repeated stress affects the subsequent acute immobilization stress-induced expression of immediate early genes but not that of NGFI-A, *Neuroscience*, 80, 763, 1997.

219. Umesono, K., Murakami, K. K., Thompson, C. C., and Evans, R. M., Direct repeats as selective response elements for the thyroid hormone, retinoic acid, and vitamin D3 receptors, *Cell*, 65, 1255, 1991.

220. van der Wees, W. J., Schilthuis, J. G., Koster, C. H., Diesveld-Schipper, H., Folkers, G. E., van der Saag, P. T., Dawson, M. I., Shudo, K., van der Burg, B. B., and Durston, A. J., Inhibition of retinoic acid receptor-mediated signalling alters positional identity in the developing hindbrain, *Development*, 125, 545, 1998.

221. Vasios, G. W., Gold, D. G., Petkovich, M., Chambon, P., and Gudas, L. J., A retinoic acid-responsive element is present in the 5'flanking region of the laminin B1 gene, *Proc. Natl. Acad. Sci. USA*, 86, 9099, 1989.

222. Vu-Dac, N., Schoonjans, K., Kosykh, V., Dallongeville, J., Heyman, R. A., Staels, B., and Auwerx, J., Retinoids increase human apolipoprotein A-11 expression through activation of the retinoid X receptor but not the retinoic acid receptor, *Mol. Cell Biol.*, 16, 3350, 1996.

223. Wagner, J., Akerud, P., Castro, D. S., Holm, P. C., Canals, J. M., Snyder, E. Y., Perlmann, T., and Arenas, E., Induction of a midbrain dopaminergic phenotype in Nurr1-overexpressing neural stem cells by type 1 astrocytes, *Nat. Biotechnol.*, 17, 653, 1999.

224. Waltz, S. E., Gould, F. K., Air, E. L., McDowell, S. A., and Degen, S. J., Hepatocyte nuclear factor-4 is responsible for the liver-specific expression of the gene coding for hepatocyte growth factor-like protein, *J. Biol. Chem.*, 271, 9024, 1996.

225. Warrell, R. P., Jr., de The, H., Wang, Z. Y., and Degos, L., Acute promyelocytic leukemia, *N. Engl. J. Med.*, 329, 177, 1993.

226. Weis, K., Rambaud, S., Lavau, C., Jansen, J., Carvalho, T., Carmo-Fonseca, M., Lamond, A., and Dejean, A., Retinoic acid regulates aberrant nuclear localization of PML-RAR alpha in acute promyelocytic leukemia cells, *Cell*, 76, 345, 1994.

227. Westin, S., Kurokawa, R., Nolte, R. T., Wisely, G. B., McInerney, E. M., Rose, D. W., Milburn, M. V., Rosenfeld, M. G., and Glass, C. K., Interactions controlling the assembly of nuclear-receptor heterodimers and co-activators, *Nature*, 395, 199, 1998.

228. White, J. A., Beckett-Jones, B., Guo, Y. D., Dilworth, F. J., Bonasoro, J., Jones, G., and Petkovich, M., cDNA cloning of human retinoic acid-metabolizing enzyme (hP450RAI) identifies a novel family of cytochromes P450, *J. Biol. Chem.*, 272, 18538, 1997.

229. Williams, G. R., Harney, J. W., Moore, D. D., Larsen, P. R., and Brent, G. A., Differential capacity of wild type promoter elements for binding and trans-activation by retinoic acid and thyroid hormone receptors, *Mol. Endocrinol.*, 6, 1527, 1992.

230. Willy, P. J., Umesono, K., Ong, E. S., Evans, R. M., Heyman, R. A., and Man-gelsdorf, D. J., LXR, a nuclear receptor that defines a distinct retinoid response pathway, *Genes Dev.*, 9, 1033, 1995.

231. Wolf, G., Multiple functions of vitamin A, *Physiol. Rev.*, 64, 873, 1984.

232. Wolf, G. and De Luca, L. M., Recent studies on some metabolic functions of vitamin A, in *Fat Soluble Vitamin Symposium*, De Luca, H. F. and Suttie, J. W., Eds., University of Wisconsin Press, Madison, 1970.

233. Woronicz, J. D., Calnan, B., Ngo, V., and Winoto, A., Requirement for the orphan steroid receptor Nur77 in apoptosis of T-cell hybridomas, *Nature*, 367, 277, 1994.

234. Wu, Q., Li, Y., Liu, R., Agadir, A., Lee, M. O., Liu, Y., and Zhang, X., Modulation of retinoic acid sensitivity in lung cancer cells through dynamic balance of orphan receptors nur77 and COUP-TF and their heterodimerization, *EMBO J.*, 16, 1656, 1997.

235. Xing, G., Zhang, L., Zhang, L., Heynen, T., Li, X. L., Smith, M. A., Weiss, S. R., Feldman, A. N., Detera-Wadleigh, S., Chuang, D. M., and Post, R. M., Rat nurr1 is prominently expressed in perirhinal cortex, and differentially induced in the hippocampal dentate gyrus by electroconvulsive vs. kindled seizures, *Brain Res. Mol. Brain Res.*, 47, 251, 1997.

236. Yamagata, K., Furuta, H., Oda, N., Kaisaki, P. J., Menzel, S., Cox, N. J., Fajans, S. S., Signorini, S., Stoffel, M., and Bell, G. I., Mutations in the hepatocyte nuclear factor-4alpha gene in maturity-onset diabetes of the young (MODY1), *Nature*, 384, 458, 1996.

237. Yamamoto, M., Drager, U. C., and McCaffery, P., A novel assay for retinoic acid catabolic enzymes shows high expression in the developing hindbrain, *Brain Res. Dev. Brain Res.*, 107, 103, 1998.

238. Yamamoto, M., Drager, U. C., Ong, D. E., and McCaffery, P., Retinoid-binding proteins in the cerebellum and choroid plexus and their relationship to region-alized retinoic acid synthesis and degradation, *Eur. J. Biochem.*, 257, 344, 1998.

239. Yamamoto, M., Fujinuma, M., Tanaka, M., Drager, U. C., and McCaffery, P., Sagittal band expression of COUP-TF2 gene in the developing cerebellum, *Mech. Dev.*, 84, 143, 1999.

240. Yamamoto, M., Ullman, D., Drager, U. C., and McCaffery, P., Postnatal effects of retinoic acid on cerebellar development, *Neurotoxicol. Teratol.*, 21, 141, 1999.

241. Yanai, K., Hirota, K., Taniguchi-Yanai, K., Shigematsu, Y., Shimamoto, Y., Saito, T., Chowdhury, S., Takiguchi, M., Arakawa, M., Nibu, Y., Sugiyama, F., Yagami, K., and Fukamizu, A., Regulated expression of human angiotensinogen gene by hepatocyte nuclear factor 4 and chicken ovalbumin upstream promoter-transcription factor, *J. Biol. Chem.*, 274, 34605, 1999.

242. Yokomori, N., Nishio, K., Aida, K., and Negishi, M., Transcriptional regulation by HNF-4 of the steroid 15alpha-hydroxylase P450 (Cyp2a-4) gene in mouse liver, *J. Steroid Biochem. Mol. Biol.*, 62, 307, 1997.

243. Yoon, J. K. and Lau, L. F., Transcriptional activation of the inducible nuclear receptor gene nur77 by nerve growth factor and membrane depolarization in PC12 cells, *J. Biol. Chem.*, 268, 9148, 1993.

244. Zechel, C., Shen, X. Q., Chen, J. Y., Chen, Z. P., Chambon, P., and Gronemeyer, H., The dimerization interfaces formed between the DNA binding domains of RXR, RAR and TR determine the binding specificity and polarity of the full-length receptors to direct repeats, *EMBO J.*, 13, 1425, 1994.

245. Zeitoun, K., Takayama, K., Michael, M. D., and Bulun, S. E., Stimulation of aromatase P450 promoter (II) activity in endometriosis and its inhibition in endometrium are regulated by competitive binding of steroidogenic factor-1 and chicken ovalbumin upstream promoter transcription factor to the same *cis*-acting element, *Mol. Endocrinol.*, 13, 239, 1999.

246. Zetterstrom, R. H., Solomin, L., Jansson, L., Hoffer, B. J., Olson, L., and Perlmann, T., Dopamine neuron agenesis in Nurr1-deficient mice, *Science*, 276, 248, 1997.

247. Zhou, C., Qiu, Y., Pereira, F. A., Crair, M. C., Tsai, S. Y., and Tsai, M. J., The nuclear orphan receptor COUP-TF-I is required for differentiation of subplate neurons and guidance of thalamocortical axons, *Neuron*, 24, 847, 1999.

14

Vitamin A and Mitochondrial Gene Expression

Helen B. Everts and Carolyn D. Berdanier

CONTENTS

14.1 Introduction 321
14.2 Mitochondrial Structure and Function..323
14.3 Oxidative Phosphorylation and the Mitochondrial Genome 324
14.4 Retinoic Acid (RA) and Mitochondrial Gene Expression...................329
14.5 Mitochondrial Gene Transcription...331
14.6 Conclusions...336
References 336

14.1 Introduction

Mitochondria are the central integrators of intermediary metabolism. Key metabolic pathways located in this organelle are the β-oxidation pathway, the TCA cycle (tricarboxylic acid cycle, Kebs cycle, citric acid cycle), and oxidative phosphorylation (OXPHOS). Mitochondria contain their own DNA (mtDNA). This deoxyribonucleic acid (DNA) encodes 13 of the 76 subunits of OXPHOS. The size of the mtDNA can vary from ~16 kb in mammals to over 300 kb in flowering plants. It is believed that originally the mtDNA contained all of the genetic information for the components needed for OXPHOS, but over time most of these genes were transferred to the nucleus.

The mtDNA has been completely sequenced and mapped for a wide variety of species including man, mouse, and rat. Shown in Fig. 14.1 is the human mt genome with each of the structural genes, the transfer ribonucleic acid (tRNAs), and the ribosomes indicated. This DNA encodes 13

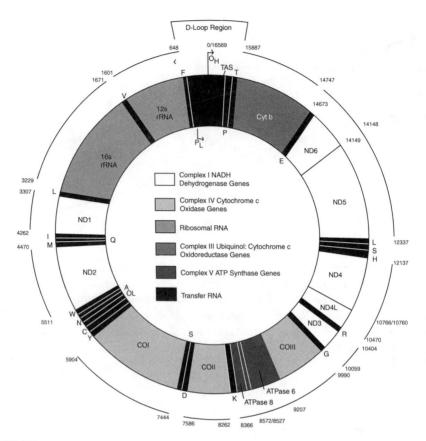

FIGURE 14.1
The human mitochondrial genome. ND1-6 = Complex I, NADH dehydrogenase genes; Cyt b
= cytochrome b, complex III, ubiquinol; Cytochrome-c oxidoreductase gene; COI-III = complex
IV, Cytochrome-c oxidase genes; ATPase 6 and 8 = Complex V, ATP synthase genes; rRNA =
ribosomal RNA; tRNA genes are listed by their single letter amino acid name. The displacement
loop (D-loop) region is indicated. P_H and P_L = promoters for the heavy and light strands; O_H
and O_L = origins of replication for the heavy and light strands, respectively.

polypeptides, 22 transfer RNAs, and 2 ribosomal RNAs. Also shown is the
D-loop which is thought to be the promoter region for most of the
genome. The regulation of its expression is only now being investigated.
Some of the steroid hormones, thyroid hormone, insulin, and retinoic acid
probably play as important a role in the expression of the mt genome as
occurs in the expression of the nuclear genome. Evidence is only now
accumulating on the roles these compounds play in mt gene expression.
In Chapter 13 of this volume is a review of the role of retinoic acid in
nuclear gene expression.[1] In this chapter, the role of retinoic acid in mt
gene expression will be described.

14.2 Mitochondrial Structure and Function

Mitochondria vary in size and shape in different cell types. Regardless of size and shape, this organelle consists of two membranes separated by an inner membrane space. The outer membrane encloses the organelle, while the inner membrane is folded into cristae. Within the cristae is the matrix. The components of OXPHOS are embedded in the inner mitochondrial membrane. This is illustrated in Fig. 14.2. The number of mitochondria within a cell can vary from a few hundred to several thousand. Their shape varies as well: They can be round or oblong, fat or slim. In brown fat cells, mitochondria are plentiful; in white fat cells, they are not. Mitochondria can be distributed by cytoskeleton motors throughout the cell in a non-random order or localized near other organelles that have a high adenine triphosphate (ATP)

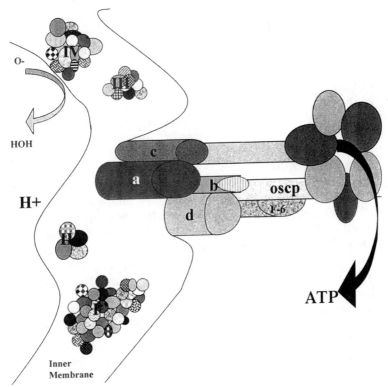

FIGURE 14.2
Schematic representation of the four respiratory complexes and the F_1F_0ATPase (complex 5). Each of the complexes have a number of subunits. Those encoded by the mitochondrial genome are shown as black; the nuclear encoded units are shaded. Note that the F_1 portion of the ATPase projects out into the matrix.

requirement. Electron microscopy studies have shown clusters of mitochondria near the ribosomes in cells undergoing high rates of protein synthesis. Clusters of mitochondria have also been found in muscle near the contracting fibers. In each instance it is supposed that these mitochondria are providing the needed ATP to support the local process. In the former, the process is protein biosynthesis; in the latter, it is muscle work.

Mitochondrial function depends not only on the metabolic fuels needed for the support of the TCA cycle and OXPHOS and on the proteins encoded by the nuclear genome and imported into the mitochondrial compartment, but also by the transcription and translation of the mt genome. This coordination of gene expression in these two organelles is of particular interest to those interested in OXPHOS.

14.3 Oxidative Phosphorylation and the Mitochondrial Genome

The mechanism of OXPHOS has been extensively reviewed.[2–21] Electrons shuttled into the mitochondrial compartment by the nicotinamide dinucleotide (NAD)-linked and flavinadinine dinucleotide (FAD)-linked shuttles are transported through inner membrane-bound respiratory chain enzyme complexes and joined to oxygen to form water. This process is linked to the formation of ATP by the $F_1F_0ATPase$. The coupled processes for water and ATP synthesis are called OXPHOS.

Mitchell in 1961 proposed that the sequential reactions of the respiratory chain generate an electrochemical gradient of H^+ ions across the inner mitochondrial membrane.[8] The energy of this gradient is captured by the F_0 portion of the $F_1F_0ATPase$ and transmitted to the F_1 portion that uses it to synthesize ATP. The newly synthesized ATP is released in the matrix only to be captured by the adenine nucleotide translocase and translocated to the cytosol. Translocation does not account for all of the ATP produced by the $F_1F_0ATPase$. Some of the newly synthesized ATP is used directly by reactions in the mitochondria. In addition, OXPHOS is not very efficient in this energy capture. Most of the energy is released as heat. The proportion of the energy released as heat vs. that used for ATP synthesis varies with the physiological and nutritional state of the animal. Under a variety of conditions (stress, cold, overeating) cells will release proteins called uncoupling proteins (UCPs). These proteins serve to dissipate the proton gradient generated by the respiratory chain such that little of the energy is converted to the high energy bond of ATP. Heat production is thus increased when UCPs are produced. The actions of the UCPs with respect to energy metabolism are reviewed by Collins et al. in this volume.[19]

In addition to those conditions that stimulate UCP production, there are dietary conditions that affect the fluidity of the inner mitochondrial membrane.

Animals fed diets containing hydrogenated coconut oil have less fluid membranes than animals fed diets containing unsaturated fatty acids, i.e., corn oil or fish oil.[20] Changing the fluidity of the inner membrane changes the environment in which the ATPase functions. The ATPase must be able to rotate within the membrane[9,13,18] and the more fluid the membrane, the greater the efficiency of OXPHOS.

There are four complexes that make up the respiratory chain and one complex, the F_1F_0ATPase, for ATP synthesis. These are as follows: nicotinamide dinucleotide, reduced (NADH)-ubiquinone (complex I) is the site of entry for NADH protons into the chain. NADH is oxidized, ubiquinone reduced and four protons are pumped from the mitochondrial matrix to the intermembrane space. In mammals there are at least 42 subunits in this complex, seven of which are encoded on mtDNA (ND1, 2, 3, 4, 4L, 5, and 6). Succinate:ubiquinone oxidoreductase (complex II) is the site of entry for $FADH_2$ protons into the chain via ubiquinone. It contains 4 subunits, all of which are nuclear encoded in mammals. No protons are pumped at this site. Ubiquinone-cytochrome-c oxidoreductase or the bc_1/ cytochrome-c reductase (complex III) accepts electrons from ubiquinone. In this reaction, ubiquinone is oxidized, electrons are transferred to cytochrome b then c_1 and four protons are pumped into the intermitochondrial space. This complex contains 11 subunits in mammals, one of which (cytochrome b) is encoded by mtDNA. Cytochrome-c oxidase (complex IV) accepts electrons through the soluble cytochrome-c and transfers them to oxygen. This process pumps four protons into the intermitochondrial space. In mammals, this complex contains 13 subunits, three of which (COX I, II, III) are encoded on mtDNA.

The pumping of protons into the intermembrane space creates a protomotive force that consists of a proton gradient and a membrane potential. This protomotive force is then used by F_1F_0ATPase, the ATP synthase or complex V to form ATP. If mutations occur in any one of the mt genes that encode any of these proteins then oxidative phosphorylation will be compromised. If the compromise is of sufficient magnitude then noticeable clinical conditions will develop. Mitochondrial diseases due to mutations in the mt DNA have been reviewed extensively in the clinical literature.[22-91] Point mutations, deletions, and duplications of this mitochondrial DNA (mtDNA) result in a variety of diseases. These diseases are degenerative in nature, maternally transmitted,[80] and all can be explained by an ATP shortfall in one or more tissues. Some of the diseases are devastating and are of early onset whereas others may take decades to develop clinical symptoms. Included in this list are diabetes, Alzheimer's disease, Parkinson's disease, and a variety of diseases involving the central nervous system, muscles, and the vital organs.

Leber's hereditary optic neuropathy (LHON) was one of the first diseases to be associated with mtDNA mutations.[22,23] LHON is a degenerative disease of the optic nerve that results in blindness between the ages of 15 and 35. This disease can be the result of a single point mutation or a combination of point mutations in one of several protein coding genes of mtDNA. The majority of these are in subunits of NADH dehydrogenase complex I-ubiquinone. In general terms, the single point mutations are in triplets that encode evolutionarily conserved amino acids in or near the active site of the enzyme, while mutations that need to be combined occur outside the active site and are less detrimental to enzyme function.

Mutations in the highly conserved leucine (nucleotide 8993) of the ATPase 6 gene can result in either neuropathy, ataxia, and retinitis pigmentosa (NARP)[24] or the more serious maternally inherited Leigh's syndrome (MILS).[25–28] Patients with this mutation are highly variable in the severity of retinitis pigmentosa and neurological manifestations. In extreme cases, severe infantile lactate acidosis and death before the age of one can occur.[27] This mutation is in the proton channel of subunit a of the F_0ATPase, near R210. Studies in lymphoblast mitochondria[29] and digitonized fibroblasts and leukocytes[27] from these patients revealed that ATP synthesis is reduced up to 50%. Oligomycin sensitive ATPase activity is also reduced.[29] In addition, subunit-b protein levels were reduced and subunit-c protein levels increased in heart and muscle, suggesting alterations in F_0-complex assembly with this mutation.[27] Through the technology of transferring mutant mitochondria into cells depleted of mtDNA and the formation of cybrids[92,93] it was shown that the T8993G mutation in the ATPase 6 gene is associated with decreased state 3 respiration and the ADP:O ratio.[81] Also, a similar mutation in *E. coli*[94] resulted in a profound inhibition of proton translocation through F_1F_0ATP synthase, reduced OXPHOS activity, and altered F_1F_0ATPase assembly or stability. A recent study found that the T8993G mutation altered catalysis rather than enzyme assembly or stability.[95]

The mutation at 8993 has also been found in patients with hypertrophic cardiomyopathy.[30] In these patients, point mutations were seen in most of the protein coding genes, as well as in tRNA and rRNA genes. Mutations in the tRNA for lysine have been associated with myoclonic epilepsy and ragged-red fiber disease (MERRF).[31,32] Mutations in the tRNA for leucine (UUR) have been shown to result in several different diseases including MERRF, mitochondrial encephalomyopathy with lactic acidosis and strokelike episodes (MELAS),[33,34] progressive kidney disease,[35] and maternally inherited diabetes and deafness (MIDD).[36,37]

A number of mutations in the mt genome can phenotype as diabetes mellitus.[36–71,86] In some cases the diabetes feature is secondary to more serious defects in CNS function or the neuromuscular system. In other instances the diabetes phenotype is the primary feature. In all cases the clinical condition of aberrant glucose homeostasis can be explained by the failure of the mitochondria to appropriately complete the oxidation of glucose to CO_2 and water with the production of ATP. Critical cells such as the pancreatic islet β cells thus experience an ATP production shortfall with the result of not only impaired glucose metabolism but also impaired insulin synthesis and release. These are the hallmarks of the diabetic state. Individuals with mt mutations typically have elevated blood lactate levels and redox states, again indicating aberrant mitochondrial metabolism that can be correlated with aberrant glucose metabolism.

Mitochondrial disease can also result from depletion, deletions, and duplications of the mitochondrial genome.[24,60,72–89] The classic example of this is seen in patients with Kearns-Sayre syndrome (KSS).[75] This is a multiorgan disease of the eye, heart, and/or brain.

Through this review of mitochondrial diseases it is seen that one disease can be the result of several independent mtDNA mutations and one mtDNA mutation can cause several different diseases. All of these diseases relate to the need for ATP generated by OXPHOS. An error or mutation in any of the genes that encode components of this system results in an ATP synthesis shortfall. In turn, this depends on where in the DNA sequence the mutation occurs. Mutations distal to the active site of the translation product will be less serious in terms of the function of that product than mutation in the DNA at or near the active site. ATP synthesis can be mildly, modestly, or severely affected depending on the mutation site. Those tissues that are highly dependent on ATP, i.e., neural cells, will have their functional capacity seriously impaired whereas adipose cells or liver cells having the same mutation burden might be more able to accommodate this mutation in the heteroplasmic state. Thus, the severity of the symptoms are related to the location of the mutation, the percent of the mutated DNA, and the dependence of each of the affected cell types on its ATP supply.

In addition, the multiplicity of disease states is attributed to the unique character of mtDNA. There are thousands of mitochondria within a cell and each mitochondrion contains 8 to 10 copies of mtDNA. Both mutant and wild type mtDNA can exist within a given cell. This phenomenon is called heteroplasmy. When a cell contains all mutant or all wild type mtDNA it is a homeoplasmic cell. It should be noted that individual cell heteroplasmy, may not be reflected by mean tissue heteroplasmy making the link between percent heteroplasmy and phenotypic expression complicated. Also, in dividing cells, selection occurs against cells with a high percent of mutant mtDNA.[72–77,79] In addition, the proportion of mutant mtDNAs can change over time such that a heteroplasmic mutation drifts towards homeoplasmy.[79] This is more of a problem in terminally differentiated cells (i.e., neurons) where rates of cell division cannot select against high percent mutant mtDNA cells and overcome this problem. Also, the inheritance of mutant vs. wild type mtDNA is random.[77,78] Thus, a pedigree can occur with family members containing various degrees of heteroplasmy and various phenotypes.

In addition to heteroplasmic mutations, homeoplasmic mutations have also been associated with mitochondrial disease. Diabetes has been reported as a homoplasmic mutation in two locations in the BHE/Cdb rat.[50,51] The diabetes is quite mild and results from a reduction (~20%) in ATP synthesis efficiency due to two mutations in the ATPase 6 gene. One of these is in the portion of the molecule that forms the proton channel while the other is in the hinge region. The latter has effects on the mobility of the subunit within the inner mitochondrial membrane whereas the former affects the ATPase function with respect to the proton channel.

Typically, heteroplasmic mutations are in highly conserved nucleotides in the active site of the enzyme or tRNA. These mutations would be lethal if homeoplasmic. In contrast, homeoplasmic mutations usually occur in less conserved nucleotides outside of the active site of the enzyme or tRNA. They are thought to result in milder OXPHOS defects and a late onset of disease. One example of this is the tRNA^{Gln} A4336G mutation associated with late-onset Alzheimer's disease and Parkinson's disease.[82,97] This nucleotide is outside the active site of the tRNA^{Gln} and is only moderately conserved throughout evolution.

Another feature of mitochondrial genetics is the threshold effect: Clinical disease occurs when mitochondrial energy output falls below some minimum threshold level. This effect has been extended to the theory that a threshold level of mutant mtDNA must exist in a cell before it can affect OXPHOS and therefore clinical disease, or severity of disease. A classical example of this is the 8993 mutation in the ATPase 6 gene.[25–27,29,78] When this mutation is present in less than 90% of mtDNA it phenotypes as NARP, but when present at greater than 90% mutant mtDNA the much more serious maternally inherited Leigh's syndrome (MILS) develops. Recently, this theory was supported by evidence that a threshold exists between % wild-type ND5 mtDNA and rotenone (complex I)-sensitive respiration.[96] In addition, it was found that (1) % wild-type ND5 DNA directly correlated to % wild-type ND5 mRNA suggesting that no compensatory upregulation of transcription or mRNA stability occurred; (2) 60 % of the normal level of wild-type mRNA was adequate to maintain normal ND5 protein synthesis; and (3) ND5 protein synthesis is near rate-limiting for complex I-dependent respiration. The results of this study suggested that the threshold effects occurred at the level of protein synthesis. It also suggested that the regulation of ND5 gene expression is an important factor in the regulation of complex I-dependent respiration.

It has also been suggested that degrees of heteroplasmy can be different between tissues leading to different phenotypes of the same genotype. This is one explanation given for the various phenotypes seen with the 3243 mutation in the tRNA$^{Leu(UUR)}$ gene. While it has been argued that other factors besides the tRNA$^{Leu(UUR)}$ mutation[98,99] contribute to the different phenotypes, extensive data point to this mutation as the sole cause of the disease in these patients.[54,56] Defects in mitochondrial protein synthesis and respiration occur in cybrids with mitochondria from patients carrying this mutation.[32,92,93] This mutation can be suppressed by a mutation in the anticodon of tRNA$^{Leu(CUN)}$ that enables it to decode UUR leucine.[96] In addition, when cybrids were compared between patients with the tRNA$^{Leu(UUR)}$ mutation genotype and MIDD vs. those with progressive kidney disease phenotypes, there was no difference in mitochondrial function, suggesting that haplotype played no role in determining phenotype.[69] Also, they found differences in the % heteroplasmy between the two distinct phenotypes. Tissue-specific threshold effects were also seen in mice who had the *Tfam* gene disrupted in heart and muscle.[96] (*Tfam* is the gene for mitochondrial transcription factor A and affects mtDNA and mtRNA levels (discussed later in depth).) This disruption produced levels of mtRNA and mtDNA that were 29 and 26% of the normal level in heart and 66 and 60% in the skeletal muscle. Only the heart had decreased ATPase-8 protein levels, and decreased respiration that lead to dilated cardiomyopathy and atrioventricular conduction blocks. Skeletal muscle had normal ATPase-8 protein levels, normal respiration, and normal morphology. This again highlights the importance of mitochondrial gene expression in the regulation of respiration and expression of mitochondrial disease.

Tissue-specific effects can also be due to different biochemical thresholds and ATP needs. Rossignol et al.[87] have shown in isolated mitochondria that different complexes within different tissues have different thresholds. For example, 60% of ATP synthase activity needs to be inhibited in brain mitochondria for respiration to be affected. But more inhibition of ATP synthase needs to occur in kidney, even more in liver, more in muscle, and yet more in heart. In contrast, inhibition of complex IV affects muscle = heart > liver > kidney = brain. Thus, the same mutation would have a very different effect on respiration in different tissues, resulting in different phenotypes. *In vivo*, different tissues can also have different thresholds due to their different respiration needs.[22,32,33,44,56,72,76–78] In this respect, brain (and optic nerve) > skeletal muscle > cardiac muscle > kidney >liver.

Thus, it is clear that mitochondrial genetics is much more complicated than nuclear genetics. The phenotypic expression of a mitochondrial mutant genotype depends on the degree of cellular heteroplasmy, tissue-specific heteroplasmy, and threshold effects due to tissue–enzyme complex interactions and tissue needs for ATP. Environmental factors, such as diet, can also play a role by altering mitochondrial mutation rate and mitochondrial gene expression. In part, nutrients can affect mitochondrial gene expression and in part can affect the environment in which the gene product functions. An example of the latter is the effect of dietary fat on the composition and fluidity of the inner mitochondrial membrane.[20] In this example, a saturated dietary fat diet reduces inner membrane fluidity and this reduction impairs the movement of the F_1F_0ATPase, reducing its efficiency in trapping the energy generated by the respiratory chain into the high energy bond of ATP. Hence, such saturated fat diets reduce OXPHOS efficiency. An example of the former is the effect retinoic acid has on mtDNA transcription.

14.4 Retinoic Acid (RA) and Mitochondrial Gene Expression

The discovery of the nuclear retinoic acid receptors, RAR and RXR, that were similar to the nuclear receptors for the steroid hormones suggested that retinoic acid could have a role in gene expression. These receptor proteins bind both retinoic acid and DNA thus playing an active role in regulating nuclear gene expression. This role is described in Chapter 13.[1]

Three genes for each of the receptors, RAR and RXR, α, β, γ have been found.[100–103] Each gene has several isoforms that arise from either different promoter usage or alternative splicing.[101–107] The differences between the receptors occur in their N-terminal region.[104,106] In addition, they have different expression patterns in both the embryo and the adult. Their synthesis and activation are regulated differently by vitamin A.[107,108] In vitamin A-deficient rats, mRNA for RAR-β is decreased with no effect on mRNA for either RARα or RARγ in lung, liver, and intestine. In the testes, $RAR\alpha_2$ expression was higher in retinol-deficient rats than retinol-sufficient rats, and this expression increased with RA feeding. RA also increased $RAR\alpha_2$ expression in the embryo. In addition, RA upregulates $RAR\alpha_1$ mRNA in the adult testes, but not lung, liver, intestine. $RAR\gamma_2$, $RAR\beta_1$, and $RAR\beta_2$ were also upregulated by RA in adult lung, liver, intestine but not testes. Embryonic tissue had a different response: RA upregulated embryonic RARα, $RAR\beta_1$, and $RAR\beta_2$ but had no effect on $RAR\gamma_2$.[105,108] The complex distribution and regulation of these receptor isoforms have led to the hypothesis that each isoform has a specific function. Studies with isoform specific null mutant mice have found that while all of the signs of vitamin A deficiency are also seen in the combination of RAR/RXR single or double null mutant mice, some redundancy does occur.[105,108–114] In some cells single-receptor isoform mutations had little or no apparent effect. This argues against the hypothesis that each receptor isoform has a unique function. These studies suggest that while we still don't know the exact function of each isoform, it is clear that RAR/RXRs play a critical role in the function of vitamin A.

Countless genes have been shown to be regulated by retinoic acid. Studies with RXRα[-/-] knockout mice have revealed that several genes involved in energy production are regulated during embryonic heart development and that RXRα is essential for energy production in the embryonic heart.[115] Mitochondrial gene expression and mitochondrial function are abnormal in these knockout mice.

Mitochondrially encoded genes have been shown to be regulated by retinoic acid. These include subunit 5 NADH dehydrogenase,[116] subunit I cytochrome-c oxidase,[117] and 16srRNA[115] and the ATPase 6 gene.[118] We have found retinoic acid receptors in the mitochondrial compartment using western blot analysis (Fig. 14.3). Antibodies against RAR β,γ-1, and γ-2 bound proteins isolated from the mitochondrial compartment.[119] However, no such reaction was found with RARα antibodies. The presence of the RARs in the mitochondrial compartment suggests that retinoic acid could have transcriptional effects with respect to mtDNA and, indeed, we have found this to be the case.

Other nutrients and hormones in addition to retinoic acid may also be involved in regulating the transcription of mtDNA. These are thought to exert some "local tuning" to the transcription process. Included in this list are thyroid hormone, insulin, vitamin D, and the glucocorticoids. All of these compounds act via their cognate receptors and all (except for the insulin receptor) of these receptors belong to a family called the steroid superfamily of receptors. A discussion of mitochondrial gene transcription follows.

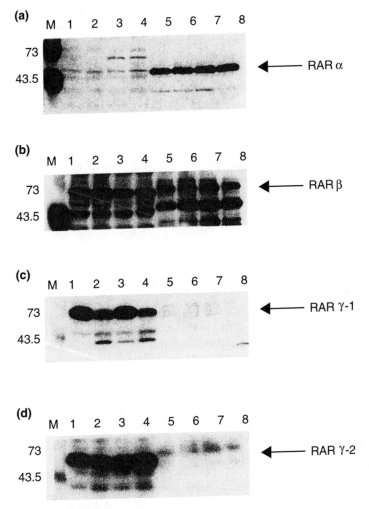

FIGURE 14.3
Western blot analysis of the retinoic acid receptors in the nucleus and the mitochondrial compartment. Cell fractions were prepared from the livers of BHE/Cdb and Sprague Dawley rats. Lanes 1, 2, 5, 6 were from BHE/Cdb rats; lanes 3, 4, 7, 8 were from Sprague Dawley rats; lanes 1 to 4 were proteins from the mitochondria; lanes 5 to 8 were proteins from the nucleus. The proteins were separated on a 10% SDS-PAGE gel. The blot was probed with a goat polyclonal IgG to Lamin B or a rabbit polyclonal antiserum to m-mtTFA.[2]

14.5 Mitochondrial Gene Transcription

Mechanisms for mitochondrial gene expression and its regulation have been studied and some aspects recently reviewed.[120–177] These mechanisms more closely resemble those of prokaryotes than do those of eukaryotes, as suggested by the endosymbiotic hypothesis of mitochondrial origin. In animals, the mtDNA exists as a double-stranded, closed circular molecule of approximately 16 Kb. These strands can be separated through a denaturing cesium chloride gradient into a light strand and a heavy strand. The heavy strand is the main coding strand and codes for 2 rRNAs, 14 tRNAs, and 12 structural genes. The light strand codes for 8 tRNAs and 1 structural gene. These genes are arranged as polycistrons, with tRNA genes interlaced between coding genes.

Early studies revealed that transcription is symmetrical[122] and is initiated within the displacement loop (D-loop, regulatory region), with the light strand moving clockwise and the heavy strand moving counterclockwise.[123–125] The light strand has a longer half life and is present in about 2 1/2 times greater quantity. The light strand is transcribed as one polycistron and the heavy strand as two.[126,127] One heavy strand polycistron encodes all of the heavy strand, while the other encodes the two rRNAs. Two distinct promoter sequences, one for the light strand (LSP) and one for the heavy strand (HSP), have been defined by deletion analysis, site-specific mutagenesis, and linker-scanning mutagenesis in an *in vitro* system.[127–134] In humans, both the LSP and the HSP contain regions near the start site containing specific nucleotides required for transcription initiation, as well as upstream regulatory regions. In the mouse, the LSP contains three domains. The first domain consists of nucleotides –10 to +9 (relative to transcription initiation) that are required for accurate transcription initiation. The second domain (nt –11 to –29) facilitates the formation of the preinitiation complex. The third domain (nt –30 to –88) affects transcriptional efficiency. In contrast, specific nucleotides are not required near or at the transcription start sites for heavy strand transcription initiation, although the start sites do make transcription more efficient.

There is an essential element upstream of the start sites in the mouse HSP. Promotor sequences are not highly conserved among species, but the mouse RNA polymerase is active on the rat mtDNA. This suggests that the rat promotor may be similar to the mouse. An additional difference between mouse and human promotors is that the two heavy strand transcription start sites are close together (near the D-loop/tRNA[Phe] border) in the mouse. In humans, the main start site is found in this location, with a minor start site found between the tRNA[Phe] and 12S genes. The main start site is thought to result in transcription of the 2 rRNA genes, while the minor one initiates transcription of the whole heavy strand. In addition, the light strand promoter also primes replication of the heavy strand[134] forming a RNA-DNA primer that is cleaved by the Rnase MRP (mitochondrial RNA processing) at the origin of heavy strand replication.[136] There are three blocks of sequences conserved among a number of species.[137] These sequences are thought to be involved in this cleavage.

At present, only two transcription factors have been identified and well studied. These are the mitochondrial transcription factor A (mtTFA) that is involved in initiation and the mitochondrial transcription termination factor (mTERF) that is involved in termination of the heavy strand.[137–140] The mTERF is active after the ribosomal RNAs are formed. *In vitro* studies have shown that mtTFA binds to both promoter regions as well as to a region between two of the conserved sequence blocks. The mtTFA condenses, unwinds, and bends mtDNA.[141,142] In addition, *in vitro*, more mtTFA is needed to promote transcription of the heavy strand than the light strand, suggesting that low levels of mtTFA may result in the activation of the light strand and be involved in replication. This suggestion is supported by the observation that mtTFA protein levels have been correlated with mtDNA copy number.[85,143]

Transgenic technology has provided further evidence for mtTFA's role in transcription and replication. First, overexpression of mtTFA in HeLa cells and in isolated liver mitochondria was shown to increase mitochondrial transcription.[143] Second, heterozygous *m-mtTFA* (also called *Tfam*) knockout mice were shown to have reduced mtDNA copy number in heart, kidney, and liver; reduced mitochondrial transcription; and reduced respiratory chain function in the heart.[144] The kidney, liver, and skeletal muscle were variable in this respect. Interestingly, the protein levels of mitochondrially encoded cytochrome-c oxidase subunit II and ATP synthase subunit 8 were normal in all tissues investigated. Using knockout mice it was found that if the gene for the mtTFA was completely absent, this absence was lethal. Thus, there are no homozygous knockout mice. These data, in combination with the *in vitro* data, support the idea that mtTFA is essential for mitochondrial replication, primed from the light strand promoter; but is not solely responsible for regulating heavy strand transcription. It is likely that mitochondrial transcription depends on the presence of other transcription factors as well.

Because genes occur in both genomes, a mechanism for the coordinated regulation of OXPHOS genes has been thought to exist. The nuclear respiratory factors (NRF) 1 and 2 and the general transcription factor Sp1 were shown to coordinate transcription by simultaneously regulating mtTFA, as well as several nuclear-encoded OXPHOS genes in some situations.[119,145–150] This is thought to be the case during rapid proliferation. But several researchers failed to find coordinated transcription in other situations, specifically in various thyroid hormone states.[150–156] In addition, mitochondrial gene expression can be regulated by growth and development in a tissue-specific manner. In the heart, regulation occurs at the level of transcription.[151,155,156] In rat heart, mitochondrial transcripts increased between 1 day and 3 months of age, then decreased between 3 months and 18 months of age. But in the liver, mRNA stability[157] and translational efficiency[158] were shown to be regulated in response to growth. They found that in neonates the half-lives of mt-mRNA were much longer than in adult liver and that translational efficiency peaked 1 hour after birth. This response to growth was also seen in nuclear-encoded OXPHOS genes.[159,160] The mechanism for this posttranscriptional regulation has been explained for the nuclear encoded F_1ATPase β subunit.[161,162] The 3′ untranslated region (UTR) of this gene contains a translational enhancer that functionally resembles an internal ribosome entry site.

During fetal development a protein (3' βFBP) binds this enhancer and inhibits translation. Within 1 hour after birth this protein no longer binds the 3' UTR, unmasking the enhancer. This produces a spike in β F_1ATPase protein levels. In the adult, this protein is present again and translation of this gene is once again inhibited. This protein has yet to be purified and characterized. It is clear that it is regulated by development, but it would be interesting to learn exactly which developmental signals are used. It is also unknown what mechanism causes the same effects on mitochondrially encoded F_0ATPase genes. Does masking also occur in the mitochondria? If so, is the same protein responsible? It has been suggested that the import of the F_1ATPase β subunit itself triggers the response of mitochondrial translation. But this has yet to be proven experimentally. This form of posttranscription regulation has also been shown to occur in cancer cells, which take on the same characterization as fetal liver.[163]

In addition to regulation during mitochondrial proliferation and differentiation, mitochondrial transcription may also be directly regulated by hormone receptors.[119] This has been called mitochondrial local tuning. Figure 14.4 shows where putative glucocorticoid (GRE), vitamin D (VDRE), thyroid hormone (TRE), and retinoic acid (RARE) response elements have been found in the D-loop.[129–131,137,164–168] The glucocorticoid receptor (GR) and a variant of the thyroid receptor (TR) have been shown to bind this region of mtDNA *in vitro*.[164,165] It was originally thought that thyroid hormone only increased mitochondrial transcription by increasing mtTFA.[170] Recently, Enriquez et al.[150] showed in isolated mitochondria that thyroid hormone directly increased the transcription of all mRNAs encoded on the heavy strand, without increasing mitochondrial rRNAs. They were unable to prove that this occurred by binding at the putative TRE. They did show protein-DNA interactions near the transcription start sites, but not at termination sites, that were affected by thyroid hormone. In addition, it was recently demonstrated that the variant form of thyroid receptor (p43) is rapidly imported into mitochondria, binds three putative TREs, and increases mitochondrial transcription in a thyroid hormone-dependent fashion.[170] Two of these putative TREs are located within the D-loop and were shown to independently increase mitochondrial transcription in the presence of p43 and thyroid hormone in a nuclear chloramphenicol acyltransferase (CAT) assay. One of these TREs is a direct repeat with two spaces. This element has also been shown to act as a RARE in other genes.[168] Thus, it is possible that retinoic acid bound to its receptor could also directly regulate mitochondrial transcription.

We have found that mitochondrial ATPase 6 gene expression is enhanced by retinoic acid *in vitro* using primary cell cultures. Using BHE/Cdb rats having a mutation in the ATPase 6 gene, we have also found that ATPase 6 gene product is increased by dietary supplements of vitamin A. Improvements in OXPHOS have also been observed in these rats in a dose-dependent manner.[119] These improvements correlated with the increase in ATPase 6 gene product. It should be noted, however, that normal Sprague Dawley rats did

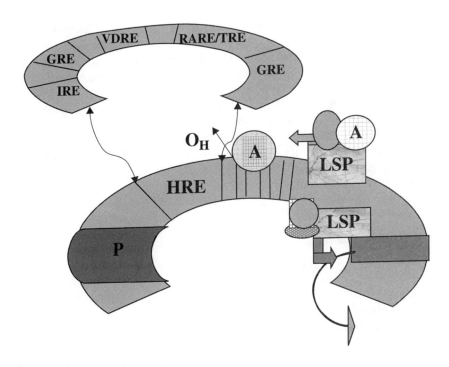

FIGURE 14.4
Putative nuclear hormone receptor response elements (HRE) found in mitochondrial D-loop (mtDNA promoter). (a) Overview of mitochondrial D-loop, highlighting the location of the putative nuclear hormone receptor response elements. O_H = origin of heavy strand replication, LSP and HSP = light and heavy strand promotors, respectively. (b) Species sequence comparison of putative glucocorticoid (GRE), vitamin D (VDRE), retinoic acid (RARE), and thyroid hormone (TRE) response elements, based on sequence alignments from Wong et al.[7] Mo = mouse, bov = bovine, hu = human, Xe = Xenopus.

not have this same response nor did rats that had not been depleted then repleted with vitamin A. Clearly, the retinoic acid effect on mt gene expression was genotype specific.

These studies suggest that the regulation of mitochondrial gene expression is a complicated tissue-specific process occurring at the levels of transcription, mRNA stability, and translation. There is a degree of coordination in the regulation of mitochondrial and nuclear OXPHOS gene expression. But, as there are many mitochondria within a given cell, direct regulation of mitochondrial gene expression by thyroid hormone, retinoic acid, and other factors may ultimately be found to be as important to this genome as they are to the nuclear genome.

The exact mechanism for hormone receptor action within mitochondria can only be speculative at this time. While mitochondria do not contain histones per se they do contain histone-like proteins.[171–174] Like histones, these proteins are rich in lysine. Since this is the site of acetylation for histones, these histone-like proteins may be acetylated during trancription activation by a similar mechanism as in the nucleus.[175] In addition, transcription activation could occur by direct interactions with the basic transcription machinery, namely, mitochondrial polymerase and/or mtTFA. Direct interactions between activators and RNA polymerase also activate transcription in prokaryotes.[176,177] Also, mitochondrial footprinting found that protein–DNA interactions near the transcription start sites were altered by thyroid hormone.[118] No known coactivators have been found within mitochondria yet, but that does not rule out their presence. Thus, the most likely mechanism would be that liganded hormone receptors bind their respective response elements and directly, or via mitochondrial specific coactivators, interact with mitochondrial polymerase and/or mtTFA. Additionally, the acetylation or phosphorylation of histone-like proteins and/or mtTFA is also a possibility.

14.6 Conclusions

Although the mt genome has been completely sequenced and mapped for several decades and although we are now accumulating information about diseases that result when this genome mutates, we have only primitive knowledge about the control of its transcription. Two transcription factors are known and several members of the steroid superfamily are suspected to play a role in this process. Current research is now focused on the possible role for the fat-soluble vitamins in mt gene expression.

References

1. McCaffery, P. et al., Vitamin A and gene regulation, in *Nutrient-Gene Interactions in Health and Disease*, N.M. Moustaïd-Moussa and C.D. Berdanier, Eds., CRC Press, Boca Raton, FL, 2001.
2. Boyer, P. D., A perspective of the binding change mechanism for ATP synthesis, *FASEB J.*, 3, 2164, 1989.
3. Boyer, P. D., The binding change mechanism for ATP synthase—some probabilities and possibilities, *Biochem. Biophy. Acta*, 1140, 215, 1993.
4. Boyer, P. D., The ATP synthase — A splendid molecular machine, *Annu. Rev. Biochem.*, 66, 717, 1997.
5. Fillingame, R. H., Jiang, W., and Dmitriev, O. Y., Coupling H^+ transport to rotary catalysis in f-type ATP synthases: Structure and organization of the transmembrane rotary motor, *J. Exp. Biol.*, 203, 9, 2000.
6. Kagawa, Y., Hamamoto, T., Endo, H., Ichida, M., Shibui, H., and Hayakawa, M., Genes of human ATP synthase: Their roles in physiology and aging, *Biosci. Rep.*, 17, 115, 1997.
7. Kell, D. B., The protonmotive force as an intermediate in electron transport-linked phosphorylation: Problems and prospects, *Curr. Top. Cell. Regulation*, 33, 279, 1992.

8. Mitchell, P., Vectorial chemistry and molecular mechanisms of chemiosmotic coupling: Power transmission by proticity, *Biochem. Soc. Trans.*, 4, 399, 1976.

9. Pederson, P. L., Frontiers in ATP synthase research: Understanding the relationship between subunit movements and ATP synthesis, *J. Bioenerg. Biomembr.*, 28, 389, 1996.

10. Racker, E., From Pasteur to Mitchell: A hundred years of bioenergetics, *Federation Proc.*, 39, 210, 1980.

11. Scheffler, I. E., *Mitochondria*, Wiley-Liss, New York, 1999.

12. Saraste, M., Oxidative phosphorylation at the fin de siecle, *Science*, 283, 1488, 1999.

13. Masaike, T., Mitome, N., Noji, H., Muneyuki, E., Yasuda, R., Kinosita, Jr., K., and Yoshida, M., Rotation of the F_1-ATPase and the hinge residues of the β subunit, *J. Exp. Biol.*, 203, 1, 2000.

14. Altendorf, K., Stalz, W.-D., Greie, J. C., and Deckers-Hebestreit, G., Structure and function of the F_0 complex of the ATP synthase from Escherichia coli, *J. Exp. Biol.*, 203, 19, 2000.

15. Capaldi, R. A., Schulenberg, B., Murray, J., and Aggeler, R., Cross-linking and electron microscopy studies of the structure and functioning of the Escherichia coli ATP synthase, *J. Exp. Biol.*, 203, 29, 2000.

16. Senior, A. E., Nadanaciva, S., and Weber, J., Rate acceleration of ATP hydrolysis by F_1F_0-ATP synthase, *J. Exp. Biol.*, 203, 35, 2000.

17. Vinogradov, A. D., Steady-state and pre-steady-state kinetics of the mitochondrial F_1F_0ATPase: Is ATP synthase a reversible molecular machine, *J. Exp. Biol.*, 203, 41, 2000.

18. Dimroth, P., Kaim, G., and Matthey, U., Crucial role of the membrane potential for ATP synthesis by F_1F_0ATP synthases, *J. Exp. Biol.*, 203, 51, 2000.

19. Collins, S., Cao, W., Dixon, T. M., Daniel, K. W., Onuma, H., and Medvedev, A.V., Body weight regulation, uncoupling proteins and energy metabolism, in *Nutrient-Gene Interactions in Health and Disease*, N.M. Moustaïd-Moussa and C.D. Berdanier, Eds., CRC Press, Boca Raton, FL, 2001.

20. Kim, M. J. C. and Berdanier, C. D., Nutrient gene interactions determine mitochondrial function, *FASEB J.*, 12, 243, 1998.

21. Berdanier, C.D. & Flatt, W.P., DHEA and mitochondrial respiration, in *Dehydroepiandrosterone: Biochemical, Physiological and Clinical Aspects*, M. Kalimi and W. Regelson, Eds., Walther de Gruyter, Berlin, 2000.

22. Brown, M. D., Voljavec, A. S., Lott, M. T., Macdonald, I., and Wallace, D. C., Leber's hereditary optic neuropathy: A model for mitochondrial neurodegenerative diseases, *FASEB J.*, 6, 2791, 1992.

23. Wallace, D. C., Singh, G., Lott, M. T., Hodge, J. A., Schurr, T. G., Lezza, A. M., Elsas II, L. J., and Nikoskelainen, E. K., Mitochondrial DNA mutation associated with Leber's hereditary optic neuropathy, *Science*, 242, 1427, 1988.

24. Holt, I. J., Harding, A. E., and Morgan-Hughes, J. A. Deletions of muscle mitochondrial DNA in patients with mitochondrial myopathies, *Nature*, 331, 717, 1988.

25. de Vries, D. D., van Engelen, B. G. M., Gabreels, F. J. M., Ruitenbeek, W., and van Oost, B. A., A second missense mutation in the mitochondrial ATPase 6 gene in Leigh's syndrome, *Ann. Neurol.*, 34, 410, 1993.

26. Pastores, G. M., Santorelli, F. M., Shanske, S., Gelb, B. D., Fyfe, B., Wolfe, D., and Willner, J. P., Leigh syndrome and hypertrophic cardiomyopathy in an infant with a mitchondrial DNA point mutation (T8993G), *Am. J. Med. Genet.*, 50, 265, 1994.

27. Houstek, J., Klement, P., Hermanska, J., Houstkave, H., Hansikova, H., Van den Bogart, C., and Zeman, J., Altered properties of mitochondrial ATP-synthase in patients with a T-G mutation in the ATPase 6 (subunit a) at position 8993 of mtDNA, *Biochim. Biophys. Acta*, 1271, 349, 1995.

28. Otabe, S., Yasuda, K., Mori, Y., Shimokawa, K., Kadowaki, H., Jimi, A., Nonaka, K., Akanuma, Y., Yazaki, Y., and Kadowaki, T., Molecular and histological evaluation of pancreata from patients with a mitochondrial gene mutation associated with impaired insulin secretion, *Biochem. Biophys. Res. Commun.*, 259, 149, 1999.

29. Tatuch, Y. and Robinson, B.H., The mitochondrial DNA mutation at 8993 associated with NARP slows the rate of ATP synthesis in isolated lymphoblast mitochondria, *Biochem. Biophys. Res. Commun.*, 192, 124, 1993.

30. Obayashi, T., Hattori, K., Sugiyama, S., Tanaka, M., Tanaka, T., Itoyama, S., Deguchi, H., Kawamura, K., Koga, Y., Toshima, H., Takeda, N., Nagano, M., Ito, T., and Ozawa T., Point mutations in mitochondrial DNA in patients with hypertrophic cardiomyopathy, *Am. Heart J.*, 124, 1263, 1992.

31. Shoffner, J. M., Lott, M. T., Lezza, A. M. S., Seibel, P., Ballinger, S. W., and Wallace, D. C., Myoclonic epilepsy and ragged-red fiber disease (MERRF) is associated with a mitochondrial DNA tRNA^{Lys} mutation, *Cell*, 61, 931, 1990.

32. Chomyn, A., Mitochondrial genetics '98: The myoclonic epilepsy and ragged-red fiber mutation provides new insights into human mitochondrial function and genetics, *Am. J. Hum. Genet.*, 62, 745, 1998.

33. Schon, E. A., Hirano, M., and DiMauro, S., Mitochondrial encephalomyopathies: Clinical and molecular analysis, *J. Bioenerg. Biomembr.*, 26, 291, 1994.

34. Schon, E. A., Koga, Y., Davidson, M., Moraes, C. T., and King, M.P., The mitochondrial tRNA$^{Leu (UUR)}$ mutation in MELAS: A model of pathogenesis, *Biochim. Biophys. Acta*, 1101, 206, 1992.

35. Jansen, J. J., Maassen, J. A., van der Woude, F. J., Lemmink, H. A. J., van den Ouweland, J. M. W., 't Hart, L. M., Smeets, H. J. M., Bruijn, J. A., and Lemkes, H. H. P. J., Mutation in mitochondrial tRNA$^{Leu (UUR)}$ gene associated with progressive kidney disease, *J. Am. Soc. Nephrol.*, 8, 118, 1997.

36. Maassen, J. A., van den Ouweland, J. M. W., 't Hart, L. M., and Lemkes, H. H. P. J., Maternally inherited diabetes and deafness: A diabetic subtype associated with a mutation in mitochondrial DNA, *Norm. Metab. Res.*, 29, 50, 1997.

37. Maassen, J. A., Jansen, J. J., Kadowaki, T., van den Ouweland, J. M. W., 't Hart, L. M., and Lemkes, H. H. P. J., The molecular basis and clinical characteristics of maternally inherited diabetes and deafness (MIDD), a recently recognized diabetic subtype, *Exp. Clin. Endochrinol. Diabetes*, 104, 205, 1996.

38. Alcolado, J. C., Majid, A., Brockington, M., Sweeney, M. G., Morgan, R., Rees, A., Harding, A. E., and Barnett, A. H., Mitochondrial gene defects in patients with NIDDM, *Diabetologia*, 37, 372, 1994.

39. Alcolado, J. C. and Thomas, A. W., Maternally inherited diabetes mellitus: The role of mitochondrial DNA defects, *Diabetic Med.*, 12, 102, 1995.

40. Ballinger, S. W., Shoffner, J. M., Gebhart, S., Koontz, D. A., and Wallace, D. C., Mitochondrial diabetes revisited, *Nature Genet.*, 7, 458, 1994.

41. Ballinger, S. W., Shoffner, J. M., Hedaya, E. V., Trounce, I., Polak, M. A., Koontz, D. A., and Wallace, D. C., Maternally transmitted diabetes and deafness associated with a 10.4 kb mitochondrial DNA deletion, *Nature Genet.*, 1, 11, 1992.

42. Chuang, L.-M., Wu, H.-P., Tsai, W.-Y., Lai, C.-S., Tai, T.-Y., and Lin, B. J., Mitochondrial gene mutations in patients with insulin-dependent diabetes mellitus in Taiwan, *Pancreas*, 12, 243, 1996.

43. Gerbitz, K.-D., Paprotta, A., Jaksch, M., Zierz, S., and Drechsel, J., Diabetes mellitus is one of the heterogeneous phenotypic features of a mitochondrial DNA point mutation within the tRNA^Leu(UUR) gene, *FEBS Lett.*, 321, 194, 1993.

44. Hanna, M. G., Nelson, I., Sweeney, M. G., Cooper, J. M., Watkins, P. J., Morgan-Hughes, J. A., and Harding, A. E., Congenital encephalomyopathy and adult-onset myopathy and diabetes mellitus: Different phenotypic associations of a new heteroplasmic mtDNA tRNA glutamic acid mutation, *Am. J. Hum. Genet.*, 56, 1026, 1995.

45. Kadowaki, T., Kadowaki, H., Mori, Y., Tobe, K., Sakuta, R., Suzuki, Y., Tanabe, Y., Sakura, H., Awata, T., Goto, Y.-I., Hayakawa, T., Matsuoka, K., Kawamori, R., Kamada, T., Horai, S., Nonaka, I., Hagura, R., Akanuma, T., and Yazaki, Y., A subtype of diabetes mellitus associated with a mutation of mitochondrial DNA, *N. Engl. J. Med.*, 330, 962, 1994.

46. Kameoka, K., Isotani, H., Tanaka, K., Azukari, K., Fujimura, Y., Shiota, Y., Sasaki, E., Majima, M., Furukawa, K., Haginomori, S., Kitaoka, H., and Ohsawa, N., Novel mitochondrial DNA mutation in tRNA^Lys (8296A→G) associated with diabetes, *Biochem. Biophys. Res. Commun.*, 245, 523, 1998.

47. Kishimoto, M., Hashiramoto, M., Araki, S., Ishida, Y., Kazumi, T., Kanda, F., and Kasuga, M., Diabetes mellitus carrying a mutation in the mitochondrial tRNA^Leu(UUR) gene, *Diabetologia*, 38, 193, 1995.

48. Kobayashi, T., Nakanishi, K., and Murase, T., Mutation at nucleotide position 3243 of the mitochondrial DNA as a cause of IDDM—A meta-analysis: Response from the authors, *Diabetologia*, 40, 1495, 1997.

49. Lynn, S., Wardell, T., Johnson, M. A., Chinnery, P. F., Daly, M. E., Walker, M., and Turnbull, D. M., Mitochondrial diabetes: Investigation and identification of a novel mutation, *Diabetes*, 47, 1800, 1998.

50. Mathews, C. E., McGraw, R. A., and Berdanier, C. D. A point mutation in the mitochondrial DNA of diabetes-prone BHE/Cdb rats, *FASEB J.*, 9, 1638, 1995.

51. Mathews, C. E., McGraw, R. A., Dean, R., and Berdanier, C. D., Inheritance of a mitochondrial DNA defect and impaired glucose tolerance in BHE/Cdb rats, *Diabetologia*, 42, 35, 1999.

52. Mathews, C. E. and Berdanier, C. D., Noninsulin-dependent diabetes mellitus as a mitochondrial genomic disease, *Proc. Soc. Exp. Biol. Med.*, 219, 97, 1998.

53. Odawara, M., Asakura, Y., Tada, K., Tsurushima, Y., and Yamashita, K., Mitochondrial gene mutation as a cause of insulin resistance, *Diabetes Care*, 18, 275, 1995.

54. Odawara, M., Sasaki, K., and Yamashita, K. Prevalence and clinical characterization of Japanese diabetes mellitus with an A-to-G mutation at nucleotide 3243 of the mitochondrial tRNA^Leu (UUR) gene, *J. Clin. Endocrinol. Metab.*, 80, 1290, 1995.

55. Odawara, M., Sasaki, K., and Yamashita, K. A G-to-A substitution at nucleotide position 3316 in mitochondrial DNA is associated with Japanese non-insulin-dependent diabetes mellitus, *Biochem. Biophys. Res. Commun.*, 227, 147, 1996.

56. Odawara, M. and Yamashita, K., Are MELAS and diabetes mellitus caused solely by the same mutation at np 3243 of the mitochondrial gene, *Diabetologia*, 38, 1488, 1995.

57. Odawara, M. and Yamashita, K., Mutation at nucleotide position 3243 of the mitochondrial DNA as a cause of IDDM—A meta-analysis, *Diabetologia*, 40, 1493, 1997.

58. Oexle, K., Oberle, J., Finckh, B., Kohlschutter, A., Nagy, M., Seibel, P., Seissler, J., and Hubner, C., Islet cell antibodies in diabetes mellitus associated with a mitochondrial tRNA^Leu (UUR) gene mutation, *Exp. Clin. Endocrinol. Diabetes*, 104, 212, 1996.

59. Poulton, J., Brown, M. S., Cooper, A., Marchington, D. R., and Phillips, D. I. W., A common mitochondrial DNA variant is associated with insulin resistance in adult life, *Diabetologia*, 41, 54, 1998.

60. Rotig, A., Bessis, J.-L., Romero, N., Cormier, V., Saudubray, J.-M., Narcy, P., Lenoir, G., Rustin, P., and Munnich, A. Maternally inherited duplication of the mitochondrial genome in a syndrome of proximal tubulopathy, diabetes mellitus, and cerebellar ataxia, *Am. J. Hum. Genet.*, 50, 364, 1992.

61. Schulz, J. B., Klockgether, T., Dichgans, J., Seibel, P., and Reichmann, H. Mitochondrial gene mutations and diabetes mellitus, *Lancet*, 341, 438, 1993.

62. Shin, C. S., Kim, S. K., Park, K. S., Kim, W. B., Kim, S. Y., Cho, B. Y., Lee, H. K., Koh, C.-S., Shin, C. H., and Lee, J. B., A new point mutation (3426, A to G) in mitochondrial NADH dehydrogenase gene in Korean diabetic patients which mimics 3243 mutation by restriction fragment length polymorphism pattern, *Endocrine J.*, 45, 105, 1997.

63. Sue, C. M., Holmes-Walker, D. J., Morris, J. G. L., Boyages, S. C., Crimmons, D. S., and Byrne, E., Mitochondrial gene mutations and diabetes mellitus, *Lancet*, 341, 437, 1993.

64. Suzuki, Y., Hinokio, Y., Hirai, S., Onoda, M., Matsumoto, M., Ohtomo, M., Kawasaki, H., Satoh, Y., Akai, H., Abe, K., Miyabayashi, S., Kawasaki, E., Nagataki, S., and Toyota, T., Pancreatic beta-cell secretory defect associated with mitochondrial point mutation of the tRNA^LEU (UUR) gene: A student in seven families with mitochondrial encephalomyopathy, lactic acidosis and stroke-like episodes (MELAS), *Diabetologia*, 37, 818, 1994.

65. 't Hart, L. M., Lemkes, H. H. P. J., Heine, R. J., Stolk, R. P., Feskens, E. J. M., Jansen, J. J., van der Does, F. E. E., Grobbee, D. E., Kromhout, D., van der Ouweland, J. M. W., and Maassen, J. A., Prevalence of maternally inherited diabetes and deafness in diabetic populations in the Netherlands, *Diabetologia*, 37, 1169, 1994.

66. Tawata, M., Ohtaka, M., Iwase, E., Ikegishi, Y., Aida, K., and Onaya, T. New mitochondrial DNA homoplasmic mutations associated with Japanese patients with type 2 diabetes, *Diabetes*, 47, 276, 1998.

67. van der Ouweland, J. M. W., Lemkes, H. H. P. J., Ruitenbeek, W., Sandkuijl, L. A., de Vijlder, M. F., Struyvenberg, P. A. A., van de Kamp, J. J. P., and Maassen, J. A., Mutation in mitochondrial tRNA^Leu (UUR) gene in a large pedigree with maternally transmitted type II diabetes mellitus and deafness, *Nature Genet.*, 1, 368, 1992.

68. van der Ouweland, J. M. W., Lemkes, H. H. P. J., Trembath, R. C., Ross, R., Velho, G., Cohen, D., Froguel, P., and Maassen, J. A., Maternally inherited diabetes and deafness is a distinct subtype of diabetes and associates with a single point mutation in the mitochondrial tRNA^Leu(UUR) gene, *Diabetes*, 43, 746, 1994.

69. van der Ouweland, J.M.W., Maechler, P., Wollheim, C.B., Attardi, G., and Maassen, J.A., Functional and morphological abrnormalities of mitochondria harbouring the tRNA$^{Leu(UUR)}$ mutation in mitochondrial DNA derived from patients with maternally inherited diabetes and deafness (MIDD) and progressive kidney disease, *Diabetologia*, 42, 485, 1999.

70. Velho, G., Byrne, M. M., Clement, K., Sturis, J., Pueyo, M. E., Blanche, H., Vionnet, N., Fiet, J., Passa, P., Robert, J.-J., Polonsky, K. S., and Froguel, P., Clinical phenotypes, insulin secretion, and insulin sensitivity in kindreds with maternally inherited diabetes and deafness due to mitochondrial tRNA$^{Leu\ (UUR)}$ gene mutation, *Diabetes*, 45, 478, 1996.

71. Wallace, D. C., Mitochondrial diseases in man and mouse, *Science*, 283, 1482, 1999.

72. Moraes, C. T., Shanske, S., Tritschler, H.-J., Aprille, J. R., Andreetta, F., Bonilla, E., Schon, E. A., and DiMauro, S., MtDNA depletion with variable tissue expression: A novel genetic abnormality in mitochondrial diseases, *Am. J. Hum. Genet.*, 48, 492, 1991.

73. Poulton, J., Deadman, M. E., and Gardiner, R. M., Duplications of mitochondrial DNA in mitochondrial myopathy, *Lancet*, 1, 236, 1989.

74. Poulton, J., Deadman, M. E., and Gardiner, R. M., Tandem direct duplications of mitochondrial DNA in mitochondrial myopathy: Analysis of nucleotide sequence and tissue distribution, *Nucl. Acids Res.*, 17, 10223, 1989.

75. Shoffner, J. M., Lott, M. T., Voljavec, A. S., Soueidan, S. A., Costigan, D. A., and Wallace, D. C., Spontaneous Kearns-Sayre/chronic external ophthalmoplegia plus syndrome associated with a mitochondrial DNA deletion: A slip-replication model and metabolic therapy, *Proc. Natl. Acad. Sci. USA*, 86, 7952, 1989.

76. Matthews, P. M., Brown, R. M., Morten, K., Marchington, D., Poulton, J., and Brown, G., Intracellular heteroplasmy for disease-associated point mutations in mtDNA: Implications for disease expression and evidence for mitotic segregation of heteroplasmic units of mtDNA, *Hum. Genet.*, 96, 261, 1995.

77. Holme, E., Tulinius, M. H., Larsson, N.-G., and Oldfors, A., Inheritance and expression of mitochondrial DNA point mutations, *Biochem. Biophy. Acta*, 1271: 249, 1995.

78. Holt, I. J., Harding, A. E., Petty, R. K. H., and Morgan-Hughes, J .A., A new mitochondrial disease associated with mitochondrial DNA heteroplasmy, *Am. J. Genet.*, 46, 428, 1990.

79. Jenuth, J. P., Peterson, A. C., Fu, K., and Shoubridge, E. A., Random genetic drift in the female germline explains the rapid segregation of mammalian mitochondrial DNA, *Nature Genet.*, 14, 146, 1996.

80. Giles, R. E., Blanc, H., Cann, H. M., and Wallace, D. C., Maternal inheritance of human mitochondrial DNA, *Proc. Natl. Acad. Sci. USA*, 77, 6715, 1980.

81. Bezold, R., Hofmann, S., Jaksch, M., Kaufhold, P., and Gerbitz, K.-D., DIDMOAD or wolfram syndrome? A mitochondrial-mediated disorder, *Diabetes Care*, 18, 583, 1995.

82. Shoffner, J. M., Brown, M. D., Torroni, A., Lott, M. T., Cabell, M. F., Mirra, S. S., Beal, M. F., Yan, C.-C., Gearing, M., Salvo, R., Watts, R. L., Juncos, J. L., Hansen, L. A., Crain, B. J., Fayad, M., Reckord, C. L., and Wallace, D. C., Mitochondrial DNA variants observed in Alzheimer disease and Parkinson disease patients, *Genomics*, 17, 171, 1993.

83. King, M.P., Koga, Y., Davidson, M., and Schon, E.A. Defects in mitochondrial protein synthesis and respiratory chain activity segregate with the tRNA[Leu(UUR)] mutation associated with mitochondrial myopathy, encephalopathy, lactic acidosis, and strokelike episodes, *Mol. Cell. Biol.*, 12, 480, 1992.

84. Ortiz, R. G., Newman, N. J., Shoffner, J. M., Kaufman, A. E., Koontz, D. A., and Wallace, D. C., Variable retinal and neurologic manifestations in patients harboring the mitochondrial DNA 8993 mutation, *Arch. Ophthalmol.*, 111, 1525, 1993.

85. Poulton, J., Morten, K., Freeman-Emmerson, C., Potter, C., Sewry, C., Dubowitz, V., Kidd, H., Stephenson, J., Whitehouse, W., Hansen, F. J., Paris, M., and Brown, G., Deficiency of the human mitochondrial transcription factor h-mtTFA in infantile mitochondrial myopathy is associated with mtDNA depletion, *Hum. Mol. Gen.*, 3, 1763, 1994.

86. Reardon, W., Ross, R. J. M., Sweeney, M. G., Luxon, L. M., Pembrey, M. E., Harding, A. E., and Trembath, R. C., Diabetes mellitus associated with a pathogenic point mutation in mitochondrial DNA, *Lancet*, 340, 1376, 1992.

87. Rossignol, R., Malgat, M., Mazat, J.-P., and Letellier, T., Threshold effect and tissue specificity: Implications for mitochondrial cytopathies, *J. Biol. Chem.*, 274, 33426, 1999.

88. Takeda, N., Tanamura, A., Iwai, T., Nakamura, I., Kato, M., Ohkubo, T., and Noma, K., Mitochondrial DNA deletion in human myocardium, *Mol. Cell. Biochem.*, 119, 105, 1993.

89. Young, C. A., Kumar, S., Young, M. J., and Boulton, A. J. M., Excess maternal history of diabetes in caucasian and afro-origin non-insulin-dependent diabetic patients suggests dominant maternal factors in disease transmission, *Diabetes Res. Clin. Pract.*, 28, 47, 1995.

90. Trounce, I., Neill, S., and Wallace, D. C., Cytoplasmic transfer of the mtDNA nt 8993 T-G (ATP6) point mutation associated with Leigh syndrome into mtDNA-less cells demonstrates cosegregation with a decrease in state III respiration and ADP/O ratio, *Proc. Natl. Acad. Sci. USA*, 91, 8334, 1994.

91. Vazquez-Memije, M. E., Shanske, S., Sanlorelli, F. M., Kranz-Eble, P., DeVivo, D. C., and DiMauro, S., Comparative biochemical studies of ATPase in cells from patients with T8993G or T8993C mitochondrial mutations, *J. Infect. Dis.*, 21, 829, 1998.

92. King, M. P. and Attardi, G., Injection of mitochondria into human cells leads to a rapid replacement of the endogenous mitochondrial DNA, *Cell*, 52, 811, 1988.

93. King, M. P. and Attardi, G., Human cells lacking mtDNA: Repopulation with exogenous mitochondria by complementation, *Science*, 246, 500, 1989.

94. Hartzog, P. E. and Cain, B. D., The $\alpha_{leu207\text{-}arg}$ mutation in F_1F_0-ATP synthase from *Escherichia coli*: A model for human mitochondrial disease, *J. Biol. Chem.*, 268, 12250, 1993.

95. Garcia, J. J., Ogilvie, I., Robinson, B. H., and Capaldi, R. A., Structure, functioning, and assembly of the ATP synthase in cells from patients with the T8993G mitochondrial DNA mutation: Comparison with the enzyme in Rho[0] cells completely lacking mtDNA, *J. Biol. Chem.*, 275, 11075, 2000.

96. Bai, Y., Shakeley, R. M., and Attardi, G., Tight control of respiration by NADH dehydrogenase ND5 subunit gene expression in mouse mitochondria, *Mol. Cell. Biol.*, 20, 805, 2000.

97. Hutchin, T. and Cortopassi, G. A., Mitochondrial DNA clone is associated with increased risk for Alzheimer's disease, *Proc. Natl. Acad. Sci. USA*, 92, 6892, 1995.
98. Meziane, A. E., Lehtinen, S. K., Hance, N., Nijtmans, L. G. J., Dunbar, D., Holt, I. J., and Jacobs, H. T., A tRNA suppressor mutation in human mitochondria, *Nature Genet.*, 18, 350, 1998.
99. Wang. J., Wilhelmsson, H., Graff, C., Li, H., Oldfors, A., Rustin, P., Bruning, J. C., Kahn, C. R., Clayton, D. A., Barsh, G. S., Thoren, P., and Larsson, N-G., Dilated cardiomyopathy and atrioventricular conduction blocks induced by heart-specific inactivation of mitochondrial gene expression, *Nature Genet.*, 21, 133, 1999.
100. Petkovich, M., Brand, N. J., Krust, A., and Chambon, P. A human retinoic acid receptor which belongs to the family of nuclear receptors, *Nature*, 220, 444, 1987.
101. Mandelsdorf, D. J., Borgmeyer, U., Heyman, R. A., Zhou, J. Y., Ong, E. S., Oro, A. E., Kakizuka, A., and Evans, R. M., Characterization of three RXR genes that mediate the action of 9-*cis* retinoic acid, *Genes Dev.*, 6, 329, 1992.
102. Mangelsdorf, D. J., Umesono, K., Kliewer, S. A., Borgmeyer, U., Ong, E. S., and Evans, R. M., A direct repeat in the cellular retinol-binding protein type II gene confers differential regulation by RXR and RAR, *Cell*, 66, 555, 1991.
103. Kastner, P., Krust, A., Mendelsohn, C., Garnier, J. M., Zelent, A., LeRoy, P., Staub, A., and Chambon, P., Murine isoforms of retinoic acid receptor γ with specific patterns of expression, *Proc. Natl. Acad. Sci. USA*, 87, 2700, 1990.
104. LeRoy, P., Nakshatri, H., and Chambon, P., Mouse retinoic acid receptor α2 isoform is transcribed from a promoter that contains a retinoic acid response element, *Proc. Natl. Acad. Sci. USA*, 88, 10138, 1991.
105. Giguere, V., Shago, M., Zirngibl, R., Tate, P., Rossant, J., and Varmuza, S., Identification of a novel isoform of the retinoic acid receptor γ expressed in the mouse embryo, *Mol. Cell. Biol.*, 10, 2335, 1990.
106. Lehmann, J. M., Hoffman, B., and Pfahl, M., Genomic organization of the retinoic acid receptor gamma gene, *Nucl. Acids Res.*, 19, 573, 1991.
107. Chambon, P., The retinoid signaling pathway: Molecular and genetic analyses, *Cell. Biol.*, 5, 115, 1994.
108. Takeyama, K., Kojima, R., Ohashi, T., Sato, T., Mano, H., Masushige, S., and Kato, S., Retinoic acid differentially up-regulates the gene expression of retinoic acid receptor α and γ isoforms in embryo and adult rats, *Biochem. Biophys. Res. Commun.*, 222, 395, 1996.
109. Haq, R.-U., Pfahl, M., and Chytil, F., Retinoic acid affects the expression of nuclear retinoic acid receptors in tissues of retinol-deficient rats, *Proc. Natl. Acad. Sci. USA*, 88, 8272, 1991.
110. Kastner, P., Grondona, J. M., Mark, M., Gansmuller, A., LeMeur, M., Decimo, D., Vonesch, J.-L., Dolle, P., and Chambon, P., Genetic analysis of RXRα developmental function: Convergence of RXR and RAR signaling pathways in heart and eye morphogenesis, *Cell*, 78, 987, 1994.
111. Grondona, J. M., Kastner, P., Gansmuller, A., Decimo, D., Chambon, P., and Mark, M., Retinal dysplasia and degeneration in RARβ2/RARγ2 compound mutant mice, *Development*, 122, 2173, 1996.
112. Lohnes, D., Kastner, P., Dierich, A., Makr, M., LeMeur, M., and Chambon, P., Function of retinoic acid receptor γ in the mouse, *Cell*, 73, 643, 1993.
113. Kastner, P., Mark, M., and Chambon, P., Nonsteroid nuclear receptors: What are genetic studies telling us about their role in real life, *Cell*, 83, 859, 1995.

114. Mendelsohn, C., Mark, M., Dolle, P., Dierich, A., Gaub, M. P., Krust, A., Lampron, C., and Chambon, P., Retinoic acid receptor β₂(RARβ₂) null mutant mice appear normal, Exp. Biol., 166, 246, 1994.
115. Krezel, W., Ghyselinck, N., Samad, T. A., Dupe, V., Kastner, P., Borrelli, E., and Chambon, P., Impaired locomotion and dopamine signaling in receptor mutant mice, *Science*, 279, 863, 1998.
116. Ruiz-Lozano, P., Smith, S. M., Perkins, G., Kubalak, S. W., Boss, G. R., Sucov, H. M., Evans, R. M., and Chien, K. R., Energy deprivation and a deficiency in downstream metabolic target genes during the onset of embryonic heart failure in RXR α⁻/⁻ embryos, *Development*, 125, 533, 1998.
117. Li, D., Desai-Yajnik, V., Lo, E., Schapira, M., Abagyan, R., and Samuels, H. H., NRIF3 is a novel coactivator mediating functional specificity of nuclear hormone receptors, *Mol. Cell. Biol.*, 19, 7191, 1999.
118. Gaemers, I. C., Van Pelt, A. M. M., Themmen, A. P. N., and De Rooij, D. G., Isolation and characterization of all-*trans*-retinoic acid-responsive genes in the rat testis, Mol. Reprod. Dev., 50, 1, 1998.
119. Everts, H. B., Effects of dietary vitamin A on mitochondrial function and gene expression in BHE/Cdb rats, PhD dissertation (C.D. Berdanier, director) University of Georgia, 2000.
120. Enriquez, J. A., Fernadez-Silva, P., and Montoya, J., Autonomous regulation in mammalian mitochondrial DNA transcriptions, *Biol. Chem.*, 380, 737, 1999b.
121. Taanman, J.-W., The mitochondrial genome: Structure, transcription, translation and replication, *Biochem. Biophy. Acta*, 1410, 103, 1999.
122. Clayton, D.A., Vertebrate mitochondrial DNA—A circle of surprises, *Exp. Cell Res.*, 255, 4, 2000.
123. Aloni, Y. and Attardi, G., Symmetrical *in vivo* transcription of mitochondrial DNA in HeLa cells, *Proc. Natl. Acad. Sci. USA*, 68, 1757, 1971.
124. Cantatore, P. and Attardi, G., Mapping the nascent light and heavy strand transcripts on the physical map of HeLa cell mitochondrial DNA, *Nucleic Acids Res.*, 8, 2605, 1980.
125. Montoya, J., Christianson, T., Levens, D., Rabinowitz, M., and Attardi, G., Identification of initiation sites for heavy-strand and light-strand transcription in human mitochondrial DNA, *Proc. Natl. Acad. Sci. USA*, 79, 7195, 1982.
126. Walberg, M. W. and Clayton, D. A., *In vitro* transcription of human mitochondrial DNA: Identification of specific light strand transcripts from the displacement loop region, *J. Biol. Chem.*, 258, 1268, 1983.
127. Montoya, J., Gaines, G. L., and Attardi, G., The pattern of transcription of the human mitochondrial rRNA genes reveals two overlapping transcription units, *Cell*, 34, 151, 1983.
128. Chang, D. D. and Clayton, D.A., Precise identification of individual promoters for transcription of each strand of human mitochondrial DNA, *Cell*, 36, 635, 1984.
129. Hixson, J. E. and Clayton, D. A., Initiation of transcription from each of the two human mitochondrial promoters requires unique nucleotides at the transcription start sites, *Proc. Natl. Acad. Sci. USA*, 82, 2660, 1985.
130. Chang, D. D. and Clayton, D. A., Precise assignment of the light-strand promoter of mouse mitochondrial DNA: A functional promoter consists of multiple upstream domains, *Mol. Cell. Biol.*, 6, 3253, 1986.

131. Chang, D. D. and Clayton, D. A., Precise assignment of the heavy-strand promoter of mouse mitochondrial DNA: Cognate start sites are not required for transcriptional initiation, *Mol. Cell. Biol.,* 6, 3262, 1986.

132. Bogenhagen, D. F., Applegate, E. F., and Yoza, B. K., Identification of a promoter for transcription of the heavy strand mtDNA: *in vitro* transcription and deletion mutagenesis, *Cell,* 36, 1105, 1984.

133. Chang, D. D., Hixson, J. E., and Clayton, D. A., Minor transcription initiation events indicate that both human mitochondrial promoters function bidirectionally, *Mol. Cell. Biol.,* 6, 294, 1986.

134. Topper, J. N. and Clayton, D. A., Identification of transcriptional regulatory elements in human mitochondrial DNA by linker substitution analysis, *Mol. Cell. Biol.,* 9, 1200, 1989.

135. Chang, D. D. and Clayton, D. A., Priming of human mitochondrial DNA replication occurs at the light-strand promoter, *Proc. Natl. Acad. Sci. USA,* 82, 351, 1985.

136. Lee, D. Y. and Clayton, D. A., RNase mitochondrial RNA processing correctly cleaves a novel R loop at the mitochondrial DNA leading-strand origin of replication, *Genes Dev.,* 11, 582, 1997.

137. Walberg, M. W. and Clayton, D. A., Sequence and properties of the human KB cell and mouse L cell D-loop regions of mitochondrial DNA, *Nucleic Acids Res.,* 9, 5411, 1981.

138. Fisher, R. P. and Clayton, D. A., A transcription factor required for promoter recognition by human mitochondrial RNA polymerase: Accurate initiation at the heavy- and light-strand promoters dissected and reconstituted *in vitro, J. Biol. Chem.,* 260, 11330, 1985.

139. Fisher, R. P. and Clayton, D. A., Purification and characterization of human mitochondrial transcription factor 1, *Mol. Cell. Biol.,* 8, 3496, 1988.

140. Kruse, B., Narasimhan, N., and Attardi, G., Termination of transcription in human mitochondria: Identification and purification of a DNA binding protein factor that promotes termination, *Cell,* 58, 391, 1989.

141. Fisher, R. P., Lisowsky, T., Parisi, M. A., and Clayton, D. A., DNA wrapping and bending by a mitochondrial high mobility group-like transcriptional activator protein, *J. Biol. Chem.,* 267, 3358, 1992.

142. Fisher, R. P., Topper, J. N., and Clayton, D. A., Promoter selection in human mitochondria involves binding of a transcription factor to orientation-independent upstream regulatory elements, *Cell,* 50, 247, 1987.

143. Larsson, N-G, Oldfors, A., Holme, E., and Clayton, D. A., Low levels of mitochondrial transcription factor A in mitochondrial DNA depletion, *Biochem. Biophys. Res. Commun.,* 200, 1374, 1994.

144. Larsson, N-G., Wang, J., Wilhelmsson, H., Oldfors, A., Rustin, P., Lewandoski, M., Barsh, G. S., and Clayton, D. A., Mitochondrial transcription factor A is necessary for mtDNA maintenance and embryogenesis in mice, *Nature Genet.,* 18, 231, 1998.

145. Tomura, H., Endo, H., Kagawa, Y., and Ohta, S., Novel regulatory enhancer in the nuclear gene of the human mitochondrial ATP synthase β-subunit, *J. Biol. Chem.,* 265, 6525, 1990.

146. Evans, M. J. and Scarpulla, R. C., NRF-1: a trans-activator of nuclear-encoded respiratory genes in animal cells, *Genes Dev.,* 4, 1023, 1990.

147. Chau, C. A., Evans, M. J., and Scarpulla, R. C., Nuclear respiratory factor 1 activation sites in genes encoding the γ subunit of ATP synthase, eukaryotic initiation factor 2α, and tyrosine aminotransferase: Specific interaction of purified NRF-1 with multiple target genes, *J. Biol. Chem.*, 267, 6999, 1992.

148. Virbasius, C. A., Virbasius, J. V., and Scarpulla, R. C., NRF-1, an activator involved in nuclear-mitochondrial interactions, utilizes a new DNA-binding domain conserved in a family of developmental regulators, *Genes Dev.*, 7, 2431, 1993.

149. Virbasius, J. V. and Scarpulla, R. C., Activation of the human mitochondrial transcription factor A gene by nuclear respiratory factors: A potential regulatory link between nuclear and mitochondrial gene expression in organelle biogenesis, *Proc. Natl. Acad. Sci. USA*, 91, 1309, 1994.

150. Enriquez, J. A., Fernadez-Silva, P., Garrido-Perez, N., Lopez-Perez, M. J., Perez-Martos, A., and Montoya, J., Direct regulation of mitochondrial RNA synthesis by thyroid hormone, *Mol. Cell. Biol.*, 19, 657, 1999a.

151. Izquierdo, J. M. and Cueza, J. M., Evidence of post-transcriptional regulation in mammalian mitochondrial biogenesis, *Biochem. Biophys. Res. Commun.*, 196, 55, 1993.

152. Luciakova, K., Li, R., and Nelson, B. D., Differential regulation of the transcript levels of some nuclear-encoded and mitochondrial-encoded respiratory-chain components in response to growth activation, *Eur. J. Biochem.*, 207, 253, 1992a.

153. Luciakova, K. and Nelson, B. D., Transcript levels for nuclear-encoded mammalian mitochondrial respiratory chain components are regulated by thyroid hormone in an uncoordinated fashion, *Eur. J. Biochem.*, 207, 247, 1992b.

154. Nelson, B. D., Luciakova, K., Li, R., and Betina, S., The role of thyroid hormone and promoter diversity in the regulation of nuclear encoded mitochondrial proteins, *Biochim. Biophys. Acta*, 1271, 85, 1995.

155. Stevens, R. J., Nishio, M. L., and Hood, D. A., Effect of hypothyroidism on the expression of cytochrome c and cytochrome c oxidase in heart and muscle during development, *Mol. Cell. Biochem.*, 143, 119, 1995.

156. Marin-Garcia, J., Ananthakrishnan, R., and Goldenthal, M. J., Mitochondrial gene expression in rat heart and liver during growth and development, *Biochem. Cell Biol.*, 75, 137, 1997.

157. Ostronoff, L. K., Izquierdo, J. M., and Cuezva, J. M., mt mRNA stability regulates the expression of the mitochondrial genome during liver development, *Biochem. Biophys. Res. Commun.*, 217, 1094, 1995.

158. Ostronoff, L. K., Izquierdo, J. M., Enriquez, J. A., Montoya, J., and Cuezva, J. M., Transient activation of mitochondrial translation regulates the expression of the mitochondrial genome during mammalian mitochondrial differentiation, *Biochem. J.*, 316, 183, 1996.

159. Izquierdo, J. M., Ricart, J., Ostronoff, L. K., Egea, G., and Cuezva, J. M., Changing patterns of transcriptional and post-transcriptional control of β-F_1 ATP synthase gene expression during mitochondrial biogenesis in liver, *J. Biol. Chem.*, 270, 10342, 1995b.

160. Luis, A. M., Izquierdo, J. M., Ostronoff, L. K., Salinas, M., Santaren, J. F., and Cuezva, J. M., Translational regulation of mitochondrial differentiation in neonatal rat liver: Specific increase in the translational efficiency of the nuclear-encoded mitochondrial β-F_1-ATPase mRNA, *J. Biol. Chem.*, 268, 1868, 1993.

161. Izquierdo, J. M. and Cuezva, J. M., Control of the translational efficiency of β-F_1-ATPase mRNA depends on the regulation of a protein that binds the 3′ untranslated region of the mRNA, *Mol. Cell. Biol.,* 17, 5255, 1997.

162. Izquierdo, J. M. and Cuezva, J. M., Internal-ribosome-entry-site functional activity of the 3′-untranslated region of the mRNA for the β subunit of mitochondrial H⁺-ATP synthase, *Biochem. J.,* 346, 849, 2000.

163. De Heredia, M. L., Izquierdo, J. M., and Cuezvas, J. M., A conserved mechanism for controlling the translation of β-F_1-ATPase mRNA between the fetal liver and cancer cells, *J. Biol. Chem.,* 275, 7430, 2000.

164. Demonacos, C. V., Karayanni, N., Hatzoglou, E., Tsiriyiotis, C., Spandidos, D. A., and Sekeris, C. E., Mitochondrial genes as sites of primary action of steroid hormones, *Steroids,* 61, 226, 1996.

165. Wrutniak, C., Cassar-Malek, I., Marchal, S., Rascle, A., Heusser, S., Keller, J. M., Flechon, J., Dauca, M., Samarut, J., and Ghysdael, J., A 43-kDa protein related to c-Erb A α1 is located in the mitochondrial matrix of rat liver, *J. Biol. Chem.,* 270, 16347, 1995.

166. Wong, J. F. H., Ma, D. P., Wilson, R. K., and Roe, B. A., DNA sequence of the Xenopus Laevis mitochondrial heavy and light strand replication origins and flanking tRNA genes, *Nucleic Acids Res.,* 11, 4977, 1983.

167. Umesono, K., Murakami, K. K., Thompson, C. C., and Evans, R. M., Direct repeats as selective response elements for the thyroid hormone, retinoic acid, and vitamin D_3 receptors, *Cell,* 65, 1255, 1991.

168. Naar, A. M., Boutin, J.-M., Lipkin, S. M., Yu, V. C., Holloway, J. M., Glass, C. K., and Rosenfeld, M. G., The orientation and spacing of core DNA-binding motifs dictate selective transcriptional responses to three nuclear receptors, *Cell,* 65, 1267, 1991.

169. Garstka, H. L., Facke, M., Escribano, J. R., and Wiesner, R. J., Stoichiometry of mitochondrial transcripts and regulation of gene expression by mitochonrial transcription factor a, *Biochem. Biophys. Res. Commun.,* 200, 619, 1994.

170. Casas, F., Rochard, P., Rodier, A., Cassar-Malek, I., Marchal-Victorian, S., Wiesner, R. J., Cabello, G., and Wrutniak, C., A variant form of the nuclear triiodothyronine receptor c-ErbAα1 plays a direct role in regulation of mitochondrial RNA synthesis, *Mol. Cell. Biol.,* 19, 7913, 1999.

171. Caron, F., Jacq, C., and Rouviere-Yaniv, J., Characterization of a histone-like protein extracted from yeast mitochondria, *Proc. Natl. Acad. Sci. USA,* 76, 4265, 1979.

172. Hillar, M. V., Rangayya, V., Jafar, B. B., Chambers, D., Vitzu, M., and Wyborny, L.E., Membrane-bound mitochondrial DNA: Isolation, transcription and protein composition, *Arch. Int. Physiol. Biochim.,* 87, 29, 1979.

173. Olszewska, E. and Tait, A., Mitochondrial chromatin in *Paramecium aurelia,* *Molec. Gen. Genet.,* 178, 453, 1980.

174. Kuroiwa, T., Ohta, T., Kuroiwa, H., and Shigeyuki, K., Molecular and cellular mechanisms of mitochondrial nuclear division and mitochondriokinesis, *Microsc.Res. Techniq.,* 27, 220, 1994.

175. Mizzen, C. A. and Allis, C. D., Linking histone acetylation to transcriptional regulation, *Cell. Mol. Life Sci.,* 54, 6, 1998.

176. Niu, W., Kim, Y., Tau, G., Heyduk, T., and Ebright, R.H., Transcription activation at Class II CAP-dependent promoters: Two interactions between CAP and RNA polymerase, *Cell,* 87, 1123, 1996.

177. Slauch, J. M., Russo, F. D., and Silhavy, T. J., Suppressor mutations in rpoA suggest that ompR controls transcription by direct interaction with the α subunit of RNA polymerase, *J. Bacteriol.*, 173, 7501, 1991.

15

Vitamin D and Gene Expression

Anthony W. Norman and Elaine D. Collins

CONTENTS
15.1 Background on Vitamin D 349
15.2 Chemistry of Vitamin D and Related Compounds 350
15.3 Metabolism of Vitamin D..352
15.4 Vitamin D Endocrine System (Generation
  of Biological Responses)..356
15.5 Signal Transduction Pathways Utilized by $1\alpha,25(OH)_2D_3$
  to Generate Biological Response..358
  15.5.1 Nuclear Receptor For $1\alpha,25(OH)_2D_3$.............................358
  15.5.2 Rapid Nongenomic Response..362
15.6 Nuclear Receptor for $1\alpha,25(OH)_2D_3$ 364
  15.6.1 Structural Domains..364
  15.6.2 Receptor Dimerization..367
  15.6.3 Hormone Response Elements 368
  15.6.4 Ligand Binding...370
15.7 Genetics and the Vitamin D Endocrine System 372
  15.7.1 Mutations in the VDR_{nuc} 372
  15.7.2 Knockout of the VDR_{nuc} 374
  15.7.3 Knockout of the 25(OH)D-24-Hydroxylase 375
15.8 Summary 376
References 377

15.1 Background on Vitamin D

In the last two decades, a new concept concerning the mode-of-action of the fat-soluble vitamin D has emerged. The cornerstone of this concept is that in terms of its availability, metabolism, and mechanism of action, it is more accurate to consider vitamin D a steroid hormone than a vitamin in the classical sense. Synthesis in the skin on exposure to ultraviolet light obviates the dietary necessity for vitamin D which is a classical part of the definition of a vitamin. The chemical transformations through which the various derivatives of vitamin D are produced are of the same kind as those that characterize the metabolism of other steroid hormones, such as the glucocorticoid and sex steroids. The close regulation of the renal production of $1\alpha,25$-dihydroxyvitamin D_3 [$1\alpha,25(OH)_2D_3$], the most potent of the naturally occurring derivatives of vitamin D, is very suggestive of its hormonal nature. The most compelling argument for the considerations of vitamin D as a steroid (pro-) hormone is the presence in classical target tissues, such as intestine, kidney, and bone of a specific, high-affinity nuclear receptor [VDR_{nuc}] for its active metabolite, $1\alpha,25(OH)_2D_3$.

The most thoroughly studied target tissue for $1\alpha,25(OH)_2D_3$ is the intestine, which depends on the hormone for adequate absorption of dietary calcium.[1,2] In the intestinal mucosa, the steroid–receptor complex induces the synthesis of a specific calcium-binding protein (mol wt = 28,000), the precise role of which in calcium absorption has yet to be elucidated.[3]

In addition to the endocrine actions of $1\alpha,25(OH)_2D_3$ in the classical target tissues of vitamin D, in which the actions of the hormone contribute to the body's maintenance of calcium homeostasis, the VDR_{nuc} has been identified in tissues not previously recognized as targets for vitamin D, such as the pancreas, pituitary, and brain[4,5] as well as the hemopoietic[6] and the immune systems.[7] Many different cell types representing these systems respond to $1\alpha,25(OH)_2D_3$, presumably through the specific receptors that have been identified in these cells, with changes in their patterns of growth and differentiation. These interactions may be of a more paracrine or autocrine nature as indicated, e.g., by the ability of activated macrophages to convert $25OHD_3$ to $1\alpha,25(OH)_2D_3$.

The actions of $1,25(OH)_2D_3$ alluded to above appear to involve changes in gene expression in the target cells.[8,10] In addition, in the intestine[11] and bone osteoblast cells,[12] components of calcium transport have been identified that respond very rapidly to $1\alpha,25(OH)_2D_3$ and are thought to be mediated by nongenomic mechanisms (see later discussion).

15.2   Chemistry of Vitamin D and Related Compounds

The molecular structure of vitamin D is closely allied to that of classical steroid hormones (see Fig. 15.1). Technically, vitamin D is a seco-steroid. Secosteroids are those in which one of the rings of the cyclopentanoperhydrophenanthrene ring structure of classic steroids has undergone fission by breakage of a carbon–carbon bond; in the instance of vitamin D, this is the 9,10 carbon bond of ring B.

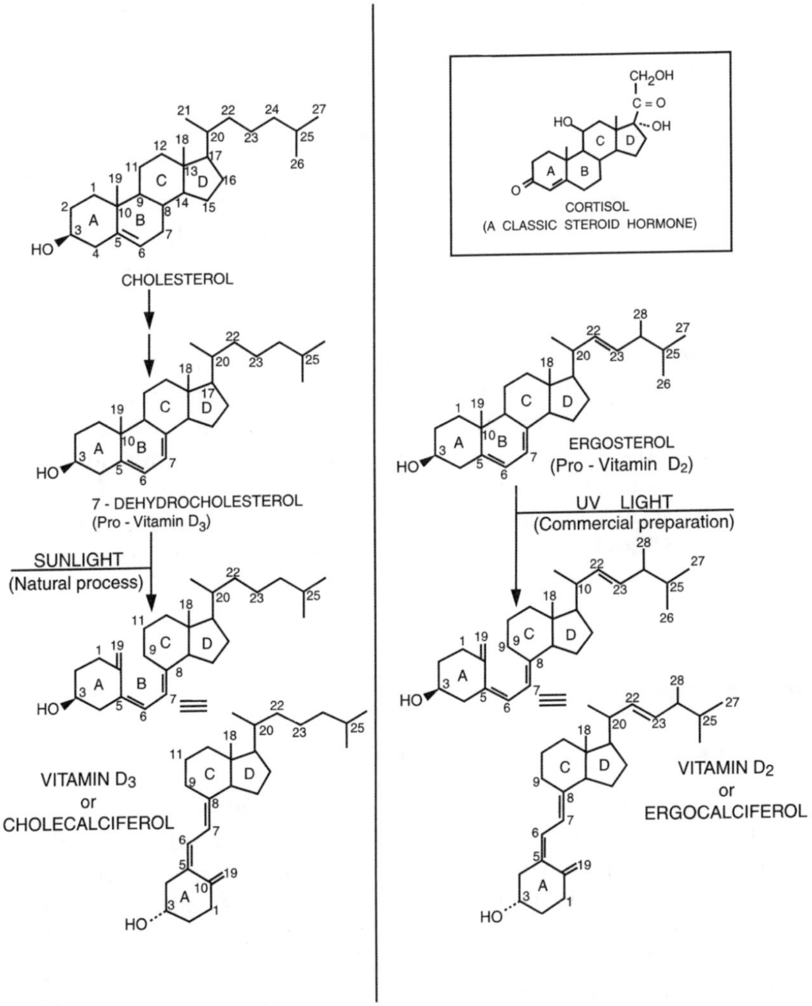

FIGURE 15.1
Structural relationship of vitamin D_3 (cholecalciferol) and vitamin D_2 (ergocalciferol) with their respective provitamins (cholesterol and ergosterol), and a classic steroid hormone, cortisol (see insert box). The two structural representations at the bottom for both vitamin D_3 and vitamin D_2 are equivalent; they are simply different ways of depicting the same molecule. It is to be emphasized that vitamin D_3 is the naturally occurring form of the vitamin; it is produced from 7-dehydrocholesterol, which is present in the skin, by the action of sunlight. Vitamin D_2 (which is equivalently potent to vitamin D_3 in humans and many mammals, but not birds) is produced commercially by the irradiation of the plant sterol ergosterol with ultraviolet light.

There is a family of vitamin D-related steroids that differ in the precise structure of the side chain attached to carbon-17. The naturally occurring form of vitamin D is that which has the side chain structure identical to that of cholesterol; this is known as vitamin D_3 or cholecalciferol. Vitamin D_2, or ergocalciferol, is not a naturally occurring form of the vitamin. Collectively, vitamin D_3 plus vitamin D_2 are the calciferols or simply vitamin D.

In the United States, the principal form of vitamin D supplementation of food was vitamin D_2 in the interval 1930–1965; since 1965 the predominant form of vitamin D supplementation has been vitamin D_3. One International Unit (IU) of vitamin D_3 is equivalent to 25 ng or 65 pmoles of the compound. In the United States the Recommended Dietary Allowance (RDA), or more recently the Reference Daily Intake* of vitamin D (either D_2 or D_3) for an adult is 200 IU, and for pregnant or lactating women or children less than 4 years of age it is 400 IU (set in 1994 by the FDA).

Although the chemical structure of vitamin D was determined in the 1930s, it was not until the 1975–1995 era that the unique structural aspects of the molecule became apparent. In contrast to other steroid hormones the vitamin D molecule has three structural features which contribute to the extreme conformational flexibility of this seco-steroid molecule; these include the presence of (i) an 8-carbon side chain, (ii) the broken B ring which "unlocks" the A-ring so that it (iii) can undergo chair–chair interchange many times per second. Figure 15.2 and its legend provide a detailed consideration of the conformational flexibility of vitamin D molecules.

15.3 Metabolism of Vitamin D

Vitamin D_3 is normally produced by exposure to sunlight of the precursor, 7-dehydrocholesterol, present in the skin. Vitamin D_2 is produced synthetically via ultraviolet irradiation of the sterol ergosterol. The chief structural prerequisite of a sterol to be classified as a provitamin D is its ability to be converted upon ultraviolet irradiation to a vitamin D; thus, it is mandatory that it have in its B ring a Δ^{5-7} conjugated double-bond system. In the skin, the principal ultraviolet irradiation product is previtamin D_3. The resulting vitamin D_3 is then transported into the general circulatory system by the vitamin D-binding protein.

A formal definition of a vitamin is that it is a trace dietary constituent required to effect normal functioning of a physiological process. Emphasis here is on *trace* and the fact that the vitamin must be supplied in the diet; this implies that the body is unable to synthesize it. Thus, cholecalciferol is only a vitamin when the animal does not have access to sunlight or ultraviolet light. Under normal physiological circumstances, all mammals, including man, can generate via ultraviolet photolysis adequate quantities of

---

* The U.S. Recommended Dietary Allowance (U.S. RDA) set in 1989 describes nutrient standards; the amounts listed represent recommendations for daily intake averaged over a 3- to 4-day interval. Effective in 1993, the U.S. RDA terminology underwent a name change to Reference Daily Intake (RDI). These RDI recommendations are used by the Food and Drug Administration (FDA) to define nutrient content guidelines for food labels.

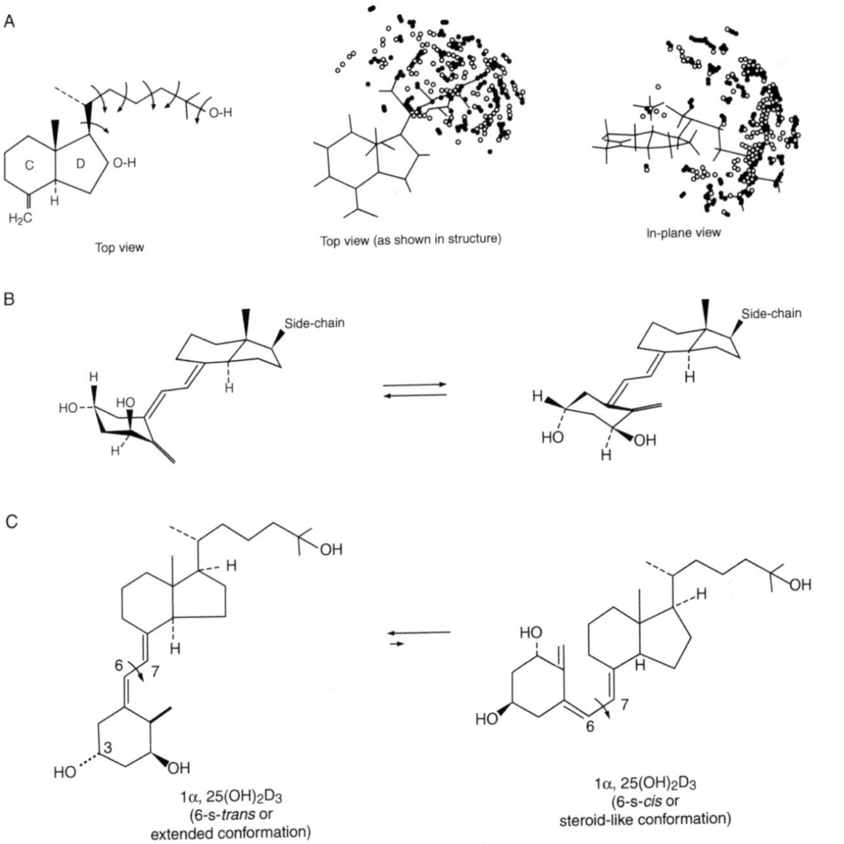

A   Top view   Top view (as shown in structure)   In-plane view

B   Side-chain   Side-chain

C   1α, 25(OH)₂D3 (6-s-*trans* or extended conformation)   1α, 25(OH)₂D3 (6-s-*cis* or steroid-like conformation)

FIGURE 15.2
Conformational flexibility of vitamin D molecules using 1α,25(OH)₂-vitamin D₃ [1α,25(OH)₂D₃] as an example. (A) Illustrates the dynamic single bond rotation of the cholesterol-like side chain of 1α,25(OH)₂D₃ (i.e., 360° rotations about the five single carbon bonds and the oxygen, as indicated by the curved arrows). The dots indicate the position in three-dimensional space of the 25-hydroxyl group for some 394 readily identifiable side-chain conformations which have been determined from energy minimization calculations. Two orientations of the C/D/side chain are presented: a top view and an in-plane view. (B) Depicts the rapid (thousands of times per second) chair-chair interconversion of the A-ring of the secosteroid which effectively equilibrates the 1α-hydroxyl between the axial and equatorial orientations. (C) Illustrates the 360° rotational freedom about the 6,7 carbon–carbon bond of the seco-β-ring which generates conformations ranging from the more steroid-like (6-s-*cis*) conformation, to the open and extended (6-s-*trans*) conformation 1α,25(OH)₂D₃.

vitamin D to meet the Recommended Dietary Allowance (RDA). It is largely through an historical accident that calciferol has been classified as a vitamin rather than as a steroid hormone. Chemists have certainly appreciated the strong structural similarity between vitamin D and other steroids but this correlation had not been widely acknowledged in the biological, clinical, or nutritional sciences until 1965–1970.

Since 1964 a totally new era in the field of vitamin D has opened with the discovery of the metabolism of vitamin D. Altogether, some 37 metabolites of vitamin D_3 have been isolated and chemically characterized (see Fig. 15.3). It is now recognized that there is an endocrine system for processing the prohormone, vitamin D, into its hormonally active daughter metabolite(s) (see Fig. 15.3).

The primary source of circulating dihydroxylated metabolites of vitamin D is the kidney, which is the vitamin D endocrine gland. In the kidney mitochondrion, $25OHD_3$, the major circulating form of vitamin D, is converted to either $1\alpha,25$-dihydroxyvitamin D_3 $[1\alpha,25(OH)_2D_3]$ or $24R,25(OH)_2$-vitamin D_3 $[24R,25(OH)_2D_3]$. The predominant dihydroxy-

VITAMIN D_3 METABOLISM

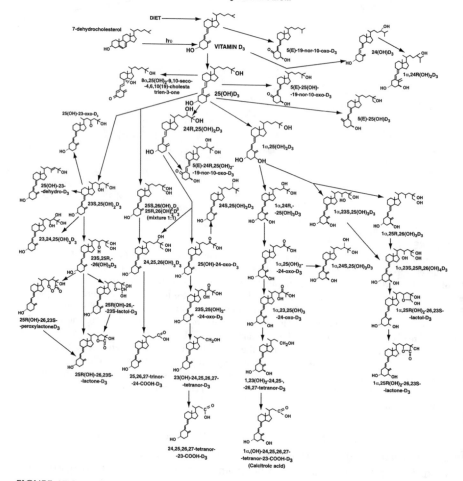

FIGURE 15.3

Metabolic pathway summarizing the conversion of vitamin D_3 (cholecalciferol) into its family of daughter metabolites. The secosteroids presented in boldface are the physiologically relevant vitamin D compounds, while the other structures are believed to be catabolites of vitamin D_3.

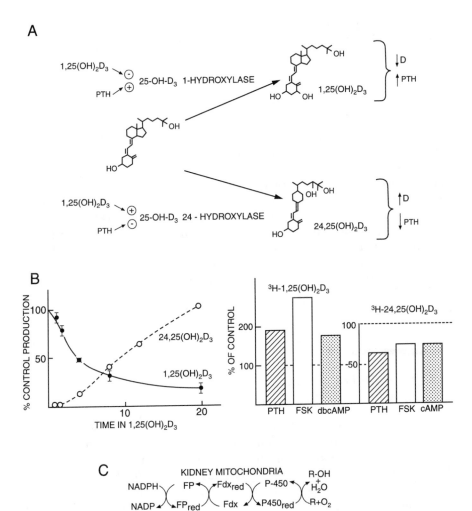

FIGURE 15.4
Regulation of vitamin D metabolism. (A) Conversion of 25OHD₃ to 1α,25(OH)₂D₃ is downregulated by 1α,25(OH)₂D₃ and upregulated by PTH. The two hormones have the opposite effects on
24R,25(OH)₂D₃ production. (B) Time course of the effect of 1α,25(OH)₂D₃ on its own production
(solid symbols and solid line) and on that of 24R,25(OH)₂D₃ (open symbols and dashed line) in
cultured chick kidney cells is shown on the left. On the right the data supporting the involvement
of the cAMP intracellular signaling cascade in the regulation of 1α,25(OH)₂D₃ and 24R,25(OH)₂D₃
production (FSK, forskolin; dbcAMP, dibutyryl cAMP) are summarized. (C) Electon transport
system supporting the reduction of O₂ to supply the hydroxl group to be incorporated into
25OHD₃. FP, ferredoxin reductase, a flavoprotein; Fdx, ferredoxin; p-450, Cytochrome P 450. (See
References 13, 129.)

lated product formed will depend on the vitamin D and parathyroid hormone (PTH) status of the individual.

In the vitamin D-deficient state, the enzymatic activity of the 1-hydroxylase
is high and of the 24-hydroxylase low (see Fig. 15.4). This is because

$1\alpha,25(OH)_2D_3$ represses the 1-hydroxylase and induces the 24-hydroxylase activity, probably through effects on the synthesis of specific proteins. Conversely, parathyroid hormone, elevated by the hypocalcemia resulting from vitamin D deficiency, increases 1-hydroxylase activity and decreases 24-hydroxylase activity. As had been shown in cell culture, cAMP mediates this effect of PTH, but protein kinase C may also be involved in $25OHD_3$ metabolisms, because 12-0-tetradecanoylphorbol-13 acetate (TPA) exerts effects opposite to those of PTH. Thus, the absence of $1,25(OH)_2D_3$ and the presence of PTH combine to keep $24R,25(OH)_2D_3$ production low. In the vitamin D-replete state, the opposite set of effects occurs, resulting in lowered $1,25(OH)_2D_3$ and elevated $24R,25(OH)_2D_3$ production (see the References 13–15).

Both the 1- and 24-hydroxylases are classical mitochondrial mixed-function oxidases involving the transfer of electrons from NADPH through a flavoprotein (renal ferredoxin reductase) and an iron sulfur protein (renal ferredoxin)[16] to cytochrome P-450.[17] All three components are located in or adjacent to the inner mitochondrial membrane. Exactly how, on a molecular level, $1\alpha,25(OH)_2D_3$ and PTH exert their effects on these enzyme systems is currently under study.[13]

15.4 Vitamin D Endocrine System (Generation of Biological Responses)

The molecule vitamin D itself has no intrinsic biological activity. All biological responses attributed to vitamin D are now known to arise only as a consequence of the metabolism of this seco-steroid into its biologically active daughter metabolites, namely, $1\alpha,25(OH)_2D_3$ and $24R,25(OH)_2D_3$.[18]

Figure 15.5 summarizes the scope of the vitamin D endocrine system. The steroid hormone $1\alpha,25(OH)_2D_3$ is produced only in accord with strict physiological signals dictated by the calcium demand of the organism; a bimodal mode of regulation has been suggested (see discussion above). Thus, under normal physiological circumstances, both renal dihydroxylated metabolites are secreted and are circulated in the plasma. There is evidence of a "short feedback loop" for both of these metabolites to modulate and/or reduce the secretion of PTH. There is also some evidence that other endocrine modulators such as estrogens, androgens, growth hormone, prolactin, and insulin may affect the renal production of $1\alpha,25(OH)_2D_3$ (see Fig. 15.5). Thus, the kidney is clearly an endocrine gland, in the classic sense, which is capable of producing in a physiologically regulated manner appropriate amounts of $1\alpha,25(OH)_2D_3$.

The plasma compartment contains a specific protein termed the vitamin D-binding protein (DBP), which is utilized to transport vitamin D seco-sterols. DBP is similar in function to the corticosteroid-binding globulin (CBG), which carries glucocorticoids, and the steroid hormone-binding globulin

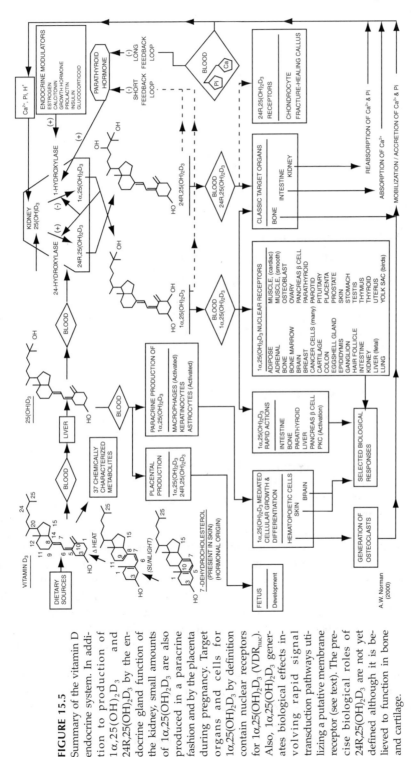

FIGURE 15.5

Summary of the vitamin D endocrine system. In addition to production of $1\alpha,25(OH)_2D_3$ and $24R,25(OH)_2D_3$ by the endocrine gland function of the kidney, small amounts of $1\alpha,25(OH)_2D_3$ are also produced in a paracrine fashion and by the placenta during pregnancy. Target organs and cells for $1\alpha,25(OH)_2D_3$ by definition contain nuclear receptors for $1\alpha,25(OH)_2D_3$ (VDR$_{nuc}$). Also, $1\alpha,25(OH)_2D_3$ generates biological effects involving rapid signal transduction pathways utilizing a putative membrane receptor (see text). The precise biological roles of $24R,25(OH)_2D_3$ are not yet defined although it is believed to function in bone and cartilage.

(SHBG), which transports estrogens or androgens. DBP is a slightly acidic (pI = 5.2) monomeric glycoprotein of 53,000 D which is synthesized and secreted by the liver as a major plasma constituent. From analysis of the cloned cDNA, it has been determined that DBP is structurally homologous to albumin and α-fetoprotein; these three plasma proteins are members of the same multigene family which likely is derived from the duplication of a common ancestral gene. DBP, originally called group-specific component (Gc), was initially studied electrophoretically as a polymorphic marker in the α-globulin region of human serum. (See References 19,20.)

15.5 Signal Transduction Pathways Utilized by $1\alpha,25(OH)_2D_3$ to Generate Biological Response

$1\alpha,25(OH)_2D_3$ is believed to mediate biological responses by interaction with its nuclear receptor, VDR_{nuc}, and also via interaction with a putative membrane receptor, VDR_{mem}, which is located on the surface of the cell of appropriate target cells; a schematic diagram of this concept is presented in Fig. 15.6. These topics will be discussed separately.

15.5.1 Nuclear Receptor For $1\alpha,25(OH)_2D_3$

The nuclear responses to $1\alpha,25(OH)_2D_3$ are generated in a manner homologous to that of classical steroid hormones, e.g., glucocorticoids, progesterone, estradiol, testosterone, and aldosterone. In the general model, the hormone is produced in an endocrine gland in response to a physiological stimulus and then circulates in the blood bound to a protein carrier (the vitamin D-binding protein or DBP), which delivers it to target tissues where the hormone enters the cell and interacts with a specific, high-affinity intracellular receptor(s). The receptor–hormone complex then localizes in the nucleus, undergoes some type of "activation" perhaps involving phosphorylation[21,25] and binds to a hormone response element (HRE) on the DNA to modulate the expression of hormone-sensitive genes. The modulation of gene transcription results in either the induction or the repression of specific mRNAs, ultimately resulting in changes in protein expression needed to produce the required biological response. High affinity receptors for $1\alpha,25(OH)_2D_3$ have been identified in at least 34 target tissues (see Fig. 15.5). A more detailed discussion of the nuclear VDR is presented below.

Identification of vitamin D-regulated transcription for specific gene products is typically supported by one or several observations. Of these, the majority of the reports present data suggesting vitamin D-dependent modulation of mRNA levels following treatment of animals, tissues, or cells with $1\alpha,25(OH)_2D_3$. Although these types of analyses are commonly accepted as

Mechanism of Action

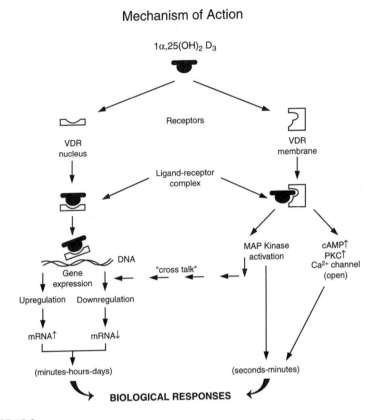

FIGURE 15.6

Pathways for generation of biological responses utilized by $1\alpha,25(OH)_2D_3$. In the genomic pathway (left side), occupancy of the nuclear receptor for $1\alpha,25(OH)_2D_3$ (VDR_{nuc}) by a ligand leads to an up- or downregulation of genes subject to hormone regulation. More than 50 proteins are known to be transcriptionally regulated by $1\alpha,25(OH)_2D_3$ [see Table 15.1 and Reference 26]. In the membrane-initiated pathway (right side), occupancy of a putative membrane receptor for $1\alpha,25(OH)_2D_3$ by a ligand is believed to rapidly lead to activation of a number of signal transduction pathways, including adenylate cyclase, phospholipase C, protein kinase C (PKC), mitogen-activated protein kinase (MAP kinase), and/or opening of voltage-gated L-type Ca^{2+} channels, which are either individually or collectively coupled to generation the biological response(s).

sufficient evidence to suggest that the protein is vitamin D-sensitive, they cannot be used exclusively to conclude that the regulation is mediated via altered gene transcription. These data do not distinguish between transcriptional regulation vs. alterations in stability of the message nor do they guarantee that the protein level is indeed altered by $1\alpha,25(OH)_2D_3$. Identification of a VDRE within the promoter region of the gene supplies additional support for vitamin D regulation but is not, in itself, indicative of altered transcription. Measurement of vitamin D-dependent nuclear transcription coupled with data supporting altered protein levels provides the best evidence of $1\alpha,25(OH)_2D_3$ regulation of a specific gene product. Unfortunately, these types of analyses have not been completed for many of the gene products presumed to be under regulation by $1\alpha,25(OH)_2D_3$. Additionally, we cannot assume that lack of such evidence indicates the gene product is not vitamin D regulated. The goal of this review is to present an updated list of proteins whose mRNA levels are known to be modulated by vitamin D status. Additionally, supporting data regarding the presence of a recognized VDRE and/or nuclear transcription data are supplied where available.

Table 15.1 lists gene products whose message levels are known to be sensitive to $1\alpha,25(OH)_2D_3$.[26] This alphabetical list contains genes associated with

TABLE 15.1

Genes Under Regulation by $1\alpha,25(OH)_2D_3$

Gene	Regulation	Evidence	Tissue/Cell	Ref.
α-tubulin	Down	mRNA	Chick intestine	130
Aldolase subunit B	Up	mRNA	Chick kidney	131
Alkaline phosphatase	Up	mRNA	Rat intestine	132
			Chick intestine	131
			TE-85 cells	133
ATP synthase	Up	mRNA	Rat intestine	134
			Chick intestine	131
	Down	mRNA	Chick kidney	131
c-FMS	Up	mRNA	HL-60 cells	135
c-FOS	Up	mRNA	MG-63 cells	136
			HL-60 cells	135
c-KI-RAS	Up	mRNA	BALB-3T3 cells	137
c-MYB	Down	mRNA	HL-60 cells	135
c-MYC	Up	mRNA	MG-63 cells	136
	Down	mRNA	U937 cells	138
			HL-60 cells	139
		Transcription	HL-60 cells	140, 141
Calbindin D_{28K}	Up	mRNA	Chick intestine	142
			Mouse kidney	143
		Transcription	Chick intestine	144
				2
Calbindin D_{9K}	Up	mRNA	Mouse kidney	144
		VDRE	Rat	145
Carbonic anhydrase	Up	mRNA	Marrow cells	146
		Transcription	Myelomonocytes	147
CD-23	Down	mRNA	PBMC	148
Collagen type I	Down	mRNA/VDRE	Rat	149
Cytochrome oxidase subunit I	Up	mRNA	Rat intestine	134
			Chick intestine	131
	Down	mRNA	Chick kidney	131
Cytochrome oxidase subunit II	Up	mRNA	Chick intestine	131
	Down	mRNA	Chick kidney	131
Cytochrome oxidase subunit III	Up	mRNA	Rat intestine	134
			Chick intestine	131
	Down	mRNA	Chick kidney	132
Cytochrome B	Down	mRNA	Chick kidney	131

TABLE 15.1 (CONTINUED)

Genes Under Regulation by $1\alpha,25(OH)_2D_3$

Gene	Regulation	Evidence	Tissue/Cell	Ref.
Fatty-acid binding protein	Down	mRNA	Chick intestine	131
Ferredoxin	Down	mRNA	Chick kidney	150
Fibronectin	Up	mRNA	MG-63,TE-85, HL-60 cells	151
γ-interferon	Down	mRNA	T-lymphocytes PBMC	152 153
Glyceraldehyde-3-phosphate dehydrogenase	Up	mRNA	BT-20 cells	154
GM-colony stimulating factor	Down	mRNA	T-lymphocytes	155
Heat shock protein-70	Up	mRNA	PBMC	156
Histone H$_4$	Down	mRNA/ Transcription	HL-60 cells	157
1α-hydroxy-vitamin D-24-hydroxylase	Up	mRNA mRNA/ Transcription	Rat kidney Rat kidney	158 159
Integrin$_{v\beta3}$	Up	mRNA/ Transcription VDRE	Avian osteoclast precursor cells Avian gene	160 161
Interleukin 6	Up	mRNA	U937	162
Interleukin 1	Up	mRNA	U937 cells	162 163
Interleukin 2	Down	mRNA	T-lymphocytes	153
Interleukin 3 receptor	Up	mRNA	MC3T3 cells	164
Matrix gla-protein	Up	mRNA	UMR106-01, ROS 25/1, ROS 25/4 cells	165
Metallothionien	Up	mRNA	Rat keratinocytes Mouse liver/kidney/skin Chick kidney	166 166 131
Monocyte derived neutrophil-activating peptide	Up	mRNA/ Transcription	HL-60 cells	167
NADH DH subunit I	Down	mRNA	Chick kidney	131
NADH DH subunit III	Up	mRNA	Chick intestine	131
NADH DH subunit IV	Up	mRNA	Chick intestine	131
Nerve growth factor	Up	mRNA	L-929 cells	168
Osteocalcin	Up	mRNA VDRE	ROS 17/2.8 ROS 25/1 ROS 17/2.8 Rat	169 165 170 171 172
Osteopontin	Up	mRNA VDRE	ROS 17/2.8 ROS 17/2.8	173 174

(continued)

TABLE 15.1 (CONTINUED)

Genes Under Regulation by $1\alpha,25(OH)_2D_3$

Gene	Regulation	Evidence	Tissue/Cell	Ref.
Plasma membrane calcium pump	Up	mRNA	Chick intestine	175
Pre-pro-PTH	Down	mRNA	Rat	176
		mRNA/ Transcription	Bovine parathyroid	177
Prolactin	Up	mRNA	GH_4C_1 cells	178
Protein kinase inhibitor	Down	mRNA	Chick kidney	179
Protein kinase C	Up	mRNA/ Transcription	HL-60 cells	180
PTH	Down	mRNA	Rat parathyroid	181
				182
PTH-related protein	Down	mRNA/ Transcription	TT cells	183
Transferrin receptor	Down	mRNA	PBMC	153
Tumor necrosis factor-α	Up	mRNA	U937 cells	162
		Transcription	HL-60 cells	184
VDR	Up	mRNA	Rat intestine	185
			Rat pituitary	186
			MG-63 cells	181
				136

^{a} Regulation by $1\alpha,25(OH)_2D_3$.

mineral homeostasis, autoregulation and vitamin D metabolism, cell differentiation and proliferation, bone matrix protein, extracellular matrix proteins, oncogenes, chromosomal proteins, growth factors, signal transduction proteins, peptide hormones, and energy metabolism. Of the 51 gene products listed, all have been reported to be $1\alpha,25(OH)_2D_3$ sensitive in terms of altered mRNA level. However, $1\alpha,25(OH)_2D_3$ regulated transcription has only been reported in 11 of the genes and the presence of a VDRE in four. Several of the genes are characterized as $1\alpha,25(OH)_2D_3$ sensitive supported by data indicating altered mRNA levels, transcription, and the presence of a VDRE: integrin$_{\alpha v \beta 3}$ and 1(OH)hydroxyvitamin-D-24-hydroxylase. It should be noted that many of these genes encode proteins whose levels are indeed sensitive to vitamin D status.

15.5.2   Rapid Nongenomic Response

Studies[27] suggest that not all of the actions of $1\alpha,25(OH)_2D_3$ can be explained by receptor–hormone interactions with the genome. Rapid actions of $1\alpha,25(OH)_2D_3$ have been observed at both the cellular (e.g., calcium transport across a tissue) and subcellular level (membrane calcium transport, changes in intracellular second messengers). Table 15.2 summarizes the cell types in which rapid responses to $1\alpha,25(OH)_2D_3$ have been shown. In comparison to our understanding of the interaction of $1\alpha,25(OH)_2D_3$ with its nuclear VDR

TABLE 15.2

Distribution of Rapid Responses to $1\alpha,25(OH)_2D_3$

Organ/Cell/System	Response Studied	Ref.
Intestine	Rapid transport of intestinal Ca^{2+} (Transcaltachia);	11, 187, 188
	CaCo-2 cells, PKC, G proteins	189
	Activation of PKC	187, 190
Colon	PKC effects subcellular distribution regulation of 25(OH)D$_3$-24-hydroxylase	191
		192, 193
		194
Fibroblasts	Accumulation of cGMP near VDR$_{nuc}$	37, 195
Osteoblast	ROS 17/2.8 cells	
	Ca^{2+} channel opening	12
	Cl$^-$ channel opening	196
	UMR-106 cells	
	Ca^{2+} channel opening by 24R,25(OH)$_2$D$_3$	191
Liver	Lipid metabolism;	197, 198
	Activation of PKC and MAP kinase	199
		199
Muscle	PKC & Ca^{2+} effects	200–203
Promyelocytic leukemic cells	Aspects of cell differentiation	204, 205
	PKC effects	206, 207
Keratinocytes	Alter PKC subcellular distribution	208
Parathyroid cells	Phospholipid metabolism	209
	Cytosolic Ca^{2+}	210
Lipid bilayer	Activation of highly purified PKC	211

Note: The reader should compare the information in this table with the concepts illustrated in Figs. 15.2 and 15.3 which summarize the vitamin D endocrine system and signal transduction pathways utilized by $1\alpha,25(OH)_2D_3$ for generation of biological responses.

and the plethora of details concerning regulation of gene transcription, it is clear at the time of preparation of this review that the field of nongenomic responses is only in its infancy.

A particularly well-studied system in the author's laboratory is the duodenum of the vitamin D-replete chick where $1\alpha,25(OH)_2D_3$ stimulates transcaltachia or "the rapid hormonal stimulation of Ca^{2+} transport" in the vitamin-D replete chick.[11] Both the chick transcaltachic response and the rat ROS 17/2.8 osteoblast cell membrane Ca^{2+} transport occur within 2 to 4 minutes after treatment with $1\alpha,25(OH)_2D_3$ in a biphasic manner.[11,12] For both systems it has been proposed that there is a membrane receptor for $1\alpha,25(OH)_2D_3$ with ligand binding properties that are different from that of the nuclear/cytosol receptor; in each system the model suggests that the ligand–receptor complex mediates the signal transduction of the hormone via opening of voltage-gated Ca^{2+} channels so as to initiate the biological response(s).[28,29]

The process of transcaltachia is not inhibited by genomic inhibitors such as actinomycin D or protein synthesis inhibitors like cycloheximide, but is inhibited by Ca^{2+} channel blockers like nifedipine. In addition, inhibitors of PKC, such as H7, and an inhibitor of phospholipase C, U73122, inhibit transcaltachia; while mastoparan, which is an activator of G-proteins, stimulates transcaltachia. Transcaltachia, induced by $1\alpha,25(OH)_2D_3$ in the intestine, appears to involve the internalization of calcium in endocytic vesicles at the brush border membrane which then fuse with lysosomes and travel along microtubules to the basal lateral membrane where exocytosis occurs.[30,31] Thus, it is not surprising that transcaltachia is inhibited both by colchicine, an antimicrotubule agent, and by leupeptin, an antagonist of lysosomal cathepsin B which is associated with lysosomal vesicles.

Other effects of $1\alpha,25(OH)_2D_3$ that do not appear to be mediated by the nuclear receptor are phosphoinositide breakdown,[32] enzymatic activity in osteoblast-derived matrix vesicles,[33] certain secretion events in osteoblasts,[34] rapid changes in cytosolic Ca^{2+} levels in primary cultures of osteoblasts and osteosarcoma cells,[12,35,36] and increases in cyclic guanosine monophosphate levels in fibroblasts.[37]

These rapid effects appear to be mediated by a membrane receptor-like protein for $1\alpha,25(OH)_2D_3$.[38] Evidence has been presented which supports the view that the VDR_{mem} is located on the external surface of the cell.[39,40] Also, a cell membrane-binding protein for $1\alpha,25(OH)_2D_3$ which has been implicated with transcaltachia has been isolated and purified approximately 4000 fold.[40] Other steroid hormones, estrogen,[41] progesterone,[42–45] testosterone,[46] glucocorticoids,[47,48] corticosteroid,[49] and thyroid[50,51] have also been shown to have similar membrane effects that result in the rapid onset of biological responses; these are reviewed by Nemere, Zhou, and Norman.[38]

Thus, the integration of the generation of the production of biological responses by the steroid hormone $1\alpha,25(OH)_2D_3$ is mediated by both genomic as well as rapid responses. Figure 15.2 provides a summary describing our current understanding of how this steroid hormone can activate the generation of second messengers in the cytosol by both a series of systems operative in the cell cytosol and plasma membrane and, in the nucleus of the cell.

15.6 Nuclear Receptor for $1\alpha,25(OH)_2D_3$

15.6.1 Structural Domains

The VDR_{nuc} belongs to a superfamily of ligand-dependent nuclear receptors[10,52,53] which includes receptors for glucocorticoids (GR), progesterone (PR), estrogen (ER), aldosterone, androgens, thyroid hormone (T_3R), hormonal forms of vitamins A (RAR, RXR) and D (VDR), and many orphan receptors (Fig. 15.7) (see References 54 and 55 for a more detailed discussion

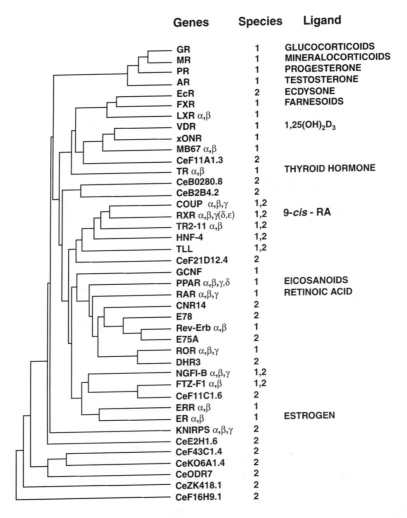

Genes	Species	Ligand
GR	1	GLUCOCORTICOIDS
MR	1	MINERALOCORTICOIDS
PR	1	PROGESTERONE
AR	1	TESTOSTERONE
EcR	2	ECDYSONE
FXR	1	FARNESOIDS
LXR α,β	1	
VDR	1	1,25(OH)$_2$D$_3$
xONR	1	
MB67 α,β	1	
CeF11A1.3	2	
TR α,β	1	THYROID HORMONE
CeB0280.8	2	
CeB2B4.2	2	
COUP α,β,γ	1,2	
RXR α,β,γ(δ,ε)	1,2	9-*cis* - RA
TR2-11 α,β	1,2	
HNF-4	1,2	
TLL	1,2	
CeF21D12.4	2	
GCNF	1	
PPAR α,β,γ,δ	1	EICOSANOIDS
RAR α,β,γ	1	RETINOIC ACID
CNR14	2	
E78	2	
Rev-Erb α,β	1	
E75A	2	
ROR α,β,γ	1	
DHR3	2	
NGFI-B α,β,γ	1,2	
FTZ-F1 α,β	1,2	
CeF11C1.6	2	
ERR α,β	1	
ER α,β	1	ESTROGEN
KNIRPS α,β,γ	2	
CeE2H1.6	2	
CeF43C1.4	2	
CeKO6A1.4	2	
CeODR7	2	
CeZK418.1	2	
CeF16H9.1	2	

FIGURE 15.7
Nuclear receptor superfamily. This figure summarizes the hypothesized evolutionary relationships for the extended family of known nuclear receptors and related orphan receptors
present in vertebrates and invertebrates (*Caenorhabditis elgans, Drosophila*). The relationships
are based on the extent of homology for the nucleotide sequence of the cDNA of the individual
protein. For further details, see References 54 and 55. (Modified from Mangelsdorf et al., *Cell*,
83, 835, 1995.)

of the evolutionary relationships). Comparative studies of these receptors
reveal that they have a common structural organization consisting of five
domains,[56] which are shown in Fig. 15.7. The different domains act as distinct
modules that can function independently of each other.[57–59]

Figure 15.8 diagrams the relationships for the VDR$_{nuc}$ among its gene,
mRNA, and receptor protein; additional information is presented in recent
reviews.[60,61] The DNA-binding domain, C, is the most conserved domain
throughout the family. About 70 amino acids fold into two zinc finger-like

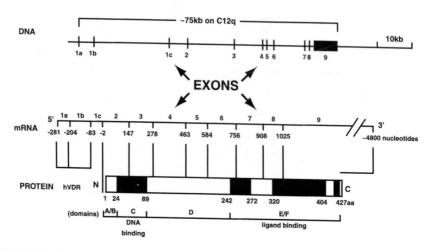

FIGURE 15.8

Schematic model of the VDR$_{nuc}$ gene, mRNA, and protein. The gene for the VDR$_{nuc}$ is located on human chromosome 12 and spans approximately 10 kb. The gene has 11 exons which are processed to yield a full-length mRNA of 4800 nucleotides. The VDR$_{nuc}$ protein is comprised of 427 amino acids. The numbers below the hVDR indicate the amino acid residue boundaries for the various domains. Nuclear receptors consist of 5 domains (A–E) based on regions of conserved amino acid sequence and function. The C domain, the most highly conserved domain, is the DNA-binding domain and it defines the superfamily. It contains two zinc finger motifs. The E domain is less conserved and is responsible for ligand binding, dimerization, and transcriptional activation. Subdomains within the domain include ligand1 and ligand2, τ_i or transcriptional inhibition, and dimerization which contains 9 heptad repeats as first described.[62] Domains A/B and D have the least sequence homology.[60,61] (Modified from Pike, *Vitamin D*, Academic Press, 1977).

motifs. Conserved cysteines coordinate a zinc ion in a tetrahedral arrangement. The first finger, which contains four cysteines and several hydrophobic amino acids, determines the DNA response element specificity. The second zinc finger, which contains five cysteines and many basic amino acids, is also necessary for DNA binding and is involved in receptor dimerization.[52,58,62,63]

The next most conserved region is the steroid-binding domain (region E). This region contains a hydrophobic pocket for ligand binding and also contains signals for several other functions including dimerization,[64,67] nuclear translocation, and hormone-dependent transcriptional activation.[57,58,68]

The A/B domain is also known as the immuno- or transactivation domain. This region is poorly conserved in amino acids and in size, and its function has not been clearly defined. The VDR has the smallest A/B domain (25 amino acids) of the known receptors; the mineralocorticoid receptor has the largest A/B domain (603 amino acids). An independent transcriptional activation function is located within the A/B region[52,58,59] which is constitutive in receptor constructs lacking the ligand-binding domain (region E). The relative importance of the transcriptional activation by this domain depends on the receptor, the context of the target gene promoter, and the target cell-type.[69]

Domain D is the hinge region between the DNA-binding domain and the ligand-binding domain. The hinge domain must be conformationally flexible because it allows the ligand-binding and DNA-binding domains some flexibility for their proper interactions. The VDR hinge region contains 65 amino acids and has immunogenic properties.[70]

15.6.2   Receptor Dimerization

The superfamily of nuclear receptors has been classified into subgroups based on their dimerization properties, DNA-binding site preferences, and cellular localization. Group I includes the receptors for glucocorticoids, estrogen, mineralocorticoids, progesterone, and androgens. These receptors bind as homodimers to palindromic DNA response elements. Group II includes the receptors for VDR_{nuc}, T_3R, RAR, RXR, ecdysone, and several orphan receptors. These receptors bind as homodimers or heterodimers to direct repeats, palindromic and inverted palindromic DNA response elements. Group III includes the receptors for reverb A, ROR, SF-1, and NGFI-B. No ligands have yet been identified for these receptors and they bind DNA response elements as monomers or heterodimers.

As a class, the group II receptors bind non-steroid conformationally flexible ligands (where vitamin D is classified as a seco-steroid rather than as a steroid). The group II receptors have more flexibility in the types of DNA response elements they can recognize and in the types of dimeric interactions they participate in than the group I receptors. All of the group II receptors can form heterodimers with RXR,[71,72] and other heterodimeric interactions have also been reported.[73] The VDR_{nuc} can bind to DNA response elements as homodimers and as heterodimers with RAR, RXR, and T_3R.[73,74] The ability to form heterodimers with other receptors allows for enhanced affinity for distinct DNA targets, generating a diverse range of physiological effects as shown in Fig. 15.9.

The first zinc finger determines the sequence specificity of the DNA element. The second zinc finger is aligned by the binding of the first finger to the DNA and is involved in the protein–protein contacts responsible for the cooperativity of binding. The spacing of nucleotides between the two half sites is important for the DNA-binding specificity because of the asymmetric dimer interface formed by the DNA-binding domains of a heterodimer pair. Ligand binding may function to modulate receptor dimerization. In fact, VDR_{nuc} has been shown to exist as a monomer in solution in either the presence or absence of ligand. When DNA is present, in the absence of ligand, the VDR_{nuc} binds to the DNA as monomers and homodimers. The addition of ligand stabilizes the bound monomer which favors the formation of VDR_{nuc}-RXR (or other) heterodimers. The presence of the ligand decreases the rate of monomer-to-homodimer conversion and enhances the dissociation of the dimer complex. The presence of the RXR ligand, 9-*cis*-retinoic acid, has the opposite effect on heterodimerization formation; it enhances the binding of

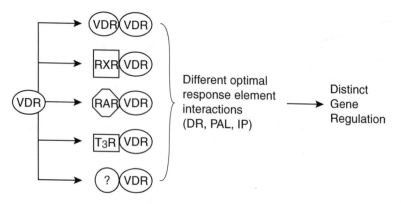

FIGURE 15.9

Schematic of possible dimeric interactions of VDR_{nuc} with other receptors. The VDR_{nuc} can bind to DNA as a homodimer or as a heterodimer with a variety of other group 2 receptors, i.e., RXR (retinoid X receptor), RAR (retinoic acid receptor), T_3R (thyroid receptor), and perhaps other receptors or factors not yet identified. Each dimer pair has an enhanced affinity for distinct DNA targets allowing a small family of receptors to generate a diverse range of physiological effects.

RXR homodimers to DR+1 elements.[75] Ligand bound to VDR_{nuc} enhances the binding of RXR-VDR_{nuc} heterodimers to DR+3 elements. There are also other possible protein–protein interactions that can involve VDR_{nuc} including association with AP-1, EE1A/TFIID, TFIIB. These protein–protein interactions can be determined by the concentration of the protein partner and/or by the concentration of ligand or both, as well as by the nature of the DNA target site itself.

15.6.3   Hormone Response Elements

Each zinc finger appears to be encoded by separate exons as shown by the genomic structure of the ER,[76] PR,[77] and the VDR_{nuc}.[78] Most of the knowledge of how zinc fingers interact with DNA response elements has been gained by studies of GR and ER. The palindromic nature of GR and ER response elements suggested that these hormone receptors would bind to DNA as symmetrical dimers. Subsequent studies have confirmed that GR and ER bind as homodimers to their response elements.[79,80] The principal ER-dimerization domain is in its ligand-binding domain.[81] Both the ER and GR contain additional residues in the DNA-binding domain that are also important for dimerization. When the GR and ER DNA-binding domains are translated, they cannot dimerize alone but in the presence of the correct palindromic response element, they bind to DNA as a dimer in a cooperative manner.[82] The five amino-acid-stretch between the first two coordinating cysteines of the second zinc finger is designated the "D" box[83] and mediates spacing requirements critical for cooperative dimer binding to palindromic HREs, probably through a dimer interface involving these residues in each monomer.[84,86]

Using the GR and ER as models of receptor–DNA interactions, the binding of VDR_{nuc} to DNA has also been examined. Since VDR_{nuc} can bind to DNA as a heterodimer, often with RXR, VDR_{nuc} and other group II receptors seem to display more variety in how they bind to their response elements.[66,78,87] The primary response element for the group II receptors is a direct repeat instead of an inverted palindrome; the protein–protein contacts are non-equivalent. There is an asymmetrical dimerization interface. Amino acid residues, designated the T/A box in the hinge region (domain D) just adjacent to the DNA-binding domain, are involved. The T/A-box residues form an α-helix making backbone and minor groove interactions which are involved in intramolecular packing against residues in the tip of the first zinc finger and determine the spacing requirements for the heterodimer pair. The P-box is the DNA-recognition helix at the C-terminal base of the first zinc finger where specific base contacts with the DNA are made. The D-box is at the N-terminal base of the second zinc finger and together with additional residues from the second zinc finger form part of the dimerization interface.[88]

Table 15.3 summarizes examples of hormone response elements for VDR_{nuc}. The natural response elements for the group II receptors appear to consist of a direct repeat of the hexamer AGGTCA. The spacing of the direct repeat determines the receptor preference: VDR_{nuc} prefers a three base pair space, T_3R prefers four base pairs, and RAR prefers five base pairs.[89] RXR, RAR, T_3R, VDR_{nuc} spacing optimum on a palindrome is no nucleotides between half-sites. Spacing on inverted palindromes depends on the overhang of the dimeric partners: 11 for VDR_{nuc}–RAR; VDR_{nuc}–RXR is predicted to be 7 to 8, but actually is 9; RXR appears to use a slightly different contact interface when it heterodimerizes with VDR_{nuc} than with other receptors.[90] Free rotation around the hinge (domain D) enables the same interaction of the ligand-binding domains of both receptors on each response element. The steric requirements of the T/A boxes give the receptor its asymmetry when binding to direct repeats and inverted palindromes and determines the optimal spacing, illustrated in Fig. 15.10.

TABLE 15.3

Hormone Response Elements for the Nuclear Vitamin D Receptor (VDR_{nuc})

Gene	Hormone Response Element	Ref.
hOsteocalcin	GGGTGA acg GGGGCA	212
rOsteocalcin	GGGTGA atg AGGACA	172
mOsteopontin	GGTTCA cga GGGTCA	174
rCalbindin D_{9k}	GGGTGA cgg AAGCCC	21
mCalbindin D_{28k}	GGGGGA tgt GAGGAG	213
24R-Hydroxylase	AGGTGA gtg AGGGCG	214
DR+3	AGGTCA agg AGGTCA	89
CONSENSUS	GGGTGA nnn <u>GGG</u>NCNAA	

Note: A comparison of reported VDREs. The two half-sites are listed as uppercase letters. The sequences are –500 to –486 of human osteocalcin, –456 to –438 of rat osteocalcin, –758 to –740 of mouse osteopontin, –488 to –474 of rat calbindin D_{9K}, and –199 to –184 of mouse calbindin D_{28K}.

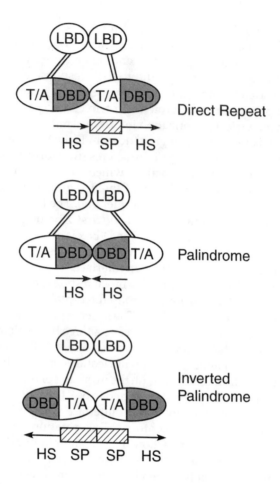

FIGURE 15.10

Mechanism of receptor dimers binding to DNA response elements. Group II receptors can bind to three types of response elements, which are direct repeats, palindromes, and inverted palindromes. The spacing (SP), number of base pairs between half-sites (HS), is determined by steric constraints of the T/A box. The orientation of the DNA half-sites is shown with arrows. The flexible hinge domain allows the formation of the same dimerization interface between ligand-binding domains (LBD) regardless of the orientation of the DNA half-sites.

15.6.4   Ligand Binding

The ligand-binding domain of group II receptors has been further dissected (see Fig. 15.8). Subdomains ligand 1 and ligand 2 are nearly identical among receptors of the same binding specificity but are different among receptors of different binding specificity.[91,93] Surprisingly, there is greater homology between the ligand binding subdomains of RAR (α, β, γ) and T_3R (α, β) than there is between RAR and RXR. The τ_i subdomain is highly conserved among all nuclear hormone receptors and is a putative transcriptional inactivating domain. Inactivation of this domain is relieved by ligand binding.

The dimerization domain consists of 8 to 9 heptad repeats of hydrophobic amino acids. The heptads contain leucine or other hydrophobic residues such as Ile, Val, Met, or Phe at positions one and eight or charged amino acids with hydrophobic side chains such as Arg or Gln in the fifth position. In an ideal coiled-coil α-helix, these amino acids would form a hydrophobic surface along one face of the helix that would act as a dimerization interface.[65] Deletion/mutation analysis of the VDR$_{nuc}$ ligand-binding domain has shown that Asp-258 and Ile-248 are involved in heterodimerization with RXR. Leu-254 and -262 are critical for heterodimerization. A mutant that is truncated at amino acid 190 becomes constituitively transcriptionally active. Other amino acids identified as being important for heterodimerization are 325–332, 383–390, and 244–263. Residues 403–427 are important for ligand binding [1α,25(OH)$_2$D$_3$].[94]

The location of the dimerization subdomain between the two ligand-binding subdomains links dimerization with ligand binding and has regulatory implications. The dimerization subdomain appears important for heterodimerization of the group II receptors.[66,67] This subdomain is similar to two known dimerization domains present in other transcription factors, the leucine zipper and helix-loop-helix motifs[87,95,96] and is sometimes called a "regulatory zipper". The group II receptors are the only members of the superfamily that have these conserved heptad repeats. The dimerization interfaces are precisely designed to accommodate the formation of homo- or heterodimers on symmetrical or asymmetrical response elements. There is considerable flexibility in response element specificity but this follows precise rules. By promiscuous dimerization, small families of structurally related proteins can result in large numbers of transcription factors with distinct functional properties such as binding affinities for specific response elements and inducibility by specific ligands.[97]

Recently, the ligand-binding domain of three steroid receptors has been determined via X-ray crystallographic techniques which have allowed for the first time a definitive view of how ligands interact with the ligand-binding domain of their cognate receptors. The new structures include the human RXR-α,[64] the rat thyroid receptor,[98] and the human estrogen receptor.[99] A striking finding is that all three structures were essentially identical. For each receptor, approximately 65% of the amino acid residues in the ligand-binding domain are arranged in 11 or 12 α-helices, forming a three-layered structure surrounding a large hydrophobic pocket which can accommodate the appropriate ligand. Thus, it seems likely that the overall topology of the VDR$_{nuc}$ ligand-binding domain will be similar to that of these three structures.

Figure 15.11 presents a schematic model of the VDR$_{nuc}$ interaction with its heterodimer partner and the subsequent interaction with the promoter of genes selected for modulation, as well with other proteins (coactivators, TATA-binding protein, etc.) to generate a competent transcriptional complex. During the past decade there has been a continuing evolution of understanding and complexity concerning the details of what constitutes a competent

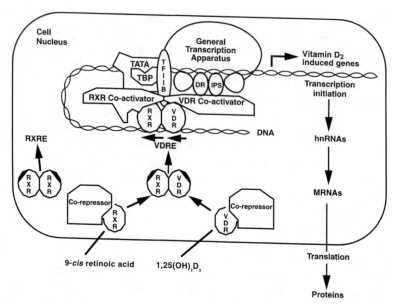

FIGURE 15.11

Model of $1\alpha,25(OH)_2D_3$ and VDR_{nuc} activation of transcription. The VDR after binding its cognate ligand $1\alpha,25(OH)_2D_3$ forms a heterodimer with RXR. This heterodimer complex then interacts with the appropriate VDRE on the promoter of genes (in specific target cells) which are destined to be up- or downregulated. The heterodimer–DNA complex then recruits necessary coactivator proteins, TATA, TBP, TFIIB, and other proteins to generate a competent transcriptional complex capable of modulating mRNA production. (Modified from Haussler et al., *Vitamin D*, Academic Press, 1977.)

transcriptional complex. Additional viewpoints and information can be found in recent review articles.[100–104]

15.7 Genetics and the Vitamin D Endocrine System

15.7.1 Mutations in the VDR_{nuc}

Vitamin D-dependent rickets-type II is a rare genetic disease. Genetic analysis has shown that it is autosomal recessive. Less than 30 kindreds have been reported. The combination of symptoms, i.e., defective bone mineralization, decreased intestinal calcium absorption, hypocalcemia, and increased serum levels of $1\alpha,25(OH)_2D_3$, suggest end-organ resistance to the action of $1\alpha,25(OH)_2D_3$. Patients do not respond to doses of vitamin D, $25(OH)D_3$ or $1\alpha,25(OH)_2D_3$.

The unresponsiveness to $1\alpha,25(OH)_2D_3$ has been demonstrated to arise from defects in the gene coding for the VDR_{nuc}. Table 15.4 summarizes the

TABLE 15.4

Genetic Analysis of the Nuclear Receptor for $1\alpha,25(OH)_2D_3$: Site of Mutation in the Nuclear Receptor for $1\alpha,25(OH)_2D_3$

VDR Domain	Mutation	Functional Consequence	Ref.
DNA-binding domain	R30Stop	Premature termination- no DNA	215
	R73Stop	binding, no ligand binding	216
	R88Stop		215
	Point mutation intron 4 results in premature stop codon		217
	R30G	Mutations occurring at highly	108
	G33D	conserved amino acid residue within	218
	H35Q	the first and second zinc fingers.	219
	K42I	Mutation interferes with the ability of	107
	K43E	the receptor to interact normally with	107
	F44I	DNA	107
	G46D		220
	R50Q		221
	R70D		108
	R73Q		218
	R80Q		222
	K91N/E92Q		223
Hinge region	148Stop	Premature termination — no ligand	216
	Q152Stop	binding	105
Ligand binding domain	Y295Stop	Premature termination — no ligand binding	106
	C190Y	Familial VDDRII	224
	S208G	Phosphorylation that modulates transcription	225
	S208A	No enhancement of transcription	
	F244G	Impaired transactivation; no RXR dimers	226
	K246G	Impaired transactivation	226
	L254G	Impaired transactivation; no RXR	226
	Q259G	dimers	
	L262G		
	C288G	Impaired ligand binding	227
	H305Q	Decreased binding (slight); decreased transactivation	228
	I314S	Impaired transactivation and RXR dimerization	229
	C337G	Impaired ligand binding	227
	C369G	Impaired transactivation and RXR	226
	R391C	dimerization	229

locations and nature of known mutations in the VDR$_{nuc}$. Two types of abnormalities have been defined by binding studies: receptor-negative and receptor-positive phenotypes. The mutations identified in the receptor-negative phenotype involve a mutation that introduces a premature stop codon in the message. The resulting truncated protein is not able to bind ligand. The receptor-positive phenotype arises from one of several missense mutations localized within the zinc finger domains of the DNA-binding domain. Several of these mutant receptors have been demonstrated to be defective in their ability to bind to DNA-cellulose and unable to mediate $1\alpha,25(OH)_2D_3$-stimulated gene transcription *in vitro*.[105–108]

15.7.2 Knockout of the VDR_{nuc}

An animal model of vitamin D-dependent rickets-type II (VDDRII) was engineered most recently by targeted disruption of DNA encoding the first and the second zinc finger of the DNA-binding domain of the VDR, respectively, by two different groups independently.[109,110] The resultant animals were phenotypically normal at birth. No defects in development and growth were observed before weaning, irrespective of reduced expression of vitamin D target genes. After weaning (3 weeks after birth), however, the VDR null mutant mice showed marked growth retardation. Such growth retardation became apparent only after weaning, even when it was either hastened or delayed. Most of the null mutant mice died by 15 weeks. No overt abnormalities, however, were found in the heterozygotes even at 6 months. All of the VDR null mutant mice developed alopecia and had few whiskers by 7 weeks. The serum levels of calcium and phosphate were reduced at 4 weeks, with markedly elevated serum alkaline phosphatase activity present in the null mutant mice while in older VDR-deficient mice, these abnormalities became more prominent. These observations in the VDR null mutant mice are similar to those in a human vitamin D-dependent rickets-type II disease, in which mutations in VDR gene have been identified in several families, although this disease is not lethal.

In the VDR null mutant mice at 3 weeks, the serum levels of $1\alpha,25(OH)_2D_3,$ $24R,25(OH)_2D_3$, and $25(OH)D_3$ were the same as those in the heterozygous and wild-type mice. However, a marked increase (10 times) in serum $1\alpha,25(OH)_2D_3$ and a clear reduction (to almost undetectable levels) in serum $24R,25(OH)_2D_3$ developed in the VDR null mutant mice at 4 weeks and persisted at 7 weeks. Immunoreactive PTH levels were also raised sharply after weaning and the size of the parathyroid glands in the 70-day-old VDR-ablated mice was increased more than 10-fold. These observations establish that VDR is essential for regulations of these enzymes by $1\alpha,25(OH)_2D_3$ after weaning, again supporting the idea that $1,25(OH)_2D_3$ (VDR) plays a critical role only after weaning. The authors suggest that a functional substitute for $1\alpha,25(OH)_2D_3$ is present in milk.

Severe bone malformation was induced by the inactivation of VDR after weaning. Radiographic analysis of VDR null mutant mice at 7 weeks revealed growth retardation with loss of bone density. A 40% reduction in bone mineral density was observed in the homozygote mutant mice. In gross appearance and on X-ray analysis of tibia and fibula, typical features of advanced rickets were observed, including widening of epiphyseal growth plates, thinning of the cortex, fraying, cupping, and widening of the metaphysis. In addition, orderly columns of hypertrophic chondrocytes were lost, and the layers of cartilage were widened with inadequate mineralization. In cancellous bone adjacent to the growth plates, marked increases in the extent and width of osteoid seams were noted, and bone surfaces were surrounded by numerous osteoblastic cells. The number of osteoclasts appeared not to be reduced in bone from VDR null mutant mice when compared to that of normal mice. These findings indicated that $1,25(OH)_2D_3$ can stimulate, but is not essential for, osteoclast formation *in vivo*, and that other factors can induce the osteoclast formation when VDR-mediated actions are absent.

The male and female VDR null mutant mice were infertile. The uterus had not matured in the female VDR knockout mice at 7 weeks. This uterine hypoplasia is not due to inability of the uterus to respond to estrogen. Only primary and secondary, but no mature, graafian follicles were observed in the null mutant mice, which indicates a lack of estrogen synthesis in the mutant overies. In contrast, male reproductive organs appeared normal in VDR null mutant mice. In addition, no obvious difference between the null mutant and wild-type mice at 3 or 7 weeks was detected in the proportional change of immunological cell population when cells from the spleen, thymus, mesenteric lymph node, and bone marrow were analyzed.

15.7.3 Knockout of the 25(OH)D-24-Hydroxylase

$24R,25(OH)_2D_3$ is the second major dihydroxylated metabolite of vitamin D_3, which is found in significant concentrations in the serum of humans,[111–113] rats,[114] and chicks.[115] Although the production of $24R,25(OH)_2D_3$ by the kidney is tightly regulated,[116] the biological importance of this compound is still the subject of uncertainty and question.[4,117] While several possible biological roles and sites of action have been suggested for $24R,25(OH)_2D_3$, including regulation of parathyroid hormone release from the parathyroid gland,[117,118] most studies concerning this vitamin D metabolite have focused on its possible actions on bone biology.[119–121] The possible existence of a nuclear or cytosolic-binding protein for $24R,25(OH)_2D_3$ was reported in the chick parathyroid gland,[122] the long bone of rat epiphysis,[123] and chick tibial fracture-healing callus;[124] however, there has been no general confirmation of these early findings. Also, several more recent reports have described specific actions or accumulation of $24R,25(OH)_2D_3$ in cartilage,[123,125] and the bone fracture-healing callus tissue.[121,126,127]

In order to address the physiological functions of $24R,25(OH)_2D_3$, a strain of mice deficient for the 25(OH)D-24-hydroxylase enzyme has been generated recently[128] through homologous recombination in embryonic stem cells. The targeted mutation effectively deleted the heme-binding domain of the cytochrome P-450 enzyme, ensuring that the mutated allele could not produce a functional protein. The analysis of the phenotype of the knockout animals revealed fascinating and previously unrecognized roles for $24R,25(OH)_2D_3$. About half of the mutant homozygote mice born from heterozygote females died before weaning. Bone development of those survivors was abnormal in homozygous mutants born of homozygous females. Histological analyses of the bones from these mice revealed an accumulation of unmineralized matrices at sites of intramembranous ossification, particularly the calvaria and exocortical surface of long bones. However, the growth plates from these mutant animals appeared normal, suggesting that $24R,25(OH)_2D_3$ is not a major regulator of chondrocyte maturation *in vivo*.

This study confirms the earlier reports that the presence of $24R,25(OH)_2D_3$ in collaboration with $1\alpha,25(OH)_2D_3$ is essential to the normal operation of the vitamin D endocrine system.

15.8 Summary

$1\alpha,25(OH)_2D_3$ is responsible for the generation of a wide array of biological responses throughout the far reaching network of its vitamin D endocrine system. In each instance, the initiation of a biological response is dependent upon the specific interaction of $1\alpha,25(OH)_2D_3$ as a ligand with the VDR_{nuc}, the VDR_{mem}, or the plasma transport-binding protein, DBP (see Fig. 15.12). While this chapter has focused upon the biological properties of only the VDR_{nuc} and the VDR_{mem}, based on evidence accumulated to date, we have concluded that DBP, VDR_{nuc}, and VDR_{mem} proteins are conformationally specific. That is, each will optimally bind a <u>different</u> shape of $1\alpha,25(OH)_2D_3$. Thus, one possible way in which the vitamin D endocrine system is able to achieve such

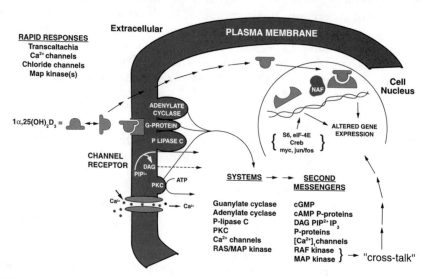

FIGURE 15.12

$1\alpha,25(OH)_2D_3$ and signal transduction; a working model. The upper left inset lists the rapid responses generated by $1\alpha,25(OH)_2D_3$ whose actions are believed to be described by this schematic model. $1\alpha,25(OH)_2D_3$ can initiate biological responses via its nuclear receptor and a putative cell membrane receptor[40] which rapidly generates the appearance of second messengers, some of which modulate via cross-talk selective events in the nucleus.

diversity in its biological responses is through utilization of receptors and transport proteins (DBP) which have evolved to be selectively responsive to different subsets within the myriad shapes available for the conformationally flexible $1\alpha,25(OH)_2D_3$. Further studies are in progress to test experimentally various ramifications of this hypothesis.

Abbreviations

$1\alpha,25(OH)_2D_3$ $1\alpha,25$-dihydroxyvitamin D_3

VDRE $1\alpha,25(OH)_2D_3$ nuclear response element

TPA 12-0-tetradecanoylphorbol-13 acetate

25OHD$_3$ 25-dihydroxyvitamin D_3

24R,25OHD$_3$ $24R,25(OH)_2$-vitamin D_3

ER estrogen nuclear receptor

GR glucocorticoid nuclear receptor

Gc group-specific component

IU International Unit

HRE nuclear receptor hormone response element

VDR$_{nuc}$ nuclear receptor for $1\alpha,25(OH)_2D_3$

PTH parathyroid hormone

PR progesterone nuclear receptor

VDR$_{mem}$ putative membrane receptor for $1\alpha,25(OH)_2D_3$

transcaltachia rapid hormonal stimulation of Ca^{2+} transport

RDA Recommended Dietary Allowance

RAR retinoid acid nuclear receptor

RXR retinoid x-nuclear receptor

T$_3$R thyroid hormone nuclear receptor

DBP vitamin D binding protein

VDDRII vitamin D-dependent rickets type II

VDR vitamin D receptor

References

1. Nemere, I. and Norman, A. W., Transport of calcium, in *Handbook of Physiology*, Field, M. and R. A. Frizzell, Eds., Amer. Physiol. Soc., Bethesda, 1991, 337.

2. Theofan, G., Nguyen, A. P., and Norman, A. W., Regulation of calbindin-D28K gene expression by 1,25-dihydroxyvitamin D_3 is correlated to receptor occupancy, *J. Biol. Chem.*, 261, 16943, 1986.
3. Leathers, V. L., Linse, S., Forsen, S., and Norman, A. W., Calbindin-D28K, a 1α,25-dihydroxyvitamin D_3-induced calcium-binding protein, binds five or six Ca_{2+} ions with high affinity, *J. Biol. Chem.*, 265, 9838, 1990.
4. Norman, A. W., Roth, J., and Orci, L., The vitamin D endocrine system: steroid metabolism, hormone receptors and biological response (calcium binding proteins), *Endocr. Rev.*, 3, 331, 1982.
5. Walters, M. R., Newly identified actions of the vitamin D endocrine system, *Endocr. Rev.*, 13, 719, 1992.
6. Reichel, H., Koeffler, H. P., and Norman, A. W., Production of 1α-25-dihydroxyvitamin D_3 by hematopoietic cells, in *Molecular and Cellular Regulation of Calcium and Phosphate Metabolism*, Peterlik, M. and F. Bronner, Eds., Liss, New York, 1990, 81.
7. Manolagas, S. C., Hustmyer, F. G., and Yu, X. P., 1,25-dihydroxyvitamin D_3 and the immune system, *Proc. Soc. Exp. Biol. Med.*, 191, 238, 1989.
8. Pike, J. W., Vitamin D_3 receptors: structure and function in transcription, *Ann. Rev. Nutr.*, 11, 189, 1991.
9. Minghetti, P. P. and Norman, A. W., 1,25(OH)$_2$-vitamin D_3 receptors: gene regulation and genetic circuitry, *FASEB J.*, 2, 3043, 1988.
10. Lowe, K. E., Maiyar, A. C., and A. W. Norman., Vitamin D-mediated gene expression, *Crit. Rev. Eukar. Gene Exp.*, 2, 65, 1992.
11. Nemere, I., Yoshimoto, Y., and Norman, A. W., Studies on the mode of action of calciferol, LIV, Calcium transport in perfused duodena from normal chicks: enhancement with 14 minutes of exposure to 1α,25-dihydroxyvitamin D_3, *Endocrinology*, 115, 1476, 1984.
12. Caffrey, J. M. and Farach-Carson, M. C., Vitamin D_3 metabolites modulate dihydropyridine-sensitive calcium currents in clonal rat osteosarcoma cells, *J. Biol. Chem.*, 264, 20265, 1989.
13. Henry, H. L., Vitamin D hydroxylases, *J. Cell. Biochem.*, 49, 4, 1992.
14. Henry, H., Dutta, L. C., Cunningham, N., Blanchard, R., Penny, R., Tang, C., Marchetto, G., and Chou, S.-Y., The cellular and molecular regulation of 1,25(OH)$_2$D$_3$ production, *J. Steroid Biochem. Mol. Biol.*, 41, 401, 1992.
15. Henry, H. L., Tang, C., Blanchard, R., and Marchetto, G. S., Regulation of the ferredoxin component of renal hydroxylases at transcriptional and posttranslational levels and of the protein inhibitor of cyclic AMP-dependent kinase, *J. Steroid Biochem. Mol. Biol.*, 53, 595, 1995.
16. Tang, C. and Henry, H. L., Overexpression in Escherichia coli and affinity purification of chick kidney ferredoxin, *J. Biol. Chem.*, 268, 5069, 1993.
17. Henry, H. L. and Norman, A. W., Studies on calciferol metabolism, IX, Renal 25-hydroxyvitamin D_3-1-hydroxylase. Involvement of cytochrome P-450 and other properties, *J. Biol. Chem.*, 249, 7529, 1974.
18. Bouillon, R., Okamura, W. H., and Norman, A. W., Structure-function relationships in the vitamin D endocrine system, *Endocr. Rev.*, 16, 200, 1995.
19. Haddad, J. G., Plasma vitamin D-binding protein (Gc-globulin): Multiple tasks, *J. Steroid Biochem. Mol. Biol.*, 53, 579, 1995.
20. Cooke, N. E. and Haddad, J. G., Vitamin D binding protein, in *Vitamin D*, Feldman, D., F. H. Glorieux, and J. W. Pike, Eds., Academic Press, San Diego, 1997, 87.

21. Darwish, H. M., Burmester, J. K., Moss, V. E., and DeLuca, H. F., Phosphorylation is involved in transcriptional activation by the 1,25-dihydroxyvitamin D$_3$ receptor, *Biochim. Biophys. Acta Lipids Lipid Metab.*, 1167, 29, 1993.
22. Hsieh, J.-C., Jurutka, P. W., Nakajima, S., Galligan, M. A., Haussler, C. A., Shimizu, Y., Shimizu, N., Whitfield, G. K., and Haussler, M. R., Phosphorylation of the human vitamin D receptor by protein kinase C. Biochemical and functional evaluation of the serine 51 recognition site, *J. Biol. Chem.*, 268, 15118, 1993.
23. Jurutka, P. W., Hsieh, J.-C., and Haussler, M. R., Phosphorylation of the human 1,25-dihydroxyvitamin D$_3$ receptor by cAMP-dependent protein kinase, *in vitro*, and in transfected COS-7 cells, *Biochem. Biophys. Res. Commun.*, 191, 1089, 1993.
24. Jurutka, P. W., Hsieh, J.-C., MacDonald, P. N., Terpening, C. M., Haussler, C. A., Haussler, M. R., and Whitfield, G. K., Phosphorylation of serine 208 in the human vitamin D receptor, *J. Biol. Chem.*, 268, 6791, 1993.
25. Ortí, E., Bodwell, J. E., and Munck, A., Phosphorylation of steroid hormone receptors, *Endocr. Rev.*, 13, 105, 1992.
26. Hannah, S. S., and Norman, A. W., 1α,25 (OH)$_2$-vitamin D$_3$-regulated expression of the eukaryotic genome, *Nutr. Reviews*, 52, 376, 1994.
27. Nemere, I. and Norman, A. W., Studies on the mode of action of calciferol. LII. Rapid action of 1,25-dihydroxyvitamin D$_3$ on calcium transport in perfused chick duodenum: effect of inhibitors, *J. Bone Miner, Res.*, 2, 99, 1987.
28. Farach-Carson, M. C., Sergeev, I. N., and Norman, A. W., Nongenomic actions of 1,25-dihydroxyvitamin D$_3$ in rat osteosarcoma cells: structure-function studies using ligand analogs, *Endocrinology*, 129, 1876, 1991.
29. Zhou, L.-X., Nemere, I., and Norman, A. W., 1,25(OH)$_2$-vitamin D$_3$ analog structure-function assessment of the rapid stimulation of intestinal calcium absorption (Transcaltachia), *J. Bone Miner. Res.*, 7, 457, 1992.
30. Nemere, I. and Norman, A. W., 1,25-Dihydroxyvitamin D$_3$-mediated vesicular transport of calcium in intestine: Time course studies, *Endocrinology*, 122, 2962, 1988.
31. Nemere, I., Leathers, V. L., Thompson, B. S., Luben, R. A., and Norman, A. W., Redistribution of calbindin-D$_{28k}$ in chick intestine in response to calcium transport, *Endocrinology*, 129, 2972, 1991.
32. Lieberherr, M., Grosse, B., Duchambon, P., and Drüeke, T., A functional cell surface type receptor is required for the early action of 1,25-dihydroxyvitamin D$_3$ on the phosphoinositide metabolism in rat enterocytes, *J. Biol. Chem.*, 264, 20403, 1989.
33. Boyan, B. D., Schwartz, Z., Bonewald, L., and Swain, L., Localization of 1,25-(OH)$_2$ D$_3$-responsive alkaline phosphatase in osteoblast-like cells (ROS 17/2.8, MG 63, and MC 3T3) and growth cartilage cells in culture, *J. Biol. Chem.*, 264, 11879, 1989.
34. Meikle, M. C., Hypercalcaemia of malignancy, *Nature*, 336, 311, 1988.
35. Cancela, L., Nemere, I., and Norman, A. W., 1α,25(OH)$_2$-Vitamin D$_3$: a steroid hormone capable of producing pleiotropic receptor-mediated biological responses by both genomic and nongenomic mechanisms, *J. Steroid Biochem. Mol. Biol.*, 30, 33, 1988.
36. Lieberherr, M., Effects of vitamin-D$_3$ metabolites on cytosolic free calcium in confluent mouse osteoblasts, *J. Biol. Chem.*, 262, 13168, 1987.
37. Barsony, J. and Marx, S. J., Rapid accumulation of cyclic GMP near activated vitamin D receptors, *Proc. Natl. Acad. Sci. USA*, 88, 1436, 1991.

38. Nemere, I., Zhou, L.-X., and Norman, A. W., Nontranscriptional effects of steroid hormones, *Receptor,* 3, 277, 1993.
39. Baran, D. T., Ray, R., Sorensen, A. M., Honeyman, T., and Holick, M. F., Binding characteristics of a membrane receptor that recognizes 1α,25-dihydroxyvitamin D₃ and its epimer, 1β,25-dihydroxyvitamin D₃, *J. Cell. Biochem.,* 56, 510, 1994.
40. Nemere, I., Dormanen, M. C., Hammond, M. W., Okamura, W. H., and Norman, A. W., Identification of a specific binding protein for 1α,25-dihydroxyvitamin D₃ in basal-lateral membranes of chick intestinal epithelium and relationship to transcaltachia, *J. Biol. Chem.,* 269, 23750, 1994.
41. Morley, P., Whitfield, J. F., Vanderhyden, B. C., Tsang, B. K., and Schwartz, J. L., A new, nongenomic estrogen action: the rapid release of intracellular calcium, *Endocrinology,* 131, 1305, 1992.
42. Aurell Wistrom, C. and Meizel, S., Evidence suggesting involvement of a unique human sperm steroid receptor/Cl⁻ channel complex in the progesterone-initiated acrosome reaction, *Dev. Biol.,* 159, 679, 1993.
43. Blackmore, P. F., Beebe, S. J., Danforth, D. R., and Alexander, N., Progesterone and 17α-progesterone: novel stimulators of calcium influx in human sperm, *J. Biol. Chem.,* 265, 1376, 1990.
44. Majewska, M. D. and Vaupel, D. B., Steroid control of uterine motility via gamma-aminobutyric acid_A receptors in the rabbit: A novel mechanism, *J. Endo.,* 131, 427, 1991.
45. Mendoza, C. and Tesarik, J., A plasma-membrane progesterone receptor in human sperm is switched on by increasing intracellular free calcium, *FEBS Lett.,* 330, 57, 1993.
46. Koenig, H., Fan, C.-C., Goldstone, A. D., Lu, C. Y., and Trout, J. J., Polyamines mediate androgenic stimulation of calcium fluxes and membrane transport in rat myocytes, *Circ. Res.,* 64, 415, 1989.
47. Gametchu, B., Watson, C. S., and Wu, S., Use of receptor antibodies to demonstrate membrane glucocorticoid receptor in cells from human leukemic patients. *FASEB J.,* 7, 1283, 1993.
48. Rehberger, P., Rexin, M., and Gehring, U., Heterotetrameric structure of the human progesterone receptor, *Proc. Natl. Acad. Sci. USA,* 89, 8001, 1992.
49. Orchinik, M., Murray, T. F., and Moore, F. L., A corticosteroid receptor in neuronal membranes, *Science,* 252, 1848, 1991.
50. Segal, J., Thyroid hormone action at the level of the plasma membrane, *Thyroid,* 1, 83, 1990.
51. Smith, T. J., Davis, F. B., and Davis, P. J., Stereochemical requirements for the modulation by retinoic acid of thyroid hormone activation of Ca²⁺-ATPase and binding at the human erythrocyte membrane, *Biochem. J.,* 284, 583, 1992.
52. Evans, R. M., The steroid and thyroid hormone receptor superfamily, *Science,* 240, 889, 1988.
53. Parker, M. G., *Molecular Mechanism, Cellular Functions, Clinical Abnormalities: Nuclear Hormone Receptors,* Academic Press, London, 1991.
54. Mangelsdorf, D. J., Thummel, C., Beato, M., Herrlich, P., Schütz, G., Umesono, K., Blumberg, B., Kastner, P., Mark, M., Chambon, P., and Evans, R. M., The nuclear receptor superfamily: The second decade, *Cell,* 83, 835, 1995.
55. Carlberg, C., The vitamin D₃ receptor in the context of the nuclear receptor superfamily: The central role of the retinoid X receptor, *Endocrine,* 4, 91, 1996.

56. Krust, A., Green, S., Argos, P., Kumar, V., Walter, P., Bornert, J. M., and Chambon, P., The chicken oestrogen receptor sequence: homology with v-erbA and the human oestrogen and glucocorticoid receptors, *Embo. J.*, 5, 891, 1986.

57. Beato, M., Gene regulation by steroid hormones, *Cell*, 56, 335, 1989.

58. Green, S. and Chambon, P., Nuclear receptors enhance our understanding of transcription regulation, *Trends Genet.*, 4, 309, 1988.

59. Ham, J. and Parker, M. G., Regulation of gene expression by nuclear hormone receptors, *Curr. Opin. Cell Biol.*, 1, 503, 1989.

60. Haussler, M. R., Whitfield, G. K., Haussler, C. A., Hsieh, J. C., Thompson, P. D., Selznick, S. H., Dominguez, C. E., and Jurutka, P. W., The nuclear vitamin D receptor: Biological and molecular regulatory properties revealed, *J. Bone Miner. Res.*, 13, 325, 1998.

61. Carlberg, C. and Polly, P., Look up, *Eukaryotic Gene Expression*, 8, 19, 1999.

62. Forman, B. M., and Samuels, H. H. Interactions among a subfamily of nuclear hormone receptors: the regulatory zipper model, *Mol. Endocrinol.*, 4, 1293, 1990.

63. Rastinejad, F., Perlmann, T., Evans, R. M., and Sigler, P. B., Structural determinants of nuclear receptor assembly on DNA direct repeats, *Nature*, 375, 203, 1995.

64. Bourguet, W., Ruff, M., Chambon, P., Gronemeyer, H., and Moras, D., Crystal structure of the ligand-binding domain of the human nuclear receptor RXR-α, *Nature*, 375, 377, 1995.

65. Fawell, S. E., Lees, J. A., White, R., and Parker, M. G., Characterization and colocalization of steroid binding and dimerization activities in the mouse estrogen receptor, *Cell*, 60, 953, 1990.

66. Forman, B. M., Yan, C.-R., Au, M., Casanova, J., Ghysdael, J., and Samuels, H. H., A domain containing leucine zipper like motifs may mediate novel *in vivo* interactions between the thyroid hormone and retinoic acid receptors, *Mol. Endocrinol.*, 3, 1610, 1989.

67. Glass, C. K., Lipkin, S. M., Devary, O. V., and Rosenfeld, M. G., Positive and negative regulation of gene transcription by a retinoic acid-thyroid hormone recptor heterodimer, *Cell*, 59, 697, 1989.

68. Picard, D., Khursheed, B., Garabedian, M. J., Fortin, M. G., Lindquist, S., and Yamamoto, K. R., Reduced levels of hsp90 compromise steroid receptor action *in vivo*, *Nature*, 348, 166, 1990.

69. Tora, L., White, J., Brou, C., Tasset, D., Webster, N., Scheer, E., and Chambon, P., The human estrogen receptor has two independent nonacidic transcriptional activation functions, *Cell*, 59, 477, 1989.

70. McDonnell, D. P., Pike, J. W., and O'Malley, B. W., The vitamin D receptor: a primitive steroid receptor related to thyroid hormone receptor, *J. Steroid Biochem.*, 30, 41, 1988.

71. Kliewer, S. A., Umesono, K., Mangelsdorf, D. J., and Evans, R. M., Retinoid X receptor interacts with nuclear receptors in retinoic acid, thyroid hormone and vitamin D_3 signalling, *Nature*, 355, 446, 1992.

72. Yu, V. C., Delsert, C., Andersen, B., Holloway, J. M., Devary, O. V., Näär, A. M., Kim, S. Y., Boutin, J.-M., Glass, C. K., and Rosenfeld, M. G., RXRβ: A coregulator that enhances binding of retinoic acid, thyroid hormone, and vitamin D receptors to their cognate response elements, *Cell*, 67, 1251, 1991.

73. Carlberg, C., RXR-independent action of the receptors for thyroid hormone, retinoid acid and vitamin D on inverted palindromes, *Biochem. Biophys. Res. Commun.*, 195, 1345, 1993.

74. Schräder, M., Bendik, I., Becker-André, M., and Carlberg, C., Interaction between retinoic acid and vitamin D signaling pathways, *J. Biol. Chem.*, 268, 17830, 1993.

75. Cheskis, B. and Freedman, L. P., Ligand modulates the conversion of DNA-bound vitamin D_3 receptor (VDR) homodimers into VDR-retinoid X receptor heterodimers, *Mol. Cell. Biol.*, 14, 3329, 1994.

76. Ponglikitmongkol, M., Green, S., and Chambon, P., Genomic organization of the human oestrogen receptor gene, *Embo. J.*, 7, 3385, 1988.

77. Huckaby, C. S., Conneely, O. M., Beattie, W. G., Dobson, D. W., Tsi, M. J., and O'Malley, B. W., Structure of the chromosomal chicken progesterone receptor gene, *Proc. Natl. Acad. Sci. USA*, 84, 8380, 1987.

78. Freedman, L. P., Anatomy of the steroid receptor zinc finger region, *Endocr. Rev.*, 13, 129, 1992.

79. Picard, D., Kumar, V., Chambon, P., and Yamamoto, K. R., Signal transduction by steroid hormones: nuclear localization is differentially regulated in estrogen and glucocorticoid receptors, *Cell Regulation*, 1, 291, 1990.

80. Schwabe, J. W., Neuhaus, D., and Rhodes, D., Solution structure of the DNA-binding domain of the oestrogen receptor, *Nature*, 348, 458, 1990.

81. Kumar, V. and Chambon, P., The estrogen receptor binds tightly to its responsive element as a ligand-induced homodimer, *Cell*, 55, 145, 1988.

82. Hard, T., Dahlman, K., Carlstedt-Duke, J., Gustafsson, J. A., and Rigler, R., Cooperativity and specificity in the interactions between DNA and the glucocorticoid receptor DNA-binding domain, *Biochemistry*, 29, 5358, 1990.

83. Umesono, K. and Evans, R. M., Determinants of target gene specificity for steroid/thyroid hormone receptors, *Cell*, 57, 1139, 1988.

84. Diamond, M. I., Miner, J. N., Yoshinaga, S. K., and Yamamoto, K. R., Transcription factor interactions: selectors of positive or negative regulation from a single DNA element, *Science*, 249, 1266, 1990.

85. Jonat, C., Rahmsdorf, H. J., Park, K. K., Cato, A. C., Gebel, S., Ponta, H., and Herrlich, P., Antitumor promotion and antiinflammation: down-modulation of AP-1, *Cell*, 62, 1189, 1990.

86. Schule, R., Rangarajan, P., Kliewer, S., Ransone, L. J., Bolado, J., Yang, N., Verma, I. M., and Evans, R. M., Functional antagonism between oncoprotein c-Jun and the glucocorticoid receptor, *Cell*, 62, 1217, 1990.

87. Jones, N., Transcriptional regulation by dimerization: two sides to an incestuous relationship, *Cell*, 61, 9, 1990.

88. Towers, T. L., Luisi, B. F., Asianov, A., and Freedman, L. P., DNA target selectivity by the vitamin D_3 receptor: Mechanism of dimer binding to an asymmetric repeat element, *Proc. Natl. Acad. Sci. USA*, 90, 6310, 1993.

89. Umesono, K., Murakami, K. K., Thompson, C. C., and Evans, R. M., Direct repeats as selective response elements for the thyroid hormone, retinoic acid, and vitamin D_3 receptors, *Cell*, 65, 1255, 1991.

90. Schräder, M., Müller, K. M., Becker-André, M., and Carlberg, C., Response element selectivity for heterodimerization of vitamin D receptors with retinoic acid and retinoid X receptors, *J. Mol. Endo.*, 12, 327, 1994.

91. Giguere, V., Ong, E. S., Segui, P., and Evans, R. M., Identification of a receptor for the morphogen retinoic acid, *Nature*, 330, 624, 1987.

92. Harrison, S. C., A structural taxonomy of DNA-binding domains, *Nature*, 353, 715, 1991.

93. Thompson, C. C., Weinberger, C., Lebo, R., and Evans, R. M., Identification of a novel thyroid hormone receptor expressed in the mammalian central nervous system, *Science*, 237, 1610, 1987.
94. Nakajima, S., Hsieh, J.-C., MacDonald, P. N., Galligan, M. A., Haussler, C. A., Whitfield G. K., and Haussler, M. R., The C-terminal region of the vitamin D receptor is essential to form a complex with a receptor auxiliary factor required for high affinity binding to the vitamin D-responsive element, *Mol. Endocrinol.*, 8, 159, 1994.
95. Abel, T. and Maniatis, T., Gene regulation. Action of lucine zippers [news], *Nature*, 341, 24, 1989.
96. Kouzarides, T., and Ziff, E., Behind the Fos and Jun leucine zipper, *Cancer Cells*, 1, 71, 1989.
97. Schräder, M., Müller, K. M., and Carlberg, C., Specificity and flexibility of vitamin D signaling. Modulation of the activation of natural vitamin D response elements by thyroid hormone, *J. Biol. Chem.*, 269, 5501, 1994.
98. Wagner, R. L., Apriletti, J. W., McGrath, M. E., West, B. L., Baxter, J. D., and Fletterick, R. J., A structural role for hormone in the thyroid hormone receptor, *Nature*, 378, 690, 1995.
99. Anstad, G. M., Carlson, K. E., and Katzenellenbogen, J. A., The estradiol pharmacophore: Ligand structure-estrogen receptor binding affinity relationships and a model for the receptor binding site, *Steroids*, 62, 268, 1997.
100. Beato, M., and Sanchez-Pacheo, A., Interaction of steroid hormone receptors with the transcription initiation complex, *Endocr. Rev.*, 17, 587, 1997.
101. Glass, C. K., Rose, D. W., and Rosenfeld, M. G., Nuclear receptor coactivators, *Curr. Opin. Cell Biol.*, 9, 222, 1997.
102. Jenster, G., Spencer, T. E., Burcin, M. M., Tsai, S. Y., Tsai, M. J., and O'Malley, B. W., Steroid receptor induction of gene transcription: A two-step model, *Proc Natl. Acad. Sci. USA*, 94, 7879, 1997.
103. Robyr, D. and Wolffe, A. P., Hormone action and chromatin remodelling, *Cell. Mol. Life Sci.*, 54, 113, 1998.
104. Weigel, N. L. and Zhang, Y. X., Ligand-independent activation of steroid hormone receptors, *J. Mol. Med.*, 76, 469, 1998.
105. Kristjansson, K., Rut, A. R., Hewison, M. H., O'Riordan, J. L., and Hughes, M. R., Two mutations in the hormone binding domain of the vitamin D receptor cause tissue resistance to 1,25 dihydroxyvitamin D_3, *J. Clin. Invest.*, 92, 12, 1993.
106. Ritchie, H. H., Hughes, M. R., Thompson, E. T., Malloy, P. J., Hochberg, Z., Feldman, D., Pike, J. W., and O'Malley, B. W., An ochre mutation in the vitamin D receptor gene causes hereditary 1,25-dihydroxyvitamin D_3-resistant rickets in three families, *Proc. Natl. Acad. Sci. USA*, 86, 9783, 1989.
107. Rut, A. R., Hewison, M., Kristjansson, K., Luisi, B., Hughes, M. R., and O'Riordan, J. L. H., Two mutations causing vitamin D resistant rickets: modelling on the basis of steroid hormone receptor DNA-binding domain crystal structures, *Clin. Endocrinol. (Oxf.)*, 41, 581, 1994.
108. Sone, T., Scott, R. A., Hughes, M. R., Malloy, P. J., Feldman, D., O'Malley, B. W., and Pike, J. W., Mutant vitamin D receptors which confer hereditary resistance to 1,25-dihydroxyvitamin D_3 in humans are transcriptionally inactive *in vitro*, *J. Biol. Chem.*, 264, 20230, 1989.

109. Yoshizawa, T., Handa, Y., Uematsu, Y., Takeda, S., Sekine, K., Yoshihara, Y., Kawakami, T., Arioka, K., Sato, H., Uchiyama, Y., Masushige, S., Fukamizu, A., Matsumoto, T., and Kato, S., Mice lacking the vitamin D receptor exhibit impaired bone formation, uterine hypoplasia and growth retardation after weaning, *Nature Genet.*, 16, 391, 1997.

110. Li, Y. C., Pirro, A. E., Amling, M., Delling, G., Baroni, R., Bronson, R., and Demay, M. B., Targeted ablation of the vitamin D receptor: An animal model of vitamin D-dependent rickets type II with alopecia, *Proc. Natl. Acad. Sci. USA*, 94, 9831, 1997.

111. Castro-Errecaborde, N., De la Piedra, C., Rapado, A., Alvarez-Arroyo, M. V., Torres, R., and Traba, M. L., Correlation between serum osteocalcin and 24,25-dihydroxyvitamin D levels in Paget's disease of bone, *J. Clin. Endocr. Metab.*, 72, 462, 1991.

112. Jongen, M. J. M., van der Vijgh, W. J. F., Netelenbos, J. C., Postma, G. J., and Lips, P., Pharmacokinetics of 24,25-dihydroxyvitamin D_3 in humans, *Horm. Metab. Res.*, 21, 577, 1989.

113. Nguyen, T. M., Guillozo, H., Garabedian, M., Mallet, E., and Balsan, S., Serum concentration of 24,25-dihydroxyvitamin D in normal children and in children with rickets, *Pediat. Res.*, 13, 973, 1979.

114. Jarnagin, K., Zeng, S.-Y., Phelps, M., and DeLuca, H. F., Metabolism and pharmacokinetics of 24,25-dihydroxyvitamin D_3 in the vitamin D_3-replete rat, *J. Biol. Chem.*, 260, 13625, 1985.

115. Goff, J. P. and Horst, R. L., Assessing adequacy of cholecalciferol supplementation in chicks using plasma cholecalciferol metabolite concentrations as an indicator, *J. Nutr.*, 125, 1351, 1995.

116. Henry, H. L. and Norman, A. W., Vitamin D: metabolism and biological action, *Ann. Rev. Nutr.*, 4, 493, 1984.

117. Norman, A. W., Leathers, V. L., Bishop, J. E., Kadowaki S., and Miller, B. E., 24R,25-dihydroxyvitamin D_3 has unique receptors (parathyroid gland) and biological responses (egg hatchability), in *Vitamin D: Chemical, Biochemical, and Clinical Endocrinology of Calcium Metabolism*, Norman, A. W., K. Schaefer, H.-G. Grigoleit, and D. Herrath, Eds., Walter de Gruyter, Berlin, 1982, 147.

118. Canterbury, J. M., Lerman, S., Claflin, A. J., Henry, H. L., Norman, A. W., and Reiss, E., Inhibition of parathyroid hormone secretion by 25-hydroxycholecalciferol and 24,25-dihydroxycholecalciferol in the dog, *J. Clin. Invest.*, 61, 1375, 1978.

119. Norman, A. W. and Hurwitz, S., The role of the vitamin D endocrine system in avian bone biology, *J. Nutr.*, 123, 310, 1993.

120. Nakamura, T., Suzuki, K., Hirai, T., Kurokawa, T., and Orimo, H., Increased bone volume and reduced bone turnover in vitamin D-replete rabbits by the administration of 24R,25-dihydroxyvitamin D_3, *Bone*, 13, 229, 1992.

121. Seo, E.-G., Einhorn, T. A., and Norman, A. W., 24R,25-dihydroxyvitamin D_3: An essential vitamin D_3 metabolite for both normal bone integrity and healing of tibial fracture in chicks, *Endocrinology*, 138, 3864, 1997.

122. Merke, J. and Norman, A. W., Studies on the mode of action of calciferol XXXII — Evidence for a 24(R),25(OH)$_2$-vitamin D_3 receptor in the parathyroid gland of the rachitic chick, *Biochem. Biophys. Res. Commun.*, 100, 551, 1981.

123. Corvol, M., Ulmann, A., and Garabedian, M., Specific nuclear uptake of 24,25-dihydroxycholecalciferol, a vitamin D_3 metabolite biologically active in cartilage, *FEBS Lett.*, 116, 273, 1980.

124. Seo, E.-G., Kato, A., and Norman, A. W., Evidence for a 24R,25(OH)$_2$-vitamin D$_3$ receptor/binding protein in a membrane fraction isolated from a chick tibial fracture-healing callus, *Biochem. Biophys. Res. Commun.*, 225, 203, 1996.

125. Seo, E.-G., Schwartz, Z., Dean, D. D., Norman, A. W., and Boyan, B. D., Preferential accumulation *in vivo* of 24R,25-dihydroxyvitamin D$_3$ in growth plate cartilage of rats, *Endocrine*, 5, 147, 1996.

126. Lidor, C., Dekel, S., Hallel, T., and Edelstein, S., Levels of active metabolites of vitamin D$_3$ in the callus of fracture repair in chicks, *J. Bone Joint Surg.*, 69, 132, 1987.

127. Seo, E.-G. and Norman, A. W., Three-fold induction of renal 25-hydroxyvitamin D$_3$-24- hydroxylase activity and increased serum 24,25-dihydroxyvitamin D$_3$ levels are correlated with the healing process after chick tibial fracture, *J. Bone Miner. Res.*, 12, 598, 1997.

128. St. Arnaud, R., Arabian, A., Travers, R., and Glorieux, F. H., Abnormal intramembranous ossification in mice deficient for the vitamin D 24-hydroxylase, in *Vitamin D: Chemistry, Biology and Clinical Application of the Steroid Hormone*, Norman, A. W., R. Bouillon, and M. Thomasset, Eds, University of California, Riverside, 1997, 635.

129. Henry, H. L. and Amdahl, L. D., Enhancement of the production of 1,25-dihydroxyvitamin D3 in chick kidney mitochondria by an extramitochondrial factor, *J. Steroid Biochem. Mol. Biol.*, 20, 645, 1984.

130. Nemere, I., Theofan, G., and Norman, A. W., 1,25-Dihydroxyvitamin D3 regulates tubulin expression in chick intestine, *Biochem. Biophys. Res. Commun.*, 148, 1270, 1987.

131. Chou, S. Y., Hannah, S. S., Lowe, K. E., Norman, A. W., and Henry, H. L., Tissue-specific regulation by vitamin D status of nuclear and mitochondrial gene expression in kidney and intestine, *Endocrinology*, 136, 5520, 1995.

132. Eliakim, R., Seetharam, S., Tietze, C. C., and Alpers, D. H., Differential regulation of mRNAs encoding for rat intestinal alkaline phosphatase, *Am. J. Physiol.*, 259, G93, 1990.

133. Kyeyune-Nyombi, E., Lau, K.-H. W., Baylink, D. J., and Strong, D. D., Stimulation of cellular alkaline phosphatase activity and its messenger RNA level in a human osteosarcoma cell line by 1,25-dihydroxyvitamin D$_3$, *Arch. Biochem. Biophys.*, 275, 363, 1989.

134. Kessler, M. A., Lamm, L., Jarnagin, K., and DeLuca, H. F., 1,25-dihydroxyvitamin-D3-stimulated messenger-RNAs in rat small-intestine, *Arch. Biochem. Biophys.*, 251, 403, 1986.

135. Brelvi, Z. S., Christakos, S., and Studzinski, G. P., Expression of monocyte-specific oncogenes c-fos and c-fms in HL- 60 cells treated with vitamin D3 analogs correlates with inhibition of DNA synthesis and reduced calmodulin concentration, *Lab. Invest.*, 55, 269, 1986.

136. Mahonen, A., Pirskanen, A., and Mäenpää, P. H., Homologous and heterologous regulation of 1,25-dihydroxyvitamin D-3 receptor mRNA levels in human osteosarcoma cells, *Biochim. Biophys. Acta Gene Struct. Expression*, 1088, 111, 1991.

137. Huh, N., Satch, M., Nose, K., Abe, E., Suda, T., Rajewsky, M. F., and Kuroki., T., 1-Alpha 25-dihydroxyvitamin-D3 induces anchorage-independent growth and c-ki-ras expression of BALB/3T3 and NIH/3T3 cells (tech. note), *Jpn. J. Canc.*, 78, 99, 1987.

138. Karmali, R., Bhalla, A. K., Farrow, S. M., Williams, M. M., Lal, S., Lydyard, P. M., and O'Riordan, J. L. H., Early regulation of c-myc mRNA by 1,25-dihydroxyvitamin D_3 in human myelomonocytic U937 cells, *J. Mol. Endo.*, 3, 43, 1989.

139. Bar-Shavit, Z., Kahn, A. J., Stone, K. R., Trial, J., Hilliard, T., Reitsma, P. H., and Teitelbaum, S. L., Reversibility of vitamin D-induced human leukemia cell-line maturation, *Endocrinology*, 118, 679, 1986.

140. Simpson, R. U., Hsu, T., Begley, D. A., Mitchell, B. S., and Alizadeh, B. N., Transcriptional regulation of the c-myc protooncogene by 1,25-dihydroxyvitamin D3 in HL-60 promyelocytic leukemia cells, *J. Biol. Chem.*, 262, 4104, 1987.

141. Simpson, R. U., Hsu, T., Wendt, M. D., and Taylor, J. M., 1,25-dihydroxyvitamin D-3 regulation of c-myc protooncogene transcription, *J. Biol. Chem.*, 264, 19710, 1989.

142. Hunziker, W., Siebert, P. D., King, M. W., Stucki, P., Dugaiczyk, A., and Norman, A. W., Molecular cloning of a vitamin D-dependent calcium-binding protein mRNA sequence from chick intestine, *Proc. Natl. Acad. Sci. USA*, 80, 4228, 1983.

143. Clemens, T. L., McGlade, S. A., Garrett, K. P., Craviso, G. L., and Hendy, G. N., Extracellular calcium modulates vitamin D-dependent calbindin-D_{28K} gene expression in chick kidney cellsm, *Endocrinology*, 124, 1582, 1989.

144. Li, H. and Christakos, S., Differential regulation by 1,25-dihydroxyvitamin D_3 of calbindin-D_{9k} and calbindin-D_{28k} gene expression in mouse kidney, *Endocrinology*, 128, 2844, 1991.

145. Darwish, H. M. and DeLuca, H. F., Identification of a 1,25-dihydroxyvitamin D_3-response element in the 5′-flanking region of the rat calbindin D-9k gene, *Proc. Natl. Acad. Sci. USA*, 89, 603, 1992.

146. Billecocq, A., Emanuel, J. R., Levenson, R., and Baron, R., $1\alpha,25$-Dihydroxyvitamin D_3 regulates the expression of carbonic anhydrase II in nonerythroid avian bone marrow cells, *Proc. Natl. Acad. Sci. USA*, 87, 6470, 1990.

147. Lomri, A., and Baron, R., $1\alpha,25$-dihydroxyvitamin D_3 regulates the transcription of carbonic anhydrase II mRNA in avian myelomonocytes, *Proc. Natl. Acad. Sci. USA*, 89, 4688, 1992.

148. Fargeas, C., Wu, C., Luo, H., Sarfati, M., Delespesse, G., and Wu, J., $1,25(OH)_2$ Vitamin D-3 inhibits the CD23 expression by human peripheral blood monocytes, *J. Immunol.*, 145, 4053, 1990.

149. Lichtler, A., Stover, M. L., Angilly, J., Kream, B., and Rowe, D. W., Isolation and characterization of the rat a1(I) collagen promoter. Regulation by 1,25-dihydroxyvitamin D, *J. Biol. Chem.*, 264, 3072, 1989.

150. Blanchard, R. K., Molecular cloning of a chick kidney ferredoxin cDNA and regulation of mRNA levels by vitamin D, Thesis/Dissertation, University California, Riverside, 1993.

151. Franceschesi, R. T., Linson, C. J., Peter, T. C., and Romano, P. R., Regulation of cellular adhesion and fibronectin synthesis by 1α, 25-dihydroxyvitamin D_3, *J. Biol. Chem.*, 262, 4165, 1987.

152. Reichel, H., Koeffler, H. P., Tobler, A., and Norman, A. W., $1\alpha,25$-Dihydroxyvitamin D_3 inhibits γ-interferon synthesis by normal human peripheral blood lymphocytes, *Proc. Natl. Acad. Sci. USA*, 84, 3385, 1987.

153. Rigby, W. F. C., Denome, S., and Fanger, M. W., Regulation of lymphokine production and human T lymphocyte activation by 1,25-dihydroxyvitamin D_3, *J. Clin. Invest.*, 79, 1659, 1987.

154. Desprez, P. Y., Poujol, D., and Saez, S., Glyceraldehyde-3-phosphate dehydrogenase (GAPDH, E.C. 1.2.1.12.) gene expression in two malignant human mammary epithelial cell lines: BT-20 and MCF-7. Regulation of gene expression by 1,25-dihydroxyvitamin D_3 (1,25-$(OH)_2D_3$), *Cancer Lett.*, 64, 219, 1992.

155. Tobler, A., Gasson, J., Reichel, H., Norman, A. W., and Koeffler, H. P., Granulocyte macrophage colony simulating factor. Sensitive and receptor mediated regulation by 1,25-dihydroxyvitamin D3 in normal human peripheral blood lymphocytes, *J. Clin. Invest.*, 79, 1700, 1987.

156. Polla, B. S., Healy, A. M., Wojno, W. C., and Krane, S. M., Hormone 1α,25-dihydroxyvitamin D_3 modulates heat shock response in monocytes, *Am. J. Physiol.*, 252, c640, 1987.

157. Brelvi, Z. S. and Studzins, G. P., Coordinate expression of c-myc, c-myb, and histone-H4 genes in reversibly differentiating HL-60 cells, *J. Cell. Physiol.*, 131, 43, 1987.

158. Akeno, N., Saikatsu, S., and Horiuchi, N., Increase of renal 25-hydroxyvitamin D_3-24-hydroxylase activity and its messenger ribonucleic acid level in 1α-hydroxyvitamin D_3-administered rats: possibility of the presence of two forms of 24-hydroxylase, *J. Nutr. Sci. Vitaminol.*, 39, 89, 1993.

159. Chen, M. L., Boltz, M. A., and Armbrecht, H. J., Effects of 1,25-dihydroxyvitamin D_3 and phorbol ester on 25-hydroxyvitamin D_3 24-hydroxylase cytochrome P450 messenger ribonucleic acid levels in primary cultures of rat renal cells, *Endocrinology*, 132, 1782, 1993.

160. Medhora, M. M., Teitelbaum, S., Chappel, J., Alvarez, J., Mimura, H. F., Ross, P., and Hruska, K. A., 1α,25-Dihydroxyvitamin D_3 up-regulates expression of the osteoclast integrin $α_3β_3$, *J. Biol. Chem.*, 268, 1456, 1993.

161. Cao, X., Ross, F. P., Zhang, L., MacDonald, P. N., Chappel, J., and Teitelbaum, S. L., Cloning of the promoter for the avian integrin $β_3$ subunit gene and its regulation by 1,25-dihydroxyvitamin D_3, *J. Biol. Chem.*, 268, 27371, 1993.

162. Taimi, M., Defacque, H., Commes, T., Favero, J., Caron, E., Marti, J., and Dornand, J., Effect of retinoic acid and vitamin D on the expression of interleukin-1b, tumour necrosis factor-a and interleukin-6 in the human monocytic cell line U937, *Immunology*, 79, 229, 1993.

163. Fagan, D. L., Prehn, J. L., Adams, J. S., and Jordan, S. C., The human myelomonocytic cell line U-937 as a model for studying alterations in steroid-induced monokine gene expression: marked enhancement of lipopolysaccharide-stimulated interleukin-1b messenger RNA levels by 1,25-dihydroxyvitamin D_3, *Mol. Endocrinol.*, 5, 179, 1991.

164. Lacey, D. L., Erdmann, J. M., Tan, H. L., and Ohara, J., Murine osteoblast interleukin 4 receptor expression: upregulation by 1,25 dihydroxyvitamin D_3, *J. Cell. Biochem.*, 53, 122, 1993.

165. Fraser, J. D., Otawara, Y., and Price, P. A., 1,25-dihydroxyvitamin D_3 stimulates the synthesis of matrix gamma-carboxygultamic acid protein by osteosarcoma cells, *J. Biol. Chem.*, 263, 911, 1988.

166. Karasawa, M., Hosoi, J. H., Hashiba, K. Nose, C., Tohyama, E., Abe, Suda, T., and Kuroki, T., Regulation of metallothionein gene expression by 1-alpha,25-dihydroxyvitamin D3 in cultured cells and in mice, *Proc. Natl. Acad. Sci. USA*, 84, 8810, 1987.

167. Kowalski, J. and Denhardt, D. T., Regulation of the mRNA for monocyte-derived neutrophil-activating peptide in differentiating HL60 promyelocytes, *Mol. Cell. Biol.*, 9, 1946, 1989.

168. Wion, D., MacGrogan, D., Neveu, I., Jehan, F., Houlgatte, R., and Brachet, P., 1,25-Dihydroxyvitamin D$_3$ is a potent inducer of nerve growth factor synthesis, *J. Neurosci. Res.*, 28, 110, 1991.

169. Ferrer, I., Tunon, T., Serrano, M. T., Casas, R., Alcantara, S., Zujar, M. J., and Rivera, R. M., Calbindin d-28k and parvalbumin immunoreactivity in the frontal cortex in patients with frontal lobe dementia of non-alzheimer type associated with amyotrophic lateral sclerosis, *J. Neurol. Neurosurg. Psych.*, 56, 257, 1993.

170. Ozono, K., Liao, J., Kerner, S. A., Scott, R. A., and Pike, J. W., The vitamin D-responsive element in the human osteocalcin gene. Association with a nuclear proto-oncogene enhancer, *J. Biol. Chem.*, 265 21881, 1990.

171. Demay, M. B., Gerardi, J. M., DeLuca, H. F., and Kronenberg, H. M., DNA sequences in the rat osteocalcin gene that bind the 1,25-dihydroxyvitamin D-3 receptor and confer responsiveness to 1,25-dihydroxyvitamin D-3, *Proc. Natl. Acad. Sci. USA*, 87, 369, 1990.

172. Terpening, C. M., Haussler, C. A., Jurutka, P. W., Galligan, M. A., Komm, B. S., and Haussler, M. R., The vitamin D-responsive element in the rat bone gla protein gene is an imperfect direct repeat that cooperates with other *cis*-elements in 1,25-dihydroxyvitamin D$_3$-mediated transcriptional activation, *Mol. Endocrinol.*, 5 373, 1991.

173. Jenis, L. G., Lian, J. B., Stein, G. S., and Baran, D. T., 1α,25-dihydroxyvitamin D$_3$-induced changes in intracellular pH in osteoblast-like cells modulate gene expression, *J. Cell. Biochem.*, 53, 234, 1993.

174. Noda, M., Vogel, R. L., Craig, A. M., Prahl, J., DeLuca, H. F., and Denhardt, D. R., Identification of a DNA sequence responsible for binding of the 1,25-dihydroxyvitamin D$_3$ receptor and 1,25-dihydroxyvitamin D$_3$ enhancement of mouse secreted phosphoprotein 1 (Spp-1 or osteopontin) gene expression, *Proc. Natl. Acad. Sci. USA*, 87, 9995, 1990.

175. Cai, Q., Chandler, J. S., Wasserman, R. H., Kumar, R., and Penniston, J. T., Vitamin D and adaptation to dietary calcium and phosphate deficiencies increase intestinal plasma membrane calcium pump gene expression, *Proc. Natl. Acad. Sci. USA*, 90, 1345, 1993.

176. Silver, J., Navehmany, T., Mayer, H., Schmeizer, H. J., and Popovtzer, M. M., Regulation by vitamin-D metabolites of parathyroid-hormone gene-transcription *in vivo* in the rat, *J. Clin. Invest.*, 78, 1296, 1986.

177. Russell, J., Lettieri, D., and Sherwood, L. M., Suppression by 1,25(OH)$_2$D$_3$ of transcription of the pre-proparathyroid hormone gene (tech. note), *Endocrinology*, 119, 2864, 1986.

178. Wark, J. D. and Tashjian, J. A. H., Regulation of prolactin messenger-RNA by 1,25-dihydroxyvitamin-D3 in GH4C1-cells (tech. note), *J. Biol. Chem.*, 258, 2118, 1983.

179. Marchetto, G. S. and Henry, H. L., mRNA levels of the inhibitor protein of cAMP-dependent protein kinase are regulated by 1α,25(OH)$_2$D$_3$ and forskolin, in *Vitamin D, A Pluripotent Steroid Hormone*, Norman, A. W., Bouillon, R., and Thomasset, N., Eds., W. de Gruyter, Berlin, 1994.

180. Obeid, L. M., Okazaki, T., Karolak, L. A., and Hannun, Y. A., Transcriptional regulation of protein kinase C by 1,25-dihydroxyvitamin D3 in HL-60 cells, *J. Biol. Chem.*, 265, 2370, 1990.

181. Naveh-Many, T., Marx, R., Keshet, E., Pike, J. W., and Silver, J., Regulation of 1,25-dihydroxyvitamin D-3 receptor gene expression by 1,25-dihydroxyvitamin D-3 in the parathyroid *in vivo*, *J. Clin. Invest.*, 86, 1968, 1990.

182. Naveh-Many, T. and Silver, J., Regulation of parathyroid hormone gene expression by hypocalcemia, hypercalcemia, and vitamin D in the rat, *J. Clin. Invest.*, 86, 1313, 1990.

183. Ikeda, K., Lu, C., Weir, E. C., Mangin, M., and Broadus, A. E., Transcriptional regulation of the parathyroid hormone-related peptide gene by glucocorticoids and vitamin D in a human C-cell line, *J. Biol. Chem.*, 264: 15743, 1989.

184. Steffen, M., Cayre, Y., Manogue, K. R., and More, M. A. S., 1,25-dihydroxyvitamin D_3 transcriptionally regulates tumour necrosis factor mRNA during HL-60 cell differentiation, *Immunology*, 63, 43, 1988.

185. Strom, M., Sandgren, M. E., Brown, T. A., and DeLuca, H. F., 1,25-dihdyroxyvitamin D-3 up-regulates the 1,25-dihydroxyvitamin D-3 receptor *in vivo*, *Proc. Natl. Acad. Sci. USA*, 86, 9770, 1989.

186. Lee, S., Szlachetka, M., and Christakos, S., Effect of glucocorticoids and 1,25-dihydroxyvitamin D_3 on the developmental expression of the rat intestinal vitamin D receptor gene, *Endocrinology*, 129, 396, 1991.

187. De Boland, A. R. and Norman, A. W., Evidence for involvement of protein kinase C and cyclic adenosine 3', 5' monophosphate-dependent protein kinase in the 1,25-dihydroxyvitamin D_3-mediated rapid stimulation of intestinal calcium transport (transcaltachia), *Endocrinology*, 127, 39, 1990.

188. De Boland, A. R. and Norman, A. W., Influx of extracellular calcium mediates 1,25-dihydroxyvitamin D_3-dependent transcaltachia (the rapid stimulation of duodenal Ca^{2+} transport), *Endocrinology*, 127, 2475, 1990.

189. Khare, S., Tien, X.-Y., Wilson, D., Wali, R. K., Bissonnette, B. M., Scaglione-Sewell, B., Sitrin, M. D., and Brasitus, T. A., The role of protein kinase-Ca in the activation of particulate guanylate cyclase by 1α,25-dihydroxyvitamin D_3 in CaCo-2 cells, *Endocrinology*, 135, 277, 1994.

190. Bissonnette, M., Tien, X.-Y., Niedziela, S. M., Hartmann, S. C., Frawley, B. P., Jr., Roy, H. K., Sitrin, M. D., Perlman, R. L., and Brasitus, T. A., 1,25(OH)₂ vitamin D_3 activates PKC-α in Caco-2 cells: A mechanism to limit secosteroid-induced rise in $[Ca^{2+}]_i$, *Am. J. Physiol. Gastrointest. Liver Physiol.*, 267, G465, 1994.

191. Bissonnette, M., Wali, R. K., Hartmann, S. C., Niedziela, S. M., Roy, H. K., Tien, X.-Y., Sitrin, M. D., and Brasitus, T. A., 1,25-dihydroxyvitamin D_3 and 12-O-tetradecanoyl phorbol 13-acetate cause differential activation of Ca^{2+}-dependent and Ca^{2+}-independent isoforms of protein kinase C in rat colonocytes, *J. Clin. Invest.*, 95, 2215, 1995.

192. Simboli-Campbell, M., Gagnon, A., Franks, D. J., and Welsh, J., 1,25-dihydroxyvitamin D_3 translocates protein kinase $C_β$ to nucleus and enhances plasma membrane association of protein kinase $C_α$ in renal epithelial cells, *J. Biol. Chem.*, 269, 3257, 1994.

193. Simboli-Campbell, M., Franks, D. J., and Welsh, J. E., 1,25(OH)₂D_3 increases membrane associated protein kinase C in MDBK cells, *Cell. Signal.*, 4, 99, 1992.

194. Mandla, S., Boneh, A., and Tenenhouse, H. S., Evidence for protein kinase C involvement in the regulation of renal 25-hydroxyvitamin D_3-24-hydroxylase, *Endocrinology*, 127, 2639, 1990.

195. Barsony, J., Pike, J. W., DeLuca, H. F., and Marx, S. J., Immunocytology with microwave-fixed fibroblasts shows 1α,25-dihydroxyvitamin D_3-dependent rapid and estrogen-dependent slow reorganization of vitamin D receptors, *J. Cell. Biol.*, 111, 2385, 1990.

196. Zanello, L. P. and Norman, A. W., 1α,25(OH)$_2$ vitamin D$_3$-mediated stimulation of outward anionic currents in osteoblast-like ROS 17/2.8 cells, *Biochem. Biophys. Res. Commun.*, 225, 551, 1996.
197. Baran, D. T., Sorensen, A. M., Honeyman, T. W., Ray, R., and Holick, M. F., Rapid actions of 1α,25-dihydroxyvitamin D$_3$ and calcium and phospholipids in isolated rat liver nuclei, *FEBS Lett.*, 259, 205, 1989.
198. Baran, D. T., Sorensen, A. M., Honeyman, R. W., Ray, R., and Holick, M. F., 1α,25-dihydroxyvitamin D$_3$-induced increments in hepatocyte cytosolic calcium and lysophosphatidylinositol: Inhibition by pertussis toxin and 1β,25-dihydroxyvitamin D$_3$, *J. Bone Miner. Res.*, 5, 517, 1990.
199. Beno, D. W. A., Brady, L. M., Bissonnette, M., and Davis, B. H., Protein kinase C and mitogen-activated protein kinase are required for 1,25-dihydroxyvitamin D$_3$-stimulated Egr induction, *J. Biol. Chem.*, 270, 3642, 1995.
200. De Boland, A. R. and Boland, R. L., 1,25-dihydroxyvitamin D$_3$ induces arachidonate mobilization in embryonic chick myoblasts, *Biochim. Biophys. Acta Mol. Cell Res.*, 1179, 98, 1993.
201. Morelli, S., De Boland, A. R., and Boland, R. L., Generation of inositol phosphates, diacylglycerol and calcium fluxes in myoblasts treated with 1,25-dihydroxyvitamin D$_3$, *Biochim. J.*, 289, 675, 1993.
202. Vazquez, G. and De Boland, A. R., Involvement of protein kinase C in the modulation of 1α,25-dihydroxy-vitamin D$_3$-induced ^{45}Ca^{2+} uptake in rat and chick cultured myoblasts, *Biochim. Biophys. Acta Mol. Cell Res.*, 1310, 157, 1996.
203. Selles, J. and Boland, R. L., Evidence on the participation of the 3′,5′-cyclic AMP pathway in the non-genomic action of 1,25-dihydroxy-vitamin D$_3$ in cardiac muscle, *Mol. Cell. Endocrinol.*, 82, 229, 1991.
204. Bhatia, M., Kirkland, J. B., and Meckling-Gill, K. A., Monocytic differentiation of acute promyelocytic leukemia cells in response to 1,25-dihydroxyvitamin D$_3$ is independent of nuclear receptor binding, *J. Biol. Chem.*, 270, 15962, 1995.
205. Bhatia, M., Kirkland, J. B., and Meckling-Gill, K. A., 1,25-dihydroxyvitamin D$_3$ primes acute promyelocytic cells for TPA-induced monocytic differentiation through both PKC and tyrosine phosphorylation cascades, *Exp. Cell Res.*, 222, 61, 1996.
206. Biskobing, D. M. and Rubin, J., 1,25-dihydroxyvitamin D$_3$ and phorbol myristate acetate produce divergent phenotypes in a monomyelocytic cell line, *Endocrinology*, 132, 862, 1993.
207. Berry, D. M., Antochi, R., Bhatia, M., and Meckling-Gill, K. A., 1,25-dihydroxyvitamin D$_3$ stimulates expression and translocation of protein kinase Cα and Cδ via a nongenomic mechanism and rapidly induces phosphorylation of a 33-kDa protein in acute promyelocytic NB4 cells, *J. Biol. Chem.*, 271, 16090, 1996.
208. Yada, Y., Ozeki, T., Meguro, S., Mori, S., and Nozawa, Y., Signal transduction in the onset of terminal keratinocyte differentiation induced by 1α,25-dihydroxyvitamin D$_3$: Role of protein kinase C translocation, *Biochem. Biophys. Res. Commun.*, 163, 1517, 1989.
209. Bourdeau, A., Atmani, F., Grosse, B., and Lieberherr, M., Rapid effects of 1,25-dihydroxyvitamin D$_3$ and extracellular Ca^{2+} on phospholipid metabolism in dispersed porcine parathyroid cells, *Endocrinology*, 127, 2738, 1990.
210. Sugimoto, T., Ritter, C., Ried, I., Morrissey, J., and Slatopolsky, E., Effect of 1,25-dihydroxyvitamin D$_3$ on cytosolic calcium in dispersed parathyroid cells, *Kidney Int.*, 33, 850, 1992.

211. Slater, S. J., Kelly, M. B., Taddeo, F. J., Larkin, J. D., Yeager, M. D., McLane, J. A., Ho, C., and Stubbs, C. D., Direct activation of protein kinase C by 1α,25-dihydroxyvitamin D₃, *J. Biol. Chem.*, 270, 6639, 1995.
212. Morrison, N. A., Shine, J., Fragonas, J.-C., Verkest, V., McMenemy, M. L., and Eisman, J. A., 1,25-dihydroxyvitamin D-responsive element and glucocorticoid repression in the osteocalcin gene, *Science*, 246, 1158, 1989.
213. Gill, R. K. and Christakos, S., Identification of sequence elements in mouse calbindin-D₂₈ₖ gene that confer 1,25-dihydroxyvitamin D₃- and butyrate-inducible responses, *Proc. Natl. Acad. Sci. USA*, 90, 2984, 1993.
214. Hahn, C. N., Kerry, D. M., Omdahl, J. L., and May, B. K., Identification of a vitamin D responsive element in the promoter of the rat cytochrome P450₂₄ gene, *Nucleic Acids Res.*, 22, 2410, 1994.
215. Mechica, J. B., Leite, M. O., Mendonca, B. B., Frazzatto, E. S., Borelli, A., and Latronico, A. C., A novel nonsense mutation in the first zinc finger of the vitamin D receptor causing hereditary 1,25-dihydroxyvitamin D₃-resistant rickets, *J. Clin. Endocr. Metab.*, 82, 3892, 1997.
216. Wiese, R. J., Goto, H., Prahl, J. M., Marx, S. J., Thomas, M., Al-Aqeel, A., and DeLuca, H. F., Vitamin D-dependency rickets type II: Truncated vitamin D receptor in three kindreds, *Mol. Cell. Endocrinol.*, 90, 197, 1993.
217. Hawa, N. S., Cockerill, F. J., Vadher, S., Hewison, M., Rut, A. R., Pike, J. W., O'Riordan, J. L. H., and Farrow, S. M., Identification of a novel mutation in hereditary vitamin D resistant rickets causing exon skipping, *Clin. Endocrinol. (Oxf.)*, 45, 85, 1996.
218. Hughes, M. R., Malloy, P. J., Kieback, D. G., Kesterson, R. A., Pike, J. W., Feldman, D., and O'Malley, B. W., Point mutations in the human vitamin D receptor gene associated with hypocalcemic rickets, *Science*, 242, 1702, 1988.
219. Haussler, M. R., Haussler, C. A., Jurutka, P. W., Thompson, P. D., Hsieh, J. C., Remus, L. S., Selznick, S. H., and Whitfield, G. K., The vitamin D hormone and its nuclear receptor: molecular actions and disease states, *J. Endocrinol.*, 154, S57, 1997.
220. Lin, N. U. T., Malloy, P. J., Sakati, N., Al-Ashwal, A., and Feldman, D., A novel mutation in the deoxyribonucleic acid-binding domain of the vitamin D receptor causes hereditary 1,25-dihydroxyvitamin D-resistant rickets, *J. Clin. Endocr. Metab.*, 81, 2564, 1996.
221. Saijo, T., Ito, M., Takeda, E., Mahbubul Huq, A. H. M., Naito, E., Yokota, I., Sone, T., Pike, J. W., and Kuroda, Y., A unique mutation in the vitamin D receptor gene in three Japanese patients with vitamin D-dependent rickets type II: Utility of single-strand conformation polymorphism analysis for heterozygous carrier detection, *Am. J. Hum. Genet.*, 49, 668, 1991.
222. Malloy, P. J., Weisman, Y., and Feldman, D., Hereditary 1α,25-dihydroxyvitamin D-resistant rickets resulting from a mutation in the vitamin D receptor deoxyribonucleic acid-binding domain, *J. Clin. Endocr. Metab.*, 78, 313, 1994.
223. Hsieh, J. C., Jurutka, P. W., Selznick, S. H., Reeder, M. C., Haussler, C. A., Whitfield, G. K., and Haussler, M. R., The T-box near the zinc fingers of the human vitamin D receptor is required for heterodimeric DNA binding and transactivation, *Biochem. Biophys. Res. Commun.*, 215, 1, 1995.
224. Thompson, E., Kristjansson, K., and Hughes, M. R., Molecular scanning methods for mutation detection: Application to the 1,25-dihydroxyvitamin D receptor, *Eighth Workshop Vitamin D*, 6, 1991.

225. Jurutka, P. W., Hsieh, J. C., Nakajima, S., Haussler, C. A., Whitfield, G. K., and Haussler, M. R., Human vitamin D receptor phosphorylation by casein kinase II at Ser-208 potentiates transcriptional activation, *Proc. Natl. Acad. Sci. USA,* 93, 3519, 1996.
226. Whitfield, G. K., Hsieh, J. C., Nakajima, S., MacDonald, P. N., Thompson, P. D., Jurutka, P. W., Haussler, C. A., and Haussler, M. R., A highly conserved region in the hormone-binding domain of the human vitamin D receptor contains residues vital for heterodimerization with retinoid X receptor and for transcriptional activation, *Mol. Endocrinol.,* 9, 1166, 1995.
227. Nakajima, S., Hsieh, J. C., Jurutka, P. W., Galligan, M. A., Haussler, C. A., Whitfield, G. K., and Haussler, M. R., Examination of the potential functional role of conserved cysteine residues in the hormone binding domain of the human 1,25-dihydroxyvitamin D_3 receptor, *J. Biol. Chem.,* 271, 5143, 1996.
228. Malloy, P. J., Eccleshall, T. R., Gross, C., Van Maldergem, L., Bouillon, R., and Feldman, D., Hereditary vitamin D resistant rickets caused by a novel mutation in the vitamin D receptor that results in decreased affinity for hormone and cellular hyporesponsiveness, *J. Clin. Invest.,* 99, 297, 1997.
229. Whitfield, G. K., Selznick, S. H., Haussler, C. A., Hsieh, J. C., Galligan, M. A., Jurutka, P. W., Thompson, P. D., Lee, S. M., Zerwekh, J. E., and Haussler, M. R., Vitamin D receptors from patients with resistance to 1,25- dihydroxyvitamin D_3: Point mutations confer reduced transactivation in response to ligand and impaired interaction with the retinoid X receptor heterodimeric partner, *Mol. Endocrinol.,* 10, 1617, 1996.
230. Pike, J. W. The vitamin D receptor and its gene, in *Vitamin D,* Feldman, D., Glorieux, F. H., and Pike, J. W., Eds., Academic Press, San Diego, 105, 1977.
231. Haussler, M. H., Jurutka, P. W., Hsieh, J.-C., Thompson, P. D., Haussler, C. A., Selznick, S. H., Remus, L. S., and Whitfield, G. K., Nuclear vitamin D receptor: Structure-Function, phosphorylation, and control of gene transcription, in *Vitamin D,* Feldman, D., Glorieux, F. H., and Pike, J. W., Eds., Academic Press, San Diego, 149, 1977.

16

Vitamin E and Gene Expression

Simin Nikbin Meydani, Kate J. Claycombe,
and Catarina Sacristán

CONTENTS

16.1 Introduction 394
    16.1.1 Tocopherol Structures, Homologs, and Bioactivity 394
    16.1.2 Tocopherol Stereoisomers: Differential Effects
    on Gene Expression 395
16.2 Modes of Vitamin E Action..396
16.3 Vitamin E and Gene Expression in Human Disease 399
    16.3.1 Vitamin E, Immune Function,
    and Immunity-Related Diseases..399
    16.3.2 Vitamin E and Control of Cellular Proliferation
    and Cancer 404
        16.3.2.1 Breast cancer 405
        16.3.2.2 Colorectal Cancer..406
        16.3.2.3 Myelodysplastic Syndromes 406
    16.3.3 Vitamin E and Cardiovascular Diseases.................................407
    16.3.4 Vitamin E and Diabetes..408
    16.3.5 Role of Vitamin E in the Reversal of Renal
    and Hepatic Tissue Damage...409
        16.3.5.1 Renal Injury and IgA Nephropathies.......................409
        16.3.5.2 Liver Injury 411
    16.3.6 Vitamin E and Neurodegenerative Conditions....................412
        16.3.6.1 Ataxias..412
        16.3.6.2 Amyotrophic Lateral Sclerosis and Other
        Neuronal Abnormalities 413
16.4 Conclusion..414
References 415

0-8493-2216-2/01/$0.00+$1.50
© 2001 by CRC Press LLC

16.1 Introduction

Free radicals and reactive oxygen species (ROS) are generated continuously in living cells, damaging cellular constituents if remaining uncontrolled. ROS cause DNA base modifications, DNA and protein cross-links, and strand breaks.[1] Proteins are also targets of ROS attack, resulting in oxidation of amino acids that can generate inactive enzymes or proteins with increased susceptibility to proteolytic attack.[2,3] In addition, oxidation of cellular membranes gives rise to peroxyl radicals and lipid epoxides.[4] Accordingly, tissues are equipped with enzymatic (catalase, superoxide dismutase, and glutathione peroxidase) and non-enzymatic (vitamins A, C, and E as well as sulfur-containing amino acids) antioxidant defense systems.

Among the dietary antioxidants, vitamin E is the most abundant and efficient scavenger of hydroperoxyl radicals in biological membranes. In addition to its effects on lipid radicals, vitamin E protects cells by regulating cellular oxido-reductive status. Recent molecular and cellular investigations have demonstrated that antioxidants such as vitamin E can directly affect redox-sensitive signal transduction cascades and, consequently, the control of gene expression. Furthermore, the beneficial effects of vitamin E in several diseases for which oxidative stress has been implicated as a contributing factor have been demonstrated. This review will discuss the interactions between vitamin E and gene expression and their implications for chronic and inflammatory diseases.

16.1.1 Tocopherol Structures, Homologs, and Bioactivity

Naturally occurring vitamin E or tocopherols have four major isoforms, each of which exerts differential biopotencies (Fig. 16.1).

These differences in biopotency are due mainly to differences in the stereospecificity of carbon atoms 2, 4' and 8', the presence of ring methyl groups,

Vitamin E homologs	Structures	Biological activity (%)*
α-Tocopherol	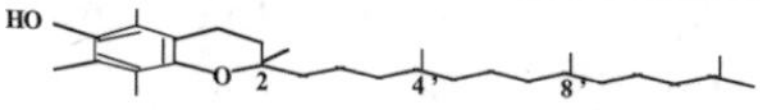	100
β-Tocopherol	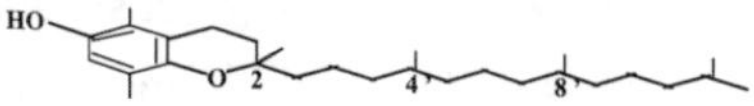	60
γ-Tocopherol	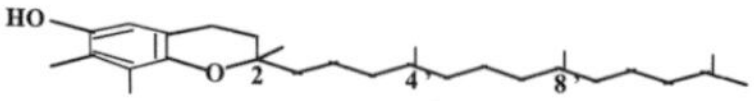	25
δ-Tocopherol	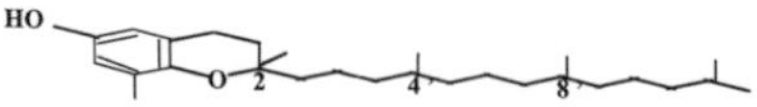	27

FIGURE 16.1
The structures and biological activities of tocopherols.
* As determined by relative activities with lipid peroxyl radicals.[5]

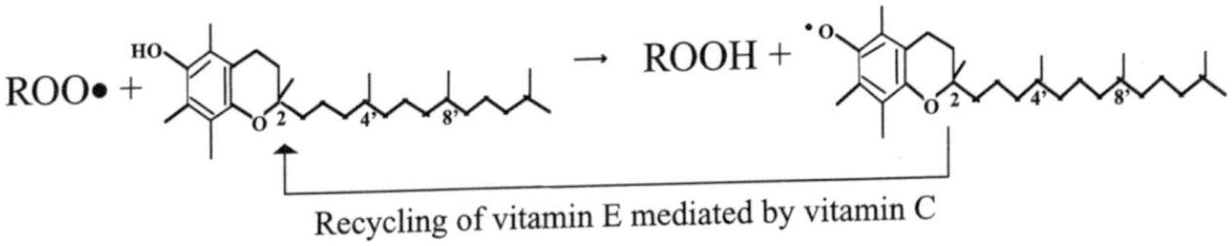

Recycling of vitamin E mediated by vitamin C

FIGURE 16.2
Peroxyl radical quenching reaction by tocopherol.

the number of carbon atoms, and the point of attachment in the side chain. Furthermore, the recycling rate, as well as differential affinity of tocopherol-binding proteins (which affect incorporation of tocopherols into lipoproteins), affects tocopherol bioavailabilty.[6] The antioxidant property of vitamin E is exerted through the phenolic hydroxyl group, which reacts with peroxyl radicals to form tocohydroxyl radicals (Fig. 16.2). This effectively interrupts the chain of peroxidation reaction, and tocopherol radicals are subsequently reduced and recycled.

16.1.2   Tocopherol Stereoisomers: Differential Effects on Gene Expression

Currently, only limited data are available for determining the relationship between tocopherol isomer bioactivity and gene expression. Even tocopherol isomers with substantially different antioxidant activity, such as α- and δ-tocopherol (Fig. 16.1, 100 and 27%, respectively), may exhibit similar influences on gene expression. For example, mRNA expression of α-tocopherol transfer protein (α-TTP), a 32 kDa protein which transports α-tocopherol to the nascent very-low-density lipoprotein (VLDL), can be induced to a similar degree by both isomers.[7]

Differential transcriptional regulation by tocopherol isomers has been demonstrated for the low-density lipoproteins (LDL)-scavenger receptor (SR) gene.[8] LDL-SR mediates the uptake of modified LDL by macrophages (Mφ). Both α-tocopherol and γ-tocopherol downregulate LDL-SR activity as well as LDL-SR mRNA expression and binding activity of transcription factor AP-1 in a dose-dependent manner. α-Tocopherol has been shown to reduce LDL-SR mRNA expression and AP-1 binding activity more significantly than γ-tocopherol. Differential regulation of gene expression by the different tocopherol isomers has also been observed in vascular smooth muscle cells, where α-tocopherol, but not β-tocopherol, downregulates proliferation of vascular smooth muscle cells. These differential effects on proliferation have been attributed to their varied effects on protein kinase C activity (PKC); α-tocopherol inhibits PKC activity whereas β-tocopherol has no effect. The inhibition of PKC activity in smooth muscle cells by α-tocopherol has been shown to occur via a decreased activation of transcription factor AP-1.[9]

Recently, we demonstrated that the concentration needed to induce maximal increases in mitogen-induced T-cell proliferation differs among tocopherol

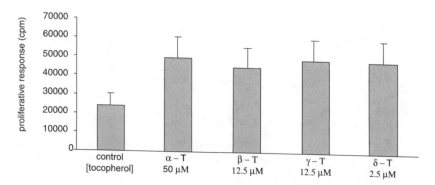

FIGURE 16.3

Effect of tocopherol homologs on concanavalin A (1.5 mg/L)-induced proliferation of mouse spleen T-cells. (From Wu et al., *Free Radic. Biol.*, 28(4), 647, 2000. With permission.)

isomers.[10] In this study, δ-tocopherol, with the lowest antioxidant capacity, required 20-fold less concentration (2.5 µM) than α-tocopherol, which has the highest antioxidant capacity (50 µM), to induce the same degree of T-cell proliferation (2-fold induction compared to control) (Fig. 16.3). Based on these data, the differential effects of tocopherol isomers on T-cell proliferation appear to be due to their regulation of gene expression through a nonantioxidant activity. At the level of gene expression, δ-tocopherol might induce a higher transient transcriptional activation than the other isomers, possibly through one or more upstream signal transduction pathways.

In the same study,[10] δ-tocopherol was also more effective in inducing cell death than was α-tocopherol. Although the mechanism of tocopherol-induced cell death is currently not known, tocopherol isomers may regulate expression of genes involved in necrosis or apoptosis differentially.

In the diet, non-α-tocopherol stereoisomers predominate; the intake of γ-tocopherol in humans is about 2 to 4 times that of α-tocopherol. Although the intestinal absorption of individual tocopherol isomers is similar, α-tocopherol is found in its highest concentration in blood and tissues, mainly because α-TTP selectively supplements nascent VLDL with α-tocopherol isomers.

α-Tocopherol, the isomer with the highest antioxidant capacity and the predominant form of tocopherol in plasma, is also preferentially incorporated into plasma lipoproteins. Consequently, most reported data demonstrating the effects of vitamin E on gene expression focus on the effects of α-tocopherol.

16.2 Modes of Vitamin E Action

Two modes of action for vitamin E on molecular physiology of cells have been proposed: antioxidant and non-antioxidant. While some studies[9,11,12] have shown that the effect of tocopherol on gene expression is mediated

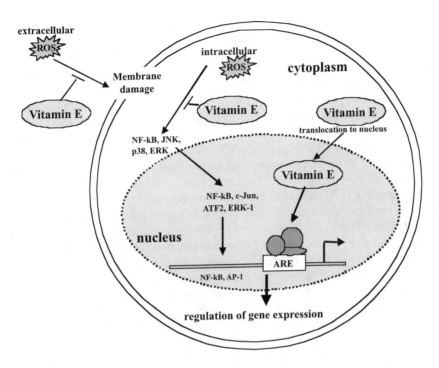

FIGURE 16.4
Proposed modes of antioxidant action of vitamin E on signal transduction. Vitamin E scavenges extracellular ROS and protects hydroperoxyl radical-induced membrane damage.[13] Intracellular ROS-induced activation of transcription factors such as NFκB and AP-1 is also inhibited by vitamin E.[14] Vitamin E can translocate to the nucleus and affect transcriptional activation by altering the RNA polymerase complex.[15] Vitamin E is proposed to regulate gene expression via the antioxidant responsive element (ARE) by interacting with ARE-associated transcription factors.

through its non-antioxidant function, most studies indicate that vitamin E alters gene expression by direct modulation of ROS, which in turn have been shown to influence signalling pathways and hence transcription factor activity (Fig. 16.4).

ROS (H_2O_2, $O_2^{\cdot-}$, and $HO^{\cdot}$) are byproducts of general metabolism in most cell types. Free radicals can originate exogenously, as seen in certain components of tobacco smoke, air pollutants, exposure to UV radiation, and through the metabolism of certain solvents, drugs, and pesticides, as well as via the oxidative respiratory chain reactions occurring in mitochondria.

ROS have been shown to induce lipid peroxidation and subsequent transactivation or repression of effector gene expression resulting in oxidative stress-induced cell damage. For example, exposure of liver cells to ROS results in the induction of lipid peroxidation accompanied by a significant increase in the constitutive expression of procollagen type I mRNA, which leads to the development of liver fibrosis.[16] This fibrogenic effect induced by ROS has been shown to be eradicated almost completely by treatment of cells with α-tocopherol.[16]

ROS are also involved in the induction of apoptosis, which can be inhibited by various antioxidants. For example, increased ROS have been shown to activate prostate apoptosis response-4 (Par-4, a product of a gene upregulated in prostate cancer cells undergoing apoptosis), and pretreatment of cultures with vitamin E can prevent Par-4 induction.[17]

Vitamin E can protect against ROS-induced vascular cell dysfunction mediated through increased adhesion molecule expression and monocyte recruitment. Intercellular adhesion molecule-1 (ICAM-1) and vascular cell adhesion molecule-1 (VCAM-1) are expressed in endothelial cells in inflammatory disease. ROS are produced in inflammatory responses and ROS-induced ICAM-1[18, 19] and VCAM-1 expression[19] are inhibited by α-tocopherol treatment.

Treatment of cells with H_2O_2[20] and ultraviolet radiation (UVA), which damages membrane lipids and reduces intracellular tocopherol[21] and glutathione[22] levels, is accompanied by a significant increase in heme oxygenase-1 (HO-1) gene expression. Free heme has been established as a source of oxidative stress capable of generating free radicals and causing cell damage. HO-1 is a rate-limiting enzyme that catalyzes the conversion of heme into carbon monoxide and biliverdin, free iron, and carbon monoxide. Thus, through catalyzing free heme, HO-1 acts as a potent antioxidant protein. Addition of α-tocopherol onto human skin fibroblasts in culture has been shown to enhance HO-1 mRNA accumulation.[23]

Vitamin E can protect proteins that are sensitive to oxidative stress. For example, vitamin E protects protein thiol-groups against oxidative damage in the maintenance of enzyme activity.[24] Thiol-groups containing amino acids (such as cysteine residues) that are located especially in DNA-binding domains of transcriptional factors[25] can be oxidized, resulting in a loss of transcriptional regulatory activity. Conserved cysteine residues and their critical role in DNA-binding activity have also been demonstrated in redox state-sensitive transcription activators such as NFκB. Mutations in the conserved residue (Cys61) within the N-terminal basic region of the p50 subunit of NFκB impair the stimulation of p50 DNA-binding activity.[26] Other transcription factors such as the *myb* protooncogene[27,28] and Jun proteins, which have been implicated in redox state-related regulation of gene expression,[29] also contain conserved cysteine sequences in the DNA-binding domain. Thus, it appears that the protective effect of vitamin E on gene expression is mediated through prevention of oxidative damage to the thiol-groups in NFκB, myb, and Jun proteins.

Vitamin E can exert its non-antioxidant effects by modulating the activity of enzymes that are involved in ROS production. For instance, in human monocytes, several subunits of NADPH-oxidase (which generate superoxide anion $O_2^{\bullet-}$) exist in two major fractions: membrane-bound (b_{558}) and cytosolic subunits (p47[phox], p67 [phox], Rac1/1, and p40 [phox]).[30] PMA-induced PKC phosphorylates the p47[phox] subunit and results in a subsequent translocation and assembly of active form of NADPH-oxidase. α-Tocopherol has been shown to inhibit phosphorylation and translocation of p47[phox] as well as PKC activity, resulting in a reduced production of $O_2^{\bullet-}$.[30] In the same study, addition of

2-carboxy-2,5,7,8-tetramethyl-6-chromanol (Trolox or CTMC), which is a water-soluble vitamin E derivative with free-radical scavenging activity, did not show any effect. Collectively, these data suggest that the inhibitory effect of vitamin E on PMA-induced $O_2^{\bullet-}$ production in human monocytes might be due to the non-antioxidant action of vitamin E. In addition, vitamin E has been shown to be localized to the nucleus[31] and to exert a non-antioxidant inhibitory effect on PMA-induced RNA-polymerase activity in isolated rat liver nuclei.[15]

The transcriptional regulation of antioxidant genes (NADPH quinone oxidoreductase, glutathione S-transferase, glutathione-S-transferase (GST) Ya subunit), are mediated by *cis*-acting elements called the antioxidant responsive element (ARE, 5′-GTGACTCAGCG-3′). The major function of these enzymes is to protect cells against oxidative radicals and against the toxic effects of xenobiotics by metabolizing them.[23,24]

Other oxidative stress-sensitive proteins such as collagenase α-1 gene[35] and HO-1[36] also contain ARE. Treatment of mice hepatocytes with α-tocopherol has been shown to inhibit basal levels of collagenase α-1[35] and phorbol ester-induced HO-1 gene expression.[36] Several transcription factors, such as Cap'n'Collar transcription factors Nrf1[37] and Nrf2[37,38] as well as Jun and Fos family proteins, recently have been shown to bind ARE.[39] Whether the inhibitory effects of α-tocopherol on collagenase α-1 and HO-1 gene expression are mediated via Jun, Fos, Nrfs, or by other transcription factors remains to be determined.

16.3 Vitamin E and Gene Expression in Human Disease

Growing evidence suggests that free radical damage contributes to the etiology of many chronic diseases, such as diabetes, emphysema, cardiovascular and inflammatory diseases, cataracts, male infertility, severe collagen diseases, lung fibrosis, neurodegenerative conditions, kidney and liver damage, and cancer. Epidemiological studies have reported an inverse correlation between increased intake of dietary antioxidants such as vitamin E and a lower risk for a number of these diseases. Below we review current findings on the effect of vitamin E on gene regulation in the progression of several human diseases.

16.3.1 Vitamin E, Immune Function, and Immunity-Related Diseases

Cells of the immune system secrete a wide variety of potent substances that, while necessary for normal host defense, can promote inflammation and tissue damage if produced in excess. Among these substances are numerous cytokines, reactive oxidant species, free radicals, and pro-inflammatory factors, including various eicosanoids, such as prostaglandins, the end products of the arachidonic acid cascade.

Many reactive oxygen intermediates (ROI) are produced by immune cells as part of their normal function of defense against the wide array of foreign antigens to which they are exposed. The oxidant/antioxidant balance is particularly important for immune function, not only for maintaining cellular integrity, but also for controlling signal transduction and gene expression. Indeed, secreted ROI contribute widely to redox changes in the milieu to which leukocytes must adjust, and have thus developed sophisticated antioxidant defense mechanisms to protect themselves from oxidative damage.

It is noteworthy that cells of the immune system are particularly sensitive to redox changes because their plasma membrane contains a higher percentage of polyunsaturated fatty acids (PUFA) relative to other cell types. Indeed, it is well established that immune cells, particularly of the myeloid lineage, contain higher levels of vitamin E than other cells.[40,41]

It is known that in T-lymphocytes, oxidative stress results in decreased IL-2 production, reduced protein tyrosine phosphorylation, and reduced intracellular calcium mobilization.[42] Moreover, it has been hypothesized that vitamin E may exert some of its immunostimulatory effects by directly or indirectly increasing IL-2 production.[43]

Numerous studies have shown vitamin E deficiency to be associated with impaired immune function. In fact, vitamin E deficiency has been shown to diminish the ability of immune cells to mount a defense against infectious microorganisms, produce adequate levels of antibodies against specific antigens, and generate delayed-type hypersensitivity reactions.[44] Interestingly, vitamin E deficiency has been linked to increased production of IL-6 in response to bacterial endotoxin.[45] Furthermore, in a study conducted on an elderly population, vitamin E supplementation was shown to inhibit IL-6 production from peripheral blood mononuclear cells.[46]

Aging is also associated with impaired T-cell-mediated function.[42,48] The age-associated changes in T-lymphocyte function are due in part to increased production of PGE_2, a macrophage (Mφ) product known to inhibit IL-2 secretion, T-cell proliferation, and T-cell cytotoxicity.[48] We have shown that the age-related increase in PGE_2 is due to increased mRNA and protein expression of the inducible form of cyclooxygenase, COX-2 (Fig. 16.5).[49,50]

In addition, we have shown that these changes contribute to the decline in T-cell-mediated function and IL-2 production by T-cells from aged animals.[47,48] Furthermore, the immunostimulatory effect of vitamin E on T-cells from aged mice is due in part to a reduction in the PGE_2 levels from Mφ of old mice (Fig. 16.6).[48,50]

The vitamin E-induced decrease in PGE_2 production is mainly mediated through inhibition of Mφ COX-2 activity.[50] The effects of vitamin E on COX-2 activity were thought to occur at a post-transcriptional level since no effect of vitamin E on COX-2 mRNA and protein levels was observed.[50] We recently showed that the post-transcriptional effect of vitamin E on COX-2 occurs through a reduction of nitric oxide (NO•) resulting in a decreased

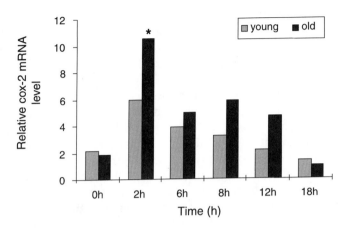

FIGURE 16.5
Relative COX-2 mRNA levels in macrophages (Mφ) from young and old C57BL/6NIA mice. Mφ from young (6 months) and old (24 months) were stimulated with 5 µg/ml LPS at the times indicated and mRNA levels were detected by RNAse protection assay. The relative values were calculated based on the expression of control β-actin mRNA using densitometry. Values are the mean of three independent experiments for 0, 2, 6, and 8 h. The other time points represent values from a single experiment. The standard deviations for 0, 2, 4, 6, and 8 h are 0.7, 0.6, 4.9, and 0.6 in young, and 0.2, 1.7, 4.8, and 2.9 in old, respectively. (From Hayek et al., *J. Immunol.*, 159(5), 2445, 1997. With permission.)
* Significantly higher than young mice at $p < 0.03$.[49]

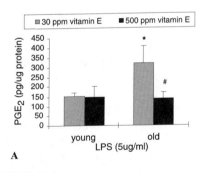

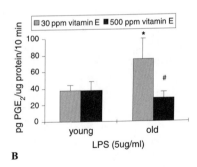

FIGURE 16.6
Effect of vitamin E on the production of accumulated PGE_2 (A) and on the activity of COX-2 (B) from peritoneal Mφ isolated from young and old mice. Young (6 months) and old (24 months) mice were fed semisynthetic diets containing adequate (30 ppm) or high (500 ppm) dl-α-tocopheryl acetate for 30 days. Peritoneal Mφ were isolated and cultured in the presence of 5 µg/ml LPS for 24 hours at 37°C. Supernatants were collected for measurement of accumulated PGE_2 production and COX activity in the presence of substrate arachidonic acid (AA). (From Wu et al., *Am. J. Physiol.*, 275, 2449, 1998. With permission.)
* Significantly higher than young mice fed 30 ppm vitamin E at $p < 0.05$. # Significantly lower than old mice fed 30 ppm vitamin E at $p < 0.05$.[50]

formation of peroxynitrite.[51] Moreover, we, as well as others, have shown that Mφ from old mice have a significantly higher production of NO•.[51] Other researchers have also found that the inducible nitric oxide synthase (iNOS) expression from murine Mφ is markedly decreased upon addition of vitamin E *in vitro*.[52,53]

The effects of oxidative stress on the transcriptional events occurring during various immune responses, although extensive, still remain controversial. For instance, one study has demonstrated that oxidation promotes a lower DNA-binding activity of the nuclear transcription factors NFAT and NFκB while increasing transactivation of the transcription factor AP-1 in T-lymphocytes.[42] In contrast, various oxidants have been shown to induce the production and secretion of prooxidative cytokines such as IL-1, IL-6, and TNFα from phagocytes in response to inflammatory stimuli mainly via activation of NFκB.[54] Another study has shown that vitamin E derivatives can decrease elevated levels of NFκB in TNF-α-stimulated Jurkat T-lymphocytes in a concentration-dependent manner.[55] Transfection studies using macrophagic TR-1 cells (derived from the THP-1 cell line) have shown that LPS-stimulated transfectants carrying the TNF-α gene promoter demonstrate decreased transcription of this gene upon culture with vitamin E succinate (50 μM concentration).[56] Gel shift assays in this study showed that NFκB DNA-binding activity of the stimulated transfectants decreased in the presence of the antioxidant. Discrepancies in NFκB binding across these studies might be explained by variations in culture conditions as well as by the biological nature and/or combination of oxidants or stimuli used.

As indicated in 16.1.2, another gene whose transcription is altered by oxidation and which is downmodulated by vitamin E is the scavenger receptor type A in Mφ. Teupser et al.[8] demonstrated that α-tocopherol (100 μM) supplementation decreased the mRNA expression of the scavenger receptor SR-A as well as its activity by 60% in a dose-dependent manner. This effect was accompanied by reduced AP-1 DNA-binding activity in these cells. γ-Tocopherol in comparison demonstrated only a weak suppression of SR-A transcription.[8]

A study involving the mRNA expression of tissue factor (blood clotting factor) in U937 and THP-1 cells has also shown that vitamin E treatment (50 μM α-tocopherol) of these cells substantially diminishes the elevated copper-induced tissue factor levels found in them.[57] These findings are interesting in that they corroborate the notion that monocytes are constantly exposed to oxidizing conditions, and that *in vitro* at least, antioxidants such as vitamin E can downmodulate at a transcriptional level the expression of various genes needed to embark on a rapid inflammatory response.

Increased cell–cell and cell–matrix interactions are hallmarks of transmigration events and leukocyte homing to vascular endothelium during inflammatory reactions. Interestingly, vitamin E (50 to 100 μM) has been shown to block the adhesion of monocytes,[58,59] Jurkat T-cells,[60] and other leukocytes to endothelial cells *in vitro*, and is correlated with the downmodulation of CD11b and VLA-4 adhesion molecule expression on leukocytes.[58]

Similarly, in three independent studies, IL-1 or TNF-α-primed U937 monocytes showed decreased adhesion to human umbilical vein endothelial cells *in vitro* upon treatment with vitamin E succinate (20 to 60 µM, 20 to 72 h) or α-tocopherol; this decrease was accompanied by a marked reduction in the monocyte expression of the VCAM-1, ICAM-1, and E-selectin adhesion molecules in a time- and dose-dependent manner.[59,61,62] However, although it is tempting to speculate that these effects are due to decreases in NFκB activation, experimental data showing the activation of NFκB in this regard have not fully supported this hypothesis.[62]

Impaired antioxidant defenses are associated with disease progression in HIV-infected individuals. Acquired immunodeficiency syndrome (AIDS), which is characterized by lymphoadenopathy, reduced cytokine levels, and overall impaired immune function, is also associated with lower tissue vitamin E levels in mice and humans compared to noninfected hosts.[63–66] Hence, the possibility of ameliorating the disease status of AIDS patients with vitamin E has been studied *in vitro* and *in vivo*.[55,67,68] Indeed, vitamin E supplementation in a murine model of AIDS (via LP-BM5 murine leukemia virus infection) has shown to decrease the retrovirus-induced increase in mononuclear phagocyte IL-6 and TNF-α production.[64] Interestingly, a study conducted by Hirano et al.[69] has shown that a particular phosphodiester compound of vitamin C and vitamin E can inhibit NFκB-dependent transcription of the HIV-1 promoter in TNF-α-treated human-cultured astrocytoma cells.

Vitamin E supplementation has become an area of therapeutic interest with regard to rheumatic diseases, which are characterized by changes in immune function. In the synovium of rheumatoid arthritis (RA) patients, transcriptional changes occur that reflect the genetic responses to a hypoxic/anoxic environment.[70] Changes in hypoxia-induced factor (HIF)-1 activation most directly involve the participation of various transcription factors and hypoxia responsive genes which ultimately play a significant role in the pathology of synovitis. The vascular endothelial growth factor (VEGF), the key to angiogenic and fibrinogenic events, is upregulated in the synovium of arthritic patients. Under hypoxic conditions, the hematopoietic factor erythropoietin is upregulated in the inflamed synovium as well. TGF-β, TNF-α, IL-1, IL-8, IL-6, NFκB, AP-1, Sp-1, collagen, ELAM-1/ICAM-1, LFA-1, VCAM-1, VLA-4 CD11a/CD18, as well as COX-2 have demonstrated increased gene expression in the arthritic synovium.[71]

Furthermore, patients with RA exhibit local vitamin E deficiencies compared to control subjects (lower vitamin E levels in the joint), and although significant anti-inflammatory effects have not been demonstrated with vitamin E administration thus far, vitamin E does have an analgesic effect in inflamed joints that appears to be independent of its antioxidant properties.[71,72]

Vitamin E might subvert inflammation by suppressing COX-2 activity. Indeed, COX-2 inhibitors are currently being tested in various animal models of experimental arthritis.[73] Another potential strategy for suppressing chronic synovitis via vitamin E includes attempts to downregulate the transcription of genes such as TNF-α.

16.3.2 Vitamin E and Control of Cellular Proliferation and Cancer

Extensive *in vitro* and *in vivo* studies have demonstrated the efficacy of vitamin E (particularly α-tocopheryl succinate or α-tocopheryl acetate) in promoting the inhibition of cell growth and proliferation in various rodent and human cells.[74,75]

Several mechanisms of action have been postulated to explain vitamin E's capability of reducing malignant cell growth. Overall, the effect of vitamin E results in a reduced expression of some transcription factors as well as reduced responses to specific growth factors, thus modulating the progression of cell-cycle events. While the exact biochemical reactions by which vitamin E modulates these pathways have not been completely delineated, it has been suggested that vitamin E's role in scavenging peroxyl radicals contributes to phosphorylation events leading to distinct changes in kinase activities that affect gene transcription. For instance, increased activity of the cyclin-dependent kinase cdc2 (cdk1) resulting in increased expression of the p53 tumor suppressor gene have been observed.[76] As described below, vitamin E has also been implicated in the regulation of TGF-β and p21 genes. Inhibition of gene expression and activity of NFAT, NFκB, or other Rel family members by vitamin E has also been noted in various human and rodent tumor cells.[74]

One of the proposed mechanisms by which vitamin E subverts cell growth is via inhibition of PKC activity. Azzi and colleagues[9,77] have shown that α-tocopherol and β-tocopherol inhibit cellular proliferation and PKC activity of Chinese hamster ovary cells (CHO). These effects, however, are not seen for HeLa cells, suggesting that there are different cell-specific pathways of cellular proliferation in which vitamin E can act. Such pathways are also likely to be differentially affected by the specific actions of the various tocopherol isoforms tested. Other important pathways where vitamin E has been shown to intervene with cell growth and proliferation involve decreases in upregulated adenylate cyclase activity, and decreased expression of the transcription factors c-myc, H-ras, and E2F.[74,78] For example, vitamin E succinate has been shown to decrease c-myc and H-ras mRNA levels in B16 melanoma cells *in vitro*.[78] In addition, d-α-tocopheryl succinate (11.3 μM) has been shown to inhibit growth and to downregulate N-myc and H-ras mRNAs in murine neuroblastoma cells (NBP2).[79]

It has been established that prostaglandins are factors that can enhance cancer development and progression, albeit in a tissue-specific as well as prostaglandin-specific manner.[80] Once again, overexpression of COX-2 mRNA and protein has been observed in numerous cancer types. Vitamin E, by downregulating the production of accumulated prostaglandins, could potentially subvert the invasive growth of cancer cells. It is noteworthy that vitamin E seems to strengthen the cytotoxic effects of various chemotherapeutic agents and NSAID on tumor cells when administered in synergistic combination.[80] Described below are several examples of the experimental evidence found for the effects of vitamin E on several types of cancer *in vitro*.

16.3.2.1 Breast cancer

Studies using the estrogen receptor negative (ER−) BT20 human breast cancer cell line showed that vitamin E decreased both the phosphorylation and the transactivation of the transcription factor E2F1 which is involved in cell cycle regulation.[81,82] Moreover, changes in increased cyclin A binding to E2F1 (which negatively regulates E2F1 function) as well as increased binding of p21 to cyclin A and to the cyclin-dependent kinase 2 (cdk2) were found, demonstrating that vitamin E is capable of activating signal transduction pathways that can prevent cell cycle arrest. In addition, these investigators showed that vitamin E could inhibit the transcriptional activation of the E2F1-responsive gene, *c-myc*.[81,82]

Yu et al.[83] reported that increases in AP-1 transactivation, prolonged c-jun N-terminal kinase (JNK) and c-jun activation (as seen by mRNA and protein levels) in MDA-MB-435 breast cancer cells can occur upon treatment with α-tocopheryl succinate. These changes paralleled the increased apoptotic events observed in the cancerous cells with vitamin E treatment.[84, 85] Studies with this cell line using α-tocopheryl succinate have also revealed increased mRNA and protein expression of the cytokines TGF-β1, TGF-β2, TGF-β3 as well as of the TGF-β type II receptor.[86] In addition, vitamin E succinate has been shown to inhibit cellular proliferation in a dose-dependent manner and to induce apoptosis of reticuloendotheliosis virus-transformed avian lymphoid cells, RECC-UTCA-1, *in vitro*. These changes are paralleled by decreased c-myc mRNA levels.[87,88] Using the ER+ human breast cancer cell line MCF-7, vitamin E succinate (19 μM) has been shown to arrest DNA synthesis, inhibit cell proliferation, and induce apoptosis. The antioxidant facilitated a persistent expression of c-jun mRNA and protein levels, as well as elevated AP-1-binding activity, suggesting that c-jun is involved in the apoptotic process induced in these cells upon vitamin E treatment.[89] Interestingly, a recent report showed that vitamin E exerts its inhibitory effect on breast cancer cell growth irrespective of ER status.[90]

Moreover, Yu et al.[84,85] have also demonstrated that treatment of murine EL4 T lymphoma cells with α-tocopheryl-succinate (20 μg/ml) can induce cells to undergo apoptotic cell death *in vitro* (95% cell death) as seen by DNA fragmentation analysis. Concomitant with these changes, reduced c-myc mRNA expression and increased bcl-2, c-fos, and c-jun mRNA levels have been observed 3 to 6 hours post-vitamin E treatment.[84,85] Additionally, gel mobility assays have shown increased AP-1 DNA-binding activity and decreased c-myc DNA-binding activity 12 to 24 hours post-vitamin E treatment.[84,85]

16.3.2.2 Colorectal Cancer

In colorectal cancer biopsies, increased ratios of arachidonic acid to eicosapentaenoic acid in mucosal tissues have been observed in diseased patients relative to controls.[91] These increased ratios are associated with the progression of adenomas to carcinomas and reflect increased substrate availability for PGE_2 synthesis. As mentioned previously, increased PGE_2 has been reported in colorectal adenomas and carcinomas. Similarly, COX-2 transcription has been shown to be elevated in most human colorectal cancers.[92,93] It is interesting that such changes in tissue fatty-acid expression reflect changes that could be caused by differences in fatty acid utilization to generate eicosanoids and could contribute to the development of tumor malignancy. It has been postulated that changes in arachidonic acid metabolism may stimulate cell proliferation via activation of PKC and other kinases.[9,94,95]

These observations strongly implicate COX-2 in the induction or progression of the malignant state of colorectal tumors, and suggest, furthermore, that PKC might be one of the important signaling pathways through which certain tumors are initiated or maintained. Since, as mentioned earlier, vitamin E exerts an inhibitory effect on COX-2 activity, vitamin E might be beneficial in circumventing colon cancer pathogenesis and/or progression via inhibition of COX-2 activity.

Vitamin E is known to induce apoptosis of colorectal cancer cells. One suggested mechanism of action for this induction involves the activation of $p21^{WAF1/CIP1}$ (cell-cycle inhibitor factor) and $c/EBP\beta$, in a manner that is independent of p53 activation.[96]

16.3.2.3 Myelodysplastic Syndromes

Myelodysplastic syndrome (MDS) patients exhibit impaired granulopoiesis and thrombopoiesis, decreased blast-forming units–erythroid progenitor cells (BFU–Es) formation and decreased responses to erythropoietin and cytokines leading to anemia. Furthermore, functional defects in mature myeloid cells have been observed in 50% of patients. α-Tocopherol has been shown to have a protective effect on erythroid progenitor cells and BFU-E growth *in vitro* (increasing number and function of mature cells through α-tocopherol treatment) and might be coupled with retinoic acid therapy to improve benefits of the treatment.[67,97] Retinoids have been shown to improve hematopoiesis and immune response against infection. Some of the effects of retinoids might be mediated through decreased gene expression and secretion of TNF-α in monocytes. Hence, it is plausible that α-tocopherol might also act in subverting myeloid defects by preventing hematopoietic failure in MDS patients via a similar mechanism of TNF-α downregulation. One study has reported a strong synergism of all trans-retinoic acid (25 to 45 mg/m2/d), G-CSF (granulocyte-colony stimulating factor) (1 mg/kg/d), erythropoietin (500 U/d), and α-tocopherol (400 mg/d) in ameliorating the number and function of hematopoietic cells of MDS patients. This study demonstrated that the combination therapy improved white blood cell counts significantly in an 8-week period, increasing hemoglobin levels in all patients, and reducing levels of TNF-α expression in a subgroup of patients.[97]

16.3.3 Vitamin E and Cardiovascular Diseases

Epidemiological studies have shown an inverse relationship between coronary artery diseases and plasma vitamin E levels,[98–100] but the precise mechanism underlying vitamin E's beneficial effects has not been elucidated fully. However, a broad range of benefits, such as promoting and modulating vascular function, has been proposed for vitamin E.

The most widely studied model of vitamin E's protective effects in atherosclerosis involves protection against low-density lipoprotein (LDL) oxidation. Vitamin E, present in the LDL as well as in the extracellular fluid of the arterial wall, protects LDL against oxidative modification. Vitamin E incorporated into subendothelial spaces also protects LDL from oxidative modification by resident vascular cells such as smooth muscle cells, endothelial cells, and Mφ. Under conditions of increased oxidative stress and in the absence of adequate antioxidant protection, accumulation of oxidized LDL (ox-LDL) occurs, resulting in monocyte chemotaxis, inhibition of Mφ egress, foam cell formation, and endothelial dysfunction.[101] In addition, ox-LDL itself induces endothelial expression and secretion of cytokines, growth factors, and several cell surface adhesion molecules, which result in the recruitment of circulating monocytes into the intima where they differentiate into Mφ and foam cells. In response to growth factors, smooth muscle cells proliferate in the intima, resulting in the narrowing of the lumen. Moreover, oxidized LDL can inhibit endothelial production of nitric oxide, a potent vasodilator.[102] Thus, vitamin E can protect against the development of atherosclerosis by retarding LDL oxidation, and inhibiting the proliferation of smooth muscle cells and monocyte adhesion to endothelial cells.

Moreover, vitamin E has been shown to prevent ox-LDL-induced endothelial cell dysfunction by inhibiting PKC activation.[103] Phorbol 12-myristate 13-acetate (PMA)-induced activation of platelet aggregation can be blocked by vitamin E supplementation via inhibition of PKC-dependent protein phosphorylation.[104] In addition, calphostin C, a potent inhibitor of PKC, has been shown to attenuate ox-LDL- induced inhibition of endothelium-dependent relaxation.[105] Furthermore, PKC can also be activated via increased DNA-binding activity of NFκB in human endothelial cells.[106]

Thus, vitamin E-induced modulation of PKC appears to play an important role in gene expression involved in endothelial dysfunction. However, the inhibitory effects of vitamin E on PKC have not been observed in some studies. For example, in human endothelial cells, vitamin E was shown to inhibit agonist-induced monocyte adhesion in a time- and concentration-dependent manner.[62] This inhibition was correlated with a decrease in steady-state levels of E-selectin mRNA and cell surface expression of E-selectin. Inhibition of E-selectin was not due to PKC activation, as vitamin E treatment did not suppress phosphorylation of PKC substrates. In addition, activation of the transcription factor NFκB was reported to be unnecessary for E-selectin expression since electrophoretic mobility shift assays failed to show vitamin E-induced decreases in activation of this transcription factor.[62]

16.3.4   Vitamin E and Diabetes

The classic markers of oxidative stress, e.g., lipid peroxides, oxidized LDL, conjugated dienes, superoxide anion, and isoprostane, are elevated in diabetes. Although the exact mechanism of oxygen-derived reactive oxygen species (ROS) generation in diabetes has not been clearly defined, elevated glucose levels appear to contribute greatly. Hyperglycemia, a classic symptom of diabetes, has been shown to increase autoxidation of glucose, to increase advanced glycation end products (AGE), and to induce NADPH-oxidase activity. AGE are formed during non-enzymatic glycation and oxidation (glycoxidation) reactions by binding of sugar molecules (aldoses) onto free amino groups of proteins or lipoproteins. This process is accelerated in diabetics due to their elevated levels of glucose (hyperglycemia) and has been implicated in the pathogenesis of diabetic vascular complications. For example, treatment with AGE has been shown to increase vascular endothelial growth factor (VEGF) mRNA with a concomitant development of retinal vascularization resulting in diabetic retinopathy.[107] Receptors for AGE (RAGE) are present on the cell membrane of endothelial cells, and blockade of RAGE by specific antibodies can correct the vascular complications observed in diabetics. AGE treatment can induce endothelial cell (EC) oxidant stress, including the generation of thiobarbituric acid reactive substances (TBARS) and activation of NFκB. NFκB has been shown to mediate AGE-induced expression of IL-6 mRNA in human bone-derived cells.[108] Moreover, AGE have been suggested to increase endothelial expression of adhesion molecules such as VCAM-1 by inducing oxidative stress with subsequent activation of nuclear transcription factor NFκB.[109]

Glycation of hemoglobin (G-Hb) in red blood cells (RBC) has been shown to increase significantly in the presence of H_2O_2 as well as with higher glucose concentrations. This increase in G-Hb can be blocked when RBC are pretreated with vitamin E. Vitamin E can also inhibit the formation of malondialdehyde (MDA), an end product of lipid peroxidation. Furthermore, treatment of RBC with MDA, or with a combination of glucose and MDA, has shown higher G-Hb formation with glucose-MDA in contrast to glucose alone.[110] In addition, hyperglycemia enhances lipid peroxidation and increases MDA accumulation.[111]

Collectively, these findings suggest that both hyperglycemia as well as hyperglycemia-induced lipid peroxidation leading to an increased formation of MDA can stimulate glycation of proteins in diabetes. Vitamin E is capable of blocking glycation of proteins by inhibiting MDA formation[110] (Fig. 16.7).

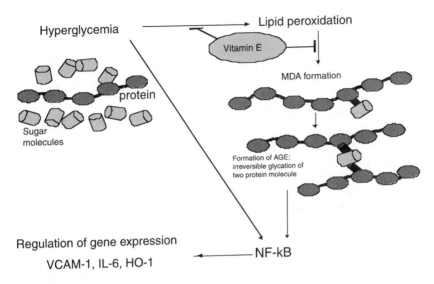

FIGURE 16.7
Hyperglycemia-induced protein glycation. Increased levels of glucose induce lipid peroxidation, and lipid peroxidation produces MDA.[110] MDA stimulates glycation of proteins leading to altered gene expression, which is mediated primarily through NFκB.[112] Hyperglycemia also directly results in activation of NFκB.[113] Vitamin E blocks the glycation of proteins by inhibiting the formation of MDA and consequently blocking hyperglycemia-associated complications.

16.3.5 Role of Vitamin E in the Reversal of Renal and Hepatic Tissue Damage

16.3.5.1 Renal Injury and Immunoglobulin A (IgA) Nephropathies

It has been established that diets deficient in vitamin E promote renal enlargement, proteinuria, mild tubulointerstitial disease, and a reduced glomerular filtration rate.[114] The mechanism of renal tissue damage is correlated to oxidative stress and increased net DNA content and synthesis in the kidney, mainly in the renal tubular epithelium. Gene transcription in damaged renal tissue is upregulated for various transcription factors, cytokines, and extracellular matrix factors. For instance, a study in which rats were fed a vitamin E-deficient diet revealed that mRNA levels were increased for factors such as c-myc, the histone H2b, TGF-β1, and collagens I, III, and IV.[114] Moreover, glutathione peroxidase mRNA expression in the kidney was also decreased with the vitamin E-deficient diet. The induction of such factors upon vitamin E deficiency in the kidney corresponds to those typically observed with oxidative stress.[114]

In vitro studies have also shown that the genes for the previously listed factors are upregulated in rodent kidney mesangial cells exposed to non-cytolytic doses of hydrogen peroxide.[114] Interestingly, in the rats fed the vitamin E-deficient diet, whole kidney catalase mRNA levels were reduced, suggesting the involvement of an additional mechanism by which clearance of hydrogen peroxide with vitamin E deficiency can be compromised in the kidney.[114]

These findings suggest that reducing the prooxidant status of renal tissue with vitamin E supplementation might lead to downregulated transcription of various oxidative stress-induced genes, thus potentially lowering tissue damage in the kidney.

Reactive oxygen species (ROS) suppress *in vitro* synthesis of erythropoietin. Vitamin A supplementation has been shown to increase erythropoietin synthesis in renal and hepatic tissue.[115] One study demonstrated that erythropoietin expression could be increased significantly relative to control tissue in a rat model of reperfused hypoxic kidney when vitamin A (retinol acetate, 0.5 µg/ml), vitamin E (α-tocopherol, 0.5 µg/ml), and vitamin C (10 µg/ml) were added in combination for 24 h.[115] In hepatoma cell cultures, while vitamin A specifically increased erythropoietin production, neither C nor E (0.05 to 500 µg/ml), when added separately, increased erythropoietin gene expression. This study suggested a strong potential for vitamins E and C to protect cells from oxidative damage but demonstrated that vitamin A was specific in stimulating erythropoietin production.[115]

In various animal species, including rodents, TNF-α levels and IL-1 renal dysfunction due to sepsis or ischemia-reperfusion injury are dramatically increased from Mφ and renal mesangial cells.[116,117] Such cytokines promote kidney parenchymal damage either directly via apoptosis, or by recruitment of neutrophils, which release ROS and proteases.[116] In such models of ischemia-reperfusion, mesangial cells have been shown to exhibit an increased activation and transcription of TNF-α, hypoxia-induced factor (HIF)-1, p38 MAPK, and JNK.[115,116,118] It has been speculated that inhibition of TNF-α production by vitamin E supplementation could be considered a therapeutic strategy to ameliorate oxidative injury in the kidney.[116]

In IgA nephropathy, it has been shown that IgA-containing immune complexes stimulate the production of oxygen free radicals in mesangial cells *in vitro*.[119] Studies conducted by Kuemmerle et al.[120,121] and by Trachtman et al.[119] have shown that α-tocopherol (100 IU/kg diet) can reduce proteinuria in experimentally induced IgA nephropathy (from bovine γ-globulin injection) in rats as early as 4 weeks of treatment and by as much as 50%. Such studies revealed that reduced renal plasma flow also was restored to normal levels upon vitamin E treatment. In addition, TGF-β mRNA expression, which was elevated with proteinuria and IgA deposition in the renal mesangium, was significantly decreased between 4 and 8 weeks of vitamin E administration. Furthermore, lipid peroxidation of LDL has also been associated with tissue damage in glomerulosclerosis. It has been shown that an important mechanism by which this might occur involves upregulation of collagen gene expression by LDL (including collagen IV) in mesangial cells. Vitamin E (at a 50 µM dose) markedly downregulated collagen mRNA expression from cultured human mesangial cells exposed to LDL.[122] Additionally, in a rat model of reflux pyelonephritis, vitamin E (24 IU/kg/day) has been proven effective in decreasing the degree of inflammation of tissue as assessed histologically.[123]

16.3.5.2 Liver Injury

In a study by Pietrangelo et al.[124] the anti-fibrinogenic properties of vitamin E were tested on gerbils to assess the molecular pathways involved in iron-induced hepatic fibrosis. With administration of an α-tocopherol-enriched diet (250 mg/kg) over 4 months, animals treated with high doses of iron (1 mg/g) showed significant decreases in collagen mRNA levels, despite exhibiting persistent liver damage. Although small, reduced levels of accumulated TGF-β mRNA produced by Mϕ and Kupffer cells were also observed.

Nonparenchymal cell proliferation (macrophagic population and fat storing cells) was arrested in contrast to control animals. Iron-dosed animals not supplemented with vitamin E developed severe hepatic cirrhosis. This study demonstrated that vitamin E supplementation could prevent liver cirrhosis by arresting fibrinogenesis during experimentally induced hepatic fibrosis by arresting collagen-mediated nonparenchymal cell proliferation.[124]

Acute liver damage in the rat can also be induced by intragastric administration of carbon tetrachloride (CCl_4).[125] In this experimental model, increased MCP-1 gene expression could be detected as early as 12 h, peaking at 48 h after lipid peroxidation events had initiated. Increased expression of MCP-1 could be detected prior to monocyte/Mϕ infiltration. Vitamin E supplementation was shown to decrease MCP-1 mRNA as well as protein levels. These changes paralleled decreased numbers of infiltrating Mϕ in the liver. The results suggested a significant role for MCP-1 in the recruitment of inflammatory cells during liver injury, and that these events could be subverted by subsequent administration of vitamin E.

Another report has demonstrated that increased DNA-binding activation of AP-1 from lipid peroxidation induced by CCl_4 can be completely blocked in the liver by treatment with α-tocopherol in rats.[126] Interestingly, in the inflammatory events taking place in hepatic cholestatic injury, NFκB and TNF-α gene expression have been shown to be upregulated in Mϕ.[127] Current investigations are focusing on the ability of vitamin E to downmodulate these genes during hepatic injury.

TGF-β1 and pro-collagen type I gene expression are also upregulated by a prooxidant status in the liver, and are considered hallmarks of liver fibrosis. Expression of these genes has been downregulated with long-term treatment of vitamin E *in vivo* in the rat.[128,129] In addition, vitamin E treatment of hepatic fat-storing cells has been shown to decrease mRNA expression of both genes in rats.[128,129]

In another report, long- and short-term supplementation with d-α-tocopherol (40 IU/day for 8 weeks or 450 IU for 48 h, respectively) of mice with hepatic injury has revealed a marked decrease in collagen-α1 type I mRNA (70 and 60%, respectively).[35] Moreover, reporter assays using hepatic stellate cells to look at collagen gene expression have allowed the characterization of an α-tocopherol responsive element in the collagen gene, suggesting that vitamin E can mitigate oxidative stress in the liver by modulating collagen gene expression *in vivo*.[35]

α-Tocopherol is metabolized in the liver with lipoproteins and is secreted into the plasma in conjunction with very low-density lipoprotein (VLDL) via the α-tocopherol transfer protein (αTTP). αTTP and its mRNA are expressed in lower levels in the plasma and liver of vitamin E-deficient rats relative to control rats, or rats given a vitamin E-enriched diet (5g/kg diet α-tocopheryl acetate).[130] In addition, it has been shown that α-tocopherol and δ-tocopherol are capable of inducing α-TTP mRNA in the liver of rats fed a vitamin E-rich diet (with either stereoisomer or with both in combination).[7,131] Interestingly, decreases in αTTP mRNA have been detected as well in tumor modules of patients with early stages of hepatic carcinogenesis,[132] suggesting that aberrant αTTP expression leading to vitamin E deficiency might lead to tumor development in the liver.

16.3.6   Vitamin E and Neurodegenerative Conditions

16.3.6.1 Ataxias

Among the inherited idiopathic ataxias, ataxia with isolated vitamin E deficiency (AVED) is an autosomal recessive disorder associated with varied neurological manifestations, including progressive ataxia, araflexia, impaired position sense, sensory loss, and pyramidal signs, and is often linked to cardiomyopathy.[133] The age of onset of this condition is 4 to 18 years of age. AVED has been linked to chromosome 8q13 in which mutations in the αTTP gene result in an impaired ability to incorporate α-tocopherol into lipoproteins that are secreted by the liver. Tamaru and colleagues have suggested that exon skipping of all transcripts for the αTTP gene results in impaired splicing mechanisms (complete inactivation of the splicing site) that lead to the inability of the αTTP protein to function correctly in the absorption of vitamin E, consequently contributing to the development of AVED ataxia.[134] α-Tocopheryl-acetate has been used therapeutically to arrest neurological loss in this as well as other ataxias.[133]

Friedreich's ataxia is also an autosomal recessive disorder with an incidence of 1 in 50,000 individuals and is associated with DNA-triplet repeat expansions (GAA) localized to chromosome 9, where the frataxin gene has been mapped. It has been suggested that this type of ataxia might be a result of defects in vitamin E metabolism. In Friedreich's ataxia, genetic abnormalities in the frataxin gene often result in a loss of function of the frataxin protein, resulting in undetectable or low levels of frataxin mRNA.[135] The function of the frataxin protein is not completely understood but it is thought that reduced frataxin in the heart and spinal cord is the primary cause of neural degeneration in these patients.[133] Interestingly, in a study conducted by Yokota et al.,[136] four individuals with Friedreich's-like ataxia accompanied by retinitis pigmentosa and with isolated vitamin E deficiency were tested. Although absorption of vitamin E was found to be normal in all four cases, decreases in serum levels of vitamin E were markedly worsened, and were associated with a specific point mutation observed in the αTTP gene, suggesting that the degree of adequate or inadequate vitamin E absorption in these individuals was dependent on the severity of genetic defects affecting the αTTP gene.[136]

16.3.6.2 Amyotrophic Lateral Sclerosis and Other Neuronal Abnormalities

Amyotrophic lateral sclerosis is a high-incidence motor neuron disease characterized by progressive neurodegeneration and cell death of lower motor neuron groups in the spinal cord and brain stem, and also of upper motor neurons in the motor cortex. The result of such neurodegenerative effects includes progressive muscle weakness and wasting. Vitamin E has been shown to retard the onset of motor neuron disease where oxidative stress contributes to the early stages of motor neuron injury.[137]

In a study conducted by Ghadge et al.,[138] mutant superoxide dismutase genes (SOD) were expressed in neuronal cells via adenoviral gene transfer and were shown to induce cell death in differentiated PC12 cells, superior cervical ganglion neurons, and hippocampal pyramidal neurons,[138] cells that displayed high rates of superoxide radicals. In contrast, cell death was prevented by administration of vitamin E (100 μM dose), copper chelators, glutathione, Z-Val-Ala-Asp-(o-methyl)-fluoromethyl Ketone (ZVAD) and Tyr-Val-Ala-Asp-aldehyde (YVAD) caspase inhibitors, as well as by the constitutive expression of bcl-2.[138]

Another study looking at mice with mutant Cu/Zn superoxide dismutase showed that neurodegeneration was slowed down markedly when these mice were cross-bred into transgenic strains overexpressing bcl-2 and thus inhibiting apoptotic pathways leading to neuronal cell death.[137,139] These findings are relevant because downregulation of Cu/Zn SOD induces apoptosis in PC12 neuronal cells,[140] and furthermore, missense mutations in the SOD1 gene (leading to impaired enzymatic activity) have been shown to contribute to the neurodegenerative effects seen in human familial amyotrophic lateral sclerosis (20% of cases). Blocking SOD1 with antisense oligonucleotides has been shown to improve neuronal cell survival. In addition, treatment of dying cells with vitamin E clearly rescues the cells from apoptosis.[141] Noteworthy is the observation that a combination of vitamin E and neural growth factor supplementation has proven to be most effective in blocking apoptosis of such cells.[138]

The effects of vitamin E on gene expression of neuronal cells exposed to oxidative stress *in vitro* were examined in a study by Post et al.[142] Clonal hippocampal HT22 cells were subjected to haloperidol (HP), a dopamine receptor antagonist that induces cell death by oxidative stress. As a result, intracellular glutathione levels were found to be reduced in parallel to increased peroxide levels, while the DNA-binding activity and transcription levels of NFκB were also increased. Treatment with α-tocopherol (200 μM) blocked NFκB activation in reporter assays, and in addition, suppressed NFκB DNA-binding activity.[142] Moreover, overexpression of IκBα suppressed NFκB transcription protecting the HT22 cells from neurotoxicity. Vitamin E thus partially protected the cells against HP oxidation, most likely by blocking lipid peroxidation events, and subsequently by suppressing HP-induced activation of NFκB.[142]

Finally, in an *in vitro* study by Noh et al.,[143] murine neuronal cortical cells subjected to zinc-mediated oxidative injury were rescued from neurotoxicity by administration of the vitamin E analog, Trolox (100 μM).[143] Although not proven directly, a mechanism by which vitamin E suppresses oxidative damage of neuronal cells indicates an inactivation of PKC. PKC can become activated upon zinc influx, leading to intracellular calcium entry and neuronal death.[143] Vitamin E is known to inhibit PKC activation.[144] Vitamin E could function in a manner very similar to that of Trolox in such cells, downregulating PKC activity and/or other kinase pathways, and leading to a consistent block of cytotoxic events resulting in prevention of neural degeneration.

Noteworthy is that COX-2 gene expression has been shown to be upregulated in various models of brain peripheral inflammation and is associated with neurodegeneration.[145,146] We have shown that vitamin E downregulates COX-2 activity in Mφ.[50] Current investigations are under way to test the ability of COX-2 inhibitors and vitamin E to downregulate the expression and activity of cyclooxygenases potentially involved in promoting apoptosis and neurodegeneration of brain cells.

16.4 Conclusion

Vitamin E is the most effective lipid-soluble antioxidant known to protect plasma and intracellular membranes against the harmful effects of free radicals. Mounting evidence points to vitamin E as an important regulator of intracellular signal transduction, and thus, an important regulator of the expression of genes coding for key metabolic proteins. Most of vitamin E's effect in this regard is mediated through its control of oxidant-sensitive transcription factors. There is, however, some evidence that vitamin E might mediate its effect through a non-antioxidant, and as yet unknown, mechanism. Vitamin E regulation of gene regulation has implications for many biologic functions including those of vascular, neuronal, and immune systems as well as the diseases related to them. There is growing interest not only in free radicals, but also in predisposing genetic factors, and the roles these might play in increasing the susceptibility of individuals to acute and chronic diseases. The ability of vitamin E to regulate gene expression directly or indirectly under physiological and pathological conditions has great implications for determining the dietary requirement of this vitamin and strongly supports the need for further research in this area.

References

1. Hong, Y. C. and Lee, K. H., Enhancement of DNA damage and involvement of reactive oxygen species after exposure to bitumen with UVA irradiation, *Mutat. Res.*, 426, 63, 1999.
2. Rivett, A. J. and Levine, R. L., Metal-catalyzed oxidation of Escherichia coli glutamine synthetase: correlation of structural and functional changes, *Arch. Biochem. Biophys.*, 278, 26, 1990.
3. Berlett, B. S. and Stadtman, E. R., Protein oxidation in aging, disease, and oxidative stress, *J. Biol. Chem.*, 272, 20313, 1997.
4. Liebler, D. C., Kaysen, K. L., and Burr, J. A., Peroxyl radical trapping and autoxidation reactions of alpha-tocopherol in lipid bilayers, *Chem. Res. Toxicol.*, 4, 89, 1991.
5. Burton, G. W. and Ingold, K. U., Autooxidation of biological molecules. I. The antioxidant activity of vitamin E and related chain-breaking phenolic antioxidants *in vitro*, *J. Am. Chem. Soc.*, 103, 6472, 1981.
6. Hosomi, A., Arita, M., Sato, Y., Kiyose, C., Ueda, T., Igarashi, O., Arai, H., and Inoue, K., Affinity for alpha-tocopherol transfer protein as a determinant of the biological activities of vitamin E analogs, *FEBS Lett.*, 409, 105, 1997.
7. Fechner, H., Schlame, M., Guthmann, F., Stevens, P. A., and Rustow, B., Alpha- and delta-tocopherol induce expression of hepatic alpha-tocopherol-transfer-protein mRNA, *Biochem. J.*, 15, 577, 1998.
8. Teupser, D., Thiery, J., and Seidel, D., Alpha-tocopherol down-regulates scavenger receptor activity in macrophages, *Atherosclerosis*, 144, 109, 1999.
9. Azzi, A., Boscoboinik, D., Fazzio, A., Marilley, D., Maroni, P., Özer, N. K., Spycher, S., and Tasinato, A., RRR-alpha-tocopherol regulation of gene transcription in response to the cell oxidant status, *Z. Ernährungswiss*, 37, 21, 1998.
10. Wu, D., Meydani, M., Beharka, A., Serafini, M., Martin, K., and Meydani, S. N., *In vitro* supplementation with different tocopherol homologues can affect the function of immune cells in old mice, *Free Radic. Biol. Med.*, 28, 643, 2000.
11. Azzi, A., Boscoboinik, D., Clement, S., Özer, N. K., Ricciarelli, R., and Stocker, A., Vitamin E mediated response of smooth muscle cell to oxidant stress, *Diabetes Res. Clin. Pract.*, 45, 191, 1999.
12. Stauble, B., Boscoboinik, D., Tasinato, A., and Azzi, A., Modulation of activator protein-1 (AP-1) transcription factor and protein kinase C by hydrogen peroxide and D-alpha-tocopherol in vascular smooth muscle cells, *Eur. J. Biochem.*, 226, 393, 1994.
13. Maiorino, M., Coassin, M., Roveri, A., and Ursini, F., Microsomal lipid peroxidation: effect of vitamin E and its functional interaction with phospholipid hydroperoxide glutathione peroxidase, *Lipids*, 24, 721, 1989.
14. Faux, S. P. and Howden, P. J., Possible role of lipid peroxidation in the induction of NF-kappa B and AP-1 in RFL-6 cells by crocidolite asbestos: evidence following protection by vitamin E, *Environ. Health Perspect.*, 105 (Suppl.), 1127, 1997.
15. Kapralov, A. A., Petrova, G. V., Vasilieva, S. M., and Donchenko, G. V., Tocopherol modulates the effects of A23187, verapamil, and phorbol myristate acetate on RNA-polymerase activity of isolated rat liver nuclei, *Biochemistry (Moscow)*, 62, 694, 1997.

16. Casini, A., Ceni, E., Salzano, R., Biondi, P., Parola, M., Galli, A., Foschi, M., Caligiuri, A., Pinzani, M., and Surrenti, C., Neutrophil-derived superoxide anion induces lipid peroxidation and stimulates collagen synthesis in human hepatic stellate cells: role of nitric oxide, *Hepatology,* 25, 361, 1997.
17. Chan, S. L., Tammariello, S. P., Estus, S., and Mattson, M. P., Prostate apoptosis response-4 mediates trophic factor withdrawal-induced apoptosis of hippocampal neurons: actions prior to mitochondrial dysfunction and caspase activation, *J. Neurochem.,* 73, 502, 1999.
18. Ikeda, M., Schroeder, K. K., Mosher, L. B., Woods, C. W., and Akeson, A. L., Suppressive effect of antioxidants on intercellular adhesion molecule-1 (ICAM-1) expression in human epidermal keratinocytes, *J. Invest. Dermatol.,* 103, 791, 1994.
19. Yoshikawa, T., Yoshida, N., Manabe, H., Terasawa, Y., Takemura, T., and Kondo, M., Alpha-tocopherol protects against expression of adhesion molecules on neutrophils and endothelial cells, *Biofactors,* 7, 15, 1998.
20. Takahashi, S., Takahashi, Y., Yoshimi, T., and Miura, T., Oxygen tension regulates heme oxygenase-1 gene expression in mammalian cell lines, *Cell Biochem. Funct.,* 16, 183, 1998.
21. Fuchs, J., Huflejt, M. E., Rothfuss, L. M., Wilson, D. S., Carcamo, G., and Packer, L., Acute effects of near ultraviolet and visible light on the cutaneous antioxidant defense system, *Photochem. Photobiol.,* 50, 739, 1989.
22. Tyrrell, R., Redox regulation and oxidant activation of heme oxygenase-1, *Free Radic. Res.,* 31, 335, 1999.
23. Basu-Modak, S., Luscher, P., and Tyrrell, R. M., Lipid metabolite involvement in the activation of the human heme oxygenase-1 gene, *Free Radic. Biol. Med.,* 20, 887, 1996.
24. Brzezinska-Slebodzinska, E. and Pietras, B., The protective role of some antioxidants and scavengers on the free radicals-induced inhibition of the liver iodothyronine 5'-monodeiodinase activity and thiols content, *J. Physiol. Pharmacol.,* 48, 451, 1997.
25. Sun, Y. and Oberley, L. W., Redox regulation of transcriptional activators, *Free Radic. Biol. Med.,* 21, 335, 1996.
26. Mitomo, K., Nakayama, K., Fujimoto, K., Sun, X., Seki, S., and Yamamoto, K., Two different cellular redox systems regulate the DNA-binding activity of the p50 subunit of NF-kappa B *in vitro, Gene,* 145, 197, 1994.
27. Guehmann, S., Vorbrueggen, G., Kalkbrenner, F., and Moelling, K., Reduction of a conserved Cys is essential for Myb DNA-binding, *Nucleic Acids Res.,* 20, 2279, 1992.
28. Grasser, F. A., LaMontagne, K., Whittaker, L., Stohr, S., and Lipsick, J. S., A highly conserved cysteine in the v-Myb DNA-binding domain is essential for transformation and transcriptional trans-activation, *Oncogene,* 7, 1005, 1992.
29. Abate, C., Baker, S. J., Lees-Miller, S. P., Anderson, C. W., Marshak, D. R., and Curran, T., Dimerization and DNA binding alter phosphorylation of Fos and Jun, *Proc. Natl. Acad. Sci. USA,* 90, 6766, 1993.
30. Cachia, O., Benna, J. E., Pedruzzi, E., Descomps, B., Gougerot-Pocidalo, M. A., and Leger, C. L., Alpha-tocopherol inhibits the respiratory burst in human monocytes. Attenuation of p47(phox) membrane translocation and phosphorylation, *J. Biol. Chem.,* 273, 32801, 1998.

31. Panin, L. E., Polyakov, L. M., Kolosova, N. G., Russkikh, G. S., and Poteryaeva, O. N., Distribution of tocopherol and apolipoprotein A-I immunoreactivity in rat liver chromatin, *Membr. Cell Biol.,* 11, 631, 1998.
32. Ng, D., Kokot, N., Hiura, T., Faris, M., Saxon, A., and Nel, A., Macrophage activation by polycyclic aromatic hydrocarbons: evidence for the involvement of stress-activated protein kinases, activator protein-1, and antioxidant response elements, *J. Immunol.,* 161, 942, 1998.
33. Talalay, P., De Long, M. J., and Prochaska, H. J., Identification of a common chemical signal regulating the induction of enzymes that protect against chemical carcinogenesis, *Proc. Natl. Acad. Sci. USA,* 85, 8261, 1988.
34. Talalay, P., Fahey, J. W., Holtzclaw, W. D., Prestera, T., and Zhang, Y., Chemoprotection against cancer by phase 2 enzyme induction, *Toxicol. Lett.,* 82, 173, 1995.
35. Chojkier, M., Houglum, K., Lee, K. S., and Buck, M., Long- and short-term D-alpha-tocopherol supplementation inhibits liver collagen alpha1(I) gene expression, *Am. J. Physiol.,* 275, G1480, 1998.
36. Prestera, T., Talalay, P., Alam, J., Ahn, Y. I., Lee, P. J., and Choi, A. M., Parallel induction of heme oxygenase-1 and chemoprotective phase 2 enzymes by electrophiles and antioxidants: regulation by upstream antioxidant-responsive elements (ARE), *Mol. Med.,* 1, 827, 1995.
37. Venugopal, R. and Jaiswal, A. K., Nrf1 and Nrf2 positively and c-Fos and Fra1 negatively regulate the human antioxidant response element-mediated expression of NAD(P)H:quinone oxidoreductase1 gene, *Proc. Natl. Acad. Sci. USA,* 93, 14960, 1996.
38. Itoh, K., Wakabayashi, N., Katoh, Y., Ishii, T., Igarashi, K., Engel, J. D., and Yamamoto, M., Keap1 represses nuclear activation of antioxidant responsive elements by Nrf2 through binding to the amino-terminal Neh2 domain, *Genes Dev.,* 13, 76, 1999.
39. Yu, R., Jiao, J. J., Duh, J. L., Gudehithlu, K., Tan, T. H., and Kong, A. N., Activation of mitogen-activated protein kinases by green tea polyphenols: potential signalling pathways in the regulation of antioxidant-responsive element-mediated phase II enzyme gene expression, *Carcinogenesis,* 18, 451, 1997.
40. Coquette, A., Vray, B., and Vanderpras, J., Role of vitamin E in the protection of the resident macrophage membrane against oxidative damage, *Arch. Int. Physiol. Biochem.,* 94, 529, 1986.
41. Hatman, L. J. and Kayden, H. J., A high-performance liquid chromatographic method for the determination of tocopherol in plasma and cellular elements of the blood, *J. Lipid Res.,* 20, 639, 1979.
42. Flescher, E., Ledbetter, J. A., Schieven, G. L., Vela-Roch, N., Fossum, D., Dang, H., Ogawa, N., and Talal, N., Longitudinal exposure of human T lymphocytes to weak oxidative stress suppresses transmembrane and nuclear signal transduction, *J. Immunol.,* 153, 4880, 1994.
43. Meydani, S. N., Meydani, M., Verdon, C. P., Blumberg, J. P., and Hayes, K. C., Vitamin E supplementation suppresses prostaglandin E2 synthesis and enhances the immune response of aged mice, *Mech. Ageing Dev.,* 34, 191, 1986.
44. Scott, M. L., Advances in our understanding of vitamin E, *Fed. Proc.,* 29, 2726, 1980.
45. Amarakoon, A. M., Tappia, P. S., and Grimble, R. F., Endotoxin induced production of IL-6 is enhanced by vitamin E deficiency and reduced by black tea extract, *Inflamm. Res.,* 44, 301, 1995.

46. Cannon, J. G., Meydani, S. N., Fielding R. A., Fitarone, M. A., Meydani, M., Farhangmher, M., Orencole, S. F., Blumberg, J. B., and Evans, W. J., The acute phase response in exercise II. Associations between vitamin E, cytokines and muscle proteolysis, *Am. J. Physiol.*, 260, R1235, 1991.

47. Hayek, M. G., Meydani, S. N., Meydani, M., and Blumberg, J. B., Age differences in eicosanoid production of mouse splenocytes: effects on mitogen-induced T-cell proliferation, *J. Gerontol.*, 49, B197, 1994.

48. Beharka, A. A., Wu, D., Han, S. N., and Meydani, S. N., Macrophage prostaglandin production contributes to the age-associated decrease in T cell function which is reversed by the dietary antioxidant vitamin E, *Mech. Ageing Dev.*, 93, 59, 1997.

49. Hayek, M. G., Mura, C., Wu, D., Beharka, A. A., Han, S. N., Paulson, K. E., Hwang, D., and Meydani, S. N., Enhanced expression of inducible cyclooxygenase with age in murine macrophages, *J. Immunol.*, 159, 2445, 1997.

50. Wu, D., Mura, C., Beharka, A. A., Han, S. N., Paulson, K. E., Hwang, D., and Meydani, S. N., Age-associated increase in PGE2 synthesis and COX activity in murine macrophages is reversed by vitamin E, *Am. J. Physiol.*, 275, C661, 1998.

51. Beharka, A. A., Serafini, M., Wu, D., Ha, W.-K., and Meydani, S. N. Vitamin E inhibits macrophage cyclooxygenase activity through peroxynitrite production. *FASEB J.*, 13, A536, 1999.

52. Hattori, S., Hattori, Y., Banba, N., Kasal, K., and Shimoda, S., Pentamethyl-hydroxychromane, vitamin E derivative, inhibits induction of nitric oxide synthase by bacterial lipopolysaccharide, *Biochem. Mol. Biol. Int.*, 35, 177, 1995.

53. Poynter, M. E. and Daynes, R. A., Age-associated alterations in splenic iNOS regulation: influence of constitutively expressed IFN-gamma and correction following supplementation with PPAR-a activators or vitamin E, *Cell. Immunol.*, 195, 127, 1999.

54. Grimble, R. F., Nutritional antioxidants and the modulation of inflammation: theory and practice, *New Horiz.*, 2, 175, 1994.

55. Packer, L. and Suzuki, Y. J., Vitamin E and alpha-lipoate: role in antioxidant recycling and activation of the NFκB transcription factor, *Mol. Aspect Med.*, 14, 229, 1993.

56. Nakamura, T., Goto, M., Matsumoto, A., and Tanaka, I., Inhibition of NF-kappa B transcriptional activity by alpha-tocopheryl succinate, *Biofactors*, 7, 21, 1998.

57. Crutchley, D. J. and Que, B. G., Copper-induced tissue factor expression in human monocytic THP-1 cells and its inhibition by antioxidants, *Circulation*, 92, 238, 1995.

58. Islam, K. N., Devaraj, S., and Jialal, I., Alpha-tocopherol enrichment of monocytes decreases agonist-induced adhesion to human endothelial cells, *Circulation*, 98, 2255, 1998.

59. Wu, D., Koga, T., Martin, K. R., and Meydani, M., Effect of vitamin E on human aortic endothelial cell production of chemokines and adhesion to monocytes, *Atherosclerosis*, 147, 297, 1999.

60. Roy, S., Sen, C. K., Kobuchi, H., and Packer, L., Antioxidant regulation of phorbol-ester induced adhesion of human Jurkat T cells to endothelial cells, *Free Radic. Biol. Med.*, 25, 229, 1998.

61. Erl, W., Weber, C., Wardemann, C., and Weber, P. C., Alpha-tocopheryl succinate inhibits monocytic cell adhesion to endothelial cells by suppressing NFκB mobilization, *Am. J. Physiol.*, 273, H634, 1997.

62. Faruqi, R., de la Motte, C., and DiCorleto, P. E., Alpha-tocopherol inhibits agonist-induced monocytic cell adhesion to cultured human endothelial cells, *J. Clin. Inv.,* 94, 592, 1994.

63. Liang, B., Ardestani, S., Chow, H.-H., Eskelson, C., and Watson, R. R., Vitamin E deficiency and immune dysfunction in retrovirus-infected C57/BL6 mice are prevented by T-cell receptor peptide treatment, *J. Nutr.,* 126, 1389, 1996.

64. Wang, Y., Huang, D. S., Liang, B. A., and Watson, R. R., Normalization of nutritional status and immune responses in mice with murine AIDS are normalized by vitamin E supplementation, *J. Nutr.,* 124, 2024, 1994.

65. Watson, R. R., Murine models for acquired deficiency syndrome, *Life Sci.,* 44, i, 1989.

66. Bogden, J. D., Baker, H., and Frank, O., Micronutrient states and human immunodeficiency virus infection, *Ann. NY Acad. Sci.,* 587, 189, 1990.

67. Geissler, R. G., Gauser, A., Ottmann, O. G., Gute, P., Morawetz, A., Guba, P., Helm, E. B., and Hoetzer, D., *In vitro* improvement of bone marrow derived hematopoietic colony formation in HIV-positive patients by alpha-tocopherol and erythropoietin, *Eur. J. Haematol.,* 53, 201, 1994.

68. Sandstrom, P. A., Roberts, B., Folks, T. M., and Buttke, T. M., HIV gene expression enhances T cell susceptibility to hydrogen peroxide-induced apoptosis, *AIDS Res. Hum. Retroviruses,* 9, 1107, 1993.

69. Hirano, F., Tanaka, H., Miura, T., Hirano, Y., Okamoto, K., Makino, Y., and Makino, I., Inhibition of NF-kappaB-dependent transcription of human immunodeficiency virus 1 promoter by a phosphodiester compound of vitamin C and vitamin E, EPC-K1, *Immunopharmacology,* 39, 31, 1998.

70. Jackson, J. R., Minton, J. A., Ho, M. L., Wie, N., and Winkler, J. D., Expression of vascular endothelial growth factor in synovial fibroblasts is induced by hypoxia and interleukin-1beta, *J. Rheumatol.,* 24, 1253, 1997.

71. Bodamyali, T., Stevens, C. R., Billingham, M. E. J., Ohta, S., and Blake, D. R., Influence of hypoxia in inflammatory synovitis, *Ann. Rheum. Dis.,* 57, 703, 1998.

72. Fairburn, K., Grootveld, M., Ward, R. J., Abiuka, C., Kus, M., and Williams, R. B., Alpha-tocopherol, lipids and lipoproteins in knee-joint synovial fluid and serum from patients with inflammatory joint disease, *Clin. Sci. (Colch),* 83, 657, 1992.

73. Crofford, L. J., COX-2 in synovial tissues, *Osteoarthr. Cartilage,* 7, 406, 1999.

74. Prasad, K. N., Kumar, A., Kochupillai, V., and Cole, W. C., High doses of multiple antioxidant vitamins: essential ingredients in improving the efficacy of standard cancer therapy, *Am. Coll. Nutr.,* 18, 13, 1999.

75. Sanders, B. G. and Kline, K., Nutrition, immunology and cancer: an overview, *Adv. Exp. Med. Biol.,* 369, 185, 1995.

76. Schwartz, J. L., Antoniades, D. S., and Zhao, S., Molecular and biochemical reprogramming of oncogenesis through the activity of prooxidants and antioxidants, *Ann. NY Acad. Sci.,* 686, 262, 1993.

77. Azzi, A., Boscoboinik, D., Marilley, D., Özer, N. K., Stäuble, B., and Tasinato, A., Vitamin E: a sensor and an information transducer of the cell oxidation state, *Am. J. Clin. Nutr.,* 62, 1337S, 1995.

78. Prasad, K. N., Cohrs, R. J., and Sharma, O. K., Decreased expressions of c-myc and H-ras oncogenes in vitamin E succinate induced morphologically differentiated murine B-16 melanoma cells in culture, *Biochem. Cell. Biol.,* 68, 1250, 1990.

79. Cohrs, R. J., Torelli, S., Prasad, K. N., Edwards-Prasad, J., and Sharma, O. K., Effect of vitamin E succinate and a cAMP-stimulating agent on the expression of c-myc and N-myc and H-ras in murine neuroblastoma cells, *Int. J. Dev. Neurosci.*, 9, 187, 1991.

80. Lupulescu, A., Prostaglandins, their inhibitors, and cancer, *Prostaglandins, Leukotrienes Essential Fatty Acids*, 54, 83, 1996.

81. Turley, J. M., Ruscetti, F. W., Kim, S. J., Fu, T., Gou, F. V., and Birchenali-Roberts, M. C., Vitamin E succinate inhibits proliferation of BT-20 human breast cancer cells: increased binding of cyclin A negatively regulates E2F transactivation activity, *Cancer Res.*, 57, 2668, 1997.

82. Turley, J. M., Fu, T., Ruscetti, F. W., Mikovits, J. A., Bertolette, D. C. R., and Birchenali-Roberts, M. C., Vitamin E succinate induces Fas-mediated apoptosis in estrogen receptor-negative human breast cancer cells, *Cancer Res,* 57, 881, 1997.

83. Yu, W., Simmons-Menchaca, M., You, H., Brown, P., Birrer, M. J., Sanders, B. G., and Kline, K., RRR-alpha-tocopheryl succinate induction of prolonged activation of c-jun amino-terminal kinase and c-jun during induction of apoptosis in human MDA-MB-435 breast cancer cells, *Mol. Carcinog.*, 22, 247, 1998.

84. Yu, W., Sanders, B. G., and Kline, K., Modulation of murine EL-4 thymic lymphoma cell proliferation and cytokine production by vitamin E succinate, *Nutr. Cancer*, 25, 137, 1996.

85. Yu, W., Sanders, B. G., and Kline, K., RRR-alpha-tocopheryl succinate inhibits EL4 thymic lymphoma cell growth by inducing apoptosis and DNA synthetic arrest, *Nutr. Cancer*, 27, 92, 1997.

86. Charpentier, A., Simmons-Menchaca, M., Yu, W., Zhao, B., Qian, M., Helm, K., Sanders, B. G., and Kline, K., RRR-alpha-tocopheryl succinate enhances TGF-beta 1, -beta 2, and -beta 3 and TGF-beta R-II expression by human MDA-MB-435 breast cancer cells, *Nutr. Cancer,* 26, 237, 1996.

87. Qian, M., Sanders, B. G., and Kline, K., RRR-alpha-tocopheryl succinate induces apoptosis in avian retrovirus-transformed lymphoid cells, *Nutr. Cancer*, 25, 9, 1996.

88. Simmons-Menchaca, M., Qian, M., Yu, W., Sanders, B. G., and Kline, K., RRR-alpha-tocopheryl succinate inhibits DNA synthesis and enhances the production and secretion of biologically active transforming growth factor-beta by avian retrovirus-transformed lymphoid cells, *Nutr. Cancer*, 24, 171, 1995.

89. Zhao, B., Yu, W., Qian, M., Simmons-Menchaca, M., Brown, P., Birrer, M. J., Sanders, B. G., and Kline, K., Involvement of activator protein (AP-1) in induction of apoptosis by vitamin E succinate in human breast cancer cells, *Mol. Carcinog.*, 19, 180, 1997.

90. Nesaretnam, K., Stephen, K., Dils, R., and Darbre, P., Tocotrienols inhibit the growth of human breast cancer cells irrespective of estrogen receptor status, *Lipids*, 33, 461, 1998.

91. Fernandez-Banares, F., Esteve, M., Navarro, E., Cabre, E., Boix, J., Abad-Lacruz, A., Klaassen, J., Planas, R., Humbert, P., Pastor, C., and Gassull, M. A., Changes of the mucosal n3 and n6 fatty acid status occur early in the colorectal adenoma-carcinoma sequence, *Gut*, 38, 254, 1996.

92. DuBois, R. N., Radhika, A., Reddy, B. S., and Entingh, A. J., Increased COX-2 levels in carcinogen-induced rat colonic tumors, *Gastroenterology,* 110, 1259, 1996.

93. Eberhart, C. E., Coffey, R. J., Radhika, A., Giardiello, F. M., Ferrenbach, S., and DuBois, R. N., Up-regulation of COX-2 gene expression in human colorectal adenomas and adenocarcinomas, *Gastroenterology*, 107, 1183, 1994.

94. Nishizuka, Y., The role of protein kinase C in cell surface signal transduction and tumor promotion, *Nature*, 308, 693, 1984.

95. Craven, P. A. and DeRubertis, F. R., Role of activation of protein kinase C in the stimulation of colonic epithelial cell proliferation by unsaturated fatty acids, *Gastroenterology*, 95, 676, 1988.

96. Chinery, R., Brockman, J. A., Peeler, M. O., Shyr, Y., Beauchamp, R. D., and Coffey, R. J., Antioxidants enhance the cytotoxicity of chemotherapeutic agents in colorectal cancer: a p53-independent function of p21WAF1/CIP1 via c/EBP beta, *Nat. Med.*, 3, 1233, 1997.

97. Maurer, A. B., Ganser, A., Seipelt, G., Ottmann, O. G., Mentsel, U., Geissler, G. R., and Hoelzer, D., Changes in erythroid progenitor cell and accessory cell compartments in patients with myelodysplastic syndromes during treatment with all-*trans* retinoic acid and haemopoietic growth factors, *Br. J. Haematol.*, 89, 449, 1995.

98. Rimm, E. B., Stampfer, M. J., Ascherio, A., Giovannucci, E., Colditz, G. A., and Willett, W. C., Vitamin E consumption and the risk of coronary heart disease in men, *N. Engl. J. Med.*, 328, 1450, 1993.

99. Stampfer, M. J., Hennekens, C. H., Manson, J. E., Colditz, G. A., Rosner, B., and Willett, W. C., Vitamin E consumption and the risk of coronary disease in women, *N. Engl. J. Med.*, 328, 1444, 1993.

100. Gey, K. F., Puska, P., Jordan, P., and Moser, U. K., Inverse correlation between plasma vitamin E and mortality from ischemic heart disease in cross-cultural epidemiology, *Am. J. Clin. Nutr.*, 53, 326S, 1991.

101. Keaney, J. F. J., Simon, D. I., and Freedman, J. E., Vitamin E and vascular homeostasis: implications for atherosclerosis, *FASEB J.*, 13, 965, 1999.

102. Blair, A., Shaul, P. W., Yuhanna, I. S., Conrad, P. A., and Smart, E. J., Oxidized low density lipoprotein displaces endothelial nitric-oxide synthase (eNOS) from plasmalemmal caveolae and impairs eNOS activation, *J. Biol. Chem.*, 274, 32512, 1999.

103. Keaney, J. F. J., Guo, Y., Cunningham, D., Shwaery, G. T., Xu, A., and Vita, J. A., Vascular incorporation of alpha-tocopherol prevents endothelial dysfunction due to oxidized LDL by inhibiting protein kinase C stimulation, *J. Clin. Invest.*, 98, 386, 1996.

104. Freedman, J. E., Farhat, J. H., Loscalzo, J., and Keaney, J. F. J., Alpha-tocopherol inhibits aggregation of human platelets by a protein kinase C-dependent mechanism, *Circulation*, 94, 2434, 1996.

105. Ohgushi, M., Kugiyama, K., Fukunaga, K., Murohara, T., Sugiyama, S., Miyamoto, E., and Yasue, H., Protein kinase C inhibitors prevent impairment of endothelium-dependent relaxation by oxidatively modified LDL, *Arterioscler. Thromb.*, 13, 1525, 1993.

106. Sugiyama, S., Kugiyama, K., Ogata, N., Doi, H., Ota, Y., Ohgushi, M., Matsumura, T., Oka, H., and Yasue, H., Biphasic regulation of transcription factor nuclear factor-kappaB activity in human endothelial cells by lysophosphatidylcholine through protein kinase C-mediated pathway, *Arterioscler. Thromb. Vasc. Biol.*, 18, 568, 1998.

107. Lu, M., Kuroki, M., Amano, S., Tolentino, M., Keough, K., Kim, I., Bucala, R., and Adamis, A. P., Advanced glycation end products increase retinal vascular endothelial growth factor expression, *J. Clin. Invest.*, 101, 1219, 1998.

108. Takagi, M., Kasayama, S., Yamamoto, T., Motomura, T., Hashimoto, K., Yamamoto, H., Sato, B., Okada, S., and Kishimoto, T., Advanced glycation endproducts stimulate interleukin-6 production by human bone-derived cells, *J. Bone Miner. Res.*, 12, 439, 1997.

109. Kunt, T., Forst, T., Wilhelm, A., Tritschler, H., Pfuetzner, A., Harzer, O., Engelbach, M., Zschaebitz, A., Stofft, E., and Beyer, J., Alpha-lipoic acid reduces expression of vascular cell adhesion molecule-1 and endothelial adhesion of human monocytes after stimulation with advanced glycation end products, *Clin. Sci. (Colch)*, 96, 75, 1999.

110. Jain, S. K. and Palmer, M., The effect of oxygen radicals, metabolites and vitamin E on glycosylation of proteins, *Free Radic. Biol. Med.*, 22, 593, 1997.

111. Roh, J. K., Hong, S. B., Yoon, B. W., Kim, M. S., and Myung, H., The effect of hyperglycemia on lipid peroxidation in the global cerebral ischemia of the rat, *J. Korean Med. Sci.*, 7, 40, 1992.

112. Yan, S. D., Schmidt, A. M., Anderson, G. M., Zhang, J., Brett, J., Zou, Y. S., Pinsky, D., and Stern, D., Enhanced cellular oxidant stress by the interaction of advanced glycation end products with their receptors/binding proteins, *J. Biol. Chem.*, 269, 9889, 1994.

113. Yerneni, K. K., Bai, W., Khan, B. V., Medford, R. M., and Natarajan, R., Hyperglycemia-induced activation of nuclear transcription factor kappaB in vascular smooth muscle cells, *Diabetes*, 48, 855, 1999.

114. Nath, K. A., Grande, J., Croatt, A., Haugen, J., Kim, Y., and Rosenberg, M. E., Redox regulation of renal DNA synthesis, transforming growth factor-beta1 and collagen gene expression, *Kidney Int.*, 52, 367, 1998.

115. Jelkmann, W., Pagel, H., Hellwig, T., and Fandrey, J., Effects of antioxidant vitamins on renal and hepatic erythropoietin production, *Kidney Int.*, 51, 497, 1997.

116. Donahoo, K. K., Shames, B. D., Harken, A. D., and Meldrum, D. R., The role of TNF in renal-ischemia-reperfusion injury, *J. Urol.*, 162, 196, 1999.

117. Brennan, D. C., Yui, M. A., Wuthrich, R. P., and Kelley, V. E., Tumor necrosis factor and IL-1 in New Zealand black/white mice. Enhanced gene expression and acceleration of renal injury, *J. Immunol.*, 143, 3470, 1989.

118. Yin, T., Sandhu, G., Wolfgang, C. D., Barrier, A., Webb, R. L., Rigel, D. F., Hai, T., and Whelan, J., Tissue-specific pattern of stress kinase activation in ischemic/reperfused heart and kidney, *J. Biol. Chem.*, 272, 19943, 1997.

119. Trachtman, H., Chan, J. C., Chan, W., Valderrama, A., Brandt, R., Wakely, P., Futterweit, S., Maesaka, J., and Ma, C., Vitamin E ameliorates renal injury in an experimental model of immunoglobulin A nephropathy, *Pediatr. Res.*, 40, 620, 1996.

120. Kuemmerle, N. B., Chan, W., Krieg, R. J. J., Norkus, E. P., Trachtman, H., and Chan, J. C., Effects of fish oil and alpha-tocopherol in immunoglobulin A nephropathy in the rat, *Pediatr. Res.*, 43, 791, 1998.

121. Kuemmerle, N. B., Krieg, R. J. J., Chan, W., Trachtman, H., Norkus, E. P., and Chan, J. C., Influence of alpha-tocopherol over the time course of experimental IgA nephropathy, *Pediatr. Nephrol.*, 13, 108, 1999.

122. Lee, H. S., Kim, B. C., Kim, Y. S., Choi, K. H., and Chung, H. K., Involvement of oxidation in LDL-induced collagen gene regulation in mesangial cells, *Kidney Int.*, 50, 1582, 1996.

123. Bennett, R. T., Mazzaccaro, R. J., Chopra, N., Melman, A., and Franco, I., Suppression of renal inflammation with vitamins A and E in ascending pyelonephritis in rats, *J. Urol.*, 161, 1681, 1999.

124. Pietrangelo, A., Gualdi, R., Casalgrandi, G., Montosi, G., and Ventura, E., Molecular and cellular aspects of iron-induced hepatic cirrhosis in rodents, *J. Clin. Invest.*, 95, 1824, 1995.

125. Marra, F., DeFranco, R., Grappone, C., Parola, M., Leonarduzzi, G., Milani, S., Pastacaldi, S., Wenzel, U., Pinzani, M., Laffi, G., Dianzani, M. U., and Gentilini, P., Expression of monocyte chemotactic protein-1 precedes monocyte recruitment in a rat model of acute liver injury, and is modulated by vitamin E, *J. Invest. Med.*, 47, 66, 1999.

126. Camandola, S., Aragno, M., Curtin, J. C., Tamagno, E., Danni, O., Chiarpotto, E., Parola, M., Leonarduzzi, G., Biasi, F., and Poli, G., Liver AP-1 activation due to carbon tetrachloride is potentiated by 1,2-dibromoethane but is inhibited by alpha-tocopherol or gadolinium chloride, *Free Radic. Biol. Med.*, 24, 1108, 1999.

127. Fox, E. S., Kim, J. C., and Tracy, T. F., NF-kappaB activation and modulation in hepatic macrophages during cholestatic injury, NF-kappaB activation and modulation in hepatic macrophages during cholestatic injury, *J. Surg. Res.*, 72, 129, 1997.

128. Parola, M., Muraca, R., Dianzani, I., Barrera, G., Leonarduzzi, G., Bendinelli, P., Piccoletti, R., and Poli, G., Vitamin E dietary supplementation inhibits transforming growth factor beta 1 gene expression in the rat liver, *FEBS Lett.*, 308, 267, 1992.

129. Parola, M., Pinzani, M., Casini, A., Albano, E., Poli, G., Gentilini, A., Gentilini, P., and Dianzini, M. U., Stimulation of lipid peroxidation or 4-hydroxynonenal treatment increases procollagen alpha 1 (I) gene expression in human liver fat-storing cells, *Biochem. Biophys. Res. Commun.*, 194, 1044, 1993.

130. Shaw, H. M. and Huang, C. J., Liver alpha-tocopherol transfer protein and its mRNA are differentially altered by dietary vitamin E deficiency and protein insufficiency in rats, *J. Nutr.*, 128, 2348, 1998.

131. Kim, H. S., Arai, H., Arita, M., Sato, Y., Ogihara, T., Inoue, K., Mino, M., and Tamai, H., Effect of alpha-tocopherol status on alpha-tocopherol transfer protein expression and its messenger RNA level in rat liver, *Free Radic. Res.*, 28, 87, 1998.

132. Wu, C. G., Hoek, F. J., Groenink, M., Reitama, P. H., van Deventer, S. J., and Chamuleau, R. A., Correlation of repressed transcription of alpha-tocopherol transfer protein with serum alpha-tocopherol during hepatocarcinogenesis, *Int. J. Cancer*, 71, 686, 1997.

133. Hammans, S. R., The inherited ataxias and the new genetics, *J. Neurol. Neurosurg. Psychiatr.*, 61, 327, 1996.

134. Tamaru, Y., Hirano, M., Kusaka, H., Ito, H., Imai, T., and Ueno, S., Alpha-tocopherol transfer protein gene: exon skipping of all transcripts causes ataxia, *Neurology*, 49, 584, 1997.

135. Rosenberg, R. N., DNA-triplet repeats and neurologic disease, *N. Eng. J. Med.*, 335, 1222, 1996.

136. Yokota, T., Shiojiri, T., Gotoda, T., Arita, M., Arai, H., Ohga, T., Kanda, T., Suzuki, J., Imai, T., Matsumoto, H., Harino, S., Kiyosawa, M., Mizusawa, H., and Inoue, K., Friedreich-like ataxia with retinitis pigmentosa caused by the His101Gln mutation of the alpha-tocopherol transfer protein gene, *Ann. Neurol.*, 41, 826, 1997.

137. Shaw, P. J., Science, medicine, and the future: motor neuron disease, *Br. Med. J.*, 318, 1118, 1999.

138. Ghadge, G. D., Lee, J. P., Bindokas, V. P., Jordan, J., Ma, L., Miller, R. J., and Roos, R. P., Mutant superoxide dismutase-1-linked familial amyotrophic lateral sclerosis: molecular mechanisms of neuronal death and protection, *J. Neurosci.*, 17, 8756, 1997.

139. Kostic, V., Jackson-Lewis, V., de Bilbao, F., Dubois-Dauphin, M., and Przedbor-ski, S., Bcl-2: prolonging life in a transgenic mouse model of familial amyo-trophic lateral sclerosis, *Science*, 277, 559, 1997.

140. Troy, C. M. and Shelanski, M. L., Down-regulation of copper/zinc superoxide dismutase causes apoptotic death in PC12 neuronal cells, *Proc. Natl. Acad. Sci. USA*, 91, 6384, 1994.

141. Gurney, M. E., Cutting, F. B., Zhai, P., Doble, A., Taylor, C. P., and Andrus, P. K., Benefit of vitamin E, riluzole, and gabapentin in a transgenic model of amyotrophic lateral sclerosis, *Ann. Neurol.*, 39, 147, 1996.

142. Post, A., Holsboer, F., and Behl, C., Induction of NF-kappaB activity during haloperidol-induced oxidative toxicity in clonal hippocampal cells: suppres-sion of NF-kappaB and neuroprotection by antioxidants, *J. Neurosci.*, 18, 8236, 1998.

143. Noh, K. M., Kim, Y. H., and Koh, J.-Y., Mediation by membrane protein kinase C of zinc-induced oxidative neuronal injury in mouse cortical cultures, *J. Neu-rochem.*, 72, 1609, 1999.

144. Ricciarelli, R., Tasinato, A., Clement, S., Ozer, N. K., Boscoboinik, D., and Azzi, A., Alpha-tcopherol specifically inactivates cellular protein kinase C α by changing its phosphorylation state, *Biochem. J.*, 334, 243, 1998.

145. Beiche, F., Scheuerer, S., Brune, K., Geisslinger, G., and Goppelt-Struebe, M., Up-regulation of cyclooxygenase-2 mRNA in the rat spinal cord following peripheral inflammation, *FEBS Lett.*, 390, 165, 1996.

146. Ichitani, Y., Shi, T., Haeggstrom, J. Z., Samuelsson, B., and Hökfelt, T., Increased levels of cyclooxygenase-2 mRNA in the rat spinal cord after peripheral in-flammation: an in situ hybridization study, *Neuro. Rep.*, 8, 2949, 1997.

17

Differential Regulation and Function of Glutathione Peroxidases and Other Selenoproteins

Xin Gen Lei

CONTENTS

17.1 Introduction 426
17.2 Characterization of Glutathione Peroxidases
      and Other Selenoproteins 426
      17.2.1 Cellular Glutathione Peroxidase (GPX1) 428
      17.2.2 Gastrointestinal Glutathione Peroxidase (GPX-GI or GPX2) 428
      17.2.3 Extracellular Glutathione Peroxidase
             (Plasma GPX or GPX3) 428
      17.2.4 Phospholipid Hydroperoxide Glutathione Peroxidase
             (PHGPX or GPX4) 429
      17.2.5 Other Selenoproteins 429
17.3 Differential Regulation of GPX1 and Other Selenoproteins
      by Selenium 430
      17.3.1 Comparisons of GPX1 with Other GPX Enzymes 430
      17.3.2 Comparisons of GPX Enzymes with Deiodinases 431
      17.3.3 Comparisons of GPX Enzymes with Selenoprotein P 432
      17.3.4 Comparisons of GPX Enzymes with Selenoprotein W 433
      17.3.5 Comparisons of GPX Enzymes
             with Thioredoxin Reductase 433
17.4 Regulation of GPX Enzymes and Other Selenoproteins
      by Non-Selenium Factors 434
17.5 Mechanisms of Selenium Incorporation and Regulation 434
      17.5.1 Co-Translation of Selenocysteine in Prokaryotes 434
      17.5.2 Comparison of Prokaryotic and Eukaryotic
             Selenoprotein Biosynthesis 436
      17.5.3 Sites of Selenium Regulation 436
17.6 Use of Gene-Knockout Approach to Study Regulation
      of Selenoprotein Expression 438
References 440

0-8493-2216-2/01/$0.00+$1.50

17.1 Introduction

A dozen of selenium (Se)-dependent proteins identified in mammals (Table 17.1) share at least two distinct features. First, Se in the polypeptide is covalently bound in a moiety of selenocysteine encoded by thymine-guanine-adenine (TGA), normally a stop codon. Second, Se availability regulates expression of not only their protein and activity, but also their mRNA levels in cells or tissues. In prokaryotes, Se is incorporated into selenocysteine co-translationally. The process is directed by a special stem-loop structure of mRNA, requiring four unique gene products. Much less is certain about the eukaryotic Se-incorporation. The dramatic impact of Se status on selenoprotein gene expression and the differential responses of various selenoproteins to Se depletion or repletion are fascinating, although the mechanism of Se regulation and the physiological implication remain largely unclear. A comprehensive understanding of selenoprotein biosynthesis in eukaryotes would help us in tackling these problems, and gene-knockout mouse models provide us with unprecedented tools. Because cellular glutathione peroxidase (EC 1.11.1.9; GPX1) is the first identified,[1,2] the most abundant,[3] and the best-studied biochemical functional form of body Se, this chapter focuses on the expression and Se regulation of GPX1 and its three family members in comparison with those of other selenoproteins.

17.2 Characterization of Glutathione Peroxidases and Other Selenoproteins

The Se-dependent GPX family consists of GPX1, GPX2, GPX3, and GPX4.[4–7] Regardless of the physiological relevance, all of these selenoperoxidases reduce H_2O_2 and hydroperoxides using reduced glutathione (GSH) *in vitro*. Only GPX4 efficiently reduces phospholipid hydroperoxides, and thus its activity is distinguishable from that of the others. In the routine assay, it is not possible to specify the precise contribution of the individual GPX enzymes to the total GPX activity using H_2O_2 as a substrate. However, total GPX activity is often interchangeably described as GPX1 activity because it numerically accounts for more than 90% of the total GPX activity in most tissues.[3] The same analogy is also used in this chapter for simplicity. Structurally, GPX4 is a monomer of 19 kDa, the other three are tetramers with respective subunits of approximately 22 to 23 kDa. In addition, GPX3 is an extracellular glycoprotein, whereas the others are intracellular enzymes.

TABLE 17.1

Characterized Mammalian Selenoproteins

Name	Size (kDa)	Role	Distribution
1. Glutathione peroxidase (GPX) family			
GPX1 or cGPX (cyotosolic, cellular, or classical GPX)	88	Antioxidative, GSH-dependent reduction of hydroperoxides	Ubiquitous
GPX2 or GPX-GI (gastrointestinal GPX)	88	GSH-dependent reduction of hydroperoxides	Mainly gastrointestinal tract
GPX3 or plasma GPX (extracellular GPX)	92	GSH-dependent reduction of hydroperoxides	Plasma and interstitial and extracellular space in lung, intestine, and kidney
GPX4 or PHGPX (phospholipid hydroperoxide GPX)	19	Reduction of phospholipid hydroperoxides	Ubiquitous, abundant in testis
2. Iodothyronine 5′-deiodinases (ID)			
ID1 (type 1)	28	Conversion of T_4 to T_3, inactivation of T_4 and T_3	Brain, kidney, liver, and thyroid
ID2 (type 2)	30	Conversion of T_4 to T_3	Adipose tissue heart, muscle, pituitary, and thyroid
ID3 (type 3)	32	Inactivation of T_4 and T_3	Brain, placenta, and skin
3. Thioredoxin reductases (TR)			
TR1	110	NADPH-dependent reduction of thioredoxin	Ubiquitous
TR2	130	NADPH-dependent reduction of thioredoxin	Adrenal, heart, kidney, testis
TR3	114	NADPH-dependent reduction of thioredoxin	Ubiquitous
4. Selenophosphate synthetase			
	48	ATP-dependent activation of selenium for biosynthesis of selenocysteine	Ubiquitous
5. Selenoproteins (Sel)			
Sel-P	57	Unknown	Plasma
Sel-W	10	Unknown	Ubiquitous
15-kD Sel	15	Unknown	Ubiquitous

17.2.1　Cellular Glutathione Peroxidase (GPX1)

As mentioned above, GPX1 was the first mammalian selenoprotein, identified in 1972 by Rotruck et al.[1] who found that H_2O_2-dependent hemolysis is no longer prevented by glucose in erythrocytes from Se-deficient rats that have low GPX1 activity. Retrospectively, two important findings in 1957 by Mills[8] on the protection of GPX against hemoglobin oxidation and by Schwarz and Foltz[9] on the essentiality of Se against liver necrosis in rats conceived this milestone discovery in Se biology. It seems that GPX1 activity is detectable in various tissues of mammals and birds studied so far. The GPX1 gene cloned from mice[10,11] is 5.2 kb and contains two exons and only one intron. There is more than 80% sequence identity in the coding region among various mammalian GPX1 genes.[5] The human GPX1 gene localizes to a single site on chromosome 3.[12] In general, GPX1 proteins consist of 201 amino acids and the selenocysteine residual locates at the 47th residual from the N-terminal of the peptides.[5] Approximately 75% of the GPX1 enzyme is found in cytosol, and the remaining 25% in mitochondria.[13] Knockout of the GPX1 gene in mice results in the disappearance of this enzyme in both of the locations.[14]

The GPX1 enzyme does not form any ternary complexes with GSH and H_2O_2 and has no fixed K_m for either substrate.[13,15,16] Because the liver GPX1 protein contains 60% of total Se in the tissue[3] and its expression fluctuates so readily and widely with alterations of Se status, GPX1 has been suggested as a Se buffer to serve a homeostatic function in Se metabolism,[5,17] instead of an antioxidant enzyme. However, we and others have generated solid evidence from the GPX1 knockout mice[11] that GPX1 is the mediator of body Se in protecting mice against acute, lethal oxidative stress.[18–21]

17.2.2　Gastrointestinal Glutathione Peroxidase (GPX-GI or GPX2)

The GPX2 cDNA isolated by Chu et al.[22] shares 61% sequence identity with GPX1. Initially, GPX2 was considered the main form of GPX activity in gastrointestinal tissues and played an important role in detoxifying hydroperoxides from digesta.[22] A recent study with the GPX1 knockout mice indicates that GPX2 is expressed in the mucosal epithelium of intestines and contributes nearly the same portion to the total GPX activity as GPX1.[23] There is relatively little information on the regulation or physiological function of GPX2 expression *in vivo*.

17.2.3　Extracellular Glutathione Peroxidase (Plasma GPX or GPX3)

Although plasma GPX3 was initially considered the same enzyme as GPX1, these two enzymes are distinctly different in their activity response to Se supply, immunological property, specific activity, heat stability, and mobility in gel electrophoresis.[24–26] The human GPX3 cDNA[27] encodes 226 amino acids and has selenocysteine at residue 73. The deduced peptide shows 44% homology with human GPX1. The human GPX3 gene consists of five exons spanning approximately 10 kb and is localized in chromosome 5, q32.[28]

The purified GPX3 has an apparent molecular mass of 92 kDa.[25] The hydrophobic core of signal peptide in rat GPX3 seems to be the first 19 deduced amino acids in the N-terminal.[29] Kidney is the primary site to produce GPX3 in humans and rodents.[29] Intestinal epithelia of both species[30] and a number of cell lines[31] also express GPX3. Although *in vitro* GPX3 reduces peroxides and even phospholipid hydroperoxides,[32] the low concentration of GSH in plasma seems to preclude its physiological action.[25] Probably, GPX3 protects against peroxides in the renal extracellular space,[33] lung epithelial lining fluid and interstitial space,[34] and intestinal intercellular space.[30] A wide antioxidant role of GPX3, including a possible role in embryogenesis, has also been speculated.[35]

17.2.4 Phospholipid Hydroperoxide Glutathione Peroxidase (PHGPX or GPX4)

The identification of GPX4 as the second intracellular GPX by Ursini et al.[36] was not fully recognized until the cloning of pig GPX4 cDNA.[37] There is 95% homology among amino acid sequences deduced from the GPX4 cDNA of rat,[5,38] mouse,[39] and human.[40] In contrast, the homology between GPX1 and GPX4 is less than 40%. Both the pig (2.8kb) and mouse (4.0 kb) GPX4 genes contain seven exons and six introns, with putative regulatory elements or binding sites for transcriptional factors.[41,42]

There are two forms of GPX4: the long form (23 kDa) with a leader sequence for transportation to mitochondria, and the short form (20 kDa) or the non-mitochondria form.[43] Although GPX4 reduces phospholipid hydroperoxides,[44] it has a relatively low rate of constant for H_2O_2. There are abundant GPX4 activity and mRNA in testis[45,46] and rat epididymal spermatozoa,[47] indicating a possible involvement in sperm maturation.[48] Recently, Flohé, Ursini, and colleagues[49] discovered that GPX4 exists as a soluble peroxidase in spermatids, but loses its activity in mature spermatozoa and persists as an oxidatively cross-linked insoluble protein. In the midpiece of mature spermatozoa, GPX4 accounts for 50% of the capsule material and is the protein previously called sperm mitochondria capsule selenoprotein.

17.2.5 Other Selenoproteins

Three types of iodothyronine deiodinases are identified as selenoenzyme.[50–52] These enzymes regulate the activity level and distribution of thyroid hormones by catalyzing step-wise deiodination. Three types of thioredoxin reductases (TR)[53–55] contain selenocysteine as an additional redox center. These pyridine nucleotide–disulfide oxidoreductases are homodimers of 55 to 57 kDa subunits containing (flavin adenine dinucleotide) FAD.[54] A human selenophosphate synthetase, equivalent to selenophosphate synthetase

(SELD) of *E. coli*, also contains selenocysteine encoded by TGA.[56] Selenoprotein P (Sel-P) contains ten TGAs in the open reading frame of the cloned cDNA.[57] Multiple forms of Sel-P are found in rat plasma[58,59] and account for 65% of the plasma Se.[60] It has been localized adjacent to endothelial cells[61] and found to be able to reduce 1-palmitoyl-2-(13-hydroperoxy-cis-9,trans-11-octadecadienoyl)-3-phosphatidylcholine hydroperoxide,[62] implying a GPX4-like antioxidant function in extracellular fluids. Selenoprotein W (Sel-W) has a molecular mass of 9.5 to 10 kDa.[63] The cDNA isolated from rat skeletal muscle contains 672 bases and the selenocysteine codon, TGA, is in the position corresponding to amino acid residual 13.[64] It exists in all the tissues tested and may relate to white muscle disease in Se-deficient animals. A prominent ^{75}Se-labeled, 15 kDa protein detected in human T-cells is also considered a new selenoprotein.[65]

17.3 Differential Regulation of GPX1 and Other Selenoproteins by Selenium

Numerous studies have demonstrated that expression of GPX1 and other selenoproteins is affected by Se status in animal tissues or cultured cells.[4–6] Animals fed Se-deficient diets for several weeks exhibit undetectable liver GPX1 activity[66–68] and a rapid exponential decline of liver GPX1 protein.[69] More strikingly, GPX1 mRNA falls dramatically in Se deficiency, as reported by all groups[70–73] except for one.[74] Apparently, Se is not used for the transcription of GPX1 mRNA. Instead, Se deficiency must exert its impact on the steady-state levels of GPX1 mRNA through regulatory pathways. In nearly all cases, GPX1 expression is modulated by Se supply more than that of any other selenoprotein and thereby is considered to be differentially regulated by Se.

17.3.1 Comparisons of GPX1 with Other GPX Enzymes

A striking difference in Se regulation of GPX1 and GPX4 expression has been observed by Weitzel et al.[75] in mice and by Lei et al.[46] in rats. While mouse liver GPX1 activity falls to near zero within 130 days of Se depletion, liver GPX4 retains 30% residual activity. In Se-deficient rats, GPX1 activity and mRNA are reduced to 1 and 6% of the Se-adequate level in liver, respectively, whereas GPX4 activity is reduced only to 25 to 50% in various tissues. Liver GPX4 mRNA is not significantly affected. Testis has 15-fold higher GPX4 activity and 45-fold higher GPX4 mRNA than liver, and testis GPX4 mRNA is almost completely resistant to Se deficiency. Similar effects of Se on GPX1 and GPX4 expression have also been shown in other studies.[76–78] In general, GPX3 activity in plasma and GPX3 mRNA in tissues respond to Se repletion quicker than those of GPX1. In patients with low Se and GPX activity in plasma and erythrocytes, supplementing Se for up to 2 weeks does not enhance the low GPX1 activity in erythrocytes,[24] but produces detectable increases in plasma GPX3 activity within 6 hours.[79] In three human cell lines, GPX3 mRNA is also more resistant to Se deprivation than that of GPX1.[31] Likewise, GPX2 seems to have a higher mRNA stability in Se deficiency and a faster protein synthesis rate upon Se repletion than that of GPX1 in cultured cells.[80] Although more research is needed to rank the Se-dependence of GPX2 expression *in vivo*, it seems clear that Se availability affects the expression of GPX1 most, GPX4 least, and GPX3 in between. The overall relative reduction of different GPX mRNA or activity levels by dietary Se deficiency in mice, summarized from six major studies conducted by us during last few years, follows the exact same pattern (Fig. 17.1).

17.3.2 Comparisons of GPX Enzymes with Deiodinases

Distinct patterns of GPX1, GPX4, and type-1 iodothyronine 5' deiodinase (ID1) expression exhibit in three tissues of rats fed diets containing Se from 0.003 to 0.405 mg/kg.[77] In liver, severe Se deficiency produces losses of GPX1 activity and mRNA by nearly 100%, GPX4 activity by 75%, ID1 activity by 95%, and ID1 mRNA by 50%. In heart, GPX1 mRNA and activity are reduced by Se deficiency to the same extent as in liver, while GPX4 activity

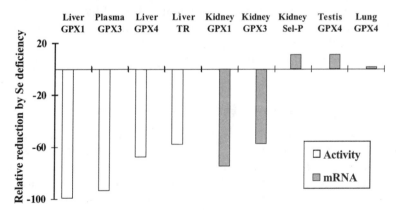

FIGURE 17.1
Relative reduction of mRNA and activity levels of GPX enzymes and other selenoproteins by dietary selenium deficiency in various mouse tissues. Data were collected from six experiments conducted in the author's laboratory during the past 4 years.[3,18–20,127,128] A total of 223 young or adult mice (3 weeks to 2 months of age) were fed a selenium-deficient (0.02 mg/kg) or a selenium-adequate (0.3 to 0.5 mg/kg) torula yeast diet for 5 to 13 weeks. Tissues were collected for different assays after these animals were anesthetized with carbon dioxide and killed by exsanguination. The reduction in mRNA or activity levels in the selenium-deficient animals is expressed as the percentage of the pertinent selenium-adequate controls within each individual experiment and then pooled among the six experiments.

is reduced only 60%. In thyroid, Se deficiency causes increases of ID1 activity by 15% and ID1 mRNA by 95%, no change in GPX4 activity, and significant decrease in GPX1 activity. Levels of GPX4 mRNA are not affected by Se deficiency in liver or heart, but increased 52% in thyroid. These data clearly indicate a tissue specificity of differential regulation of GPX enzymes from that of ID1.

In second generation Se- or iodine-deficient rats, Se deficiency results in changes of GPX1, GPX4, and ID1 expression in liver and thyroid similar to or slightly different from those seen in the first generation rats.[81] When iodine deficiency induces mRNA of the three enzymes from 2- to 5-fold in thyroid, only GPX1 and ID1 activities are increased. In contrast, GPX4 activity is decreased. In the combined deficiency of Se and iodine, ID1 activity is increased, GPX1 activity is unaltered, and GPX4 is decreased while mRNA levels of all three enzymes are increased. Thus, iodine deficiency may act as an oxidative stress in thyroid to induce mRNA expression of selenoenzymes at limited Se supply, and Se is preferentially used by ID1 and GPX1 to maintain thyroid function. Iodine deficiency also increases brain type-2 ID or ID2 activity by up to 3-fold in 4 to 11 day old rats, regardless of Se status.[82] However, Se or iodine deficiency has little effect on the expression of these three enzymes in most brain regions studied.[83] At excessive Se supply (2 mg/kg), hepatic ID1 and GPX1 activities are not elevated in rats.[84] A lower dietary Se level is required to maximize tissue ID1 activity than that of GPX1.[85]

Differential regulation of ID1 and GPX1 expression has also been illustrated in cultured porcine kidney epithelial cell line LLC-PK1.[86] Thyroid-stimulating hormone induces a larger increase in ID1 expression in Se-deficient FRTL-5 cells than that in the Se-repleted cells, indicating an interaction of Se and hormone in the regulation of selenoenzyme expression.[87]

17.3.3   Comparisons of GPX Enzymes with Selenoprotein P

Plasma concentration of Sel-P falls at approximately the same rate as GPX3 activity in rats fed a Se-deficient diet.[88] When rats are fed graded levels of dietary Se from 0.01 to 2.0 mg/kg, the elevations of plasma Sel-P concentration precede those of plasma GPX3 and liver GPX1 activities and reach a plateau at a lower level of Se. The GPX enzymes do not seem to respond to an injection of Se as strongly as Sel-P.[89] When an intraperitoneal injection of Se at 50 µg/kg body weight in Se-deficient rats enhances Sel-P from 7 to 43% of the Se-adequate control level by 12 hours, there is only a 2 to 3% increase in liver GPX1 and plasma GPX3 activities. In Se-deficient rats, Sel-P mRNA is 19% of the control while GPX1 mRNA is only 3% of the control.[71] There is also a tissue dependence of differential regulation of Sel-P from GPX1 or ID1.[66] When Se deficiency reduces rat liver GPX1 mRNA by 89%, abolishes GPX1 activity, and reduces ID1 mRNA and activity by 69 and 70%, respectively, Sel-P mRNA is lowered by only 14%. Thus, Sel-P is more resistant to Se deprivation than GPX1 or ID1 in rat liver. However, Sel-P mRNA is decreased more by Se deficiency than that of ID1 mRNA in rat kidney. Similar resistance of Sel-P expression to dietary Se deficiency has also been illustrated in our recent mouse studies (Fig. 17.1). Compared with the Se-adequate controls, the Se-deficient mice have slightly increased levels of Sel-P mRNA in kidney, just as those of GPX4 mRNA in lung and testis, while GPX1 and GPX3 mRNA levels in kidney are reduced by 74 and 57%, respectively.

17.3.4 Comparisons of GPX Enzymes with Selenoprotein W

Differences in Se regulation of the Sel-W protein from that of the GPX activities in several tissues have been illustrated in rats fed diets containing Se ranged from 0.004 to 4.0 mg/kg.[90] The GPX1 activity is saturated at 0.1 mg Se/kg in the brain, and at 0.06 mg Se/kg in both testes and spleen. In muscle, GPX1 activity increases further when 1.0 and 2.0 mg Se/kg are fed. In contrast, the amounts of Sel-W protein in muscle do not change until 0.06 mg Se/kg is fed and increase rapidly up to the plateau level at 1.0 mg Se/kg. Both brain and spleen Sel-W levels increase linearly with the Se concentration up to 0.1 mg Se/kg. Marked increase of Sel-W in testis occurs at 0.01 mg Se/kg with no further elevation beyond that level. In Se-deficient sheep, brain Se content and GPX1 activity are reduced by 50 and 30%, respectively, whereas Sel-W level remains unaltered.[91] Thus, Sel-P may be preferentially protected than GPX1 in brain in Se deficiency.

17.3.5 Comparisons of GPX Enzymes with Thioredoxin Reductase

When rats are fed Se-deficient diets for 14 weeks following weaning, thioredoxin reductase (TR) activity in liver and kidney are decreased to 4.5 and 11% of the controls, respectively, without change in brain.[92] Meanwhile, plasma GPX3 and Sel-P are reduced to 0.9 and 7.1%, respectively, and GPX1 reduced to 1.2, 4.3, and 70% of the controls in liver, kidney, and brain, respectively. At 12 or 48 hours after an intraperitoneal injection of Se at 50 µg/kg body weight, TR activity in liver is replete to a relatively higher level than those of liver GPX1 and plasma GPX3, but to a lower level than that of the Sel-P concentration.[92] In mice, hepatic TR activity is also more resistant to dietary Se deficiency than that of GPX enzymes (Fig. 17.1). In contrast, TR in four human cell lines have consistently lower responses to Se than GPX1,[93] indicating the possible existence of a Se-unresponsive isoenzyme or a residual disulfide reductase activity in the Se-free truncated protein produced in Se deficiency. In another study, the increased TR activity in cells[94] is not directly related to the increase in protein amount but rather the increase in the specific activity of the enzyme. Primary human fibroblasts express greater TR and GPX4 proteins than those of melanocytes, and keratinocytes express little of these two enzymes.[95]

17.4 Regulation of GPX Enzymes and Other Selenoproteins by Non-Selenium Factors

Many factors other than Se can influence expression of selenoproteins. As discussed above, iodine modulates expression of three selenoenzymes in thyroid at least as much as Se. In cultured cardiomyocytes, α-tocopherol (200 μM) increases GPX1 activity and mRNA levels up to 2-fold, and this action is independent of oxygen tension, Se, and *de novo* synthesis of GPX1 transcripts.[96] A marginal effect of high levels of α-tocopherol on tissue GPX4 or GPX1 activity has also been seen in mice under acute oxidative stress.[97] Expression of GPX1 mRNA, protein, and activity are reduced by as much as 60% by iron deficiency in various tissues[98] or copper deficiency in liver of rats.[99]

Female rats have 1- to 2-fold higher levels of GPX1 activity and mRNA than the males,[100] but no such difference in mice. There are two potential estrogen-regulatory elements in the upstream sequences of GPX1 gene.[101] Testis GPX4 expression depends on gonadotropin as hypophysectomy causes a rapid decline of the activity and gonadotropin treatment partially restores the activity.[45] However, the age or gonadotropin-dependent expression of GPX4 in testis is due to differentiation stage-specific expression in late spermatids, rather than from a direct gene transcriptional activation by testosterone.[48] There are oxygen responsive elements in the 5′ flanking region of human GPX1 gene,[102] and oxygen tension induces GPX1 expression in cultured cells.[103] Liver GPX1 mRNA, protein, or activity in rodents is affected by nafenopin,[104] paraquat,[19,21] and many factors related to redox status.[6] In addition, GPX1 and other selenoproteins are affected by development.[105]

17.5 Mechanisms of Selenium Incorporation and Regulation

There are two apparent ways in which Se can influence selenoprotein expression. As a cofactor, Se is incorporated into these proteins through the co-translational synthesis of selenocysteine. As a regulator, Se affects the expression of selenoprotein genes at different levels. However, it is difficult to distinguish these two types of Se action in many studies reported. To understand the hierarchy of Se used for the synthesis of various mammalian selenoproteins, we need to know the eukaryotic Se-incorporation system. That system in prokaryotes has been well characterized and may serve as a good reference.

17.5.1 Co-Translation of Selenocysteine in Prokaryotes

Using a series of *E. coli* mutants unable to synthesize Se-dependent formate dehydrogenases, Böck and his colleagues discovered four genes and their

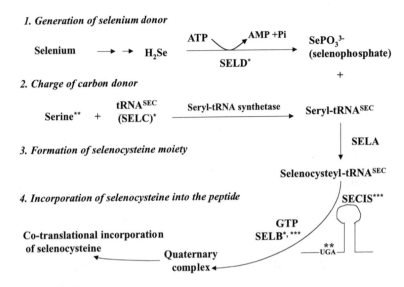

FIGURE 17.2
Schematic pathways of selenoprotein biosynthesis by prokaryotes. The process requires four unique gene products (SELA, SELB, SELC, and SELD) and two special mRNA sequence elements: the UGA codon for selenocysteine and an immediate downstream stem-loop selenocysteine insertion sequence (SECIS) for directing the co-translation of selenocysteine at UGA. Single asterisk (') indicates that the eukaryotic equivalents of SELB, SELC, and SELD have been identified: the SECIS-binding protein to serve as a translational regulator, the selenocysteine tRNA, and the selenophosphate synthetase to generate activated selenium donor. Double asterisks (") indicate that both prokaryotic and eukaryotic selenocysteines are encoded by UGA and their carbon sources are from serine. Triple asterisks (") indicate that (1) the stem-loop SECIS required for selenocysteine translation is located in the 3'untranslated region of eukaryotic selenoprotein mRNA instead of the open read frame of prokaryotic selenoprotein mRNA; and (2) there is more than one SECIS-binding protein in eukaryotes and the elongation mechanism is probably much more sophisticated than the action of SELB in prokaryotes. Eukaryotic selenoprotein genes cannot be directly expressed in prokaryotic hosts.

products required for the synthesis and insertion of Se into selenoproteins (Fig. 17.2).[7,106] The four genes are named *selA*, *selB*, *selC*, and *selD* and encode selenocysteyl-tRNA synthetase, an elongation factor, selenocysteyl-tRNA (tRNA[SEC]), and selenophosphate synthetase, respectively. Biosynthesis of selenocysteine is initiated by the generation of an active Se donor (selenophosphate) and carbon source (serine). The active form of Se is formed from selenide and ATP under the catalysis of selenophosphate synthetase (SELD), and serine is esterified to the 3' terminal of the novel selenocysteyl-tRNA (SELC) that contains the anti-codon for uracil-guanine-adenine (UGA), by the normal seryl-tRNA synthetase. Selenocysteyl-tRNA synthetase (SELA) catalyzes the dehydration of L-serine in the seryl-tRNA to form aminoacrylyl-tRNA[sec], and selenophosphate replaces the side-chain oxygen in serine and produces selenocysteine moiety (still esterified to the tRNA[sec]). The novel elongation factor (SELB) specifically recognizes the selenocysteyl-tRNA, presumably by binding to the stem-loop structure of 3' untranslated region (UTR) of mRNA. These three components, plus guanosin-triphosphate (GTP), form a functional quaternary complex on the ribosome, and selenocysteine is incorporated into the growing peptide at the position corresponding to that of UGA in the mRNA.

17.5.2   Comparison of Prokaryotic and Eukaryotic Selenoprotein Biosynthesis

Because selenoprotein biosynthesis requires highly species-specific translation machinery, mammalian selenoprotein genes cannot be directly expressed in *E. coli* and vice versa. Nevertheless, these two types of organisms seem to share common features in the overall biosynthesis of selenoproteins. First, selenocysteine in both organisms is encoded by UGA. Second, both require a stem-loop structure of the mRNA for distinguishing UGA as the selenocysteine codon from that of termination codon, although the stem-loop is located immediately downstream the UGA codon in *E. coli* and in the 3'UTR of mRNA in mammals. Deletion of this conserved stem-loop mRNA, called selenocysteine insertion sequence motif (SECIS) in human GPX1, completely abolishes selenocysteine insertion.[107] This motif is functionally interchangeable among various seleno-protein genes[108] and is able to direct selenocysteine integration at predetermined positions of heterologous gene.[109] Third, the carbon source of eukaryotic selenocysteine is also from serine.[110] Last, the identified components of the eukaryotic selenocysteine incorporation machinery may be similar to three respective gene products in *E. coli*.[111–113]

A special tRNA, the SELC equivalent, is essential for early embryonic development[114] (see below). Two selenophosphate synthetases,[56,112,115] the SELD equivalent, have been identified from mice and human. Thus, Se may be activated in the same way in eukaryotes as in prokaryotes. One of the enzymes is Se-dependent, indicating a possible autoregulation mechanism.[56] Two SECIS-binding proteins, the SELB equivalent, have also been identified,[113,116] although the role and complexity of these binding proteins in eukaryotic selenocysteine insertion may exceed those of SELB in prokaryotes.[116] Moreover, high levels of rat TR can be expressed in *E. coli* when the open reading frame of the gene is fused with the SECIS element of the bacterial selenoprotein formate dehydrogenase H.[117] Co-expression with *selA*, *selB*, and *selC* genes further enhances the production of and the specific activity of the recombinant protein. Thereby, the species-specific translation of seleno-proteins is probably dictated by the characteristics of the pertinent SECIS motif. In spite of this, there is a good similarity in selenoprotein expression between eukaryotes and prokaryotes, and *E. coli* can be used as an efficient host to produce recombinant selenoproteins of mammalian sources.

17.5.3   Sites of Selenium Regulation

Although the tissue specificity of GPX1 and other selenoprotein expression is determined mainly at the transcriptional level,[118] transcription rate of GPX1 mRNA, as well as other selenoprotein mRNA, is not affected by Se deficiency.[66,73,77] Thus, the loss of GPX1 mRNA in Se deficiency is post-transcriptional, probably due to accelerated degradation.[5,76]

It appears that GPX1 mRNA has the lowest stability in Se deficiency because it is reduced more dramatically than that of any other selenoprotein at this circumstance. A recent study by Moriarty et al.[119] indicates that Se deprivation does not alter levels of either nuclear pre-mRNA or nuclear mRNA, but reduces the level of cytoplasmic mRNA in a nonsense codon-mediated and translational-dependent way.

Overall, Se-dependent differential mRNA stability does not account for the complete changes of selenoprotein expression with the alteration of Se status. For example, reductions of enzyme activity or protein often exceed that of mRNA.[4,119] Activities of GPX1 and GPX4 are reduced by Se deficiency in rat testes without comparable changes in their mRNA levels.[46] In addition, the chemical form of supplemental Se affects the nature of selenoprotein synthesis.[120] Based on these observations and the assumption that eukaryotic selenoprotein biosynthesis follows pathways similar to those of prokaryotes, the rate of synthesis would depend on the availability of selenocysteine-loaded tRNA^{sec}. For each individual selenoprotein, this availability could be decided by its characteristic mRNA stability and SECIS efficiency at different status of Se.[6] As there are possibly multiple forms of SECIS-binding proteins in eukaryotes,[113,116] the same availability may also be regulated by the structural specificity and distribution of these proteins and their ability to form functional complexes with different SECIS.

Because the UGA-mediated translation of selenocysteine is a rather inefficient process,[121] there would be a strong competition between termination (production of truncated proteins) and elongation (co-translation of selenocysteine) at the UGA codon under limited Se supply. Although different SECIS elements are functionally interchangeable, their efficiencies in directing Se incorporation are not equal. The SECIS element from ID1 is more efficient than that of GPX1, but less efficient than that of Sel-P in directing the expression of ID1.[108] The GPX4 SECIS element is more efficient than that of ID1 or Sel-P in suppression of UGA by reporter-gene assays.[122] Among three GPX enzymes, SECIS efficiency ranks in the order of GPX4 > GPX1 > GPX2 and the augmentation of SECIS efficiency by Se is highest for GPX1, marginal for GPX2, and intermediate for GPX4.[80] Consistently, the tentative efficiency order of different SECIS elements matches well the relative susceptibility of the pertinent protein and mRNA to Se deficiency.[6]

Based on the above described Se-dependent differential mRNA stabilities and different SECIS efficiencies of selenoproteins, Flohé et al.[6] have proposed that the differential response of any given selenoprotein to Se availability can be achieved by the formation of complex among the translational factor SELB (binding protein), selenocysteine-loaded tRNA^{sec}, and the specific mRNA. If the binding of tRNA^{sec} to SELB is determined by Se availability, this binding would specifically affect the affinity of a particular SECIS motif to SELB or the binary complex SELB-tRNA^{sec}. Conceivably, the alteration of affinity may determine the feasibility in forming the three components complex. Those mRNAs that form productive ternary complex first because of the largest affinity increases would be translated efficiently and resistant to degradation. Therefore, the Se-dependent mRNA stability and SECIS efficiency of the individual selenoprotein dictate its own fate in the preferential biosynthesis at limited Se supply. Experimentally, Se regulation of GPX1 mRNA in cultured cells requires the presence of intact SECIS,[123,124] although its presence, along with the UGA codon, does not necessarily confer an efficient selenocysteine biosynthesis.[125] In Se deficiency, more GPX1 mRNA may be released from polysomes and degraded than that of GPX4 mRNA because of its greater decrease in translation.[76]

Two important recent findings[116] should be added to the above-discussed model. First, there is more than one SECIS-binding protein in eukaryotes and specific association of homologous or heterologous factors may be presented in the RNA-protein binding functional complex. Second, a minimal binding site in the 3′UTR of selenoprotein mRNA is necessary. However, only binding itself seems to be insufficient for selenocysteine incorporation.

17.6 Use of Gene-Knockout Approach to Study Regulation of Selenoprotein Expression

Two gene knockout mouse models have been used in Se research. One is the targeted disruption of the mouse selenocysteine tRNA gene (*Trsp*) in chromosome 7.[114] The heterozygous mutants have 50 to 80% of the wild-type levels of tRNA[sec] in most organs, but exhibit normal viability, fertility, and expression of GPX1. However, the homozygous mutants die shortly after implantation, and the embryos are resorbed before 6.5 days post coitum. Thus, the haploid amount of tRNA[sec] is not limiting in selenoprotein expression, but *Trsp* expression is essential for early embryonic development. To study the role of *Trsp* expression at other stages of development in selected tissues, conditional knockout of the gene is in progress.[126]

The other knockout model is the disruption of the GPX1 gene in mice. Using this model, we have demonstrated that:

1. GPX1 represents 60% of liver Se and the most abundant selenoprotein in the organ.[3,127]

2. The expression of GPX3, GPX4, Sel-P, or TR in Se-deficient or adequate mice is independent of GPX1, and there is no change in Se channeled to the expression of these proteins by altering GPX1 expression.[3,20,97,127–129]

3. GPX1 is the major metabolic form of body Se in protecting mice against acute,[18–20,129] lethal oxidative stress induced by prooxidants and high levels of vitamin E do not replace that role of GPX1.[97]

4. GPX1 knockout has no significant impact on mouse fertility or susceptibility to low levels of oxidative stress or other antioxidant enzymes.[11,18,129]

These unequivocal data cannot be obtained using conventional approaches. With more selenoprotein gene knockout models being developed, our understanding of the regulation and function of selenoprotein expression will be significantly enhanced.

Acknowledgments: Work in the author's laboratory has been supported by a National Institutes of Health grant DK53018.

Abbreviations

FAD   flavin adenine dinucleotide

GPX1   cellular glutathione peroxidase

GPX2 (GPX-GI)   gastrointestinal glutathione peroxidase

GPX3   plasma or extracellular glutathione peroxidase

GPX4 (PHGPX)   phospholipid hydroperoxide glutathione peroxidase

GSH   reduced glutathione

ID1   type-1 iodothyronine 5′ deiodinase

Se   selenium

SECIS   selenocysteine insertion sequence motif

Sel   selenoprotein

Sel-P   selenoprotein P

Sel-W   selenoprotein W

TR   thioredoxin reductase

Trsp   selenocysteine tRNA gene

UTR   untranslated region

Glossary

Glutathione peroxidases: Intra- or extra-cellular selenoenzymes, homotetramer (~88 kDa) or monomer (19 kDa), catalyzing the reduction or removal of H_2O_2, lipid peroxides, or phospholipid hydroperoxides using reduced glutathione

Iodothyronine 5′ deiodinases: Selenoenzymes (~28 to 30 kDa), catalyzing the conversion of T_4 to T_3 and the inactivation of both hormones, three different types based on distribution and function

Selenium: An essential trace element for animals and humans

Selenoproteins: Proteins containing selenium in the form of selenocysteine

Selenoenzymes: Enzymes containing selenium in the form of selenocysteine

Selenoperoxidases: Refer to four different selenium-dependent glutathione peroxidases that use reduced glutathione to reduce hydroperoxides

Selenocysteine insertion sequence (SECIS): A well-conserved stem-loop mRNA sequence in the 3′ untranslated region of selenoprotein genes that directs selenium incorporation into the peptide

selA: Prokaryotic gene of selenocysteine synthetase (SELA) that catalyzes the formation of selenocysteine moiety from seryl-tRNA and selenophosphate

selB: Prokaryotic gene of an elongation factor (SELB) needed for co-translation of selenocysteine

selC: Prokaryotic gene of selenocysteine tRNA (SELC) that contains the anticodon for UGA that encodes selenocysteine

selD: Prokaryotic gene of selenophosphate synthetase (SELD) that activates selenium for co-translation of selenocysteine

Selenoprotein P: A selenium-dependent glycoprotein of 57 kDa, accounting for 65% of plasma selenium in rodents

Selenoprotein W: A selenium-dependent protein of 10 kDa, relatively high in muscle, low expression in selenium-deficient animals with white muscle disease

Thioredoxin reductases: Pyridine nucleotide-disulfide oxidoreductases, homodimers of 55 to 65 kDa subunits, catalyzing NADPH-dependent reduction of thioredoxin

tRNA[SEC]: A novel tRNA that contains the anticodon for UGA and carries serine for the biosynthesis of selenocysteine

---

References

1. Rotruck, J. T., Pope, A. L., Ganther, H. E., Swanson, A. B., Hafeman, D. G., and Hoekstra, W. G., Selenium: biochemical role as a component of glutathione peroxidase, *Science*, 179, 585, 1973.

2. Flohé, L., Günzler, W. A., and Schock, H. H., Glutathione peroxidase: a selenoenzyme, *FEBS Lett.*, 32, 132, 1973.
3. Cheng, W.-H., Ho, Y.-S., Ross, D. A., Valentine, B. A., Combs, Jr., G. F., and Lei, X. G., Cellular glutathione peroxidase knockout mice express normal levels of selenium-dependent plasma and phospholipid hydroperoxide glutathione peroxidases in various tissues, *J. Nutr.*, 127, 1445, 1997.
4. Burk, R. F. and Hill, K. E., Regulation of selenoproteins, *Ann. Rev. Nutr.*, 13, 65, 1993.
5. Sunde, R. A., Intracellular glutathione peroxidases - structures, regulation, and functions, in *Selenium in Biology and Human Health*, Burk, R. F., Ed., Springer-Verlag, New York, NY, 1994, 47.
6. Flohé, L., Wingender, E., and Brigelius-Flohé, R., Regulation of glutathione peroxidase, in *Oxidative Stress and Signal Transduction*, Forman, H. J. and Cadenas, E., Eds., Chapman & Hall, New York, NY, 1997, 415.
7. Stadtman, T. C., Selenocysteine, *Ann. Rev. Biochem.*, 65, 83, 1996.
8. Mills, G. C., Hemoglobin catabolism. I. Glutathione peroxidase, an erythrocyte enzyme which protects hemoglobin from oxidative breakdown, *J. Biol. Chem.*, 229, 189, 1957.
9. Schwarz, K. and Foltz, C. M., Selenium as an integral part of Factor 3 against dietary necrotic liver degeneration, *J. Am. Chem. Soc.*, 79, 3292, 1957.
10. Chambers, I., Frampton, J., Goldfarb, P., Affara, N., McBain, W., and Harrison, P. R., The structure of the mouse glutathione peroxidase gene: the selenocysteine in the active site is encoded by the termination codon, TGA, *EMBO J.*, 5, 1221, 1986.
11. Ho, Y.-S., Magnenat, J. -L., Bronson, R. T., Cao, J., Gargano, M., Sugawara, M., and Funk, C. D., Mice deficient in cellular glutathione peroxidase develop normally and show no increased sensitivity to hyperoxia, *J. Biol. Chem.*, 272, 16644, 1997.
12. Chada, S., Le Beau, M. M., Casey, L., and Newburger, P. E., Isolation and chromosomal localization of the human glutathione peroxidase gene, *Genomics*, 6, 268, 1990.
13. Flohé, L., The selenoprotein glutathione peroxidase, in *Glutathione: Chemical, Biochemical, and Medical Aspects-Part A*, Dolphin, D., Poulson, R., and Avramovic, O., Eds., John Wiley & Sons, New York, NY, 1989, 644.
14. Esworthy, R. S., Ho, Y.-S., Chu, F. F., The Gpx1 gene encodes mitochondrial glutathione peroxidase in the mouse liver, *Arch. Biochem. Biophys.*, 340, 59, 1997.
15. Flohé, L., Loschen, G., Günzler, W. A., and Eichole, E., Glutathione peroxidase. V. The kinetic mechanism. Hoppe-Seyler's, *Physiol. Chem.*, 353, 987, 1972.
16. Wendel, A., Glutathione peroxidase, *Methods Enzymol.*, 77, 325, 1981.
17. Burk, R. F., Molecular biology of selenium with implications for its metabolism, *FASEB J.*, 5, 2274, 1991.
18. Cheng, W.-H., Ho, Y.-S., Valentine, B. A., Ross, D. A., Combs, Jr., G. F., and Lei, X. G., Cellular glutathione peroxidase is the mediator of body selenium to protect against paraquat lethality in transgenic mice, *J. Nutr.*, 128, 1070, 1998.
19. Cheng, W.-H., Fu, Y. X., Porres, J. M., Ross, D. A., and Lei, X. G., Selenium-dependent cellular glutathione peroxidase protects mice against a pro-oxidant-induced oxidation of NADPH, NADH, lipids, and protein, *FASEB J.*, 13, 1467, 1999.
20. Fu, Y. X., Cheng, W.-H., Porres, J. M., Ross, D. A., and Lei, X. G., Knockout of cellular gluathione peroxidase gene renders mice susceptible to diquat-induced oxidative stress, *Free Radic. Biol. Med.*, 27, 605, 1999.

21. de Haan, J. B., Bladier, C., Griffiths, P., Kelner, M., O'Shea, R. D., Cheung, N. S., Bronson, R. T., Silvestro, M. J., Wild, S., Zheng, S. S., Beart, P. M., Hertzog, P. J., and Kola, I., Mice with a homozygous null mutation for the most abundant glutathione peroxidase, Gpx1, show increased susceptibility to the oxidative stress-inducing agents paraquat and hydrogen peroxide, *J. Biol. Chem.*, 273, 22528, 1998.

22. Chu, F.-F., Doroshow, J. H., and Esworthy, R. S., Expression, characterization, and tissue distributions of a new cellular selenium-dependent glutathione peroxidase, GSHPX-GI, *J. Biol. Chem.*, 268, 2571, 1993.

23. Esworthy, R. S., Swiderek, K. M., Ho, Y.-S., and Chu, F. F., Selenium-dependent glutathione peroxidase-GI is a major glutathione peroxidase activity in the mucosal epithelium of rodent intestine, *Biochim. Biophys. Acta*, 1381, 213, 1998.

24. Cohen, H. J., Chovaniac, M. E., Mistrerra, D., and Baker, S. S., Selenium repletion and glutathione peroxidase differential effects on plasma and red blood cell enzyme activity, *Am. J. Clin. Nutr.*, 41, 735, 1985.

25. Cohen, H. J. and Avissar, N., Extracellular glutathione peroxidase: a distinct selenoprotein, in *Selenium in Biology and Human Health*, Burk, R. F., Ed., Springer-Verlag, New York, NY, 1994, 81.

26. Takahashi, K. and Cohen, H. J., Selenium-dependent glutathione peroxidase protein and activity: immunological investigations on cellular and plasma enzymes, *Blood*, 68, 640, 1986.

27. Takahashi, K., Akasaka, M., Yamamoto, Y., Kobayashi, C., Mixoguchi, J., and Koyama, J., Primary structure of human plasma glutathione peroxidase deduced from cDNA sequences, *J. Biochem. (Tokyo)*, 108, 145, 1990.

28. Yoshimura, S., Suemizu, H., Taniguchi, Y., Arimori, K., Kawabe, N., and Moriuchi, T., The human plasma glutathione peroxidase-encoding gene: organization, sequence and localization to chromosome 5q32, *Gene*, 145, 293, 1994.

29. Yoshimura, S., Watanabe, K., Suemizu, H., Onozawa, T., Mizoguchi, J., Tsuda, K., Hatta, H., and Moriuchi, T., Tissue specific expression of the plasma glutathione peroxidase gene in rat kidney, *J. Biochem.*, 109, 918, 1991.

30. Tham, D. M., Whitin, J. C., Kim, K. K., Zhu, S. X., and Cohen, H. J., Expression of extracellular glutathione peroxidase in human and mouse gastrointestinal tract, *Am. J. Physiol.*, 275, G1463, 1998.

31. Avissar, N., Kerl, E. A., Baker, S. S., and Cohen, H. J., Extracellular glutathione peroxidase mRNA and protein in human cell lines, *Arch. Biochem. Biophys.*, 309, 239, 1994.

32. Esworthy, R. S., Chu, F.-F., Geiger, P., Girotti, A. W., and Doroshow, J. H., Reactivity of plasma glutathione peroxidase with hydroperoxide substrates and glutathione, *Arch. Biochem. Biophys.*, 307, 29, 1993.

33. Maser, R. L., Magenheimer, B. S., and Calvet, J. P., Mouse plasma glutathione peroxidase, *J. Biol. Chem.*, 269, 27066, 1994.

34. Avissar, N., Finkelstein, J. N., Horowitz, S., Willey, J. C., Coy, E., Frampton, M. W., Watkins, R. H., Khullar, P., Xu, Y.-L., and Cohen, H. J., Extracellular glutathione peroxidase in human lung epithelial lining fluid and in lung cells, *Am. J. Physiol.*, 270, L173, 1996.

35. Kingsley, P. D., Whitin, J. C., Cohen, H. J., and Palis, J., Developmental expression of extracellular glutathione peroxidase suggests antioxidant roles in deciduum, visceral yolk sac, and skin, *Mol. Reprod. Develop.*, 49, 343, 1998.

36. Ursini, F., Maiorino, M., and Gregolin, C., The selenoenzyme phospholipid hydroperoxide glutathione peroxidase, *Biochim. Biophys. Acta*, 839, 62, 1985.

37. Schuckelt, R., Brigelius-Flohé, R., Maiorino, M., Roveri, A., Reumkens, J., Strassburger, W., Ursini, F., Wolf, B., and Flohé, L., Phospholipid hydroperoxide glutathione peroxidase is a selenoenzyme distinct from the classical glutathione peroxidase as evident from cDNA and amino acid sequencing, *Free Radic. Res. Commun.*, 14, 343, 1991.

38. Pushpa-Rekha, T. R., Burdsall, A. L., Oleksa, L. M., Chisolm, G. M., and Driscoll, D. M., Rat phospholipid-hydroperoxide glutathione peroxidase: cDNA cloning and identification of multiple transcription and translation start sites, *J. Biol. Chem.*, 270, 26993, 1995.

39. Knopp, E. A., Arndt, T. L., Eng, K. L., Caldwell, M., LeBoeuf, R. C., Deeb, S. S., and O'Brien, K. D., Murine phospholipid hydroperoxide glutathione peroxidase: cDNA sequence, tissue expression, and mapping, *Mamm. Genome*, 10, 601, 1999.

40. Esworthy, R. S., Doan, K., Doroshow, J. H., and Chu, F.-F., Cloning and sequencing of the cDNA encoding a human testis phospholipid hydroperoxide glutathione peroxidase, *Gene*, 144, 317, 1994.

41. Brigelius-Flohé, R., Aumann, K. D., Blöcker, H., Gross, G., Kiess, M., Klöppel, K. D., Maiorino, M., Roveri, A., Schuckelt, R., Ursini, F., Wingender, E., and Flohé, L., Phospholipid-hydroperoxide glutathione peroxidase: Genomic DNA, cDNA and deduced amino acid sequence, *J. Biol. Chem.*, 269, 7342, 1994.

42. Borchert, A., Schnurr, K., Thiele, B. J., and Kühn, H., Cloning of the mouse phospholipid hydroperoxide glutathione peroxidase gene, *FEBS Lett.*, 446, 223, 1999.

43. Arai, M., Imai, H., Koumura, T., Yoshida, M., Emoto, K., Umeda, M., Chiba, N., and Nakagawa, Y., Mitochondrial phospholipid hydroperoxide glutathione peroxidase plays a major role in preventing oxidative injury to cells, *J. Biol. Chem.*, 274, 4924, 1999.

44. Maiorino, M., Gregolin, C., and Ursini, F., Phospholipid hydroperoxide glutathione peroxidase, *Meth. Enzymol.*, 186, 448, 1990.

45. Roveri, A., Casasco, A., Maiorino, M., Dalan, P., Calligaro, A., and Ursini, F., Phospholipid hydroperoxide glutathione peroxidase of rat testis, *J. Biol. Chem.*, 267, 6142, 1992.

46. Lei, X. G., Evenson, J. K., Thompson, K. T., and Sunde, R. A., Glutathione peroxidase and phospholipid hydroperoxide glutathione peroxidase are differentially regulated by dietary selenium, *J. Nutr.*, 125, 1438, 1995.

47. Godeas, C., Tramer, F., Micali, F., Soranzo, M., Sandri, G., and Panfili, E., Distribution and possible novel role of phospholipid hydroperoxide glutathione peroxidase in rat epididymal spermatozoa, *Biol. Reprod.*, 57, 1502, 1997.

48. Maiorino, M., Wissing, J. B., Brigelius-Flohé, R., Calabrese, F., Roveri, A., Steinert, P., Ursini, F., and Flohé, L., Testosterone mediates expression of the selenoprotein PHGPx by induction of spermatogenesis and not by direct transcriptional gene activation, *FASEB J.*, 12, 1359, 1998.

49. Ursini, F., Heim, S., Kiess, M., Maiorino, M., Roveri, A., Wissing, J., and Flohé, L., Dual function of the selenoprotein PHGPx during sperm maturation, *Science*, 285, 1393, 1999.

50. Berry, M. J., Banu, L., and Larsen, P. R., Type 1 iodothyronine deiodinase is a selenocysteine-containing enzyme, *Nature (London)*, 349, 438, 1991.

51. Croteau, W., Davey, J. C., Galton, V. A., and St. Germain, D. L., Cloning of the mammalian type II iodothyronine deiodinase. A selenoprotein differentially expressed and regulated in human and rat brain and other tissues, *J. Clin. Invest.*, 98, 405, 1996.

52. Salvatore, D., Low, S. C., Berry, M., Mai, A. L., Harney, J. W., Croteau, W., St. Germain, D. L., and Larsen, P. R., Type 3 iodothyronine deiodinase: cloning, *in vitro* expression, and functional analysis of the placental selenoenzyme, *J. Clin. Invest.*, 96, 2421, 1995.

53. Sun, Q. A., Wu, Y., Zappacosta, F., Jeang, K.-T., Lee, B. Y., Hatfield, D. L., and Gladyshev, V. N., Redox regulation of cell signaling by selenocysteine in mammalian thioredoxin reductases, *J. Biol. Chem.*, 274, 24522, 1999.

54. Tamura, T. and Stadtman, T. C., A new selenoprotein from human lung adenocarcinoma cells: purification, properties, and thioredoxin reductase activity, *Proc. Natl. Acad. Sci. USA*, 93, 1006, 1996.

55. Gromer, S., Arscott, L. D., Williams, Jr., C. H., Schirmer, R. H., and Becker, K., Human placenta thioredoxin reductase, *J. Biol. Chem.*, 273, 20096, 1998.

56. Kim, I. Y., Guimaraes, M. J., Zlotnik, A., Bazan, J. F., and Stadtman, T. C., Fetal mouse selenophosphate synthetase 2 (SPS2): Characterization of the cysteine mutant form overproduced in a baculovirus-insect cell system, *Proc. Natl. Acad. Sci. USA*, 94, 418, 1997.

57. Hill, K. E., Lloyd, R. S., Yang, J. G., Read, R., and Burk, R. F., The cDNA for rat selenoprotein P contains ten TGA codons in the open reading frame, *J. Biol. Chem.*, 266, 10050, 1991.

58. Himeno, S., Chittum, H. S., and Burk, R. F., Isoforms of selenoprotein P in rat plasma. Evidence for a full-length form and another form that terminates at the second UGA in the open reading frame, *J. Biol. Chem.*, 271, 15769, 1996.

59. Chittum, H. S., Himeno, S., Hill, K. E., and Burk, R. F., Multiple forms of selenoprotein P in rat plasma, *Arch. Biochem. Biophys.*, 325, 124, 1996.

60. Read, R., Bellew, T., Yang, J.-G., Hill, K. E., Palmer, I. S., and Burk, R. F., Selenium and amino acid composition of selenoprotein P, the major selenoprotein in rat serum, *J. Biol. Chem.*, 265, 17899, 1990.

61. Hill, K. E., Boeglin, M. E., Chittum, H. S., and Burk, R. F., Immunohistochemical location of selenoprotein P in rat tissues, *FASEB J.*, 10, A558, 1996.

62. Saito, Y., Hayashi, T., Tanaka, A., Watanabe, Y., Suzuki, M., Saito, E., and Takahashi, K., Selenoprotein P in human plasma as an extracellular phospholipid hydroperoxide glutathione peroxidase, *J. Biol. Chem.*, 274, 2866, 1999.

63. Vendeland, S. C., Beilstein, M. A., Chen, C. L., Jensen, O. N., Barofsky, E., and Whanger, P. D., Purification and properties of selenoprotein W from rat muscle, *J. Biol. Chem.*, 268, 17103, 1993.

64. Vendeland, S. C., Beilstein, M. A., Yeh, J.-Y., Ream, W., and Whanger, P. D., Rat skeletal muscle selenoprotein W: cDNA clone and mRNA modulation by dietary selenium, *Proc. Natl. Acad. Sci. USA*, 92, 8749, 1995.

65. Gladyshev, V. N., Jeang, K.-T., Wootton, J. C., and Hatfield, D. L., A new human selenium-containing protein, *J. Biol. Chem.*, 273, 8910, 1998.

66. Christensen, M. J., Cammack, P. M., and Wray, C. D., Tissue specificity of selenoprotein gene expression in rats, *J. Nutr. Biochem.*, 6, 367, 1995.

67. Hafeman, D. G., Sunde, R. A., and Hoekstra, W. G., Effect of dietary selenium on erythrocyte and liver glutathione peroxidase in the rat, *J. Nutr.*, 104, 580, 1974.

68. Knight, S.A.B. and Sunde, R. A., Effect of selenium repletion on glutathione peroxidase protein level in rat liver, *J. Nutr.*, 118, 853, 1988.

69. Knight, S.A.B. and Sunde, R. A., The effect of progressive selenium deficiency on antiglutathione peroxidase antibody reactive protein in rat liver, *J. Nutr.*, 117, 732, 1987.

70. Baker, R. D., Baker, S. S., LaRosa, K., Whitney, C., and Newburger, P. E., Selenium regulation of glutathione peroxidase in human hepatoma cell line Hep3B, *Arch. Biochem. Biophys.*, 304, 53, 1993.

71. Hill, K. E., Lyons, P. R., and Burk, R. F., Differential regulation of rat liver selenoprotein mRNAs in selenium deficiency, *Biochem. Biophys. Res. Commun.*, 185, 260, 1992.

72. Saedi, M. S., Smith, C. G., Frampton, J., Chambers, I., Harrison, P. R., and Sunde, R. A., Effect of selenium status on mRNA levels for glutathione peroxidase in rat liver, *Biochem. Biophys. Res. Commun.*, 153, 855, 1988.

73. Toyoda, H., Himeno, S., and Imura, N., Regulation of glutathione peroxidase mRNA level by dietary selenium manipulation, *Biochim. Biophys. Acta*, 1049, 213, 1990.

74. Li, N-Q., Reddy, P. S., Thyagaraju, K., Reddy, A. P., Hsu, B. L., Scholz, R. W., Tu, C.-P. D., and Reddy, C. C., Elevation of rat liver mRNA for selenium-dependent glutathione peroxidase by selenium deficiency, *J. Biol. Chem.*, 265, 108, 1990.

75. Weitzel, F., Ursini, F., and Wendel, A., Phospholipid hydroperoxide glutathione peroxidase in various mouse organs during selenium deficiency and repletion, *Biochim. Biophys. Acta*, 1036, 88, 1990.

76. Bermano, G., Arthur, J. R., and Hesketh, J. E., Selective control of cytosolic glutathione peroxidase and phospholipid hydroperoxide glutathione peroxidase mRNA stability by selenium supply, *FEBS Lett.*, 387, 157, 1996.

77. Bermano, G., Nicol, F., Dyer, A. A., Sunde, R. A., Beckett, G. J., Arthur, J. R., and Hesketh, J. E., Tissue-specific regulation of selenoenyzme gene expression during selenium deficiency in rats, *Biochem. J.*, 311, 425, 1995.

78. Lei, X. G., Dann, H. M., Ross, D. A., Cheng, W. H., Combs, Jr., G. F., and Roneker, K. R., Dietary selenium supplementation is required to support full expression of three selenium-dependent glutathione peroxidases in various tissues of weanling pigs, *J. Nutr.*, 128, 130, 1998.

79. Cohen, H. J., Brown, M. R., Hamilton, D., Lyons, J. M., Patterson, J., Avissar, N., and Liegey, P., Glutathione peroxidase and selenium deficiency in patients receiving home parenteral nutrition, time course for development of deficiency and repletion of enzyme activity in plasma and blood cells, *Am. J. Clin. Nutr.*, 49, 132, 1989.

80. Wingler, K., Böcher, M., Flohé, L., Kollmus, H., and Brigelius-Flohé, R., mRNA stability and selenocysteine insertion sequence efficiency rank gastrointestinal glutathione peroxidase high in the hierarchy of selenoproteins, *Eur. J. Biochem.*, 259, 149, 1999.

81. Mitchell, J. H., Nicol, F., Beckett, G. J., and Arthur, J. R., Selenoenzyme expression in thyroid and liver of second generation selenium- and iodine-deficient rats, *J. Mol. Endocr.*, 16, 259, 1996.

82. Mitchell, J. H., Nicol, F., Beckett, G. J., and Arthur, J. R., Selenoprotein expression and brain development in preweanling selenium- and iodine-deficient rats, *J. Mol. Endocr.*, 20, 203, 1998.

83. Mitchell, J. H., Nicol, F., Beckett, G. J., and Arthur, J. R., Selenium and iodine deficiencies: effects on brain and brown adipose tissue selenoenzyme activity and expression, *J. Endocrin.*, 155, 255, 1997.

84. Behne, D., Kyriakopoulos, A., Gessner, H., Walzog, B., and Meinhold, H., Type I iodothyronine deiodinase activity after high selenium intake, and relations between selenium and iodine metabolism in rats, *J. Nutr.*, 122, 1542, 1992.

85. Vadhanavikit, S. and Ganther, H. E., Selenium requirements of rat for normal hepatic and thyroid 5'-deiodinase (Type I) activities, *J. Nutr.*, 123, 1124, 1993.

86. Gross, M., Oertel, M., and Kohrle, J., Differential selenium-dependent expression of type I 5'-deiodinase and glutathione peroxidase in the porcine epithelial kidney cell line LLC-PK$_1$, *Biochem. J.*, 306, 851, 1995.

87. Villette, S., Bermano, G., Arthur, J. R., and Hesketh, J. E., Thyroid stimulating hormone and selenium supply interact to regulate selenoenzyme gene expression in thyroid cells (FRTL-5) in culture, *FEBS Lett.*, 438, 81, 1998.

88. Yang, J. G., Hill, K. E., and Burk, R. F., Dietary selenium intake controls rat plasma selenoprotein P concentration, *J. Nutr.*, 119, 1010, 1989.

89. Cockell, K. A., Brash, A. R., and Burk, R. F., Influence of selenium status on activity of phospholipid hydroperoxide glutathione peroxidase in rat liver and testis in comparison with other selenoproteins, *J. Nutr. Biochem.*, 7, 333, 1996.

90. Yeh, J.-Y., Vendeland, S. C., Gu, Q.-P., Butler, J. A., Ou, B.-R., and Whanger, P. D., Dietary selenium increases selenoprotein W levels in rat tissues, *J. Nutr.*, 127, 2165, 1997.

91. Yeh, J.-Y., Gu, Q.-P., Beilstein, M. A., Forsberg, N. E., and Whanger, P. D., Se influences tissue levels of Se-W in sheep, *J. Nutr.*, 127, 394, 1997.

92. Hill, K. E., McCollum, G. W., Boeglin, M. E., and Burk, R. F., Thioredoxin reductase activity is decreased by selenium deficiency, *Biochem. Biophy. Res. Commun.*, 234, 293, 1997.

93. Marcocci, L., Flohé, L., and Packer, L., Evidence for a functional relevance of the selenocysteine residue in mammalian thioredoxin reductase, *BioFactors*, 6, 351, 1997.

94. Gallegos, A., Berggren, M., Gasdaska, J. R., and Powis, G., Mechanisms of the regulation of thioredoxin reductase activity in cancer cells by the chemopreventive agent selenium, *Cancer Res.*, 57, 4965, 1997.

95. Rafferty, T. S., McKenzie, R. C., Hunter, J.A.A., Howie, A. F., Arthur, J. R., Nicol, F., and Beckett, G. J., Differential expression of selenoproteins by human skin cells and protection by selenium from UVB-radiation-induced cell death, *Biochem. J.*, 332, 231, 1998.

96. Li, R.-K., Cowan, D. B., Mickle, D.A.G., Weisel, R. D., and Burton, G. W., Effect of vitamin E on human glutathione peroxidase (GSH-PX1) expression in cardiomyocytes, *Free Radic. Biol. Med.*, 21, 419, 1996.

97. Cheng, W.-H., Valentine, B. A., and Lei, X. G., High levels of dietary vitamin E do not replace cellular glutathione peroxidase in protecting mice from acute oxidative stress, *J. Nutr.*, 129, 1951, 1999.

98. Moriarty, P. M., Picciano, M. F., Beard, J. L., and Reddy, C. C., Classical selenium-dependent glutathione peroxidase expression is decreased secondary to iron deficiency in rats, *J. Nutr.*, 125, 293, 1995.

99. Prohaska, J. R., Sunde, R. A., and Zinn, K. R., Livers from copper-deficient rats have lower glutathione peroxidase activity and mRNA levels but normal liver selenium levels, *J. Nutr. Biochem.*, 3, 429, 1992.

100. Prohaska, J. R. and Sunde, R. A., Comparison of liver glutathione peroxidase activity and mRNA in female and male mice and rats, *Comp. Biochem. Physiol.*,105B, 111, 1993.

101. Moscow, J. A., Morrow, C. S., He, R., Mullenbach, G. T., and Cowan, K. H., Structure and function of the 5'-flanking sequence of the human cytosolic selenium-dependent glutathione peroxidase gene (hgpx1), *J. Biol. Chem.*, 267, 5949, 1992.

102. Cowan, D. B., Weisel, R. D., Williams, W. G., and Mickle, D. A., Identification of oxygen responsive elements in the 5'-flanking region of the human glutathione peroxidase gene, *J. Biol. Chem.*, 268, 26904, 1993.

103. Jornot, L. and Junod, A. F., Differential regulation of glutathione peroxidase by selenomethionine and hyperoxia in endothelial cells, *Biochem. J.*, 306, 581, 1995.

104. Garberg, P. and Thullberg, M., Decreased glutathione peroxidase activity in mice in response to nafenopin is caused by changes in selenium metabolism, *Chem. Biol. Interact.*, 99, 165, 1996.

105. Lei, X. G., Ross, D. A., and Roneker, K. R., Comparison of age-related differences in expression of phospholipid hydroperoxide glutathione peroxidase mRNA and activity in various tissue of pigs, *Comp. Biochem. Physiol.*, 117B, 109, 1997.

106. Böck, A., Forchhammer, K., Heider, J., Leinfelder, W., Sawers, G., Veprek, B., and Zinoni, F., Selenocysteine: the 21st amino acid, *Mol. Microb.*, 5, 515, 1991.

107. Shen, Q., Chu, F.-F., and Newburger, P. E., Sequences in the 3'-untranslated region of the human cellular glutathione peroxidase gene are necessary and sufficient for selenocysteine incorporation at the UGA codon, *J. Biol. Chem.*, 268, 11463, 1993.

108. Berry, M. J., Banu, L., Harney, J. W., and Larsen, P. R., Functional characterization of the eukaryotic SECIS elements which direct selenocysteine insertion at UGA codons, *EMBO J.*, 12, 3315, 1993.

109. Leonard, J. L., Leonard, D. M., Shen, Q., Farwell, A. P., and Newburger, P. E., Selenium-regulated translation control of heterologous gene expression: normal function of selenocysteine-substituted gene products, *J. Cell Biochem.*, 61, 410, 1996.

110. Sunde, R. A. and Evenson, J. K., Serine incorporation into the selenocysteine moiety of glutathione peroxidase, *J. Biol. Chem.*, 262, 933, 1987.

111. Lee, B. J., Rajagopalan, M., Kim, Y. S., You, K. H., Jacoson, K. B., and Hatfield, D. L., Selenocysteine tRNA[Ser]Sec gene is ubiquitous within the animal kingdom, *Mol. Cell. Biol.*, 10, 1940, 1990.

112. Low, S. C., Harney, J. W., and Berry, M. J., Cloning and functional characterization of human selenophosphate synthetase, an essential component of selenoprotein synthesis, *J. Biol. Chem.*, 270, 21659, 1995.

113. Shen, Q., Wu, R., Leonard, J. L., and Newburger, P. E., Identification and molecular cloning of a human selenocysteine insertion sequence-binding protein, *J. Biol. Chem.*, 273, 5443, 1998.

114. Bösl, M. R., Takaku, K., Oshima, M., Nishimura, S., and Taketo, M. M., Early embryonic lethality caused by targeted disruption of the mouse selenocysteine tRNA gene (Trsp), *Proc. Natl. Acad. Sci. USA*, 94, 5531, 1997.

115. Guimaraes, M. J., Peterson, D., Vicari, A., Cocks, B. G., Copeland, N. G., Gilbert, D. J., Jenkins, N. A., Ferrick, D. A., Kastelein, R. A., Bazan, J. F., and Zlotnik, A., Identification of a novel selD homolog from eukaryotes, bacteria, and archaea: Is there an autoregulatory mechanism in selenocysteine metabolism? *Proc. Natl. Acad. Sci. USA*, 93, 15086, 1996.

116. Copeland, P. R., and Driscoll, D. M., Purification redox sensitivity, and RNA binding properties of SECIS-binding protein 2, a protein involved in selenoprotein biosynthesis, *J. Biol. Chem.*, 274, 25447, 1999.

117. Arner, E.S.J., Sariouglu, H., Lottspeich, F., Holmgren, A., and Bock, A., High-level expression in Escherichia coli of selenocysteine-containing rat thioredoxin reductase utilizing gene fusions with engineered bacterial-type SECIS elements and co-expression with the selA, selB, and selC genes, *J. Mol. Biol.*, 292, 1003, 1999.

118. Himeno, S., Takekawa, A., Toyoda, H., and Imura, N., Tissue-specific expression of glutathione peroxidase gene in guinea pigs, *Biochim. Biophys. Acta,* 1173, 283, 1993.

119. Moriarty, P. M., Reddy, C. C., and Maquat, L. E., Selenium deficiency reduces the abundance of mRNA for Se-dependent glutathione peroxidase 1 by a UGA-dependent mechanism likely to be nonsense codon-mediated decay of cytoplasmic mRNA, *Mol. Cell. Biol.,* 18, 2932, 1998.

120. Brigelius-Flohé, R., Lötzer, K., Maurer, S., Schultz, M., and Leist, M., Utilization of selenium from different chemical entities for selenoprotein biosynthesis by mammalian cell lines, *BioFactors,* 5, 125, 1996.

121. Berry, M. J., Harney, J. W., Ohama, T., and Hatfield, D. L., Selenocysteine insertion or termination: factors affecting UGA codon fate and complementary anticodon: codon mutations, *Nucleic Acids Res.,* 22, 3753, 1994.

122. Kolmus, H., Flohé, L., and McCarthy, J.E.C., Analysis of eukaryotic mRNA structure directing cotranslational incoporation of selenocysteine, *Nucleic Acids Res.,* 24, 1195, 1996.

123. Weiss, L. S. and Sunde, R. A., Selenium regulation of classical glutathione peroxidase expression requires the 3'-untranslated region in Chinese hamster ovary cells, *J. Nutr.,* 127, 1304, 1997.

124. Bermano, G., Arthur, J. R., and Hesketh, J. E., Role of the 3' untranslated region in the regulation of cytosolic glutathione peroxidase and phospholipid-hydroperoxide glutathione peroxidase gene expression by selenium supply, *Biochem. J.,* 320, 891, 1996.

125. Wen, W., Weiss, L. S., and Sunde, R. A., UGA codon position affects the efficiency of selenocysteine incorporation into glutathione peroxidase-1, *J. Biol. Chem.,* 273, 28533, 1998.

126. Gladyshev, V. N. and Hatfield, D. L., Selenocysteine-containing proteins in mammals, *J. Biomed. Sci.,* 6, 151, 1999.

127. Cheng, W.-H., Combs, Jr., G. F., and Lei, X. G., Knockout of cellular glutathione peroxidase affects selenium-dependent parameters similarly in mice fed adequate and excessive dietary selenium, *BioFactors,* 7, 31, 1998.

128. Cheng, W.-H., Ho, Y.-S., Ross, D. A., Han, Y., Combs, Jr., G. F., and Lei, X. G., Overexpression of cellular glutathione peroxidase does not affect expression of plasma glutathione peroxidase or phospholipid hydroperoxide glutathione peroxidase in mice offered diets adequate or deficient in selenium, *J. Nutr.,* 127, 475, 1997.

129. Fu, Y. X., Cheng, W. H., Ross, D. A., and Lei, X. G., Cellular glutathione peroxidase protects mice against lethal oxidative stress induced by various doses of diquat, *Proc. Soc. Exp. Biol. Med.,* 222, 164, 1999.

18

Ferritin: A Novel Human Ferritin Heavy-Chain MRNA is Predominantly Expressed in the Adult Brain

Madhu S. Dhar

CONTENTS

18.1 Introduction 449
18.2 Role of Iron in Brain Disorders...450
18.3 Role of Ferritin, Transferrin, and Iron Regulatory Proteins in Iron
      Homeostasis 450
18.4 A Novel Ferritin H Chain mRNA in the Human Brain 452
18.5 Ferritin H Chain mRNA in Aging..453
18.6 Conclusions..454
References 455

18.1 Introduction

Ferritin, a 480-kDa protein, is composed of 24 subunits of a 21-kDa heavy chain (FTH) and a 19-kDa light chain. It is a multifunctional molecule involved in detoxification, storage, and transport of iron. Transferrin is a serum glycoprotein involved in iron transport. Free intracellular iron regulates the rates of synthesis of ferritin and transferrin receptors. The accumulation of iron and synthesis of ferritin are developmentally regulated. Both ferritin and transferrin also store and transport aluminum. Studies aimed toward the characterization of the effects of aging and of certain neurodegenerative diseases, for example, Alzheimer's disease (AD), which is associated with the accumulation of iron, aluminum, ferritin, and transferrin, give information about the regulation and contribution of genes involved in iron homeostasis.

The present chapter describes the work involving molecular identification and characterization of a novel ferritin H chain cDNA from the adult and fetal human brains. New findings and a possible role of this human FTH cDNA in normal and AD brains are discussed.

18.2 Role of Iron in Brain Disorders

The brain is a highly compartmentalized organ. An adult human brain weighs about 1.5 kg. and constitutes only about 2% of the body weight. It is aerobic and gets its energy primarily by the oxidation of glucose. Several enzyme reactions involved in the oxidation of glucose require oxidation and/or reduction of Fe^{+2} and Fe^{+3}. About 20% of the oxygen consumed by the body is used by the brain. Brain cells undergo limited or regeneration, and thus, the brain has a perfect environment for the accumulation of various toxins such as aluminum. The brain is also the primary target for diseases arising due to overloading of iron as well as of iron metabolism. For example, Alzheimer's disease (AD) is a neurological disorder that affects primarily older people. AD is characterized by altered memory, cognition, and behavior. In AD, nerve cells in specific areas of the brain degenerate. Besides AD, Parkinson's disease (PD), Huntington's disease (HD), and Hallervorden-Spatz disease are some of the other neurodegenerative diseases associated with the accumulation of iron in the brain.[1-4] The basal ganglia contain the highest levels of iron in the brain. Iron metabolism is disrupted in patients with AD and HD. Overloading of iron in the brain also leads to oxidative damage in the brain cells. However, Bartzokis and Tishler, using Magnetic Resonance Imaging (MRI) to suggest that the increase in the levels of iron in the basal ganglia in AD and HD may be regulated by independent pathways and thus the presence of these high levels of iron at the onset of the disease, propose iron to be a risk factor rather than the result of the disease.[5] In addition to aberrations in the metabolism of iron in the AD brain, defects are also observed in the central nervous system and plasma.[6,7]

18.3 Role of Ferritin, Transferrin, and Iron Regulatory Proteins in Iron Homeostasis

Ferritin is a ubiquitous iron-storage protein with a molecular weight of about 480,000. It is composed of two types of subunits: heavy (H, Mr 21,000) and light (L, Mr 19,000) chains.[8,9] Ferritin is ubiquitously expressed in the tissues like heart, brain, liver, lung, etc. Isoferritins varying in subunit composition exist in different tissues. The H and L subunits of ferritin are genetically and functionally distinct. The H chain subunit is predominantly found in cells and tissues (the heart and the brain) that have high levels of oxidative phosphorylation, while the L subunit is present in the tissues (the liver and the spleen) that store iron.[10] Furthermore, ferritin H and L subunits are independently regulated and are differentially regulated in response to the intracellular iron. Han et al. have recently shown that severe iron deficiency reduced brain ferritin H protein levels significantly in all the regions of the brain, whereas ferritin L levels only in the striatum, substantia nigara, and pons were affected. Exogenously added iron in the diet increased both the H and L subunits. These data suggest post-transcriptional regulation of the two subunits in response to iron.[11]

Ferritin binds several metal ions *in vitro* and *in vivo*.[12] An expanded role for ferritin in metal toxicity is suggested.[13–15] Ferritin–aluminum complexes have been isolated from the brains of two AD patients. Furthermore, ferritin isolated from two AD and one normal brain had from 2 to 4 moles of aluminum bound per mole of protein (Fleming and Joshi, unpublished). It has been shown that in AD brains, the total concentration of iron and ferritin is significantly higher than their age-matched controls. Ferritin is also found to be a component of the senile plaques in the dementia of AD.[16] Taken together, data show that there are elevated levels of ferritin in AD brains, aluminum–ferritin complexes could be isolated *in vitro*, and the rate of iron uptake by ferritin is reduced by aluminum.[17,18]

Transferrin(s) is a family of glycoproteins of MW 80,000. It is a single polypeptide chain and has two metal binding sites, one each at the N- and C-terminal ends. It is the major serum protein involved in iron transport. In the brain, besides being present in the iron-containing cells, transferrin is also found in oligodendrocytes, which are important in myelin synthesis. Transferrin receptor is highly expressed on blood vessels, large neurons in the cortex, striatum, and the hippocampus.[19,20]

In higher organisms, iron bound to transferrin and ferritin constitutes more than 90% of non-heme iron.[21] Both the proteins also sequester other metal ions including aluminum.[22]

Intracellular concentration of iron regulates the synthesis of ferritin and the stability of the transferrin receptors. This translational regulation is due to a conserved sequence (termed as the Iron Responsive Element, IRE) of 28 nucleotides in the 5' untranslated region of ferritin mRNA and the 3' untranslated region of the transferrin receptor RNA.[19,23]

Two iron regulatory proteins (IRPs), IRP1 and IRP2, have been isolated from both rodent and human tissues. These interact with the IRE and modulate the expression of ferritin and transferrin at the mRNA level. Pinero et al. hypothesized that the alterations in the IRP/IRE binding are the event which is altered in the AD brains. They showed a change in the stability of the IRP1/IRE complex in normal vs. AD brain extracts. They propose that relatively high endogenous ribonuclease activity in the AD brain may be one of the mechanisms by which iron homeostasis is disrupted.[24]

18.4   A Novel Ferritin H Chain mRNA in the Human Brain

Ferritin is an important protein involved in the regulation of iron and it is evident that the H subunit (FTH) is of major significance in the central nervous system. Thus, an in-depth characterization of FTH from the human brain was undertaken. A major portion of this project was carried out in collaboration between the laboratories of Dr. J.G. Joshi (Department of Biochemistry, University of Tennessee, Knoxville, TN, USA) and Dr. Marie Percy (Department of Physiology, University of Toronto and Surrey Place Center, Toronto, Ontario, Canada).

High performance liquid chromatography (HPLC) of human brain ferritin revealed five distinct molecular species of brain FTH but, only one major species of ferritin L chain was identified. There is more of the ferritin H subunit than the L in the human brain. Protein chemistry of human brain ferritin from normal and AD brains revealed no differences.[8,21] Thus, molecular studies were initiated to address these observations. A human liver ferritin heavy chain cDNA (a gift from Dr. R. Klausner, NIH, Bethesda, MD) was used as a probe to screen a normal adult human brain cDNA library (Clonetech, Palo Alto, CA, USA). Northern blot analysis of the poly(A)[+] RNAs from human brain and liver showed two transcripts of 1.4 and 1.1 kb, respectively.[25] The 1.4 kb transcript was ubiquitously expressed in the human heart, brain, liver, kidney, lung, skeletal muscle, placenta, and pancreas. The level of expression, however, in each tissue was different. The 1.4 kb RNA is predominantly expressed in the brain, while its level of expression in the liver is 10 times lower.[26] On the other hand, the 1.1 kb RNA is predominantly expressed in the liver. Sequence analysis showed that the 1.1kb transcript is identical to the previously characterized RNA from liver and lymphoctes.[27] The larger transcript contained an additional 279 bp sequence at the 3′ end. A genomic clone containing the 279 bp sequence was obtained.[28] Sequence comparison of the cDNA and the genomic clones showed that in the larger transcript, the 279 bp sequence is a part of the transcribed sequence and hence of the mature mRNA, whereas in the smaller one, it is a part of the non-transcribed sequence present only in the genomic clone.

These data suggested that differential processing of the primary transcript of the FTH mRNA in human tissues generates two mature mRNAs of 1.4 and 1.1 kb. This is due to the utilization of an alternative polyadenylation site in the precursor mRNA. Sequencing of the cDNAs confirmed this observation, wherein, one polyadenylation site is identical to the one reported to be in the liver, and the other is a part of the 279 bp fragment and is found to be 16 bp upstream to the poly(A) tract.[29] Primer extension and reverse-transcriptase polymerase chain reaction (RT-PCR) were used to obtain full-length cDNAs from both the normal as well as AD brains. Sequence analysis showed that the IRE and the 279 bp sequence coexist in at least one of the FTH transcripts in the brain.[8] Search for an L chain mRNA consisting of the 279 bp sequence was unsuccessful (Dhar and Joshi, unpublished). Thus, it is possible that the novel H chain mRNA identified in the human brain has a special role in brain homeostasis.

Percy et al. (1998) showed tissue- as well as region-specific expression of the novel FTH message within the brain — the level of expression was the highest in the amygdala, caudate nucleus, putamen, substantia nigra, and spinal cord, and lowest in the cerebellum.[30]

In AD, hippocampus is often the most seriously affected structure. To determine whether the observed elevated levels of ferritin in the AD brain are area specific and disease dependent, and if the concentration of H chain parallels the changes in the 279 bp containing message, ribonuclease protection assays (RPA) were carried out using total RNA from human liver and brain as well as from the hippocampal regions of normal and the AD-affected brains. Furthermore, tissue *in situ* RT-PCR analysis was also carried out to visualize relative levels of only FTH mRNA containing the 279 bp sequence in its 3'UTR in different cell types. Preliminary data showed lower concentrations of the mRNA in the liver compared to the brain. However, the concentrations were identical in both the normal and the AD brains.[8,30,31] In the normal adult hippocampus, this new message localizes strongly to non-neuronal cells, capillary endothelial cells, and to the granule cells of the dentate gyrus.[33] Future experiments involving Northern blotting, RPA analysis, and primer extension analysis are required to study the expression of the novel H chain mRNA in AD tissues.

18.5 Ferritin H Chain mRNA in Aging

The accumulation of iron and the synthesis of ferritin in the human brain is developmentally regulated. A human fetal brain contains low levels of iron and ferritin.[32] By contrast, an adult human brain contains large quantities of iron and about one third of its total nonheme iron is stored in ferritin.[33]

An 11-week-old human fetal brain (FB) cDNA library (a gift from Dr. Swaroop, University of Michigan, Ann Arbor, MI) was screened using the human liver ferritin H-chain cDNA as the probe. Northern blot analysis together with sequencing showed that one type of cDNA corresponded to the FTH transcript reported in liver while the other was identical to the novel FTH transcript identified in the adult human brain.[29,34] The relatively low level of the 279 bp carrying transcript in the fetal brain observed in quantitative *in situ* hybridization experiments is indicative of developmental regulation of this message. The iron responsive element could not be detected, instead a new 54 bp sequence is observed. The role of this 54 bp sequence is not yet known. [30,34]

18.6 Conclusions

Our understanding of the mechanisms of iron transport and homeostasis in the brain is still limited. A large number of experiments to delineate the role of these new biological tools have to be carried out. Percy et al. (1998) reported some interesting features from the predicted secondary structures of FTH RNAs containing the IRE in the 5′UTR and the novel 279 bp sequence in the 3′UTR. The residues 999–1120 (located in the novel 279 bp 3′UTR) formed three stem-loop structures. Blast sequence similarity search showed about 88% homology between the positions 1013 and 1095 of this stem-loop region and a region in the 3′UTR of human endopeoxide synthase type II cyclooxygenase-2 (COX 2).[30] These enzymes are rate-limiting in the synthesis of prostaglandins, which are mediators of inflammation. A role of COX-2 is also suggested in arthritis rheumatoid.[35,36] Even though there is some homology between the 279 bp sequence and another gene not related to ferritin, the 279 bp sequence seems to be associated with the functional FTH gene and mRNA. This novel FTH cDNA maps exclusively to human chromosome 11. It maps to the same locus as the functional liver FTH cDNA.[31] These observations suggest that it is unlikely that this entire sequence exists in any other human gene including the FTH pseudogenes, the gene for human liver ferritin L, or its pseudogenes that map to other human chromosomes than 11.

The interactions between iron, the iron-responsive element (IRE) in the 5′UTR of H and L-ferritin mRNA, and in the 3′UTR of the transferrin receptor mRNA as well as the IRE-binding protein (IRE-BP) are now well documented.[19] The role of the novel FTH cDNAs from human adult and fetal brains is still unknown. Henderson et al. reported a second IRE-binding protein, IRF, an Iron Regulatory Factor, in mammalian tissues, with the highest levels in the brain.[37] Though the affinity of IRE to IRF is similar to that of IRE-BP, the role of IRF is still under investigation. The identification of a novel cDNA for ferritin H subunit along with a new iron-binding protein, both highly expressed in human brains, may be functionally relevant rather than a coincidence. Their roles in ferritin synthesis are unknown; however, a few interesting questions can open new avenues for exciting research — do the IRE-BP and the IRF bind to the 279 bp sequence? If yes, how does this affect the translation of ferritin H chain? Why is a part of the 279 bp sequence conserved/present in human COX-2? What is the biological role of this conserved sequence? Is there any differential transcription of the liver-like ferritin H chain vs. the longer brain-like message? Is the elongated form of FTH expressed in other animal species? Are there any factors or conditions like stress or disease that favor one form over the other? What, if any, is the role of the elongated message in AD brain? Does it influence the expression of the FTH gene differentially in the AD brain vs. the normal human brain? If so, what triggers this differential expression? Future experiments to study the biological function and role of this novel elongated FTH cDNA have to be carried out.

Acknowledgments: The author acknowledges the Council of Tobacco Research for funding her postdoctoral project involving the molecular characterization of the ferritin H chain in human adult and fetal brains. The author also extends her gratitude to Dr. J. G. Joshi and to all the students, staff, and faculty of the biochemistry dept., University of Tennessee at Knoxville for their valuable discussions, guidance, and support throughout this project.

References

1. Bouras, C., Giannakopoulos, P., Good, P. F., Hsu, A., Hof, P. R., and Perl, D. P., A laser microprobe mass analysis of brain aluminum and iron in dementia pugilistica: comparison with Alzheimer's disease, *Eur. Neurol.*, 38, 53, 1997.
2. Logroscino, G., Marder, K., Graziano, J., Freyer, G., Slavkovich, V., LoIacono, N., Cote, L., and Mayeux, R., Altered systemic iron metabolism in Parkinson's disease, *Neurology*, 49, 714, 1997.
3. Dexter, D. T., Jenner, P., Shapira, A. H., and Marsden, C. D., Alterations in levels of iron, ferritin, and other trace metals in neurodegenerative diseases affecting basal ganglia. *Ann. Neurol.*, 32, (Suppl.), S94, 1992.
4. Taylor, T. D., Litt, M., Kramer, P., Pandolfo, M., Angelini, L., Nardocci, N., Davis, S., Pineda, M., Hattori, H., Flett, P. J., Cilio, M. R., Bertini, E., and Hayflick, S. J., Homozygosity mapping of Hallervorden-Spatz syndrome to chromosome 20p12.3-p13, *Nat. Genet.*, 14, 479, 1996.
5. Bartzokis, G. and Tishler, T. A., MRI evaluation of basal ganglia ferritin iron and neurotoxicity in Alzheimer's and Huntington's disease, *Cell. Mol. Biol. (Noisy-le-grand)*, 46, 821, 2000.
6. Feldman, H., Kennard, M., Yamada, T., Adams, S., and Jefferies, W., *Alzheimer's Disease: Biology, Diagnosis and Therapeutics*, Iqbal, K., Winblad, B., Nishimura, T., Takaeda, M., and Wisniewski, H. M., Eds., Wiley, New York, 1997.
7. Fischer, P., Gotz, M. E., Danielczyk, W., Gsell, W., and Riederer, P., Blood transferrin and ferritin in Alzheimer's disease, *Life Sci.*, 60, 2273, 1997.
8. Joshi, J. G., Fleming, J. T., Dhar, M., and Chauthaiwale, V., A novel ferritin heavy chain messenger ribonuleic acid in the human brain, *J. Neurol. Sci.*, 134 (Suppl.), 52, 1995.
9. Beard, J. L., Dawson, H., and Pinero, D. J., Iron metabolism: a comprehensive review, *Nutr. Rev.*, 54, 295, 1996.
10. Connor, J. R., Boeshore, K. L., Benkovic, S. A., and Menzies, S. L., Isoforms of ferritin have a specific cellular distribution in the brain, *J. Neurosci. Res.*, 37, 461, 1994.
11. Han, J., Day, J. R., Thomson, K., Connor, J. R., and Beard, J. L., Iron deficiency alters H- and L-ferritin expression in rat brain, *Cell. Mol. Biol. (Noisy-le-grand)*, 46, 517, 2000.
12. Price, D. J. and Joshi, J. G., Ferritin. Binding of beryllium and other divalent metal ions, *J. Biol. Chem.*, 258, 10873, 1983.

13. Lindenschmidt, R. C., Sendelbach, L. E., Witschi, H. P., Price, D. J., Fleming, J., and Joshi, J. G., Ferritin and *in vivo* beryllium toxicity, *Toxicol. Appl. Pharmacol.*, 82, 344, 1986.
14. Joshi, J. G., Goodman, S., Deshpande, V. V., and Price, D. J., in *Proteins of Iron Storage and Transport*, Spike, G., Montreuil, J., Crichton, R. R., and Mazurier, J., Eds., Elsevier, Amsterdam, 1985, 93.
15. Fleming, J. T. and Joshi, J. G., Ferritin: the role of aluminum in ferritin function, *Neurobiol. Aging*, 12, 413, 1991.
16. Grundke-Iqbal, I., Fleming, J. T., Tung, Y. C., Lassmann, H., Iqbal, K., and Joshi, J. G., Ferritin is a component of the neuritic (senile) plaque in Alzheimer dementia, *Acta Neuropathol. (Berl.)*, 81, 105, 1990.
17. Cochran, M. and Chawtar, V., Interaction of horse-spleen ferritin with aluminum citrate, *Clin. Chim. Acta*, 178, 79, 1984.
18. Fleming, J. and Joshi, J. G., Ferritin: Isolation of aluminum-ferritin complex from brain, *Proc. Natl. Acad. Sci. USA*, 84, 7866, 1987.
19. Theil, E. C., Regulation of ferritin and transferrin receptor mRNAs, *J. Biol. Chem.*, 265, 4771, 1990.
20. Connor, J. R. and Menzies, S. L., Cellular management of iron in the brain, *J. Neurol. Sci.*, 134 (Suppl.), 33, 1995.
21. Aisen, P., and Listowsky, I., Iron transport and storage proteins, *Ann. Rev. Biochem.*, 49, 357, 1980.
22. Joshi, J. G. and Clauberg, M., Ferritin: An iron storage protein with diverse function, *BioFactors*, 1, 207, 1988.
23. Joshi, J. G., Dhar, M., Clauberg, M., and Chauthaiwale, V., Iron and aluminum homeostasis in neural disorders, *Environ. Health Perspect.*, 102 (Suppl. 3), 207, 1994.
24. Pinero, D. J., Hu, J., and Connor, J. R., Alterations in the interaction between iron regulatory proteins and their iron responsive element in normal and Alzheimer's diseased brains, *Cell. Mol. Biol. (Noisy-le-grand)*, 46, 761, 2000.
25. Joshi, J. G., Fleming, J. T., Dhar, M., and Chauthaiwale, V., A novel ferritin heavy chain messenger ribonucleic acid in the human brain, *J. Neurol. Sci.*, 134 (Suppl.), 52, 1995.
26. Dhar, M. S. and Joshi, J. G., Detection and quantitation of the novel ferritin heavy chain message in human tissues, *BioFactors*, 4, 147, 1994.
27. Chou, C., Gatti, R. A., Fuller, M. L., Concannon, P., Wong, A., Chada, S., David, R. C., and Salser, W. A., Structure and expression of ferritin gene in a human promyelocytic cell line that differentiates *in vitro*, *Mol. Cell. Biol.*, 6, 566, 1986.
28. Costanzo, F., Colombo, M., Staempfli, S., Santor, C., Marone, M., Frank, R., Delius, H., and Cortese, R., Structure of gene and pseudogenes of human apoferritin H, *Nucleic Acids Res.*, 14, 721, 1986.
29. Dhar, M. S. and Joshi, J. G., Differential processing of the ferritin heavy chain mRNA in human liver and adult human brain, *J. Neurochem.*, 61, 2140, 1993.
30. Percy, M. E., Wong, S., Bauer, S., Liaghati-Nasseri, N., Perry, M. D., Chauthaiwale, V. M., Dhar, M., and Joshi, J. G., Iron metabolism and human ferritin heavy chain cDNA from adult brain with an elongated untranslated region: new findings and insights, *Analyst*, 123, 41, 1998.
31. Percy, M. E., Bauer, S. J., Rainey, S., McLachlan, D. R., Dhar M. S., and Joshi, J. G., Localisation of a new ferritin heavy chain sequence present in human brain mRNA to chromosome 11, *Genome*, 38, 450, 1995.

32. Hallgren, B. and Sourander, P., The effect of age on the nonheme iron in the human brain, *J. Neurochem.*, 3, 41, 1958.
33. Hill, J. M., The distribution of iron in the brain, in *Brain Iron: Neurochemical and Behavioral Aspects*, Youdin, M.B.H., Ed., Taylor and Francis, London, 1988, 1.
34. Dhar, M., Chauthaiwale, V., and Joshi, J. G., Sequence of a cDNA encoding the ferritin H-chain from an 11-week-old human fetal brain, *Gene*, 126, 275, 1993.
35. O'Neill, G. P. and Ford-Hutchinson, A. W., Expression of mRNA for cyclooxygenase-1 and cyclooxygenase-2 in human tissues, *FEBS Lett.*, 330, 156, 1993.
36. Ristimaki, A., Narko, K., and Hla, T., Down-regulation of cytokine-induced cyclooxygenase-2 transcript isoforms by dexamethasone: evidence for post-transcriptional regulation, *Biochem. J.*, 318, 325, 1996.
37. Henderson, B. R., Menotti, E., and Kuhn, L. C., Iron regulatory proteins 1 and 2 bind distinct sets of RNA target sequences, *J. Biol. Chem.*, 271, 4900, 1996.

Index

A

AA. *See* Arachidonic acid
Abbreviations, 119, 151, 301–302, 377, 439
Aberrant crypt focus (ACF), 235
AC. *See* Adenylyl cyclase
ACC. *See* Acetyl CoA-carboxylase
Acetyl CoA, 3
Acetyl CoA-carboxylase (ACC), 2–3, 52
Acetyl/malonyl transferase, 3
Acquired immunodeficiency syndrome
    (AIDS), 403
acrp30. *See* Adipocyte complement related
    protein
ACS1. *See* Acyl-CoA synthetase 1
Acyl-CoA dehydrogenase, 93
Acyl-CoA esters, 93–94
Acyl-CoA synthetase 1 (ACS1)
    function, 77–78
    gene expression
        disease state-specific regulation, 87–94
        nutritional and hormonal regulation,
            82–87, 94
        tissue distribution and developmental
            regulation, 79–80
    gene family, 81–82
    structure, 78–79
ADD-1. *See* Adipocyte determination and
    differentiation factor
Adenine nucleotide translocase, 93
Adenosine monophosphate (AMP), 78
Adenosine receptor, 145
Adenosine triphosphate (ATP), 78
    in apoptosis, 274
    mitochondrial respiration and, 263, 323,
        324, 327
    threshold effects of mutant mtDNA and,
        328–329
Adenylyl cyclase (AC), 133, 143, 145, 147,
    266–267
Adhesion molecules, 398, 402, 403
Adipocyte complement related protein
    (acrp30), 27

Adipocyte determination and differentiation
    factor (ADD-1)
    in adipocyte gene expression, 28–30, 71
    general characteristics, 37–38
    nutritional considerations, 38–39
    role in insulin transcription, 10–11
Adipocytes
    cascade of transcriptional events, 28–30
    de-differentiation, 88
    differentiation, 28–30, 41, 65–71
    fatty acid binding protein regulation in,
        103, 111, 117–118
    gene expression
        and dietary fatty acid, 68–71
        and nutrition, 30–41
    pleiotropic functions, 26–28
    3T3-L1 cell line. *See* 3T3-L1 adipocytes
Adipose tissue. *See* Brown adipose tissue;
    White adipose tissue
Adipsin, 27
β-Adrenergic receptor
    effects of adenylyl cyclase, 266–267
    as fat-specific gene, 264
    novel signaling properties, 269–270
    selective agonists, 268–269
    thermogenesis by, 264–265, 266
Adrenocorticotropin receptor, 213
Advanced glycation end products (AGE), 408
Aging
    adenosine receptors, 145
    ferritin H chain mRNA, 453
    T-lymphocyte function, 400
    in vivo response time, 7
Agouti
    antagonist for melanocortin receptors, 178
    effects on calcium, 16, 212, 217–220
    gene mutations, 206–208
    interactions with leptin, 215–217
    interactions with mahogany and
        mahoganoid, 215–216
    molecular characteristics, 209–212
    obesity and, 205–222
    peripheral actions, 217
    regulation of FAS gene, 6, 16

role of melanocortin receptors in signaling, 212–214
Agouti related protein (AGRP), 214, 215
ALA. *See* α-Linoleic acid
Alcohol
    fetal alcohol syndrome, 148–149
    gene expression in the central nervous system and, 131–150
    prevalence of use, U.S., 132
Aluminum, 449, 451
Alzheimer's disease, 449
    aluminum and, 451
    effects on the hippocampus, 453
    ferritin and, 450, 451, 453
    from mtDNA mutations, 325
γ-Aminobutyric acid receptors (GABA), 133, 135, 137–139
Amphetamine, 141, 146
Amyotrophic lateral sclerosis, 413–414
Angiotensin II, 6, 15
Angiotensinogen (AGT), 27
Anorexia, murine mutation model, 190
Antioxidant defense systems, 399
Antioxidant response element (ARE), 399
Antioxidants, modes of action, 394, 396–398, 405
APC gene, 235–240, 249
Apoptosis, 273–274
    of colorectal cancer cells, and vitamin E, 406
    induction by reactive oxygen species, 398
    NUR77 and, 298
Arachidonic acid (AA)
    effects on adipocyte differentiation, 66
    effects on lipogenesis, 12, 13
    vs. N-3 fatty acids, 245, 246, 249
ARE. See Antioxidant response element; AU-rich elements
Aspirin, 248
Ataxias and vitamin E, 412–413
Ataxia with isolated vitamin E deficiency (AVED), 412
ATB-BMPA, 170
Atherosclerosis
    ACS1 esters and, 94
    SCD regulation and, 50
    vitamin E and, 407
ATP-citrate lyase, 2
AU-rich elements (ARE), 57

B

BDNF. *See* Brain-derived neurotrophic factor

Beef tallow, 64
Behavior, food intake, 178, 186
Blood clotting factor, 402
Brain
    ferritin H chain mRNA in, 452–453
    fetal, iron and ferritin in, 453
    percent of oxygen consumed by the body, 450
    role of iron in disorders, 450
    role of uncoupling proteins, 274
    seizures and induction of NUR77, 298
Brain-derived neurotrophic factor (BDNF), 148, 150
Breast cancer, 405
BRL49653, 92
Brown adipose tissue, 262. *See also* Uncoupling proteins

C

Calcium, dietary
    absorption and vitamin D, 350
    modulation of intracellular calcium by, 220–222
Calcium, intracellular
    effects of agouti, 16, 212, 217–220
    L-type channels, 140–141
    mediation of acyl-CoA, 92
    modulation by dietary calcium, 220–222
    in rapid nongenomic response to vitamin D_3, 363–364, 376
    reduced mobilization with oxidative stress, 400
cAMP. *See* 3',5'-Cyclic monophosphate
cAMP responsive element-binding protein (CREBP), 133, 147–148, 149
Cancer
    breast, and vitamin E, 405
    chemotherapeutic agents, 404–405
    colorectal, 231–250, 406
    control of cellular proliferation by vitamin E, 404–407
    epithelial, 284
    prostate, 398
    SCD regulation and, 50
    tumor regression, 239
Carbacyclin, 66
Carboxypeptidases, 178, 184
Cardiovascular disease, 26, 407–408
Carnitine palmitoyl transferase 1, 93
Catecholamines, 266
β-Catenin, 237–238
Caveolin-1, 105

CCAAT/enhancer binding proteins (C/EBP)
in adipocyte gene expression, 28–30, 41,
70–71
cooperative functions, 36
enoyl reductase, 3
general characteristics, 34–35
nutritional considerations, 36–37
translational and post-translational
modifications, 35
Cell-cycle inhibitor factor, 406
Cellular glutathione peroxidase, 428,
430–434, 436–439
Cellular membranes, effects of reactive
oxygen species, 394
Cellular rapid nongenomic responses to
vitamin D_3, 363, 376
Cellular retinoic acid binding proteins
(CRABP), 290
Cellular retinol binding proteins (CRBP),
284–287, 290
Central nervous system (CNS)
alcohol and gene expression in the,
131–150
disease from mtDNA mutations, 325
obesity as disease of the, 178
Chemotherapeutic agents, 404–405
Chick ovalbumin upstream promotor-
transcription factors (COUP-TF),
293, 294–296, 298–299, 301
Chloramphenical acetyl transferase (CAT),
6–7
Cholecalciferol. *See* Vitamin D_3
Chromosomal DNA (cDNA)
ferritin H chain, 450, 452, 453
structural effects of reactive oxygen
species, 394
vitamin D_3 nuclear receptor binding to,
368–370
Chromosome 9, 412
Chromosome 8q13, 412
Cirrhosis, 17, 411
CLA. *See* Conjugated linoleic acid
Clonidine, 144
Cloning
β-adrenergic receptor gene, 269
agouti gene, 205
brown adipose fat uncoupling proteins,
262, 263, 264
hippocampal HT22 cells, 413
quantitative trait locus analysis for, 195
vitamin D-binding protein, 358
Clozapine, 143
Cocaine, 141, 146
Coconut oil, 64, 65, 325
Collagen, 410, 411

Colorectal cancer, 231–250, 406
Conjugated linoleic acid (CLA), 53, 240–243
Copper, regulation of fatty acid synthase
gene, 16–17
Copper chelators, 413
Corn oil, 15, 325
Corn starch, 64
COUP-TF. *See* Chick ovalbumin upstream
promotor-transcription factors
COX. *See* Cyclooxygenases; Cytochrome-c
oxidase complex
CPE mutations, 186–188, 191, 193, 194
CRABP. *See* Cellular retinoic acid binding
proteins
CRBP. *See* Cellular retinol binding proteins
CTMC, 399
3',5'-Cyclic monophosphate (cAMP)
acyl-CoA synthetase I, 83
dibutyryl, 8
effects of β-adrenergic receptor gene, 269
effects on lipogenesis, 13–14
Cyclohexamide, 8
Cyclooxygenases (COX), 13, 233–234
characteristics, 235
effects of aging, 400–401
effects of vitamin E, 406, 414
interaction with GLA, 247
role in rheumatoid arthritis, 454
role in tumorigenesis, 248
upregulation, 238–239
Cysteine residues, 398
Cytochrome b_5, 49
Cytochrome-c oxidase complex (COX), 325
Cytochrome P-450, 356, 375

D

$1\alpha24(OH)_2D_3$. *See* Vitamin D_3
DAT. *See* Dopamine transporter
D-box, 368, 369
DBP. *See* Vitamin D-binding protein
Dehydratase, 3
Dementia, 274
Δ-6 Desaturase, 245, 247
Developmental regulation, acyl-CoA
synthetase 1, 79–80
DHA. *See* Docosahexaenoic acid
25(OH)D-24-hydroxylase, 375–376
Diabetes, 25, 30
ACS1 gene mechanism, 92, 93
atherosclerosis with, 94
maternally inherited, and deafness, 326,
328
from mtDNA mutations, 325, 326, 327

reversal, 264
transient gestational, 191
Type II, 193, 273
vitamin E and, 408–409
Diacylglycerol, 133
Diet
    calcium, and modulation of intracellular
        calcium, 220–222
    effects of amount and type of fatty acid,
        64–65
    fat body mass and, 63
    fat-free, 7
    fat intake and intestinal tumorigenesis,
        231–250
    food intake behavior control, 178, 186
    high-calcium, 220–222
    high-fat, 64
    selenium-deficient, 437
    trends, 17
    typical American, 17
    typical Western, 5, 102, 239
    vitamin A-deficient, 286
    vitamin D-deficient, 355–356
    vitamin E-deficient, 400, 409, 412
Dietary regulation
    of fatty acid synthase gene, 1–17
    of stearoyl-CoA desaturase, 49–58
    of uncoupling protein expression,
        270–271
Disease. *See also specific diseases*
    associated with prohormone processing
        defects, 190–193
    energy homeostasis disorders, 185–195
    mitochondrial, due to mtDNA mutations,
        325–328
    -specific regulation of acyl-CoA
        synthetase 1, 87–94
    vitamin E and gene expression, 399–414
Distribution. *See* Tissue distribution
DNA. *See* Chromosomal DNA;
        Mitochondrial DNA
Docosahexaenoic acid (DHA), 240–243
Domains of fatty acid synthase, 3
Dopamine receptors, 141–143
Dopamine transporter (DAT), 146
Drug-related disorders, 132, 141, 145, 146

E

Eating behavior, 178, 186
E-boxes, 9–10, 171
Eicosanoids, 34, 41, 53, 400
Eicosapentaenoic acid (EPA), 240–243, 245,
        246

(n-9)-Eicosatrienoic acid, 51–52
Encephalomyopathy, 326
Endocrine functions of adipocytes, 27
Endocrine system of vitamin D
    generation of biological responses,
        356–358
    genetics, 372–376
Endocrinopathy, multiple, 191
Endoproteases, 183–184
Energy homeostasis
    adipocyte gene expression and, 30
    distal effects on, 193–195
    food intake behavior and, 178, 186
    prohormone processing and disorders of,
        177–195
Enhancer binding proteins. *See*
        CCAAT/enhancer binding
        proteins
EPA. *See* Eicosapentaenoic acid
Epidemiological studies, vitamin E, 399, 407
Epinephrine, 267
Epithelial cancer, 284
Epithelial tissue, differentiation and vitamin
        A deficiency, 284
Ergocalciferol. *See* Vitamin D₂
ERK pathway, 269–270
Erythropoietin, 410
Estrogen, regulation of glutathione
        peroxidases, 434
Estrogen receptors, 300, 371, 405
Ethanol, effects on gene expression in the
        CNS, 131–150
Eumelanin, 206
Evolutionary aspects, 179, 365
Extracellular glutathione peroxidase,
        428–429, 430–431
Eyes, disorders of the, 287, 412

F

FABPpm transport protein, 103–104
Familial adenomatous polyposis (FAP), 235
FAP. *See* Familial adenomatous polyposis
FAR. *See* Fatty acid receptor
FAS. *See* Fatty acid synthase
Fasting
    effects on acyl-CoA synthetase I, 82
    effects on insulin, 5
    effects on lipogenesis, 5, 7, 13–14
    in vivo effects, 7
FAT/CD36. *See* Fatty acid translocase
fat mutation, 186–188
FATP. *See* Fatty acid transport proteins

Fatty acid
    deficiency, 52, 63
    effects of amount and type, 64–65
    flux across plasma membrane, 102–105,
        114. *See also* Fatty acid transport
        proteins
    metabolites, 69–70
    molecular sensors of, 68–69
    saturated *vs.* unsaturated, 64
    stimulation of uncoupling proteins,
        271–272
Fatty acid binding proteins (FABP), 103,
        106–107
    regulation by PPARs, 117–118
    regulation of gene expression, 107,
        108–112
Fatty acid receptor (FAR), 105
Fatty acid synthase (FAS)
    effects of type of dietary fat, 64–65
    organization and function, 3–4
    rat *vs.* human, 3
    role in fatty acid synthesis, 2–3
    SCD gene expression and production of,
        51–52
    tissue distribution, 4, 68
Fatty acid synthase gene
    dietary regulation, 1–17
    5'-flanking region, 6–7
        binding by SREBPs, 9–10
        deletion experiments, 8, 14
    intracellular calcium and, 218
    regulation, 5–7
        by glucose, 5–7, 11–12
        by insulin, 5, 8–11, 14, 15–16
        obesity genes, 15–16
        by other factors, 16–17
        by PUFA, 12–13
        by thyroid hormone, 6, 14
    structure, 4
    transcription initiation sites, 4
Fatty acid translocase (FAT/CD36), 104, 108
Fatty acid transport proteins (FATP)
    effects of PPARs on, 116–118
    mechanisms of flux across plasma
        membrane, 101–107
    molecular mechanism of regulation,
        113–118
    nutrient regulation of gene expression,
        107–119
    types and tissue distribution, 103
Fenofibrate, 86
Ferritin
    characteristics, 449, 450
    role in iron homeostasis, 450–451
    role in metal toxicity, 451

Ferritin H chain (FTH)
    cDNA in humans, 450, 452, 454
    mRNA, in the human brain, 452–453
Fetal alcohol syndrome, 148–149
Fibrates, 34, 68
Fibroblasts, 36
    PPAR-expressing, 68, 69, 70
    rapid nongenomic responses to vitamin
        D_3, 363
    skin, effects of vitamin E, 398
Fibrosis, 397, 411
Fish oil
    -derived n-3 fatty acids, 240–243
    diet containing, 325
5HT receptors. *See* Serotonin receptors
5-HTT. *See* Serotonin transporter
Food intake behavior, 178, 186
Frataxin gene, 412
Free fatty acid (FFA), 27
Free radicals, 394, 397, 399. *See also* Reactive
        oxygen species
Friedreich's ataxia, 412
Fructose, 165
FTH. *See* Ferritin H chain

G

GABA. *See* γ-Aminobutyric acid
Gastrointestinal glutathione peroxidase, 428,
        437, 438
Gene transcription, mitochondrial DNA,
        331–336
Genetic mapping, quantitative trait loci,
        194–195
GH. *See* Growth hormone
GLA. *See* γ-Linoleic acid
Glinbenclamide, 220
Glomerulosclerosis, 410
Glossary, 439–440
Glucocorticoid response element (GRE), 334,
        335
Glucocorticoids, effects on lipogenesis, 5,
        13–14
Glucokinase, 93
Glucose
    effects of deprivation, 164–165
    insulin-stimulated, nutrient control of,
        163–171
    metabolism by adipocytes, 27
    regulation of lipogenesis, 5–7, 11–12
Glucose-6-phosphatase, 93
Glucose-6-phosphate (G-6-P), 11, 12
Glucose-6-phosphate dehydrogenase
        (G6PDH), 2

Glucose response-binding protein (GRBP), 12
Glucose transporter family, 164
GLUT1, 164, 166
GLUT4, 36–37, 67, 166–171
Glutamate, 132–133
Glutathione, 413, 426
Glutathione peroxidases (GPX), 409, 439
    characterization, 426–430
    differential regulation and function,
        430–439
    enzyme comparisons with deiodinases,
        431–432
    regulation by non-selenium factors, 434
    tissue specificity, 436–437
Glutathione S-transferase, 399
Glycemic index, 17
Glycine receptors, effects of alcohol on gene
        expression, 135, 139–140
Golgi apparatus, 180–181
G-6-P. *See* Glucose-6-phosphate
G6PDH. *See* Glucose-6-phosphate
        dehydrogenase
GPCR. *See* G-protein-coupled receptor
G-protein-coupled receptor (GPCR), 133,
        141–146, 264
G-proteins, 147
GPX. *See* Glutathione peroxidases
Granulopoiesis, 406–407
Growth factors (GF), 150
Growth hormone (GH), 16
Guanine nucleotides, 147, 271–272
Guanosin-triphosphate, 436

H

Hallervorden-Spatz disease, 450
Haloperidol, 413
Heart fatty acid binding protein, 103, 111–112
Heat production. *See* Thermogenesis
Heme oxygenase-1 gene, 398
Hemoglobin glycation with diabetes, 408
Hepatic fatty acid binding protein (HABP),
        103, 109–110, 117–118
Hepatic lipogenesis, 5, 88–91
Hepatic retinol, 287
Hepatic tissue damage, role in vitamin E in
        reversal, 411–412
Hepatocyte nuclear factor-4 (HNF-4), 293,
        298–299, 300
Hereditary nonpolyposis colorectal cancer
        (HNPCC), 235–236
High-density microsomal fraction (HDM),
        GLUT4, 168–169
Histone-like proteins, 335

HMG CoA reductase, 93
HNF-4. *See* Hepatocyte nuclear factor-4
HO-1 gene, 399
HODE. *See* Hydroxyoctadecadienoic acid
Hormone response element (HRE), 358,
        368–370
Human immunodeficiency virus (HIV), 403
Huntington's disease, 450
Hydrogen peroxide, 398, 410, 426
Hydroxyoctadecadienoic acid (HODE), 33
Hyperglycemia, 408–409
Hyperinsulinemia, 25–26
Hyperlipidemia, 30
Hyperplasia, 64
Hypersensitivity reaction, 400
Hypertension, 25
Hypertrophy, 64
Hypothyroidism, 14
Hypoxia-induced factor-1, 403

I

Ibuprofen, 78
ICAM-1. *See* Intercellular adhesion molecule-1
ID. *See* Iodothyronine 5'-deiodinases
IEG. *See* Immediate early genes
IL. *See specific interleukins*
Immediate early genes (IEG), 148, 149
Immune function
    tissue distribution of uncoupling proteins
        and, 272–273
    vitamin E and, 399–404
Immunoglobulin A nephropathies, 409, 410
Indomethacin, 248
Inflammation and vitamin E, 399–400
Inflammatory reaction, 402
Inositoltriphosphate, 133
Insulin
    acyl-CoA synthetase 1 and, 83–87, 92, 93
    control of food intake behavior, 178
    effects of fasting. *See* Fasting, effects on
        insulin
    effects on lipogenesis, 5, 8–11, 14
    effects on PPAR mRNA levels, 34
    interaction with agouti, 218–219
    mediation by ADD-1, 37–39
    mediation by tumor necrosis factor α, 88
    nutrient control of glucose transport,
        163–171
    regulation of lipogenesis, 5–7
    transcription factors, 9–11
    upstream stimulatory factors, 9, 11, 12
Insulin-like growth factor I (IGF-1), 80

Insulin responsive sequences (IRS), 8–9, 14, 107
Intercellular adhesion molecule-1 (ICAM-1), 398, 403
Interferon-γ, 40
Interleukin-1, 88, 90, 403, 410
Interleukin-2, 400
Interleukin-4, 40
Interleukin-6, 27, 400, 403
Intestinal fatty acid binding protein, 110–111, 130
Intestinal glutathione peroxidase. *See* Gastrointestinal glutathione peroxidase
Intestine
    rapid nongenomic responses to vitamin D$_3$, 363
    tumorigenesis and dietary fat, 231–250
Iodothyronine 5'-deiodinases (ID)
    characteristics, 427
    selenium and patterns of expression, 431–432, 437
IRE. *See* Iron-responsive element
IRF. *See* Iron regulatory factor
Iron
    homeostasis, 450–451, 454
    role in brain disorders, 450
Iron regulatory factor (IRF), 454
Iron regulatory proteins (IRP), 451
Iron-responsive element (IRE), 451, 454
IRP. *See* Iron regulatory proteins
Isoprostane, 408
Isoproterenol, 269

J

Janus kinases (JAK), 39

K

Kearns-Sayre syndrome, 327
β-Ketoacyl synthase, 3
Kexin, 179
Kunitz protein inhibitor (KPI), 185

L

LAP. *See* Liver activator protein
Leber's hereditary optic neuropathy (LHON), 325–326
Leigh's syndrome, 326, 328
Leptin
    control of food intake behavior, 178

    interactions with agouti, 215–217
    obesity and gene mutations, 178
    regulation by PPARs, 116
    regulation of acyl-CoA synthetase 1 gene, 15–16
    regulation of FAS gene, 15–16
Leucine, 326, 328
Ligand-gated receptors, 132–140
Ligands
    β-adrenergic, 264
    of PPAR, 32–34, 69, 113–115, 271
    of vitamin D$_3$ nuclear receptor, 359, 370–372
α-Linoleic acid (ALA), 240–243, 247
γ-Linoleic acid (GLA), 240–244
LIP. *See* Liver inhibitor protein
Lipogenesis, 2
    activation by calcium, 218–219
    effects of fasting, 5, 7, 13–14
    enzymatic process, 2–3
    hepatic vs. adipose tissue, 5
    human, 5
    lipoprotein lipase vs. *de novo*, 2, 7
    sites, 5
Lipopolysaccharide (LPS), 88–89
Lipoprotein lipase (LPL)
    deficiency, 17, 63
    vs. *de novo* lipogenesis, 2, 7
Liver activator protein (LAP), 35
Liver inhibitor protein (LIP), 35
Long-chain fatty acids (LCFA)
    effects on adipocyte differentiation, 66–67, 71
    metabolism, 77
    regulation of acyl-CoA synthase 1 gene expression, 85–86
Low-density lipoprotein (LDL), 395, 407
Low-density lipoprotein scavenger receptor (LDL-SR), 395
Low-density microsomal fraction (HDM), 168, 170, 171
LPL. *See* Lipoprotein lipase
L-type calcium channels, 140–141

M

Mahogany/mahoganoid mutations, 215–216
Malic enzyme (ME), 2
Malonyl CoA, 3, 49, 92
MAP. *See* Mitogen-activated protein kinase
Maternally inherited diabetes and deafness (MIDD), 326, 328
MDS. *See* Myelodysplastic syndrome
Melanin-concentrating hormone, 186

Melanin stimulating hormone (MSH), 178
Melanocortin receptors (MCR), 178
    POMC-derived peptides and, 214–215
    role in agouti signaling, 212–214
α-Melanocyte-stimulating hormone (α-
        MSH), 206, 214–215
Membranes. *See* Cellular membranes; Plasma
        membranes
Menhaden oil, 7
Mesenchymal tissues, 284
Metabolic rate
    effects of type of dietary fat, 65
    in heat production by brown adipose
        tissue, 262
    SCD regulation and, 50
1-Methyl-3-isobutylxanthine, 83
Mitochondria
    D-loop, 334, 335
    respiratory chain, 325
    structure and function, 321, 323–324
Mitochondrial DNA (mtDNA)
    gene transcription, 331–336
    human genome, 322
    local tuning of transcription process, 330,
        334
    mutant vs. wildtype, 327
    overview, 321–322, 327
Mitochondrial termination factor (mTERF),
        333
Mitochondrial transcription factor A
        (mtTFA), 332–333
Mitochondrial uncoupling, 263
Mitogen-activated protein kinase (MAP),
        269, 270
Morphine, 145
mRNA
    acyl-CoA synthetase I, 83, 85–86, 88–91
    β-adrenergic receptor, 265, 266
    blood clotting factor, 402
    collagen, 410, 411
    cyclooxygenases, 400–401
    cytokines, 405
    dopamine receptors, 141, 143
    fatty acid binding proteins, 117–118
    fatty acid synthase, 3
    fatty acid transport proteins, 107–108, 116
    ferritin H chain, 452–453
    GABA receptor, 135, 138–139
    gene products sensitive to vitamin D₃,
        360–362
    GLUT1, 166
    GLUT4, 166–170
    glutathione peroxidase, 430, 436–437
    immediate early genes, 148
    lipoproteins, and vitamin E, 395

MC4-R, 217
    NMDA receptors, 134–135, 136
    opioid receptors, 145
    procollagen type 1, 397, 411
    retinoic acid receptors, 149
    selenium-dependent stability, 437–438
    stearoyl-CoA desaturase, 56–57
    uncoupling proteins, 270–271
    vascular endothelial growth factor, 408
    vitamin D₃ nuclear receptor, 366
MSH. *See* Melanin stimulating hormone
α-MSH. *See* α-Melanocyte-stimulating
        hormone
mtDNA. *See* Mitochondrial DNA
mTERF. *See* Mitochondrial termination factor
MTII, 214
mt TFA. *See* Mitochondrial transcription
        factor A
Multiple endocrinopathy, 191
Murine anorexia mutation, 190
Murine fatty acid synthase, 4
Murine 3T3-L1 adipocytes. *See* 3T3-L1
        adipocytes
Muscarinergic acetylcholine receptor, 145
Myelodysplastic syndrome (MDS), 406–407
Myoclonic epilepsy and ragged-red fiber
        disease (MERRF), 326

N

NADPH-dependent cytochrome b₅
        reductase, 49
NADPH-oxidase, 398
Naltrexone, 145
Naproxen, 78
National Health and Nutrition Examination
        Survey (NHANES II), 221
Nerve growth factor (NGF), 150
Neurodegenerative conditions and vitamin
        E, 412–414
Neuro-endocrine peptides, 179–185, 193–195
Neuronal protein, 178
Neuron-deprived orphan receptor (NOR-1),
        297
Neuropathy, ataxia, and retinitis pigmentosa
        (NARP), 326
Neuropeptide Y receptor family (NPY), 179,
        186, 190
Neurotensin receptor, 145–146
Neurotransmitter transporters, 142, 146–147
NF-Y protein, 56
NGF. *See* Nerve growth factor
[³H]Nitrendipine-binding-site densities, 140
Nitric oxide synthase, 402

NMDA receptors, 132–137, 295
Non-insulin-dependent diabetes mellitus
    (NIDDM), 193, 326
Non-steroidal anti-inflammatory drugs
    (NSAIDS), 78, 247–248, 405
NOR-1. *See* Neuron-deprived orphan
    receptor
Noradrenergic receptors, 142, 144–145
NPY. *See* Neuropeptide Y receptor family
Nuclear receptor superfamily, 365, 367
Nuclear respiratory factors (NRF), 333
NUR77 orphan receptor, 293, 297–298
NURR1 orphan receptor, 293, 297–298

O

Obesity
    agouti gene and, 205–222
    gene regulatory effects, 15–16
    health risks, 25–26
    high-calcium diet and reduction of,
        220–222
    impaired adipose tissue adrenergic
        signaling, 265–268
    Quebec Family Study, 213–214
    reversal, 264
    SCD regulation and, 50
    single-gene mutations, 178, 186–190
    therapy with selective β-adrenergic
        receptor agonists, 268–269
    thermogenesis defects, 262–263
    trends, 17
Olanzapine, 143
Oleate, 49, 50
Olive oil, 64
Opioid receptors, 142, 145
Opioids, 141, 179
Orphan receptors, 179
    discovery of new, 300
    effects on retinoic acid receptors, 293–299
Orphanins, 179
Oxidative phosphorylation (OXPHOS),
        324–325, 328, 333
Oxidative stress
    effects on neuronal cells, 413
    effects on T-lymphocytes, 400, 401
    effects on transcriptional events, 402
    from LDL oxidation, 407
    reduced calcium mobilization with, 400
Oxidized low-density lipoproteins (oxLDL),
        33, 34
OXPHOS. *See* Oxidative phosphorylation
Oxygen responsive elements, glutathione
    peroxidases, 434

Oxytocin, 179

P

PAI-1. *See* Plasminogen activator inhibitor
    type 1
Palm oil, 64
Palmitate, 3–4, 49–50
Palmitoleate, 49, 50
Parathyroid hormone (PTH), 355, 356
Parkinson's disease, 325, 450
P-Box, 369
PC1 mutations, 191–192
PC2 mutations, 188–189, 193, 195
Peptides
    neuro-endocrine, 179–185
    of polyprotein precursors, 181–182
    POMC-derived, 214–215
Perilla oil, 64
Peroxisome proliferator activated receptors
    (PPAR), 12, 64
    in acyl-CoA synthase 1 gene expression,
        86–87
    in adipocyte gene expression, 28–30, 41,
        68–71
    in β-adrenergic receptor gene expression,
        269
    crystal structure, 69
    general characteristics, 31–32
    interaction with retinoic acid signaling,
        293, 299–300, 301
    natural and synthetic ligands, 32–34
    nutritional considerations, 34
    regulation of fatty acid transport proteins,
        113–118
    types, 113
Peroxisome proliferator response element
    (PPRE), 86–87, 113, 114, 116–117
Pertussis toxin, 269
Phaeomelanin, 206
Phosphate, inorganic, 78
Phosphatidylinositol 3-kinase (PI3-K), 9–10
Phosphoinositolbiphosphate, 133
Phosphoinositoldiphosphate, 147
Phospholipase, 133, 237
Phospholipid hydroperoxide glutathione
    peroxidase, 429, 430, 431, 437, 438
Phospholipid production, 50, 52
PI3-K. *See* Phosphatidylinositol 3-kinase
Piroxicam, 248
PKC. *See* Protein kinase C
Plasma glutathione peroxidase, 428–429,
        430–431, 432

Plasma membranes
   fatty acid transport protein flux across,
      101–107, 114
   GLUT4 in the, 168–169, 170, 171
Plasminogen activator inhibitor type 1
   (PAI-1), 27
PLZF. See Promyelocytic leukemia zinc-
   finger protein
PML. See Promyelocytic leukemia protein
Polyadenylation site, human vs. other
   animals, 4
Polyps, 235
Polyunsaturated fatty acid responsive
   element (PUFA-RE), 53–54
Polyunsaturated fatty acids (PUFA)
   in immune system cells, 400
   as ligand for PPAR, 33, 34
   metabolism, 232–233
   N-3, 240–244, 245, 246
   regulation of lipogenesis, 6–7, 12–13
   role in stearoyl-CoA desaturase
      regulation, 49–58
POMC. See Proopiomelanocortin
Positron emission tomography (PET), 146
Post-mortem studies, serotonin transporter
   levels, 146
PPAR. See Peroxisome proliferator activated
   receptors
PPRE. See Peroxisome proliferator response
   element
Procholecystokinin, 182, 185, 186
Procollagen type 1, 397, 411
Proenkephalons, 181
Proglucagon, 182
Prohormone processing
   animal models with defects, 185–190
   disorders of energy homeostasis and,
      177–195
   human disease associated with defects,
      190–193
   pathway, 181–182
   regulation, 184–185
Promyelocytic leukemia protein (PML), 292
Promyelocytic leukemia zinc-finger protein
   (PLZF), 292
Proopiomelanocortin (POMC), 179, 180–181,
   182, 186
   deficiency from genetic defects, 192–193
   role of POMC-derived peptides, 214–215
Prostacyclin, 66
   in COX pathway, 234
   as ligand for PPAR, 69–70, 71
Prostaglandin E, 147, 248–250, 400, 401, 406
Prostaglandins, 13, 69, 233–234, 246, 247–249,
   400, 404–405

Prostanoid pathway, 12
Prostate cancer, 398
Protein kinase C (PKC), effects of vitamin E,
   395, 399, 404, 407–408, 414
Protein kinases, 9–10, 133, 185, 269, 270, 356,
   364. See also Protein kinase C
Proteins
   effects of reactive oxygen species, 394
   protective effect of vitamin E, 398
   regulation of fatty acid synthase gene,
      16–17
   selenium-dependent. See Glutathione
      peroxidases; Selenoproteins
Provasoactive intestinal peptide, 182
PTH. See Parathyroid hormone
PUFA. See Polyunsaturated fatty acids
Pyruvate dehydrogenase, 93
Pyruvate kinase, 12

Q

Quantitative trait locus (QTL), 194–195,
   263–264
Quebec Family Study, 213–214

R

RAR. See Retinoic acid receptors
RARE. See Retinoic acid response elements
RBP. See Retinol binding protein
Reactive oxygen intermediates (ROI), 400
Reactive oxygen species (ROS), 272–273, 274
   action of vitamin E, 396–399, 408
   effects of antioxidants, 394, 396–398
   generation in diabetes, 408
   role in apoptosis, 398
   suppression of erythropoietin synthesis,
      410
Refeeding
   effects on acyl-CoA synthetase I, 82
   in vivo effects, 7
Renal disorders, 326, 409–410
Restriction fragment length polymorphisms
   (RLFP), 213
Retinal, oxidation of retinol to, 285
Retinitis pigmentosa, 412
Retinoic acid (RA), 32, 285, 288, 300–301
Retinoic acid receptors (RAR;RXR), 115,
   148–149
   binding to response elements, 289, 292
   effects of orphan receptors on, 293–299
   gene transcription regulation by, 288–299,
      301

mitochondrial gene expression and, 329–331
role in vitamin A homeostasis, 285, 286–287
vitamin D nuclear receptor binding, 367–368, 369
Western blot analysis, 331
Retinoic acid response elements (RARE;RXRE), 288–289, 290–291, 296, 301, 334, 335
Retinoids
improvement of hematopoiesis with, 406
topical therapy, 284
Retinol. *See* Vitamin A
Retinol binding protein (RBP), 287
Reverse endocrinology, 300
Rheumatoid arthritis, 403, 454
Rickets-type II, 372–373, 374–375
ROI. *See* Reactive oxygen intermediates
ROR/RZR orphan receptors, 293, 296–297
ROS. *See* Reactive oxygen species
RXR. *See* Retinoic acid receptors

S

Safflower oil, 64, 65
Satiety signals, 63
Saturated fats, vs. unsaturated, 64
Scavenger receptor type A, 402
SCD. *See* Stearoyl-CoA desaturase
SECIS. *See* Selenocysteine insertion sequence
Second messenger systems, 147, 185
Seco-steroids, 350, 367
E-Selectin, 403
Selective serotonin reuptake inhibitors (SSRI), 144
Selenium
bioavailability, 426
deficiency, 437
differential regulation of selenoproteins by, 430–433
mechanisms of incorporation, 434–436
sites of regulation, 436–438
Selenocysteine, 434–435, 437
Selenocysteine insertion sequence (SECIS), 435, 436, 437–438
Selenocysteine tRNA gene, 438–439
Selenocystyl-tRNA, 435, 436
Selenoenzymes, 429–430
Selenophosphate synthetase, 427
Selenoprotein P, 430, 432–433, 438
Selenoprotein W, 430, 433

Selenoproteins
characteristics, 427
characterization, 426–430
knockout approach to study expression, 438–439
mechanism of selenium incorporation, 434–436
prokaryotic vs. eukaryotic biosynthesis, 435, 436
regulation by non-selenium factors, 434
Serotonin receptors, 133, 142, 143–144
Serotonin transporter (5-HTT), 146
7B2 mutations, 189–190, 195
Signal transducers and activators of transcription (STAT)
in adipocyte gene expression, 28–30
general characteristics, 39–40
nutritional considerations, 40
Signal transduction
importance of oxidant/antioxidant balance, 400
vitamin D_3 and, 358–364, 376
Single photon emission computer tomography (SPECT), 146
Skin
cancer, 284
fatty acid binding protein, 103, 112
vitamin D synthesis, 350
Soybean oil, 64
SREBP. *See* Sterol regulatory element-binding proteins
SSRI. *See* Selective serotonin reuptake inhibitors
STAT. *See* Signal transducers and activators of transcription
Stearoyl-CoA desaturase (SCD)
post-transcriptional control, 56–57
regulation by PUFA, 49–58
transcriptional control, 53–56
Sterol regulatory element (SRE), 54
Sterol regulatory element-binding proteins (SREBP)
ADD-1 and function, 37–38, 71
effects on FAS gene expression, 13
role in insulin transcription, 9–11, 28–30
in SCD gene expression, 54–56
Streptozotocin (STZ), 8
Subtilisin, 179
Sulfonylurea receptor (SUR), 220
Sulindac, 239, 248
Superoxide dismutase, 413
SUR. *See* Sulfonylurea receptor
Synovitis, 404

T

TAG. *See* Triacylglycerols
Tallow, 64
TATA-binding protein, 115
Testosterone, regulation of glutathione
    peroxidases, 434
Thermogenesis, 64
  by β-adrenergic receptor, 264–265,
    266–269
  by brown adipose tissue, 262
  defects in, and obesity, 262–263
Thermogenin, 262
Thiazolidinedione (TZD), 32, 33, 69, 92
Thioesterase, 3
Thioredoxin reductase (TR)
  characteristics, 427, 429–430
  comparison with glutathione
    peroxidases, 433
3T3-L1 adipocytes, 4
  acyl-CoA synthetase I gene expression,
    83, 84–85
  β-adrenergic receptor expression in, 265
  effect of insulin, 8, 40
  insulin-stimulated glucose transport,
    163–171
  post-transcriptional control of SCD, 56
  preadipocytes, 28
  SCD gene expression, 52, 67
  STAT activation, 40
Thrombopoiesis, 406–407
Thromboxanes, 234
Thyroid hormone (T3). *See* Triiodothyronine
Thyroid hormone receptor (TR), 14, 371
Thyroid hormone response element (TRE),
    14, 334, 335
Tissue damage
  hepatic, role in vitamin E in reversal,
    411–412
  renal, role in vitamin E in reversal,
    409–410
Tissue distribution
  acyl-CoA synthetase 1, 79–80
  fatty acid binding proteins, 103
  fatty acid synthase, 4, 68
  fatty acid transport proteins, 103
  HNF-4, 298
  rapid nongenomic responses to vitamin
    D$_3$, 363
  ROR/RZR orphan receptors, 297
  threshold effects of mutant mtDNA and,
    329
  uncoupling proteins, 272–273
T-lymphocytes
  impaired function with aging, 400
  induction by vitamin E, 395–396
  oxidative stress reaction, 400
  transcriptional events, 402
TNFα. *See* Tumor necrosis factor α
Tocopherols. *See* Vitamin E
TR. *See* Thioredoxin reductase; Thyroid
    hormone receptor
Transcaltachia, 364
Transcription factors
  binding of antioxidant responsive
    elements, 399
  chick ovalbumin upstream promoter, 293,
    294–296, 298–299, 301
  effects of ethanol, 147–149
  effects of oxidative stress, 402, 403,
    413–414
  reduction of expression, and malignant
    cell growth, 404
Transfer RNA (tRNA)
  effects of mtDNA mutations and, 328
  in human mitochondrial genome, 322
  in mitochondrial DNA gene transcription,
    332–336
  selenocystyl, 435
Transferrin
  characteristics, 449, 451
  role in iron homeostasis, 450–451
Transthyretin (TTR), 287
TRE. *See* Thyroid hormone response element
Triacsin C, 80, 92
Triacylglycerols (TAG)
  daily intake in typical Western diet, 102
  effects of refeeding, 7
  production, 50
  storage by adipocytes, 27
Triiodothyronine (T3), 6, 14, 83, 86
tRNA. *See* Transfer RNA
Troglitazone, 92–93
Trolox, 399, 414
T3. *See* Triiodothyronine
TTR. *See* Transthyretin
Tumor growth factor, 409, 410, 411
Tumor necrosis factor α (TNFα)
  antibody, effects on uncoupling protein
    mRNA, 272–273
  effects of vitamin E, 402, 403, 410, 411
  and myelodysplastic syndromes, 406–407
  production and function, 27, 87–88, 90
Tumor regression, 239
Tumorigenesis
  control by vitamin E, 404–407
  intestinal, and dietary fats, 231–250
TZD. *See* Thiazolidinedione

U

UCP. *See* Uncoupling proteins
Ultraviolet radiation, effects on vitamin E, 398
Uncoupling proteins (UCP)
　dietary regulation of expression, 270–271
　future research, 273–274
　homologs, 263–264
　metabolic rate and energy metabolism, 261–274
　modulators of activity, 271–272
　overview, 262–264
　production during oxidative phosphorylation, 324
　role in apoptosis, 273–274
3'-untranslated region (UTR), 57, 333–334, 435, 438, 453, 454
Upstream stimulatory factors, 171

V

Vasopressin, 179
Very-low-density lipoprotein (VLDL), 395, 396, 412
Vitamin A
　deficiency, 284, 286
　gene expression and, 283–301
　homeostasis, 284–287
　induction of erythropoietin synthesis, 410
　ligands from, 32
　metabolism, 284–285
　mitochondrial gene expression and, 321–336
　prenatal deficiency syndrome, 148–149
Vitamin C, and erythropoietin synthesis, 410
Vitamin D
　chemistry and related compounds, 350–352
　conformational flexibility of molecules, 353
　deficiency, 355–356
　endocrine system, 356–358
　gene expression and, 349–377
　overview, 349–350
　production and metabolism, 352–356
　recommended daily intake, 352
　stimulation of calcium influx by, 220, 221, 222
　structure, 351
　supplements, 352
Vitamin D_2, 351–352
Vitamin D_3, 350, 351–352, 376
　endocrine system of, 356–358

　mRNA of gene products sensitive to, 360–362
　nuclear receptor for, 364–372
　rapid nongenomic responses to, 362–364, 376
　role in bone development, 375–376
　signal transduction pathways for biological responses, 358–364, 376
Vitamin D-binding protein (DBP), 356, 358, 376
Vitamin D-dependent rickets-type II (VDDRII), 372–373, 374–375
Vitamin D_3 nuclear receptor (VDR_{nuc}), 350, 376
　activation and transcription, 371–372
　dimerization, 367–368, 371
　interactions with other receptors, 368
　knockout of the, 372–375
　mutations, 372–374
　schematic model, 366
　structural domains, 364–367, 368
Vitamin D receptor, 115
Vitamin D response element (VDRE), 334, 335, 359, 362
Vitamin E
　bioavailability, 395, 396
　deficiency, 400, 409, 412
　gene expression and, 393–414
　immune function and immunity-related diseases, 399–404
　modes of action, 396–399
　non-antioxidant effects, 398–399, 414
　regulation of glutathione peroxidases, 434
　role in reversal of hepatic tissue damage, 411–412
　role in reversal of renal tissue damage, 409–410
　stereoisomers, 396
　structures and homologs, 394–395
　supplementation, 403
Voltage-operated channels, effects of alcohol on gene expression, 140–141

W

White adipose tissue (WAT), 64–65
Wnt-signaling pathway, 237–238

Y

Yeast, acyl-CoA synthetases, 81

Z

Zinc-mediated oxidative injury, 414